Psychiatry: Advanced Researches and Practices

Psychiatry: Advanced Researches and Practices

Edited by **Harvey Wilson**

hayle medical

New York

Published by Hayle Medical,
30 West, 37th Street, Suite 612,
New York, NY 10018, USA
www.haylemedical.com

Psychiatry: Advanced Researches and Practices
Edited by Harvey Wilson

International Standard Book Number: 978-1-63241-387-1 (Hardback)

Printed in the United States of America.

Contents

Preface

This book traces the progress of psychiatry as a discipline and highlights some of its key concepts and applications. It presents researches and studies performed by experts across the globe. Mental health issues are generally affective or behavioral. Psychiatry aims to study, diagnose and treat usual as well as rare mental disorders. It is a field of medicine which encompasses subfields such as geriatric psychiatry, child adolescent psychiatry, forensic psychiatry, addiction psychiatry, clinical neurophysiology, etc. This book will provide interesting topics for research which readers can take up. It includes some of the vital pieces of work being conducted across the world, on various aspects related to psychiatry. This book is appropriate for students seeking detailed information in this area as well as for experts. The extensive content of this book provides readers with a thorough understanding of this subject.

This book has been the outcome of endless efforts put in by authors and researchers on various issues and topics within the field. The book is a comprehensive collection of significant researches that are addressed in a variety of chapters. It will surely enhance the knowledge of the field among readers across the globe.

It gives us an immense pleasure to thank our researchers and authors for their efforts to submit their piece of writing before the deadlines. Finally in the end, I would like to thank my family and colleagues who have been a great source of inspiration and support.

Editor

Screening for Psychiatric Disorders in Bariatric Surgery Candidates with the German Version of the Patient Health Questionnaire

Ulrich Palm,[1] Wolfgang E. Thasler,[2] Peter Rittler,[2] Ann Natascha Epple,[3] Martin Lieb,[4] Rabee Mokhtari-Nejad,[1] Susanne Rospleszcz,[1] Larissa de la Fontaine,[1] Felix M. Segmiller,[1] and Daniela Eser-Valeri[1]

[1] Department of Psychiatry, Psychotherapy and Psychosomatics, Ludwig-Maximilians University Munich, Nußbaumstraße 7, 80336 Munich, Germany
[2] Department of General, Visceral, Transplantation, Vascular, and Thoracic Surgery, Ludwig-Maximilians University Munich, Marchioninistraße 15, 81377 Munich, Germany
[3] KBO Heckscher Clinic for Childhood and Adolescent Psychiatry, Deisenhofener Straße 28, 81539 Munich, Germany
[4] Privatklinik Meiringen, Willigen, 3860 Meiringen, Switzerland

Correspondence should be addressed to Ulrich Palm; ulrich.palm@med.uni-muenchen.de

Academic Editor: Xingguang Luo

Objective. Obesity has been linked to psychiatric disorders in several studies. Prevalence and severity of psychiatric disorders are high in patients undergoing bariatric surgery. Thus, psychiatric assessment of bariatric surgery candidates has become a standard procedure. However, socially desirable responding leads to biased results in self-reported questionnaires. Here, bariatric surgery candidates were screened with the Patient Health Questionnaire (PHQ-D) additionally to the psychiatric examination. *Method.* 355 bariatric surgery candidates filled in the PHQ-D before the psychiatric examination as a part of the surgery assessment procedure. PHQ-D results were compared to psychiatric diagnoses and body mass index (BMI). *Results.* Gender ratio, mean BMI, and age were comparable to earlier studies. Depressive and somatization symptoms did not correlate to BMI. However, females showed higher prevalence of psychiatric disorders with elevated syndrome severity in depressive and somatization disorders, as well as more frequent antidepressant intake. Eating disorders and addiction disorders were rarely reported. *Conclusion.* The findings suggest a socially desirable responding when filling in the PHQ-D before bariatric surgery. The use of the PHQ-D in this patient sample could be augmented by psychometric tests with internal correction and validation scales. Furthermore, psychiatric examination should be separated from the surgery evaluation process.

1. Introduction

Obesity has become a relevant socioeconomic and medical problem in developed and new industrialized countries, leading to a 10% increase of obesity rates per decade in the USA [1] and an even greater increase in European countries [2, 3]. In people with a body mass index (BMI) ranging from 30 to 35 kg/m^2, expectancy of life declines by 2–4 years, in people with a BMI ranging from 40 to 45 kg/m^2 even by 8–10 years [4]. Obese persons, especially women, show higher rates of psychiatric disorders, that is, depressive disorders [5], and they have a higher risk of lifetime depression than normal weight controls [6–12]. Furthermore, prevalence of psychiatric disorders is correlated to increasing BMI [13–15]. Morbidly obese patients (obesity III°) undergoing bariatric surgery show higher prevalence and severity of psychiatric disorders than people with lower degree of obesity (I-II°) [16] or normal weight controls [17–23]. With increasing rates of obesity, bariatric surgery has emerged as an important treatment option in severely obese patients as they do not sufficiently respond to standard weight loss programs [24, 25]. Psychiatric assessment of bariatric surgery candidates has become a standard procedure before undergoing bariatric surgery, due to high rates of psychiatric comorbidity [26]. However, a tendency to dissimulation has been observed during the assessment process for bariatric surgery [12, 27, 28]. Depressive symptoms among bariatric surgery candidates are higher when they are assured that their diagnostic assessment is independent from the suitability rating before bariatric surgery, suggesting that rates of depression are much higher than reported in the respective literature [26, 29–31]. As the preoperative diagnosis of depressive or anxiety disorders as well as binge eating disorder is associated with lower weight loss after surgery [32–36], concomitant screening for depressive and other psychiatric disorders during assessment process and follow-up phases has been fostered by additional use of self-reported symptom screening questionnaires, for example, Beck Depression Inventory [23, 37–39]. The PHQ (Patient Health Questionnaire) has been investigated in bariatric surgery candidates in only one study so far. Cassin et al. suggested an elevated cut-off for depression rating in bariatric surgery candidates with the PHQ-9 (module for depressive disorders) due to the interference with somatization symptoms, leading to a false positive result of depressive symptoms [40], and they found a lower sensitivity and specificity of each 0.75 compared to the earlier PHQ studies, suggesting socially desirable responding by the candidates. Here, we aimed at evaluating psychiatric symptoms in a sample of German bariatric surgery candidates with the full German version of the PHQ (PHQ-D) for several reasons: the full PHQ version delivers a clearer discrimination between depressive and somatoform disorders due to the items assessed in the somatoform disorder category. It provides information on additional symptoms relevant for the evaluation process of suitability, for example, eating disorders, alcoholism, stress symptoms, and medication intake. These additional factors are relevant for weighing up absolute/relative contraindications and for screening for socially desirable responding. To our knowledge, the PHQ-D has not been applied in bariatric surgery candidates yet.

2. Materials and Methods

2.1. Subjects.
All participants were bariatric surgery candidates from the Department of Surgery of the Ludwig-Maximilians University. Before undergoing surgery, candidates were examined by the Psychiatric Liaison Service of the Department of Psychiatry and gastroenterologic as well as cardiologic evaluation for their suitability. The criteria for considering bariatric surgery were BMI $\geq 40 \, \text{kg/m}^2$ or a BMI $\geq 35 \, \text{km/m}^2$ with at least one comorbidity, for example, diabetes mellitus II, hyperlipidemia, sleep apnea, and orthopedic problems [41]. Before the psychiatric examination, subjects were asked to fill in the PHQ-D questionnaire as an additional examination to the standard assessment procedure. They were assured that refusal would not have consequences in terms of the psychiatric assessment and that

the collected data were anonymized for scientific use. However, subjects were not informed in advance that the PHQ-D had no impact to the psychiatric assessment procedure. Between 2006 and 2011, more than 700 bariatric surgery candidates were evaluated and a total of 355 patients agreed to fill in the questionnaire.

2.2. PHQ-D.
The PHQ-D is the German translation of the PRIME-MD Patient Health Questionnaire [42]. The questionnaire has been validated in several studies and showed sufficient validity, sensitivity, specificity, and internal consistency (Cronbach's α for depression scale: 0.88; for somatization scale: 0.79) [43–45]. The PHQ-D covers somatization disorders (q. 1), depressive disorders (q. 2), anxiety disorders (q. 3–5), eating disorders (q. 6–8), alcohol abuse (q. 9-10), psychosocial functioning (q. 11), stress symptoms (q. 12), posttraumatic stress disorder (q. 13), intake of psychopharmacologic drugs (q. 15), and questions on premenstrual dysphoric disorder (q. 16). In this study, depressive, somatization, and stress symptoms are calculated by a sum score; all other items are calculated by a cut-off/threshold or a dichotomous criterion (yes/no). Additionally, depressive symptoms are clustered in groups of severity according to the PHQ-D manual [46]. Free answers (q. 14) and the question on psychosocial functioning (q. 11) were excluded for lacking reliability. Premenstrual dysphoric syndrome was assessed dichotomously by q. 16b.

2.3. Psychiatric Assessment.
After filling in the questionnaire, patients underwent a standardized psychiatric examination by an experienced psychiatrist. The semistructured interview included a psychopathological examination, medical and psychiatric history, history of weight gain, eating and drinking characteristics, calculation of actual BMI, former pharmacological and psychotherapeutic treatments, and sociodemographic and economic properties. Additionally, compliance, resilience, and motivational factors for bariatric surgery as well as subjective risk estimation were assessed. If applicable, PHQ-D results were discussed with the patients and they were told that the PHQ-D had no impact on the recommendation or rejection of bariatric surgery. Finally, up to three psychiatric diagnoses were made according to ICD-10 criteria and diagnoses were sorted by their relevance. If there was no relevant psychopathology, no psychiatric diagnosis was made. In addition, obesity was assessed by the ICD-10 categories (degrees I–III). Recommendation for or rejection of bariatric surgery was reported to the department of surgery and the patients.

2.4. Statistical Analyses.
Demographic data were measured as mean and standard deviation, where applicable, or median and interquartile range. Incomplete data sets ($n = 13$) or values exceeding two standard deviations were not excluded from analysis to reflect the whole spectrum of results. A level of significance ≤ 0.05 was accepted. Fisher's exact test was used for detecting gender differences in the PHQ-D categories. Pearson's correlation coefficient was used for correlations between BMI and age, BMI and somatization scale, BMI and

stress symptoms, stress symptoms and somatization, BMI and depression score, and depression score and stress symptoms. ANOVA was applied to assess the correlation between BMI and depression categories of the PHQ-D, the BMI and the psychiatric diagnoses, and stress symptoms and depression categories. Unadjusted t-tests were used for BMI differences in the groups with and without binge eating disorder or bulimia, depression score and antidepressant intake, somatization score and antidepressant intake, and depression score and premenstrual syndrome. The correlation between depression category and antidepressant intake was assessed by a chi-square test. Bonferroni correction was applied where necessary. The statistical program R 2.15.2 (Institute for Statistics and Mathematics, Vienna, Austria) was used for all statistical analyses.

3. Results

3.1. Demographic Data and Psychiatric Diagnoses. Overall, 355 bariatric surgery candidates completed the PHQ-D; 271 (76%) were female. Mean age was 41.8 ± 12.3 years with a range of 17–72 years. Mean BMI was $47.8 \pm 8.4 \, \text{kg/m}^2$ with a range of 27–80 kg/m^2. Mean age of female candidates was 41.2 years compared to 43.7 years in male candidates ($P = 0.2$). BMI in males was significantly higher ($50.2 \pm 11.3 \, \text{kg/m}^2$) than in females ($47.0 \pm 9.0 \, \text{kg/m}^2$) ($P = 0.0054$). 190 (71%) female candidates showed a premenstrual syndrome due to PHQ. Obesity categories showed a high prevalence of BMI $\geq$ 40 kg/m^2 (morbid obesity, ICD-10: E66.02) in 309 candidates (87%), followed by BMI 35–39.9 kg/m^2 (ICD-10: E66.01) in 33 candidates (9%) and BMI 30–34.9 kg/m^2 (ICD-10: E66.00) in 11 candidates (3%). Two male patients had a Prader-Willi syndrome (ICD-10: Q87.1).

Psychiatric diagnoses were clustered to depressive disorders including (recurrent) major depressive disorder and adjustment disorder (ICD-10: F32.x, F33.x, F43.2), eating disorders including bulimia, binge eating disorder, and other eating disorders (ICD: F50.2, F50.4, F50.9), and other psychiatric disorders including addiction disorders, personality disorders, delusional disorders, anxiety disorders, obsessive-compulsive disorders, and posttraumatic stress disorders (ICD-10: F1x.x, F2x.x, F40.x, F41.x, F42.x, F43.1, F60.x). 127 candidates (36%) had no psychiatric diagnosis at all, 228 subjects (64%) had at least one psychiatric diagnosis, 23 candidates had a second psychiatric diagnosis, and 4 candidates had a third psychiatric diagnosis. At the first psychiatric diagnosis 161 subjects (70%) showed a depressive disorder, 44 subjects (20%) were diagnosed with an eating disorder, and 23 subjects (10%) had other psychiatric diagnoses. The second psychiatric diagnosis showed eating disorders in 10 patients (43%) and other psychiatric disorders in 13 patients (57%). The third psychiatric diagnosis consisted in other disorders ($n = 4$). Overall, 161 subjects had a depressive disorder as primary diagnosis; 54 showed an eating disorder and 40 had other psychiatric disorders as primary or concomitant diagnoses. Women had significantly more diagnoses of depressive disorders (48%) than men (36%) ($P = 0.011$). Further details are reported in Table 1.

3.2. PHQ-D Results. For the whole sample, PHQ-D depression categories showed no depressive symptoms in 104 candidates (29%), mild depressive symptoms in 119 candidates (34%), moderate depressive symptoms in 86 candidates (24%), moderate-severe depressive symptoms in 32 candidates (9%), and severe depressive symptoms in 13 candidates (4%). Panic disorder occurred in 23 patients (6%) and anxiety disorder occurred in 25 subjects (7%). 26 patients (7%) reported bulimia symptoms and 25 patients (7%) reached the cut-off for binge eating disorder. Alcohol abuse was reported by only 11 subjects (3%). PTSD symptoms occurred in 10 patients (3%). 56 candidates (16%) reported use of psychopharmacologic medication. Median somatization score was 11 ± 9 points (range 0–28) and median stress score was 7 ± 6 points (range 0–24).

In male candidates, the category "no depression" was significantly more frequent (39%) than in female subjects (26%) ($P = 0.046$) and men showed less severe depressive syndromes (0%) than women (5%). The somatization scale was significantly increased in female subjects (median 12 ± 8; range 0–28) compared to male subjects (9 ± 9; range 0–23) ($P = 0.0005$) and females showed a significantly more frequent antidepressant intake (18%) than males (7%) ($P = 0.015$). All other PHQ-D measures did not show significant gender differences (Table 1).

3.3. Correlation Analyses. Pearson's correlation coefficient showed no significance for BMI and age, BMI and somatization, BMI and stress symptoms, BMI and score of depressive symptoms, BMI and depression categories, BMI and psychiatric diagnoses, BMI and binge eating disorder, and BMI and bulimia. However, women showed a higher (but not significant) correlation coefficient between BMI and clinical relevant depression score (threshold disorder; 5–29 points) than the whole sample ($r = 0.099$; $P = 0.174$). Furthermore, in women, BMI increased corresponding to the depression categories "mild," "moderate," and "moderate-severe" ($P = 0.4$), but not to the category "severe."

Correlation between stress symptoms and somatization was statistically significant ($r = 0.592$; $P < 0.01$); also stress symptoms and score of depressive symptoms showed a highly significant correlation ($r = 0.667$; $P < 0.001$). Score of stress symptoms was significantly correlated with the depression categories ($P < 0.001$). Depressive symptom scores were associated with medication intake ($P < 0.001$) and showed a mean score of 7.6 in the drug-naive group compared to a mean score of 11.8 in the medicated group. Furthermore, depression categories and antidepressant intake were correlated ($P < 0.001$). Somatization scores were associated with antidepressant intake ($P < 0.001$) and showed a mean score of 10.6 in the drug-naive group compared to a mean score of 14.1 in the medicated group.

4. Discussion

In this trial, the German version of the Patient Health Questionnaire was used for screening for psychiatric disorders in a sample of 355 bariatric surgery candidates.

TABLE 1: Demographic and clinical characteristics.

	Whole sample	Male	Female	P value
N	355	84 (24%)	271 (76%)	
Age (years)	41.8 ± 12.3	43.7 ± 23.5	41.2 ± 17.0	$P = 0.2$
BMI (kg/m^2)	47.8 ± 8.4	50.2 ± 11.3	47.0 ± 9.0	$P = 0.0054$*
Somatic ICD-10 diagnoses				
E66.00	11 (3%)	1 (1%)	10 (4%)	
E66.01	33 (9%)	6 (7%)	27 (10%)	$P = 0.11$[a]
E66.02	309 (88%)	75 (90%)	234 (86%)	
Q87.1	2 (1%)	2 (2%)	0 (0%)	
Psychiatric disorders				
Depressive disorders	161 (54%)	30 (36%)	131 (48%)	
Eating disorders	44 (12%)	8 (10%)	36 (13%)	$P = 0.011$*[a]
Other disorders	23 (6%)	3 (4%)	20 (7%)	
No disorder	127 (36%)	43 (51%)	84 (31%)	
PHQ depression category				
No depression	105 (29%)	33 (39%)	72 (26%)	
Mild depression	119 (34%)	24 (29%)	95 (35%)	
Moderate depression	86 (24%)	18 (21%)	68 (25%)	$P = 0.046$*[a]
Moderate-severe depression	32 (9%)	9 (11%)	23 (9%)	
Severe depression	13 (4%)	0 (0%)	13 (5%)	
PHQ other categories				
Somatization	11.2 ± 9.0	9.3 ± 7.5	11.8 ± 8.0	$P = 0.0005$*
Stress symptoms	7.8 ± 6.0	7.0 ± 6.0	8.1 ± 6.0	$P = 0.063$
Panic	23 (6%)	5 (6%)	18 (7%)	$P = 1$
Anxiety	25 (7%)	5 (6%)	20 (7%)	$P = 0.81$
Bulimia	26 (7%)	4 (5%)	22 (8%)	$P = 0.47$
Binge eating	25 (7%)	3 (4%)	22 (8%)	$P = 0.22$
Alcoholism	11 (3%)	6 (7%)	5 (2%)	$P = 0.025$*
PTSD	10 (3%)	1 (1%)	9 (3%)	$P = 0.46$
Medication	56 (16%)	6 (7%)	50 (18%)	$P = 0.015$*

*Significance ≤0.05.
[a]Significant difference between male and female patients in at least one diagnostic category.

The sociodemographic results of our study are in line with the findings in earlier trials, that is, similar percentage of women (3/4 of the study population), median BMI and age [37, 40, 47, 48]. Krukowski et al. [37] found a similar BMI (49 kg/m^2) in predominantly female patients (84%) with a mean age of 43 years, but higher rates of minimal and mild depression in their investigation on the utility of Beck's Depression Inventory in bariatric patients. Cassin et al. [40] found similar BMI (48 kg/m^2) and a mean age (44 years), as well as a high proportion of female gender (77%). The elevated proportion of female gender, associated with higher depression severity, has been shown in various studies [37, 40, 49, 50] and could be confirmed in our analysis. However, BMI was not correlated to depression severity or somatization in our study. This correlation has been found in most of the studies, and also a negative result has been reported [47]. The prevalence of at least one psychiatric diagnosis in bariatric surgery patients is 64% in our study and comparable to the respective literature [12]. The prevalence of a second or third psychiatric diagnosis in our sample is lower than in

other studies [6, 8–12, 18, 51]. Furthermore the low rate of eating disorders, addiction disorders, and medication intake in our sample is in contrast to other studies [52–54]. This discrepancy could point to a strict preselection of bariatric surgery candidates before psychiatric assessment. However, socially desirable responding which has also been reported in other studies [27, 28, 48] cannot be fully excluded.

The lacking correlation of depression severity and BMI could be not only due to distortion in responding, but also due to the treatment of severe depressive disorders with psychopharmacologic medication, especially in women. This group showed more drug intake than male candidates, higher severity of depressive and somatization symptoms, and increasing depression severity with higher BMI, except for the category of severe depression. Although this correlation did not reach significance, it could be speculated that females with severe depression are more likely medicated with antidepressants, masking a correlation between depression and BMI that probably could be seen if there was no antidepressant intake. The illness severity may be underlined by the elevated score of depressive and somatization symptoms which is higher despite drug intake compared to patients without medication. Overall, the medicated group presented a median depression score of 11.8 points (moderate depression), indicating a potentially higher depression severity without antidepressant intake.

The significant correlations between somatization × stress, depression score × stress, and depressive, respectively, somatization symptoms × medication intake confirms the good internal consistency of the questionnaire and shows a higher prevalence and severity of psychiatric syndromes in female candidates despite having lower BMI than males. Females with premenstrual dysphoric syndrome show higher depression score than females without, and females are more likely to be medicated with psychotropic drugs.

4.1. Limitations.
The lack of a correlation between BMI and psychopathologic symptoms in our study is rather surprising in regard to several studies showing clear correlation between BMI and psychiatric disorders. Thus, elevated BMI is supposed to provoke more physical restraints and disabilities, leading to increased somatization symptoms. Social stigmatization following elevated BMI could also be responsible for depressive feelings. However, there are some studies without a clear correlation between BMI and psychiatric disorders, pointing to a socially desirable responding in bariatric surgery candidates. It is possible that socially desirable responding in the self-administered PHQ could have led to our results. This bias in responding is probably most prominent in the categories of eating disorders and alcohol syndrome, where the prevalence is quite lower than in the respective literature, and also the categories with stress-related questions and somatization/depression could be biased. Another proposed explanation for potential bias is the diagnostic process made by the psychiatrist, bearing in mind that anamnesis underlies subjective statements and the psychiatric assessment process is probably too short to investigate discrepancies [12]. Although our evaluation process was standardized and executed by experienced psychiatrists, this potential bias cannot be fully ruled out. For this reason the use of psychometric rating instruments with internal correction and validity scales like the *Minnesota Multiphasic Personality Inventory-2* (MMPI-2) has been suggested [55]. Furthermore the PHQ did not reach the same diagnostic sensitivity compared to other psychometric tests [56, 57], especially regarding dysthymia [57]. This could lead to a distortion of the prevalence of depressive disorders.

Other more psychodynamic mechanisms could involve an unconscious neglect of physical and psychological burden or an altered subjective cause-effect relationship without mandatory conjunction of weight and burden. This could be an explanation for the finding that somatization/depression score and psychosocial stress showed significant correlation, whereas physical burden (expressed by BMI) and psychological burden showed no correlation. Additionally, socioeconomic and culture-bound heterogeneity of the sample could have influenced subjective rating of obesity and psychological burden [58]. Another possible explanation could be an adaptation process of obese patients, leading to neutral subjective rating of objectively severe restraints and impairments [49].

4.2. Implications for the Use of the PHQ.
The PHQ-D can easily be used as a screening tool for psychiatric disorders in bariatric surgery candidates. The questionnaire is comprehensible for patients, the summary is made quickly, and the results can be used for further distinct questions on abnormalities. However, bearing in mind the lack of sensitivity in the depression/dysthymia domain and the problem of socially desirable responding, the use of the PHQ as an indicator for the direction of the psychiatric assessment is by no means sufficient. Contrarily, the psychiatric interview should cover all relevant topics at first; afterwards the PHQ could be used to screen for additional symptoms or to discuss discrepancies between the psychiatric assessment and the PHQ result. Due to the lack of internal correction and validation scales in the PHQ, additional psychometric tests could be used. Recent investigations showed that even standardized assessments (e.g., Structured Clinical Interview for DSM-IV - SCID) had low concordance with diagnoses made by subjective psychiatric exploration [59, 60]. Thus, a standardized assessment process with reliable diagnostic tools has been recommended, leading to reduced bias by both patients and psychiatrists and yielding sufficient discriminatory power between the different syndromes. Additionally, the evaluation process for bariatric surgery could be separated from the psychiatric interview in order to achieve less bias in reporting severe symptoms [61]. If the fear of being rejected from bariatric surgery could be reduced by a separated evaluation process, the bias in self-reported symptom severity could decline as well. In this case, the PHQ(-D) might be useful as a screening instrument before and in the follow-up of bariatric surgery.

5. Conclusion

The PHQ-D has been investigated to screen for psychiatric disorders in a large sample of bariatric surgery candidates. Depression, somatization severity, and medication intake were more frequent in female than in male patients. However, BMI was not correlated to depression and somatization score. This could be due to biases in self-reporting psychiatric symptoms, a also due to a lack of concordance in psychiatric diagnoses and test results. The lack of correlation between PHQ categories and BMI hampers the use of the PHQ as a standard or first line assessment tool in bariatric surgery candidates. Thus, psychiatric evaluation should rely on the diagnostic interview and psychometric tests with internal correction and validation scales. A future standardized procedure for the assessment of bariatric surgery candidates could split the evaluation rating from the psychiatric diagnosis, leading to the reduction of bias in self-reporting due to the fear of rejection from surgery. In this case, the PHQ could be used to screen before and after bariatric surgery for depicting the course of psychiatric disorders. However, further studies are needed to elucidate the use of the PHQ(-D) in bariatric surgery candidates.

Conflict of Interests

The authors declare that there is no conflict of interests.

Acknowledgments

This work is part of the M.D. degree thesis of Ann Natascha Epple. The authors thank Angela Poeller for data collection.

References

[1] K. M. Flegal, M. D. Carroll, C. L. Ogden, and C. L. Johnson, "Prevalence and trends in obesity among US adults, 1999-2000," *Journal of the American Medical Association*, vol. 288, no. 14, pp. 1723–1727, 2002.

[2] R. Hyde, "Europe battles with obesity," *The Lancet*, vol. 371, no. 9631, pp. 2160–2161, 2008.

[3] G. B. M. Mensink, T. Lampert, and E. Bergmann, "Overweight and obesity in Germany 1984–2003," *Bundesgesundheitsblatt-Gesundheitsforschung-Gesundheitsschutz*, vol. 48, no. 12, pp. 1348–1356, 2005.

[4] K. R. Fontaine, D. T. Redden, C. Wang, A. O. Westfall, and D. B. Allison, "Years of life lost due to obesity," *Journal of the American Medical Association*, vol. 289, no. 2, pp. 187–193, 2003.

[5] L. De Wit, F. Luppino, A. van Straten, B. Penninx, F. Zitman, and P. Cuijpers, "Depression and obesity: a meta-analysis of community-based studies," *Psychiatry Research*, vol. 178, no. 2, pp. 230–235, 2010.

[6] K. A. Halmi, M. Long, A. J. Stunkard, and E. Mason, "Psychiatric diagnosis of morbidly obese gastric bypass patients," *American Journal of Psychiatry*, vol. 137, no. 4, pp. 470–472, 1980.

[7] M. Q. Werrij, S. Mulkens, H. J. Hospers, and A. Jansen, "Overweight and obesity: the significance of a depressed mood," *Patient Education and Counseling*, vol. 62, no. 1, pp. 126–131, 2006.

[8] R. Gertler and G. Ramsey-Stewart, "Pre-operative psychiatric assessment of patients presenting for gastric bariatric surgery (surgical control of morbid obesity)," *Australian and New Zealand Journal of Surgery*, vol. 56, no. 2, pp. 157–161, 1986.

[9] J. Glinski, S. Wetzler, and E. Goodman, "The psychology of gastric bypass surgery," *Obesity Surgery*, vol. 11, no. 5, pp. 581–588, 2001.

[10] F. Larsen, "Psychosocial function before and after gastric banding surgery for morbid obesity. A prospective psychiatric study," *Acta Psychiatrica Scandinavica, Supplement*, vol. 82, no. 359, pp. 1–57, 1990.

[11] P. S. Powers, A. Rosemurgy, F. Boyd, and A. Perez, "Outcome of gastric restriction procedures: weight, psychiatric diagnoses, and satisfaction," *Obesity Surgery*, vol. 7, no. 6, pp. 471–477, 1997.

[12] D. B. Sarwer, N. I. Cohn, L. M. Gibbons et al., "Psychiatric diagnoses and psychiatric treatment among bariatric surgery candidates," *Obesity Surgery*, vol. 14, no. 9, pp. 1148–1156, 2004.

[13] M. Heo, A. Pietrobelli, K. R. Fontaine, J. A. Sirey, and M. S. Faith, "Depressive mood and obesity in US adults: comparison and moderation by sex, age, and race," *International Journal of Obesity*, vol. 30, no. 3, pp. 513–519, 2006.

[14] G. E. Simon, M. Von Korff, K. Saunders et al., "Association between obesity and psychiatric disorders in the US adult population," *Archives of General Psychiatry*, vol. 63, no. 7, pp. 824–830, 2006.

[15] H. Baumeister and M. Härter, "Mental disorders in patients with obesity in comparison with healthy probands," *International Journal of Obesity*, vol. 6, pp. 1–10, 2007.

[16] C. U. Onyike, R. M. Crum, H. B. Lee, C. G. Lyketsos, and W. W. Eaton, "Is obesity associated with major depression? Results from the third National Health and Nutrition Examination Survey," *American Journal of Epidemiology*, vol. 158, no. 12, pp. 1139–1147, 2003.

[17] D. W. Black, W. R. Yates, J. H. Reich, S. Bell, R. B. Goldstein, and E. E. Mason, "DSM-III personality disorder in bariatric clinic patients," *Annals of Clinical Psychiatry*, vol. 1, no. 1, pp. 33–37, 1989.

[18] D. W. Black, R. B. Goldstein, and E. E. Mason, "Prevalence of mental disorder in 88 morbidly obese bariatric clinic patients," *American Journal of Psychiatry*, vol. 149, no. 2, pp. 227–234, 1992.

[19] S. Herpertz, R. Burgmer, A. Stang et al., "Prevalence of mental disorders in normal-weight and obese individuals with and without weight loss treatment in a German urban population," *Journal of Psychosomatic Research*, vol. 61, no. 1, pp. 95–103, 2006.

[20] L. Sjostrom, B. Larsson, L. Backman et al., "Swedish obese subjects (SOS). Recruitment for an intervention study and a selected description of the obese state," *International Journal of Obesity*, vol. 16, no. 6, pp. 465–479, 1992.

[21] M. Sullivan, J. Karlsson, L. Sjöström et al., "Swedish obese subjects (SOS)—an intervention study of obesity. Baseline evaluation of health and psychosocial functioning in the first 1 743 subjects examined," *International Journal of Obesity and Related Metabolic Disorders*, vol. 17, no. 9, pp. 503–512, 1993.

[22] T. A. Wadden, D. B. Sarwer, L. G. Womble, G. D. Foster, B. G. McGuckin, and A. Schimmel, "Psychosocial aspects of obesity and obesity surgery," *Surgical Clinics of North America*, vol. 81, no. 5, pp. 1001–1024, 2001.

[23] T. A. Wadden, M. L. Butryn, D. B. Sarwer et al., "Comparison of psychosocial status in treatment-seeking women with class III vs. Class I-II obesity," *Surgery for Obesity and Related Diseases*, vol. 2, no. 2, pp. 138–145, 2006.

[24] C. Ayyad and T. Andersen, "Long-term efficacy of dietary treatment of obesity: a systematic review of studies published between 1931 and 1999," *Obesity Reviews*, vol. 1, no. 2, pp. 113–119, 2000.

[25] G. K. Goodrick and J. P. Foreyt, "Why treatments for obesity don't last," *Journal of the American Dietetic Association*, vol. 91, no. 10, pp. 1243–1247, 1991.

[26] M. A. Kalarchian, M. D. Marcus, M. D. Levine et al., "Psychiatric disorders among bariatric surgery candidates: relationship to obesity and functional health status," *American Journal of Psychiatry*, vol. 164, no. 2, pp. 328–334, 2007.

[27] S. Ambwani, A. G. Boeka, J. D. Brown et al., "Socially desirable responding by bariatric surgery candidates during psychological assessment," *Surgery for Obesity and Related Diseases*, vol. 9, no. 2, pp. 300–305, 2003.

[28] A. N. Fabricatore, D. B. Sarwer, T. A. Wadden, C. J. Combs, and J. L. Krasucki, "Impression management or real change? Reports of depressive symptoms before and after the preoperative psychological evaluation for bariatric surgery," *Obesity Surgery*, vol. 17, no. 9, pp. 1213–1219, 2007.

[29] B. Mühlhans, T. Horbach, and M. de Zwaan, "Psychiatric disorders in bariatric surgery candidates: a review of the literature and results of a German prebariatric surgery sample," *General Hospital Psychiatry*, vol. 31, no. 5, pp. 414–421, 2009.

[30] M. Mauri, P. Rucci, A. Calderone et al., "Axis I and II disorders and quality of life in bariatric surgery candidates," *Journal of Clinical Psychiatry*, vol. 69, no. 2, pp. 295–301, 2008.

[31] P. H. Rosenberger, K. E. Henderson, and C. M. Grilo, "Psychiatric disorder comorbidity and association with eating disorders in bariatric surgery patients: a cross-sectional study using structured interview-based diagnosis," *Journal of Clinical Psychiatry*, vol. 67, no. 7, pp. 1080–1085, 2006.

[32] Y. Averbukh, S. Heshka, H. El-Shoreya et al., "Depression score predicts weight loss following roux-en-Y gastric bypass," *Obesity Surgery*, vol. 13, no. 6, pp. 833–836, 2003.

[33] P. Brunault, D. Jacobi, V. Miknius et al., "High preoperative depression, phobic anxiety, and binge eatings scores and low medium-term weight loss in sleeve gastrectomy obese patients: a preliminary cohort study," *Psychosomatics*, vol. 53, pp. 363–370, 2012.

[34] M. De Zwaan, J. Enderle, S. Wagner et al., "Anxiety and depression in bariatric surgery patients: a prospective, follow-up study using structured clinical interviews," *Journal of Affective Disorders*, vol. 133, no. 1-2, pp. 61–68, 2011.

[35] T. Legenbauer, M. de Zwaan, A. Benecke, B. Mühlhans, F. Petrak, and S. Herpertz, "Depression and anxiety: their predictive function for weight loss in obese individuals," *Obesity Facts*, vol. 2, no. 4, pp. 227–234, 2009.

[36] T. Legenbauer, F. Petrak, M. de Zwaan, and S. Herpertz, "Influence of depressive and eating disorders on short- and long-term course of weight after surgical and nonsurgical weight loss treatment," *Comprehensive Psychiatry*, vol. 52, no. 3, pp. 301–311, 2011.

[37] R. A. Krukowski, K. E. Friedman, and K. L. Applegate, "The utility of the beck depression inventory in a bariatric surgery population," *Obesity Surgery*, vol. 20, no. 4, pp. 426–431, 2010.

[38] D. J. Munoz, E. Chen, S. Fischer et al., "Considerations for the use of the beck depression inventory in the assessment of weight-loss surgery seeking patients," *Obesity Surgery*, vol. 17, no. 8, pp. 1097–1101, 2007.

[39] M. J. Hayden, W. A. Brown, L. Brennan, and O. 'Brien PE, "Validity of the Beck Depression Inventory as a screening tool for a clinical mood disorder in bariatric surgery candidates," *Obesity Surgery*, vol. 22, pp. 1666–1675, 2012.

[40] S. Cassin, S. Sockalingam, R. Hawa et al., "Psychometric properties of the Patient Health Questionnaire (PHQ-9) as a depression screening tool for bariatric surgery candidates," *Psychosomatics*, vol. 54, pp. 352–358, 2013.

[41] NIH (National Institutes of Health) Consensus Statement, "Gastrointestinal surgery for severe obesity," *Consens Statement*, vol. 279, pp. 1–20, 1991.

[42] R. L. Spitzer, K. Kroenke, and J. B. W. Williams, "Validation and utility of a self-report version of PRIME-MD: The PHQ Primary Care Study," *Journal of the American Medical Association*, vol. 282, no. 18, pp. 1737–1744, 1999.

[43] K. Gräfe, S. Zipfel, W. Herzog, and B. Löwe, "Screening psychischer Störungen mit dem, Gesundheitsfragebogen für Patienten (PHQ-D)," *Ergebnisse der Deutschen Validierungsstudie. Diagnostica*, vol. 50, pp. 171–181, 2004.

[44] B. Löwe, K. Gräfe, S. Zipfel, S. Witte, B. Loerch, and W. Herzog, "Diagnosing ICD-10 depressive episodes: superior criterion validity of the Patient Health Questionnaire," *Psychotherapy and Psychosomatics*, vol. 73, no. 6, pp. 386–390, 2004.

[45] B. Löwe, R. L. Spitzer, K. Gräfe et al., "Comparative validity of three screening questionnaires for DSM-IV depressive Disorders and physician's diagnoses," *Journal of Affective Disorders*, vol. 78, pp. 131–140, 2004.

[46] B. Löwe, R. L. Spitzer, and W. Herzog, *PHQ-D: Gesundheitsfragebogen Für Patienten*, Pfizer, Karlsruhe, Germany, 2002.

[47] M. R. Ali, J. J. Rasmussen, J. B. Monash, and W. D. Fuller, "Depression is associated with increased severity of co-morbidities in bariatric surgical candidates," *Surgery for Obesity and Related Diseases*, vol. 5, no. 5, pp. 559–564, 2009.

[48] L. R. Jones-Corneille, T. A. Wadden, D. B. Sarwer et al., "Axis i psychopathology in bariatric surgery candidates with and without binge eating disorder: results of structured clinical interviews," *Obesity Surgery*, vol. 22, no. 3, pp. 389–397, 2012.

[49] G. M. Papageorgiou, A. Papakonstantinou, E. Mamplekou, I. Terzis, and J. Melissas, "Pre- and postoperative psychological characteristics in morbidly obese patients," *Obesity Surgery*, vol. 12, no. 4, pp. 534–539, 2002.

[50] R. L. Kolotkin, R. D. Crosby, R. Pendleton, M. Strong, R. E. Gress, and T. Adams, "Health-related quality of life in patients seeking gastric bypass surgery vs non-treatment-seeking controls," *Obesity Surgery*, vol. 13, no. 3, pp. 371–377, 2003.

[51] H. Ø. Lier, E. Biringer, B. Stubhaug, H. R. Eriksen, and T. Tangen, "Psychiatric disorders and participation in Pre- and postoperative counselling groups in bariatric surgery patients," *Obesity Surgery*, vol. 21, no. 6, pp. 730–737, 2011.

[52] M. De Zwaan, J. E. Mitchell, L. Michael Howell et al., "Characteristics of morbidly obese patients before gastric bypass surgery," *Comprehensive Psychiatry*, vol. 44, no. 5, pp. 428–434, 2003.

[53] J. E. Mitchell and M. P. Mussell, "Comorbidity and binge eating disorder," *Addictive Behaviors*, vol. 20, no. 6, pp. 725–732, 1995.

[54] C. F. Telch and E. Stice, "Psychiatric comorbidity in women with binge eating disorder: prevalence rates from a non-treatment-seeking sample," *Journal of Consulting and Clinical Psychology*, vol. 66, no. 5, pp. 768–776, 1998.

[55] S. Walfish, D. Vance, and A. N. Fabricatore, "Psychological evaluation of bariatric surgery applicants: procedures and reasons for delay or denial of surgery," *Obesity Surgery*, vol. 17, no. 12, pp. 1578–1583, 2007.

[56] K. A. Wittkampf, H. van Ravesteijn, K. D. Baas et al., "The accuracy of Patient Health Questionnaire-9 in detecting depression and measuring depression severity in high-risk groups in primary care," *General Hospital Psychiatry*, vol. 31, no. 5, pp. 451–459, 2009.

[57] S. M. Eack, C. G. Greeno, and B.-J. Lee, "Limitations of the patient health questionnaire in identifying anxiety and depression in community mental health: many cases are undetected," *Research on Social Work Practice*, vol. 16, no. 6, pp. 625–631, 2006.

[58] J. F. Kinzl, C. Maier, and A. Bösch, "Morbidly obese patients: psychopathology and eating disorders—results of a preoperative evaluation," *Neuropsychiatr*, vol. 26, pp. 159–165, 2012.

[59] A. Schlick, S. A. Wagner, B. Mühlhans et al., "Agreement between clinical evaluation and structured clinical interviews (SCID for DSM-IV) in morbidly obese pre-bariatric surgery patients," *Psychotherapie Psychosomatik Medizinische Psychologie*, vol. 4, pp. 640–646, 2010.

[60] J. E. Mitchell, K. J. Steffen, M. de Zwaan, T. W. Ertelt, J. M. Marino, and A. Mueller, "Congruence between clinical and research-based psychiatric assessment in bariatric surgical

candidates," *Surgery for Obesity and Related Diseases*, vol. 6, no. 6, pp. 628–634, 2010.

[61] R. I. Berkowitz and A. N. Fabricatore, "Obesity, psychiatric status, and psychiatric medications," *Psychiatric Clinics of North America*, vol. 34, no. 4, pp. 747–764, 2011.

Missing Motherhood: Jordanian Women's Experiences with Infertility

Hala Mahmoud Obeidat,[1] Adlah M. Hamlan,[2] and Lynn Clark Callister[3]

[1] *Maternal Child Health Nursing Department, Princess Muna College of Nursing, Mutah University, Amman, Jordan*
[2] *Jordan University, Amman, Jordan*
[3] *Brigham Young University College of Nursing, Provo, UT 84602, USA*

Correspondence should be addressed to Lynn Clark Callister; callister-lynn@comcast.net

Academic Editor: Takahiro Nemoto

Aim, Background, and Introduction. Bearing and rearing children are an important part of life in nearly all cultures and are a central role for Jordanian Muslim women. Infertility can create anxiety, stress, and depression for couples who are infertile. Women frequently bear the emotional stigma of a couple's infertility. There is a paucity of literature focusing on Jordanian Muslim women experiencing infertility and failed assistive reproductive technology. Therefore, this study explored these women's lived experience. *Methods.* Qualitative data were collected through interviews with 30 Jordanian Muslim women who experienced failed assistive reproductive technology for infertility. Perceptions of experiences with failed treatment of infertility were documented and analyzed. *Results.* Major themes were identified: missing out on motherhood and living with infertility, experiencing marital stressors, feeling social pressure, experiencing depression and disappointment, having treatment associated difficulties, appreciating support from family and friends, using coping strategies, and fear of an unknown future. *Discussion, Conclusion, and Implications for Clinical Practice.* Being infertile significantly influences the physical, emotional, social, and spiritual health of Jordanian Muslim women as well as their quality of life. Perceived social support and personal coping strategies were used by study participants to mediate failed attempts to conceive. Designing and implementing culturally appropriate interventions for Muslim women globally who are experiencing infertility are essential.

1. Introduction

Children provide their parents the existential role of participating in the continuity of the family, the culture, and the community. Most societies, especially in developing countries, are structured to rely on children for the future care and maintenance of older family members [1]. The United Nations (UN) Declaration of Human Rights recognizes that adults, without any limitations due to race, nationality, or religion, have the right to marry and have a family [2]. Infertility has been recognized by WHO as a public health issue, and the right to infertility treatment is part of Millennium Development Goal number 5 [3].

Infertility is a condition in which pregnancy has not occurred after one year of unprotected, well-timed intercourse [4]. Infertility is a reproductive health indicator, such as maternal mortality rates. It is an important global issue where infertility is perceived as a tragedy for many women who may be ostracized and stigmatized in their sociocultural environment [5].

Impaired fertility affects approximately 80 million people globally, with rates ranging from less than 5% to over 30% [2]. The rates of infertility worldwide are estimated to be at least 15% in women of childbearing age, with an estimated 40.5 million women seeking treatment [6]. Even with the advancement in reproductive technology, the incidence of infertility is expected to increase to 7.7 million by 2025 [7]. In Jordan, the primary infertility rate is estimated to be 3.5% and the secondary infertility rate 13.5% [8]. A more recent source concludes that the prevalence of infertility in Jordan is not definitive which may be related to differing definitions of infertility [9].

Women frequently bear the emotional stigma of a couple's infertility even though infertility is shared by both men and women. In 35% of infertile couples the woman is infertile, in 35% the man is infertile, and in the remaining 30% the problem is either shared by both partners or of undetermined origin [4].

Islam is the second largest religion in the world, with 25% of the global population espousing these religious beliefs and practices [10]. In Jordan, which is an Arab Muslim nation, marriage is strongly linked to procreation and family formation. Adoption is not a choice for infertile couples due to religious prohibitions. Therefore, diagnosis of infertility itself is stigmatizing and may lead to significant levels of emotional distress. Women for whom child bearing is a major object of their lives may be hesitant to reveal their infertility problems even to their closest friends and relatives. In Muslim communities, Islam encourages family formation and assisted reproduction, when indicated, within the frame of a committed legal marital relationship [11, 12].

2. Significance and Background

The medicalization of infertility may lead to a disregard of the feelings infertility may engender, including depression, anger, anxiety, emotional distress, loss of control, shame, stigmatization, and feelings of isolation [13–16]. Regardless of the cause of the infertility, women bear the burden of invasive procedures related to diagnosis and management of infertility [4]. Health care providers may view infertility as a medical condition rather than taking a holistic approach to caring for couples who are infertile.

Qualitative approaches can describe the lived experience of women who are experiencing infertility. No published studies could be found in the literature focusing on the infertility experience of Jordanian Muslim women. Such research can guide health care providers in planning and developing holistic care that addresses the cultural and psychosocial needs of women who are infertile. The aim of the study was to explore Jordanian Muslim women's lived experience of infertility.

The Biopsychosocial Theory of Infertility conceptualizes infertility as an acute life crisis with long-term implications for the individual, his or her partner, their relationship, and family and friends [17]. The stressors of infertility are categorized as psychological, physical, and interpersonal. According to this theory, social support and other coping strategies mediate the effect of infertility. This theory was used to guide data collection and analysis.

Social stressors of infertility may differ according to societal norms. In developed societies, voluntary childlessness is viewed as a more viable and legitimate option and women without children are often presumed to be voluntarily childfree. However, in developing countries like Jordan, bearing and rearing children are central to women's power and wellbeing and stigma related to infertility may be greater [18, 19].

The central role of motherhood for Jordanian Muslim women has been described. For example, a 39-year-old mother of seven children noted, "Our prophet Mohammed said, 'Reproduce and have children as I am in the life after. I will be proud of you in front of the nations'" [20]. In another

study, a Jordanian Muslim primipara said, "People start asking after the first month of marriage whether you "save anything inside your abdomen" meaning, "are you pregnant yet?" So is the nature of life. I got pregnant after two months of marriage" [21].

According to Islamic tradition, having children is the most important Muslim religious injunction [22]. Procreation is encouraged, and a bride's status is not ensured until she demonstrates proven fertility. Pressure to have children includes cultural traditions, familial expectations, and religious injunctions. In addition to Islamic beliefs about the sacred nature of bearing children, children are highly valued for social prestige as well as the potential for future economic and physical support of their parents [23–26].

The impact of infertility on marital relationships depends on the sociocultural context. In settings where women's roles are more closely tied to having children, where producing children for one's family is considered an important obligation and where marriage is defined in terms of producing and raising children, infertility is likely to have a greater negative impact on the couple's relationship [18]. There are gender differences in response to infertility. In a study of Dutch couples experiencing infertility, women had lower levels of quality of life than their partners [27].

Social support and coping are considered to be mediators of infertility stress experience. Studies on psychological interventions for infertile couples suggest that psychosocial interventions could reduce negative effect associated with infertility [28, 29]. Women receiving assisted reproductive technologies cope with the stress of infertility by using their social support resources [28, 30].

One of the coping strategies that women use in their experience of infertility is making a conscious effort to create a new life that created a space to move forward by shifting from grief to focusing their energy toward the future [31]. However, coping strategies which are beneficial to one individual may be problematic for his or her partner. Couples with men using high amounts of distancing, while their partner used low amounts of distancing, reported higher levels of distress [32].

3. Methodology

This descriptive qualitative study has qualitative phenomenological components [33]. Such research is useful in increasing our understanding of complex life experiences such as infertility. The study participants were thirty Muslim women experiencing infertility with age range from 26 to 42 years with mean age of 32 ± 5.2 years. Table 1 presents the demographic characteristics of study participants. They were selected purposively by using snowball sampling technique through professional and social networking. The participants met the inclusion criteria including failure to conceive after at least one year of unprotected sex, identification of self as being infertile, having underwent failed treatment of infertility, and being willing to share their experience.

The study participants were educated with a minimal educational level of secondary school through having graduate

TABLE 1: Demographics.

Demographic variable	Frequency	Percentage
Employment status		
Employed	12	40
Homemaker	18	60
Education		
Primary	20	66.7
Secondary	10	33.3
University		
Demographic variable	Mean	Standard deviation
Age	32	
Years of infertility	7	2.1

degrees. They had primary infertility and experienced five to eight failed assistive reproductive procedures in infertility centers in Jordan. They were married for seven to ten years with an upper middle class income and were all employed outside the home.

3.1. Data Collection and Analysis. The data were generated by using digitally recorded interviews in the home of the participants. The interview was started with the question, "Please tell me about your experience of not having children." In addition, the interview included questions based on a review of the literature, the researcher's clinical experience, and the Biopsychosocial Theory of Infertility.

Data analysis was concurrent with data collection. Data collection continued until saturation was reached. The interviews were transcribed into text by the interviewer shortly after it was conducted. Before the translation of text into English, the digitally taped interviews were compared with transcript. The confirmed transcripts were translated to English language by the researcher and then back translated into Arabic by another bilingual person. Three researchers analyzed the data separately and then compared the results.

Colaizzi's [34] method of analysis and interpretation was utilized to identify the significant statement, subthemes, and major themes. Data analysis began with the researcher rereading the participant's descriptions frequently and putting herself in their place in order to understand their concepts. Reading and rereading of transcripts were used to identify the significant statements. After that, this information was grouped in meaningful units that comprise the themes clusters (subthemes). These subthemes were grouped together to provide the major themes which were supported by the researcher citing specific excerpts from the interviews [33]. Also, the nonverbal expressions of participants were used to support the meaning of emerged significant statements. Individual data analyses were compared and consensus was reached on the final themes by the research team (Figure 1).

3.2. Trustworthiness of the Data. Data rigor in qualitative research (trustworthiness) is how accurately the study discovers and represents the participants' experience. Immersion of researcher in the data by recurrent reading of the transcript

and constant comparative of significant information was used to enhance the dependability of data. Member check was used as a potential contributor to data credibility. Also, using multiple researchers on data analysis was used to ensure the data confirmability.

3.3. Ethical Consideration. The study was approved by the Ethical Committee of Jordan Royal Medical Services. Participants provided written informed consent upon recruitment as well as a process consent which was used throughout the interviews. Confidentiality and privacy were ensured.

4. Study Findings

Study participants were Jordanian Muslim women who had not become pregnant after at least one year of unprotected sex. They were all employed and had five to eight failed trials of assistive reproductive technology procedures.

The results are expressed in major themes that reflect the Biopsychosocial Theory assumptions. The overriding theme is missing motherhood and living with infertility. Others include experiencing marital stressors, feeling social pressure, experiencing depression and disappointment, feeling treatment associated difficulties, appreciating support from family and friends, and fearing an unknown future. Figure 2 presents the model of Biopsychosocial Theory showing related major themes emerging from study findings.

5. Missing Motherhood and Living with Infertility

The overriding theme of participants experiences with infertility was missing motherhood. Study participants described their dreams of having children and their pain at not being as other women who seemed to become pregnant so easily. One woman said, "*Every one of us dreams of having children. I married at age 23. Everyone dreams that when she arrives in her thirties she* [will have] *one or two children. Every one of us dreams of being a mother.*" She described being a mother as "*life's sinew*" and said her seven years of seeking to become pregnant seemed so long.

The participants spoke with deep emotion about seeing other women pregnant, "*Sometimes you see women who complain about the pregnancy: 'ooh, my abdomen is large. I am tired' and at the same time you wish to be just like them for just one day, and I couldn't. Of course this hurts, hurting my* [heart] *more than any other thing.*"

5.1. Experiencing Marital Stressors. The participants reported marital stressors such as "querying the social questioning," "lack of relation intimacy," and "feeling guilt." They described social questioning regarding their situation with the intrusion into a very personal and painful experience. One study participant said, "*People around us still pressure us and still ask, 'Why?' What did you do?' When somebody talks about the issue, we start to argue* [with each other]." Participants felt that infertility contributed to a lack of intimacy in the marital

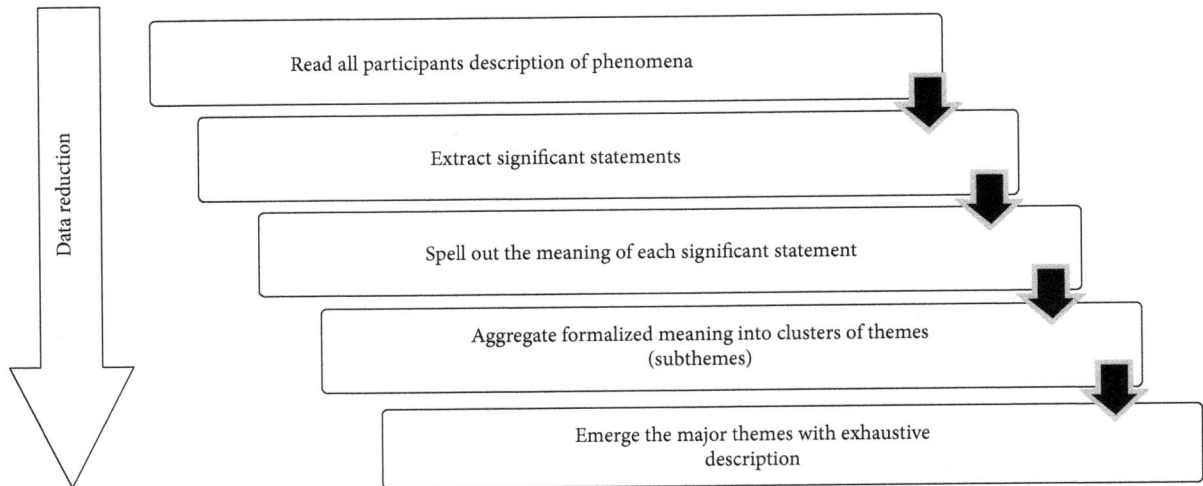

FIGURE 1: Data analysis.

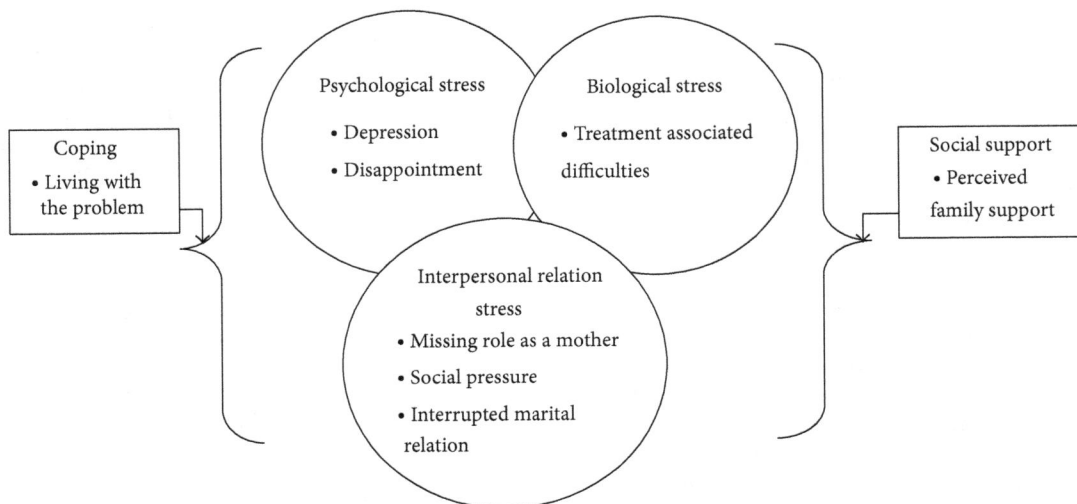

FIGURE 2: Study results as within the framework of the Biopsychosocial Theory of Infertility.

relationship since sexual relations were focused on getting pregnancy rather than as an expression of love.

Feelings of guilt emerged when they spoke of their inability to provide a child for their husbands as expressed by one wife, "*You are affected when you see your husband playing with other people's children. You feel that he also has a desire to have a child. You feel guilty.*"

Also, feeling of failure resulted from the participant's response to treatment failure and inability to reach the optimum goal considered as a stressor that affects the marital relationship. Some study participants feared the future, expecting their husband may divorce them or marry another woman. One woman said, "*even though my husband loves me, he may decide to divorce me or marry another women to reach his goal of being a father.*"

5.2. Feeling Social Pressure. Social pressure was described as social questioning and social stigma. Social questioning

increases stress, "*of course these questions started. These questions let you still think about the issue. Every time you try to forget the issue—to live with it—people are still remembering.*" The participants also spoke of the social stigma as if the situation were their fault when treatment did not succeed, "*They said, 'strange—everyone succeeded but you. This is hurting me a lot because it's out of my hands.*"

5.3. Experiencing Depression and Disappointment. Depression was expressed as recurrent suffering and sadness. The women reported that their suffering recurred monthly with each menstrual period signaling no pregnancy again and failed treatment, "*Every month when menstruation occurs—its like a moment of suffering and sorrow because this month no pregnancy occurs.*" After a failed insemination procedure, with again no pregnancy, they reported weeping, crying, refusing to eat, and sleeplessness in response to treatment failure.

Study participants repeatedly asked "*why do I not become pregnant?*"

Study participants spoke about having feelings of uncertainty and failure, wondering whether or not treatment would be successful in conceiving, "*You are nervous, upset, afraid: maybe yes, maybe no. The days and nights passed and I was thinking [only] God knows.*" They wanted so much to please their husband and their parents by becoming pregnant and bearing a child. They said with pain, "*Again I did not reach my goal.*"

5.4. Having Treatment Associated Difficulties. The participants spoke of the physiological side effects of infertility treatment, "*When you take injections and hormones you have tiredness, increase in heart rate, and [rapid] breathing. You feel hot because all of your hormones are disturbed.*"

The women described the financial burdens associated with infertility treatment, since it was not covered by health insurance, saying, "*you still pay and pay and at last no results.*" Recurrent work leaves were required, contributing to time lost from their employment.

Infertility was ameliorated by social support and using coping strategies in order to live with infertility. Coping strategies included turning to God by intensified religious practices, exercising avoidance, and continuing to pursue having a child.

5.5. Appreciating Support from Friends and Families. Most of the participants noted they had their thoughtful and sensitive colleagues in the workplace who "*comfort me and this reduces my stress.*" Family support, both emotional and instrumental, proved very helpful. The participants reported that their family supported them emotionally by being considerate of their feelings and by advocating for them when others asked about the situation, "*When anyone talked about the issue, my father in law said, 'do not pressure them. It's enough, the pressure they already have.'*" Instrumental support was provided by the family helping to bear the costs of the medical procedures, "*My family and my husband's family were helping when we have a critical situation of no money.*" They expressed their gratitude that their families did not give up on helping them.

5.6. Using Coping Strategies. The women lived with the problem by turning to God, utilizing avoidance strategies, and problem focused strategies. They found their spiritual beliefs in God and the practice of religious rituals helpful in coping with infertility as well as increasing their religious faith, "*It's well known that we are Muslims. Always we leave everything in God's hands. First the person should trust in God. Second is to turn to prayer, invocation, and reading the Quran.*" They repeated that in spite of their belief that "*everything is in God's hands,*" they could not hide their feelings of disappointment and a sense of sadness in not becoming pregnant.

Avoidance helped the couples to escape from the constant focus on having a child, "*My husband and I try to change the situation. We travel especially after any procedure or when menstruation occurs.*" Problem focused strategies included continuing to participate actively in assisted reproductive technologies, as well as trying complementary and alternative interventions.

6. Discussion

Study findings document stressors associated with infertility in Jordanian Muslim women. These women described the social stressors experienced living in a society that highly values bearing children. This finding is consistent with those of Fido and Zahid [35], who reported that childlessness resulted in social stigmatization for Kuwaiti women who are infertile, placing them at risk of serious social and emotional consequences.

Social relationships may be strained as a result of infertility. In the current study lack of relationship intimacy was reported as one of the effects of infertility related to concentrating on having sexual relation to become pregnant. Consistently, in a study of Turkish women, the respondents reported negative influence of fertility problems on the sexual relationships within couples as change in the patterns of their relationships, tension and arguments between partners [36].

The assumptions of Biopsychosocial Theory and the literature indicate that the negative psychological effects of infertility can damage an individual's self-image, especially when achieving pregnancy is failed and the individual starts regarding himself or herself as worthless as well as the generating depression and self-destructive thoughts [37]. Study findings supported theoretical assumptions with reports of depression, feelings that emerged through sadness, and recurrent suffering especially when conventional medical interventions fail.

Most of the studies reported that infertile women experienced psychopathological consequences like depression, anger, anxiety, social isolation, and feelings of guilt [14–16]. Infertile Kuwaiti women exhibited a significant higher psychopathology in the form of tension, hostility, anxiety, depression, self-blame, and suicidal ideation [35]. However, participants in the current study did not disclose self-destructive thoughts, which could be related to their religious beliefs and faith as a Muslim.

Regarding the physical stressors of infertility, Gerrity [37] stated that physical effect of infertility is more direct for women because of available medical interventions. Current study findings indicated that difficulties associated with medical treatment of infertility include physiological side effects, compounded by overwhelming financial expenses and time losses.

The literature as well as the women in this study reported that the physiological side effects of infertility treatment are one of the most challenging physical stressors women experience [38].

One of the factors mediating the pain of infertility is social support. In this case, study participants reported receiving emotional support from extended family as well as instrumental support to overcome the financial burden of infertility treatment costs. Jordanian Muslim cultural values include strong family adherence.

Appraisal of the situation resulted in the use of different coping strategies. Findings of the current study indicate that learning to live with infertility was the major theme when assisted reproductive technology failed. Trust in God was a powerful coping strategy for these women experiencing infertility. Islamic spiritual beliefs and religious rites strengthened these women's trust in God and helped them cope with this challenge. These women also utilized problem focused strategies, seeking medical solutions for infertility. This is also reflected in a study of infertile Kuwaiti women who sought medical treatment [35].

On the other hand, some study participants used avoidance as a coping strategy after failed medical treatment. Peterson and associates [39] also reported that couples who use active avoidance coping seek relief from stress through actively avoiding problematic situations and reminders of infertility.

Bardaweel and associates [9] found among 1,031 Jordanian individuals struggling with infertility, 45% used spiritual healing and herbal medicine in addition to mainstream medical interventions. The use of complementary medicine is common in developing countries including Jordan and may be associated with strong religious beliefs.

Limitations of the Study. The study has limitations including recruitment methods used to generate a convenience sample. Participants were both educated and economically secure. The inclusion of Muslim women exclusively in this study was essential in order to identify the lived experience for those in the same cultural and religion background. The generalizability of the findings is limited but transferability to other populations of women with infertility is ensured by the trustworthiness of the data.

7. Implications for Clinical Practice and Research

Jordanian Muslim women experiencing infertility report this having a profound impact on all aspects of their lives. This research highlights several important implications for clinical practice with global dimensions since Muslim women live throughout the world. The findings of qualitative research can be translated into clinical practice guidelines [40]. The Low Cost *In Vitro* Fertilization Foundation (http://www.lowcost-ivf.org/) was established in 2006 to overcome the lack of cost-effective ART available in the developing world [41]. Such noteworthy initiatives are essential to implement if Millennium Development Goal number 5 is to be met by 2015. This may ameliorate the financial burden of infertility treatment.

Little is known about the effectiveness of complementary and alternative methods (CAM) in treating infertility, but perhaps the use of complementary methods may help couples feel that they have attempted all treatment options [9]. Nurses need to be aware of the psychosocial and emotional impact of women's experience with infertility within their sociocultural context [42, 43]. Thus, designing and conducting supportive

programs play an important role in providing quality care for them [29]. Culturally sensitive assessment of the woman's partner, extended family, and social support network is important as a means to ascertain levels of social support that may mediate the experience's effects and enhance their sense of wellbeing [26–28].

Future research is recommended to identify the lived experience of infertility by further studying the marital dyad as a unit of analysis in order to enrich our knowledge of the social perspective of the infertility experience. Longitudinal studies measuring changes over time are also recommended [15].

Conflict of Interests

No conflict of interests has been declared by the authors.

References

[1] I. Hassanin, T. Abd-El-Raheem, and A. Shahin, "Primary infertility and health-related quality of life in Upper Egypt," *International Journal of Gynecology and Obstetrics*, vol. 110, no. 2, pp. 118–121, 2010.

[2] World Health Organization, *Reproductive Health Indicators: Guidelines for their Generation, Interpretation and Analysis for Global Monitoring*, World Health Organization, Geneva, Switzerland, 2006.

[3] United Nations, "Millennium Development Goals," 2000, http://www.un.org/millennium/declaration/ares552e.

[4] Centers for Disease Control, *Outline for a National Action Plan for the Prevention, Detection and Management of Infertility*, Centers for Disease Control, Atlanta, Ga, USA, 2010.

[5] L. C. Callister, "Global infertility: are we caring yet?" *The American Journal of Maternal Child Nursing*, vol. 35, no. 3, p. 174, 2010.

[6] M. C. Inhorn, "Right to assisted reproductive technology: overcoming infertility in low-resource countries," *International Journal of Gynecology and Obstetrics*, vol. 106, no. 2, pp. 172–174, 2009.

[7] M. N. Mascarenhas, S. R. Flaxman, T. Boerma, S. Vanderpoel, and G. A. Stevens, "National, regional and global trends in infertility prevalence since 1990. Health surveys," *PLoS Medicine*, vol. 9, no. 12, Article ID e 1001356.

[8] S. Rutstein and I. Shah, *Infecundity, Infertility, and Childlessness in Developing Countries*, DHS Comparative Reports No. 9, ORC Macro and the World Health Organization, Calverton, Md, USA, 2004.

[9] S. K. Bardaweel, M. Shehadeh, G. A. R. Y. Suaifan, and M. V. Z. Kilani, "Complementary and alternative medicine utilization by a sample of infertile couples in Jordan for infertility treatment: clinics-based survey," *BMC Complementary and Alternative Medicine*, vol. 13, article 35, 2013.

[10] M. C. Inhorn and G. I. Serour, "Islam, medicine, and Arab-Muslim refugee health in America after 9/11," *The Lancet*, vol. 378, no. 9794, pp. 935–943, 2011.

[11] M. C. Inhorn, "Making Muslim babies: IVF and gamete donation in Sunni versus shi'a Islam," *Culture and Medicine and Psychiatry*, vol. 30, no. 4, pp. 427–450, 2006.

[12] G. Serour, "Islamic perspectives in human reproduction," *Reproductive BioMedicine*, vol. 17, no. 3, pp. 34–38, 2008.

[13] T. Cousineau and A. Domar, "Psychological impact of infertility," *Best Practice and Research: Clinical Obstetrics and Gynaecology*, vol. 21, no. 2, pp. 293–308, 2007.

[14] A. Galhardo, M. Cunha, and J. Pinto-Gouveia, "Psychological aspects in couples with infertility," *Sexologies*, vol. 20, no. 4, pp. 224–228, 2011.

[15] B. D. Peterson, C. S. Sejback, L. Pieritana, and L. Schmidt, "Are severe depressive symptoms associated with infertility-related distress in individuals and their partners?" *Human Reproduction*, vol. 29, no. 1, pp. 76–82, 2014.

[16] L. Schmidt, "Infertility and assisted reproduction in Denmark: epidemiology and psychosocial consequences," *Danish Medical Bulletin*, vol. 53, no. 4, pp. 390–417, 2006.

[17] L. A. Pasch and C. Dunkel-Schetter, "Fertility problems: complex issues faced by women and couples," in *Health Care for Women: Psychological, Social, and Behavioral Influences*, S. J. Gallant, G. P. Keita, and R. Royak-Schaler, Eds., American Psychological Association, Washington, DC, USA, 1997.

[18] A. Greil, K. Slauson-Blevins, and J. McQuillan, "The experience of infertility: a review of recent literature," *Sociology of Health and Illness*, vol. 32, no. 1, pp. 140–162, 2010.

[19] P. Jennings, "God had something else in mind: family, religion, and infertility," *Journal of Contemporary Ethnography*, vol. 39, no. 2, pp. 215–237, 2010.

[20] I. A. Khalaf, F. Abu-Moghli, L. C. Callister, and R. Rasheed, "Jordanian women's experiences with the use of traditional family planning," *Health Care for Women International*, vol. 29, no. 5, pp. 527–538, 2008.

[21] I. Khalaf and L. C. Callister, "Cultural meanings of childbirth: muslim women living in Jordan," *Journal of Holistic Nursing*, vol. 15, no. 4, pp. 373–388, 1997.

[22] A. Y. Ali, *An English Interpretation of the Holy Quran*, Ashraf Printing, Lahore, Pakistan, 1992.

[23] M. Farsoun, N. Khoury, and C. Underwood, *In Their Own Words: A Qualitative Study of Family Planning in Jordan*, IEC Field Report no. 6, John Hopkins University Center for Communication Programs, Baltimore, Md, USA, 1996.

[24] S. A. Kridli and K. Libbus, "Contraception in Jordan: a cultural and religious perspective," *International Nursing Review*, vol. 48, no. 3, pp. 144–151, 2001.

[25] S. A. Kridli, "Health beliefs and practices among Arab women," *The American Journal of Maternal Child Nursing*, vol. 27, no. 3, pp. 178–182, 2002.

[26] J. Schmid, S. Kirchengast, E. Vytiska-Binstorfer, and J. Huber, "Infertility caused by PCOS—Health-related quality of life among Austrian and Moslem immigrant women in Austria," *Human Reproduction*, vol. 19, no. 10, pp. 2251–2257, 2004.

[27] A. S. Huppelschoten, A. J. C. M. van Dongen, C. M. Verhaak, J. M. J. Smeenk, J. A. M. Kremer, and W. L. D. M. Nelen, "Differences in quality of life and emotional status between infertile women and their partners," *Human Reproduction*, vol. 28, no. 8, pp. 2168–2176, 2013.

[28] M. V. Martins, B. D. Peterson, V. Almeida, L. Mesquita-Guimaraes, and M. C. Costa, "Dyadic dynamics of perceived social support in couples facing infertility," *Human Reproduction*, vol. 29, no. 1, pp. 85–89, 2014.

[29] T. Wischmann, "Implications of psychosocial support in infertility a critical appraisal," *Journal of Psychosomatic Obstetrics and Gynecology*, vol. 29, no. 2, pp. 83–90, 2008.

[30] D. Gibson and J. Myers, "The effect of social coping resources and growth-fostering relationships on infertility stress in women," *Journal of Mental Health Counseling*, vol. 1, pp. 1–6, 2005.

[31] P. McCarthy, "Women's lived experience of infertility after unsuccessful medical intervention," *Journal of Midwifery and Women's Health*, vol. 53, no. 4, pp. 319–324, 2008.

[32] B. Peterson, C. Newton, K. Rosen, and R. Schulman, "Coping processes of couples experiencing infertility," *Family Relations*, vol. 55, no. 2, pp. 227–239, 2006.

[33] H. S. Speziale, H. J. Streubert, and D. Carpenter, *Qualitative Research in Nursing*, Lippincott Williams & Wilkins, Philadelphia, Pa, USA, 2011.

[34] P. Colaizzi, *Reflection and Research in Psychology*, Kendall Kent, Dubque, IL, USA, 1973.

[35] A. Fido and M. A. Zahid, "Coping with infertility among Kuwaiti women: cultural perspectives," *International Journal of Social Psychiatry*, vol. 50, no. 4, pp. 294–300, 2004.

[36] F. B. van Rooij, F. van Balen, and J. Hermanns, "The experiences of involuntarily childless Turkish immigrants in the Netherlands," *Qualitative Health Research*, vol. 19, no. 5, pp. 621–632, 2009.

[37] D. Gerrity, "A biopsychosocial theory of infertility," *The Family Journal*, vol. 9, no. 2, pp. 151–158, 2001.

[38] V. Madge, "Infertility, women and assisted reproductive technologies: an exploratory study in Pune, India," *Indian Journal of Gender Studies*, vol. 18, no. 1, pp. 1–26, 2011.

[39] B. Peterson, M. Pirritano, J. Block, and L. Schmidt, "Marital benefit and coping strategies in men and women undergoing unsuccessful fertility treatments over a 5-year period," *Fertility and Sterility*, vol. 95, no. 5, pp. 1759–1763, 2011.

[40] P. S. Hinds, J. S. Gattuso, E. Barnwell et al., "Translating psychosocial research findings into practice guidelines," *Journal of Nursing Administration*, vol. 33, no. 7-8, pp. 397–403, 2003.

[41] I. D. Cooke, L. Gianaroli, O. Hovatta et al., "Affordable ART and the Third World: difficulties to overcome," *Human Reproduction*, vol. 10, no. 1, pp. 93–96, 2008.

[42] H. Azaizeh, B. Saad, E. Cooper, and O. Said, "Traditional Arabic and Islamic medicine: a re-emerging health aid," *Evidence-based Complementary and Alternative Medicine*, vol. 7, no. 4, pp. 419–424, 2010.

[43] A. Oweis, "The Hashemite Kingdom of Jordan," in *Cultural Health Assessment*, A. Polyanskaya, Ed., Elsevier, New York, NY, USA, 4th edition, 2008.

3

Factors in Mental Health Problems among Japanese Dialysis Patients Living in Heavily Damaged Prefectures Two Years after the Great East Japan Earthquake

Hidehiro Sugisawa,[1] Hiroaki Sugisaki,[2] Seiji Ohira,[3] Toshio Shinoda,[4] Yumiko Shimizu,[5] and Tamaki Kumagai[6]

[1] *Graduate School of Gerontology, J. F. Oberlin University, Machida-shi 194-0294, Japan*
[2] *Hachioji Azumacho Clinic, Hachioji-shi 192-0082, Japan*
[3] *Sapporo Kita Clinic, Sapporo-shi 001-0018, Japan*
[4] *Kawakita General Hospital, Suginami-ku 166-0001, Japan*
[5] *School of Nursing, Jikei University, Chofu-shi 182-08570, Japan*
[6] *Faculty of Health Care and Nursing, Juntendo University, Urayasu-shi 279-0023, Japan*

Correspondence should be addressed to Hidehiro Sugisawa; sugisawa@obirin.ac.jp

Academic Editor: Kai G. Kahl

This study examined the prevalence of mental health problems and related factors among dialysis patients living in prefectures that were heavily damaged by the Great East Japan Earthquake. Research was conducted two years following the disaster, and data of 1500 residents of the prefectures were analyzed. This study examined disaster related stressors, gender, socioeconomic status, health problems prior the earthquake, and social support, all of which have been identified as aggravating/mitigating factors in previous research on disaster survivors. We also examined advanced awareness of emergency planning as a dialysis specific factor. Mental health problems after the disaster were categorized into three types: PTSD and depression comorbidity, PTSD only, and depression only. Results indicated that people with comorbidity, PTSD, and depression comprised 7.5%, 25.0%, and 2.9% of the sample, respectively. Not only disaster related stressors but also health problems prior to the disaster had an aggravating direct effect on comorbidity and PTSD. In addition, social support and advanced awareness of disaster planning had a mitigating effect on comorbidity. These results suggest that advanced awareness of disaster planning is a dialysis specific factor that could decrease the occurrence of comorbidity among dialysis patients following a disaster.

1. Introduction

The earthquake known as the Great East Japan Earthquake occurred on March 11, 2011. The temblor, which was registered at a magnitude of 9.0, triggered a massive tsunami that struck the northeastern coastline, which in turn resulted in a catastrophic failure at the Fukushima Daiichi nuclear power plant, seriously damaging the reactor cooling systems and releasing radioactivity. The compound nature of the disaster—the earthquake, tsunami, and release of radiation—devastated vast areas of northeastern Japan. Many parts of this region have not fully recovered. According to the national police agency, as of November 2012 the death toll from the earthquake and related events stands at 15,883, with a separate number of 2,651 listed as missing [1].

Effects of natural disasters on certain aspects of mental health in survivors have been identified in most studies reviewed by Norris and Elrod [2]. In Japan, the influence of disaster on survivors' mental health has been examined in relation to previous earthquakes [3–9]. The impact of the Great East Japan Earthquake (also known as the 3/11 earthquake) on mental health has been examined in various groups: people evacuated in shelters [10], young people [11–13], and others [14]. Hemodialysis patients are among those that have a higher risk of developing mental health problems in the aftermath of natural disasters for the following reasons. First, there is the possibility of disruptions in maintaining regular treatments because many dialysis units might be disabled in the aftermath of a disaster, which can have a harmful impact on the health of hemodialysis patients [15–18]. Second, the available diet in evacuation shelters, which is high in sodium and potassium, could worsen the conditions of patients with chronic renal failure, who are usually on special diets [15, 19]. Third psychological stress, which can have serious health consequences such as triggering heart attacks or strokes, can be more severe in hemodialysis patients than in the general population [20]. However, information on conditions affecting this population following natural disasters is scarce [21]. Hyre et al. [22] reported that 24% of hemodialysis patients who received treatment in New Orleans during the week before Hurricane Katrina reported symptoms consistent with a diagnosis of PTSD a full year later. In a separate study, Hyre et al. [23] also reported that 46% of hemodialysis patients in post-Katrina New Orleans reported symptoms consistent with a diagnosis of major depression.

Mental health problems have been shown to be important indicators of related factors such as the deterioration of physical health and greater usage of medical resources [24]. Therefore, this study, conducted approximately two years after the 3/11 earthquake, examined the prevalence of mental health problems and related factors among dialysis patients living in the heavily damaged prefectures.

2. Methods

2.1. Analytic Framework.
In this study, both exposure to the 3/11 earthquake and life strains after the event were employed as disaster related stressors. This is because life strains after a catastrophic event can be as influential on mental health as the exposure to the disaster itself [25, 26]. A number of variables have been identified as aggravating/mitigating factors in the mental health of survivors. Many studies have shown that gender, lower social status, and the presence or absence of health problems prior to a disaster are factors related to whether individuals develop serious mental health problems following disasters. Additionally, survivors with higher social support are at reduced risk of developing serious mental health disorders in the future [26]. Moreover, higher awareness of advance emergency planning, specifically, the steps that dialysis patients should take to prepare for a disaster, has been identified as a mitigating factor; the Kidney Community Emergency Response Coalition recommends that dialysis patients be familiar with the emergency renal diet and maintain a list of health problems [27].

The mental health issue most often assessed and observed in research on survivors of natural disasters is Posttraumatic Stress Disorder [2]. A number of previous studies assessing mental health problems of survivors have also reported the prevalence of depression in this population [2]. The present study uses both PTSD and depression in assessing the mental health of survivors and investigated factors related

to the comorbidity of PTSD and depression. Tracy et al. [28] suggested that PTSD and depression might be different predictors. Additionally, there are high comorbidity rates between PTSD and depression, and other mental disorders have been reported [29, 30], and the presence of depressive disorders in patients with PTSD has been associated with greater functional impairment [31–34]. However, little is known about risk factors involved in comorbidity [32, 34].

2.2. Data Sources.
Respondent candidates were all members of the Japan Association of Kidney Disease Patients. At the time of the survey they were living in Fukushima, Miyagi, and Iwate, the three prefectures most heavily affected by the earthquake (N = 4,085). According to a survey of all dialysis facilities in Japan conducted by the Japanese Society for Dialysis Therapy [35], the number of dialysis patients living in these three prefectures in December 31, 2012, was 12,679, 32.2% of whom were members of Dialysis Therapy Patient's Association. The questionnaires described below were hand-delivered to members of dialysis facilities. The number of questionnaires returned by mail was 1,845. However, not all patients that returned the questionnaire were included in the effective sample. As the earthquake occurred in March of 2011 and the survey was conducted in March 2013, patients who began hemodialysis therapy after the earthquake were included as candidate respondents. The questionnaires included a question about the frequency of skipping dialysis treatment due to disruptions caused by the earthquake. Participants (n = 100) who indicated that this question was not applicable or did not respond to the question were excluded from the analysis. In addition, the actual number of participants in our analysis was smaller than 1,745 because, as described below, some participants had missing values for variables used in this study.

2.3. Assessments

2.3.1. Disaster Related Stressors.
Traumatic experiences resulting from the earthquake were measured by a scale that was developed based on scales used in research by Tohyama [36] and other studies [37, 38]. The scale comprised 10 items that evaluated the number of traumatic experiences resulting from the disaster itself (e.g., "suffering injury or burns") that participants may have faced. To quantify the responses, we added up the number of traumatic experiences reported by the participants. The number of traumatic experiences for participants with missing values less than or equal to 20% of the total traumatic experiences was obtained by calculating individual mean scores for all items other than those with missing values and then calculating the total score by multiplying the individual mean score by 10. This method has been suggested as a reliable way to handle missing values in surveys using multiple instruments [39, 40].

The scale to assess life strains after the earthquake was developed based on the scale used in research by Tohyama [36]. Life strains were defined as "having more difficulties in each life dimension at the time of this survey as compared to one's situation before the disaster." The scale consisted of seven life dimension items, assessing variables such as decreasing frequency of contact with friends and neighbors. Participants responded by using the two response choices provided for each item, either "Yes" or "No." Results indicated that, among the 1795 participants in this study, the highest percentage of participants (55.6%) did not feel any increased difficulties in any of the life dimensions after the disaster, whereas the next highest percentage of participants (11.9%) felt increased difficulties in only one life dimension. Therefore, life strain was evaluated by whether or not participants felt more difficulty in at least one dimension after the disaster, as compared to before the disaster. Basically, participants who had one and more missing items on this scale were excluded from the analysis. However, even in these participants, respondents who indicated that following the earthquake they felt more difficulty in at least one dimension were used in the analysis.

2.3.2. Other Aggravating/Mitigating and Control Factors. Psychiatric problems prior to the earthquake were retrospectively assessed using the instrument developed by Johannesson et al. [41]. This scale evaluates whether participants suffered from psychiatric problems prior to the earthquake. Traumatic experiences prior to the earthquake were measured using an indicator based on that in research by the Hurricane Katrina Community Advisory Group [42]. Using this indicator, participants were asked if they had experienced any of six different types of traumatic events, such as "psychical, or sexual assault" prior to the 3/11 earthquake. Results indicated that the largest number of traumatic experiences experienced by participants was one (47.6%) in participants ($n = 1,795$), followed by zero (39.8%). Therefore, traumatic experiences prior to the earthquake were evaluated on the basis of whether participants had experienced at least one traumatic event or had no experience of traumatic events. Basically, participants who had one or more missing items on this scale were excluded from the analysis. However, even in these participants, data of those who had experienced at least one traumatic event were used in the analysis.

Activities of daily living (ADL) prior to the earthquake were retrospectively assessed by one item in which participants were asked about their ADL one month prior to the disaster. Response choices comprised five levels, 1 (I could go anywhere by myself without any difficulty) to 5 (I was in bed almost all day) [43] and the total score was calculated. Annual household income during the year prior to the 3/11 earthquake was assessed by measuring the total annual household income. Participants were asked to indicate the approximate total annual income of all household members from all sources of income before tax deductions during the year before the earthquake. There were eight levels of income, from which respondents could choose the most appropriate (e.g., the lowest level was "under 1.2 million yen" and the highest level was "over 10 million yen"), and the midpoint of each category was used for quantification. The midpoint of each category was divided by the square root of the number of people living in the household to adjust for the influence of household size on income. The monetary amount was indicated in units of one million yen.

The two factors that were classified as aggravating/mitigating indicators at the time of this survey were social support and awareness of advance emergency planning. Finally, gender and education were included as sociodemographic factors. The indicator that we termed social support was developed based on questions developed by Americans' Changing Lives [44]. Respondents made assessments regarding three aspects: informational, instrumental, and emotional. The participants were told, "Please indicate the level of support you think that you received from each relationship, such as your spouse, for each aspect of support using the four-point scale." To quantify the response, each response on the scale was assigned a separate value from 1 to 4. The highest score for resources of social support was used to measure the level of each dimension of social support [45]. Total scores for support were obtained from the sum of the score for each dimension of social support.

Currently, no scale exists to assess advanced awareness of emergency planning among dialysis patients. For the present study, we developed a scale based on recommendations from both the Kidney Community Emergency Response Coalition [46] and a number of dialysis physicians. The scale comprised five items, including items such as the following: "Are there hemodialysis facilities where you can receive dialysis if your current facility is not available due to a disaster?" Participants responded with a "Yes" or "No" to each question. To quantify the responses, we added the number of "Yes" responses by the participants. Missing values on items on the scale were handled in the same manner as in the scale used for exposure to the disaster. To assess education, participants were asked to indicate the highest degree received or most recent educational institution attended. To quantify the responses, the minimum number of years needed to obtain each degree was calculated. In the item for gender, the choices "male" and "female" were assigned the numbers 1 and 0, respectively. Additionally, age and the length of time an individual had been receiving dialysis treatment were employed as control factors.

2.3.3. Mental Health Problems. The present study employed two indicators to assess mental health problems at the time of the survey: the Impact of Event Scale-Revised (IES-R) as an indicator of PTSD [47, 48] and K6 as an indicator of depression [49, 50]. Responses to both IES-R and K6 had missing items; however, no methodology exists for handling missing items on these scales. Thus, in the current study, missing values on questionnaires were handled in the same way as on the scale of exposure to the disaster. Participants were categorized into four types (PTSD and depression comorbidity (hereafter comorbidity), PTSD only, depression only, and neither PTSD nor depression) to examine factors related to comorbidity. Categorization into the four types was conducted using a clinical cutoff point for each K6 and PTSD scale to screen for persons with a high possibility of metal health problems (13 for K6 and 25 for ISE-R separately).

2.4. Statistical Analysis. Multinomial logistic regression analysis was used to examine related factors in mental health problems. Among the four categories, the classification of neither PTSD nor depression was used as a reference. The effects of aggravating/mitigating factors on mental health problems were examined by entering these factors and control factors as independent variables in the equation. Data of participants without missing values (89.4%) for the dependent variables were used in the analysis. The highest percentage of missing values for independent variables was in the indicator of life strains after the earthquake (11.6%), which was followed by adjusted household income (10.9%). The percentage of missing values for other independent variables was less than 10%. If we had analyzed only the data of participants without missing values for the independent variables, the effective sample of this study would have been 1,253 because deletions would have reduced the sample size. Therefore, in this study, 1,540 participants with missing values less than or equal to 20% of the total were included in the analysis through the use of multiple imputation methods. We created 20 data sets that were input to estimate values in items with missing values. The data were analyzed with SPSS version 19.

2.5. Ethical Considerations. This study was conducted according to the guidelines in the Helsinki Declaration. All the procedures of the study were approved by the Research Ethics Board of J. F. Oberlin University. A letter of invitation explaining the content of the study and the questionnaire was handed to each potential participant in this survey. Data collection procedures assured confidentiality by the use of self-administered, anonymous questionnaires. Participation in this study was completely voluntary.

3. Results

Table 1 shows the distributions of PTSD, depression, aggravating/mitigating, and control factors. Of the participants, 32.5% and 10.4%, respectively, showed PTSD and depression. Table 2 shows percentages of different disaster induced traumatic experiences reported by the participants. The highest percentage of participants (82.2%) felt fairly or very afraid, which was followed by participants who felt strong anxiety about the safety of their family (46.1%). Figure 1 shows the distribution of participants with comorbidity (7.5%), PTSD only (25.0%), depression only (2.9%), and neither PTSD nor depression (64.7%) at the time of the survey. The rate of comorbidity with depression among participants with PTSD was 23.1% as calculated by the following formula: [comorbidity/(comorbidity + PTSD only) × 100].

Table 3 shows the direct effects of aggravating/mitigating factors on mental health problems. There were similar effects of aggravating/mitigating factors on comorbidity and PTSD only. The number of traumatic experiences resulting from the disaster, experiences of life strains after the disaster, gender, health problems prior to the earthquake, and social support had significant impacts on whether participants developed comorbidity or only PTSD. In addition, levels of advanced awareness of emergency planning had significant impact on comorbidity. The number of traumatic experiences due to the disaster, experience of prior (preearthquake) depression,

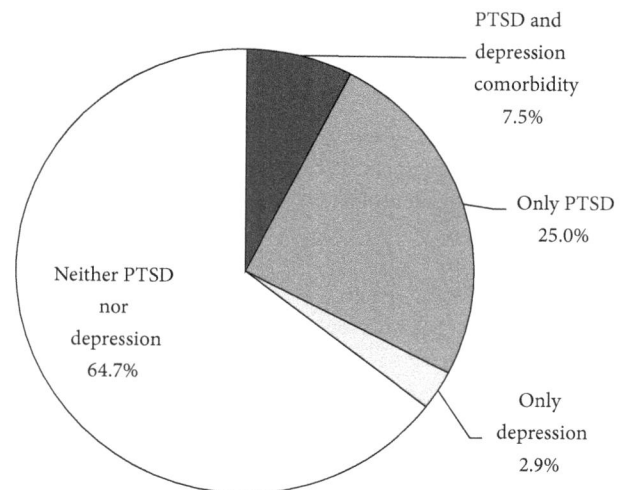

FIGURE 1: Prevalence of PTSD and depression at the time of the survey.

and prior difficulties of ADL had significant impacts on depression only.

4. Discussion

It is rather difficult to compare the above findings with prevalence of PTSD reported in previous studies, as methodologies and referenced sources of population from previous studies were different from those used here [51]. However, according to a systematic review by Neria et al. [52], studies of survivors of natural disasters overall report PTSD prevalence ranging from 3.7% to 60% in the first one to two years after an event, with most studies reporting prevalence estimates in the lower half of this range. In addition, estimates of higher prevalence of PTSD have been reported in specific groups such as clinical samples and populations in areas heavily affected by a disaster. As this study included participants who did not directly experience the earthquake and/or tsunami, it should be noted that prevalence of PTSD in participants with exposure to disaster was 32.5%. Hyre et al. [22] reported that 91.8% of hemodialysis patients in their sample were evacuated after Hurricane Katrina and 42.2% of these individuals reported symptoms consistent with PTSD or partial PTSD one year following the disaster. These results suggest that hemodialysis patients not only are vulnerable to the immediate physical effects of disaster but also may experience longer term mental health issues; this is despite the fact that the period during which these factors occur, that is, the disaster and the aftermath, is seen as being short term [26]. As K6 is a global indicator, comparison with prevalence of depression in a reference group is needed to evaluate whether prevalence of depression among the dialysis patient sample is high or low. Kuriyama et al. [53] reported that the prevalence of depression measured using K6 among a population of persons living in Japan aged 40 and over was 6.7%. Prevalence of depression among the dialysis patients in our sample after the earthquake was 10.4%, twice that of

TABLE 1: Descriptive statistics of variables under investigation[a].

Variable		
Prevalence rate of PTSD	(%)	32.5
Prevalence rate of depression	(%)	10.4
Number of traumatic experiences resulting from the earthquake	Mean (SD)	2.217 (1.474)
Rate of experiencing life strains after the earthquake	(%)	36.1
Gender	Male (%)	42.7
	Female (%)	57.3
Education (number of years)	Mean (SD)	12.042 (2.159)
Income (in units of one million yen)	Mean (SD)	2.027 (1.413)
Rate of experiencing depression prior to the earthquake	(%)	17.0
Rate of traumatic experiences prior to the earthquake	(%)	61.6
Levels of disability of ADL (activity of daily living) prior to the disaster	Mean (SD)	2.148 (1.176)
Levels of awareness of advanced planning	Mean (SD)	2.695 (1.421)
Social support	Mean (SD)	10.769 (1.909)
Age (years)	Mean (SD)	64.688 (10.670)
Period undergoing dialysis (number of years)	Mean (SD)	11.420 (8.280)

[a]Numbers were calculated by using 20 data sets for inputting estimated values instead of missing values $N = 1,540$.

TABLE 2: Percentage of different traumatic experiences caused by the disaster[a].

Kind	(%)
Feeling fairly or very afraid	82.2
Strong anxieties about family safety	46.1
Finding shelter	35.7
Partial or complete destruction of home	19.1
Suffering from a permanent physical injury	14.3
Helping to rescue victims of the disaster	9.0
Seeing dead or seriously injured people	7.3
Death of a family member	3.3
Suffering from injury or burns	2.9
Injury or permanent physical damage to a family member	1.4

[a]A database for inputting estimated values for missing values was used ($n = 1,540$). Missing values were input to the scale indicating the number of traumatic experiences caused by the disaster. However, missing values for each type of traumatic experience caused by the disaster were not input. Percentages of the types of disaster were calculated by excluding each case with missing values.

the general population. However, it has been widely claimed that depression is the most common mental health problem among dialysis patients; this is not only because dialysis patients may have experienced multiple difficulties at home and work, for example, fatigue and sexual dysfunction, but also due to multiple stressors such as dietary constraints and dependency upon treatment [54].

Previous studies have reported that rates of comorbid depression among participants with PTSD were over 40% [30, 34, 55]. The rate of comorbid depression among participants with PTSD in this sample (23.1%) was lower than that found in other studies of disaster survivors. As the current study is the first to examine comorbidity following a disaster in dialysis patients, this finding may not be conclusive. However, if these results prove to be valid, differences in each risk

factor for PTSD and depression after a disaster among dialysis patients could be wider than in the risk factors among the general population. As depression among dialysis patients is often related to dialysis specific stressors, such as role changes at home and in the workplace [54], it is possible that the factors related to depression differ largely from other disaster related stressors that cause PTSD. Factors related to comorbidity and PTSD only in our sample of dialysis patients are similar to factors related to mental health problems in disaster survivors found in previous research [2]. Tracy et al. [28] point to certain stressors during and following a natural disaster that play a central role in PTSD and also cite postevent nontraumatic stressors that are associated with risk of depression. In this study, disaster related stressors had a lower impact on depression than on comorbidity and PTSD. Dialysis specific causes of depression among patients may have had an influence on our results.

While awareness of advance emergency planning is important in reducing deaths among dialysis patients in the event of a natural disaster [21], in empirical research only Hyre et al. [23] have demonstrated that a lack of evacuation plan awareness was related to poor psychosocial health following a disaster. The results in this study provide support for the effectiveness of advance emergency planning and awareness of measures that can be taken in preventing mental health problems among dialysis patients.

There are some limitations in the present research. First, assessments of changes in depression were not possible as preearthquake data from this region were not available. Second, assessments of recovery from the acute phase immediately following the earthquake were not possible as the study interviews were conducted only once, two years after the events of 3/11. Third, it is difficult to examine the causal linkage of these factors to an appearance of mental health problems as several factors prior to the earthquake were collected through a retrospective survey. Finally, a low response rate (here 45.2%) is thought to provide an underestimation

TABLE 3: Direct effects of aggravating/mitigating factors on mental health problems[a].

	PTSD and depression[b] Odds ratio[c] (95% CI)	PTSD only[b] Odds ratio[c] (95% CI)	Depression only[b] Odds ratio[c] (95% CI)
The number of traumatic experiences caused by disaster	1.494 (1.288–1.733)[***]	1.425 (1.293–1.572)[***]	1.299 (1.037–1.626)[*]
Experience of life stressors after the earthquake	3.858 (2.307–6.452)[***]	2.096 (1.560–2.816)[***]	1.151 (0.566–2.339)
Gender (male = 1, female = 0)	0.655 (0.420–1.021)	0.735 (0.562–0.963)[*]	1.473 (0.764–2.840)
Education	0.916 (0.820–1.024)	0.922 (0.863–0.986)[*]	1.052 (0.907–1.221)
Income	0.934 (0.781–1.117)	0.912 (0.820–1.015)	0.810 (0.623–1.051)
Experience of depression prior to the earthquake	4.971 (3.062–8.069)[***]	2.058 (1.454–2.912)[***]	5.032 (2.606–9.717)[***]
Experience of trauma prior to the earthquake	1.520 (0.950–2.432)	1.517 (1.151–2.000)[**]	0.527 (0.282–0.986)[*]
Levels of disability in activities of daily living prior to the earthquake	1.579 (1.313–1.899)[***]	1.200 (1.066–1.351)[**]	1.330 (1.026–1.724)[*]
Levels of awareness of disaster planning	0.751 (0.634–0.891)[**]	1.049 (0.954–1.153)	0.810 (0.642–1.020)
Social support	0.862 (0.776–0.959)[**]	0.927 (0.864–0.994)[*]	0.963 (0.825–1.124)
Age	1.022 (1.000–1.045)	1.021 (1.007–1.035)[**]	0.969 (0.942–0.998)[*]
Period of taking dialysis	1.011 (0.983–1.038)	0.997 (0.981–1.013)	0.998 (0.960–1.037)

[a]$n = 1,540$.
[b]Reference category was "neither PTSD nor depression."
[c]Odds ratio means changes in odds ratio if each factor increases by one point.
[*]$P < .05$; [**]$P < .01$; [***]$P < .001$.

of the rates of PTSD or depression, as patients with more serious mental health problems have a higher possibility of not responding to this type of survey. Although these limitations need to be noted, the present research has several important features that should be noted: (1) this is the second quantitative study to examine the effects of a natural disaster on a population of dialysis patients, the first being the previously mentioned study following Hurricane Katrina; (2) this study uncovered related factors in comorbidity, a very important mental health issue following a disaster; and (3) previous studies on survivors of earthquakes and other natural disasters have been conducted with selective samples that were not representative of the affected population [56]. While this study had a selective sample, the sample was obtained from members of patient groups, which comprised one-third of all patients living in the affected prefectures. Evidence based on convenience sampling or snowballing methods tends to show substantially higher rates of PTSD and other mental disorders than seen in representative groups recruited using random sampling methods [57]. Evidence from this study has smaller bias of prevalence of mental health problems than that found in other researches using convenience sampling.

5. Conclusion

People with comorbidity, PTSD only, and depression only comprised 7.5%, 25.0%, 2.9% of the sample, respectively. Not only disaster related stressors but also health problems prior to the disaster had an aggravating direct effect on comorbidity and PTSD. In addition, social support and advanced awareness of disaster planning had a mitigating effect on comorbidity. Results of this study suggest that the awareness

of disaster planning in advance could mitigate the occurrence of comorbidity. Disaster related stressors had a weaker impact on depression than on comorbidity and PTSD. Dialysis specific stressors may have played a large part in depression among patients after the disaster and mental and physical health prior to the disaster.

Conflict of Interests

All the authors declare no competing interests.

Acknowledgments

The authors acknowledge the help from the board members of Iwate, Miyagi, and Fukushima of Japan Association of Kidney Disease Patients. This study was supported by the research fund for fiscal 2013 of the Japanese Association of Dialysis Physicians.

References

[1] National Police Agency of Japan Emergency Disaster Counter-measures Headquarters, *Damage Situation and Police Counter-measures*, 2014, http://www.npa.go.jp/archive/keibi/biki/higa-ijokyo.pdf.

[2] F. H. Norris and C. L. Elrod, "Psychological consequences of disaster," in *Methods for Disaster Mental Health*, F. H. Norris, S. Galea, M. J. Friedman, and P. J. Watson, Eds., pp. 20–42, The Guilford Press, New York, NY, USA, 2006.

[3] T. Fujimori and K. Fujimori, "Mental health of victims of 1993 Hokkaido Nanseioki Earthquake," *Psychiatry Diagnosis*, vol. 7, pp. 65–76, 1993.

[4] M. Tanaka and O. Takagi, "A study of the victims in the temporary housing built outside of the stricken disaster area of

the Great Hanshin-Awaji Earthquake I: the impact on physical and mental health of the people in the temporary housing a year after the Earthquake," *The Japanese Journal of Experimental Social Psychology*, vol. 37, no. 1, pp. 76–84, 1997 (Japanese).

[5] T. Fujimori, "Prolong mental health problems due to natural disaster: a study of Hokkaido Nanseioki Earthquake victims," *The Japanese Journal of Personality*, vol. 7, no. 1, pp. 11–21, 1998 (Japanese).

[6] S. Fukuda, K. Morimoto, K. Mure, and S. Maruyama, "Posttraumatic stress and change in lifestyle among the Hanshin-Awaji earthquake victims," *Preventive Medicine*, vol. 29, no. 3, pp. 147–151, 1999.

[7] S. Fukuda, K. Morimoto, K. Mure, and S. Maruyama, "Effect of the Hanshin-Awaji earthquake on posttraumatic stress, lifestyle changes, and cortisol levels of victims," *Archives of Environmental Health*, vol. 55, no. 2, pp. 121–125, 2000.

[8] S.-I. Toyabe, T. Shioiri, H. Kuwabara et al., "Impaired psychological recovery in the elderly after the Niigata-Chuetsu Earthquake in Japan: a population-based study," *BMC Public Health*, vol. 6, article 230, 2006.

[9] S.-I. Toyabe, T. Shioiri, K. Kobayashi et al., "Factor structure of the General Health Questionnaire (GHQ-12) in subjects who had suffered from the 2004 Niigata-Chuetsu Earthquake in Japan: a community-based study," *BMC Public Health*, vol. 7, article 175, 2007.

[10] J. Tayama, T. Ichikawa, K. Eguchi, T. Yamamoto, and S. Shirabe, "Tsunami damage and its impact on mental health," *Psychosomatics*, vol. 53, no. 2, pp. 196–197, 2012.

[11] Y. Kotozaki and R. Kawashima, "Effects of the Higashi-Nihon earthquake: posttraumatic stress, psychological changes, and cortisol levels of survivors," *PloS one*, vol. 7, no. 4, 2012.

[12] M. Usami, Y. Iwadare, M. Kodaira et al., "Relationships between traumatic symptoms and environmental damage conditions among children 8 months after the 2011 Japan Earthquake and tsunami," *PLoS ONE*, vol. 7, no. 11, Article ID e50721, 2012.

[13] T. Takeda, M. Tadakawa, S. Koga, S. Nagase, and N. Yaegashi, "Premenstrual symptoms and posttraumatic stress disorder in Japanese high school students 9 months after the great east-Japan earthquake," *Tohoku Journal of Experimental Medicine*, vol. 230, no. 3, pp. 151–154, 2013.

[14] M. Fushimi, "Posttraumatic stress in professional firefighters in Japan: rescue efforts after the Great East Japan earthquake (Higashi Nihon Dai-Shinsai)," *Prehospital and Disaster Medicine*, vol. 27, no. 5, pp. 416–418, 2012.

[15] A. Inui, H. Inoue, M. Uemoto, M. Kasuga, and H. Taniguchi, "Kobe earthquake and the patients on hemodialysis," *Nephron*, vol. 74, no. 4, article 733, 1996.

[16] S. J. Hwang, K. H. Shu, J. D. Lain, and W. C. Yang, "Renal replacement therapy at the time of the Taiwan Chi-Chi earthquake," *Nephrology Dialysis Transplantation*, vol. 16, supplement 5, pp. 78–82, 2001.

[17] M. S. Sever, E. Erek, R. Vanholder et al., "Features of chronic hemodialysis practice after the Marmara Earthquake," *Journal of the American Society of Nephrology*, vol. 15, no. 4, pp. 1071–1076, 2004.

[18] A. H. Anderson, A. J. Cohen, N. G. Kutner, J. B. Kopp, P. L. Kimmel, and P. Muntner, "Missed dialysis sessions and hospitalization in hemodialysis patients after Hurricane Katrina," *Kidney International*, vol. 75, no. 11, pp. 1202–1208, 2009.

[19] S. Ochi, V. Murray, and S. Hodgson, "The Great East Japan Earthquake disaster: a compilation of published literature on health needs and relief activities, March 2011–September 2012," *PLOS Currents Disasters*, vol. 5, 2013.

[20] N. Haga, J. Hata, K. Ishibashi, M. Nomiya, N. Takahashi, and Y. Kojima, "Blood pressure in hemodialysis patients after Great East Japan earthquake in Fukushima: the effect of tsunami and nuclear power accident," *Journal of Hypertension*, vol. 31, no. 8, pp. 1724–1726, 2013.

[21] R. C. Vanholder, W. A. van Biesen, and M. S. Sever, "Hurricane Katrina and chronic dialysis patients: better tidings than originally feared?" *Kidney International*, vol. 76, no. 7, pp. 687–689, 2009.

[22] A. D. Hyre, A. J. Cohen, N. Kutner, A. B. Alper, and P. Muntner, "Prevalence and predictors of posttraumatic stress disorder among hemodialysis patients following Hurricane Katrina," *American Journal of Kidney Diseases*, vol. 50, no. 4, pp. 585–593, 2007.

[23] A. D. Hyre, A. J. Cohen, N. Kutner et al., "Psychosocial status of hemodialysis patients one year after Hurricane Katrina," *American Journal of the Medical Sciences*, vol. 336, no. 2, pp. 94–98, 2008.

[24] D. Edmondson, C. Gamboa, A. Cohen et al., "Association of posttraumatic stress disorder and depression with all-cause and cardiovascular disease mortality and hospitalization among hurricane katrina survivors with end-stage renal disease," *American Journal of Public Health*, vol. 103, no. 4, pp. e130–e137, 2013.

[25] C. R. Brewin, B. Andrews, and J. D. Valentine, "Meta-analysis of risk factors for posttraumatic stress disorder in trauma-exposed adults," *Journal of Consulting and Clinical Psychology*, vol. 68, no. 5, pp. 748–766, 2000.

[26] F. H. Norris, M. J. Friedman, P. J. Watson, C. M. Byrne, E. Diaz, and K. Kaniasty, "60,000 disaster victims speak: part I. An empirical review of the empirical literature, 1981–2001," *Psychiatry*, vol. 65, no. 3, pp. 207–239, 2002.

[27] J. B. Kopp, L. K. Ball, A. Cohen et al., "Kidney patient care in disasters: emergency planning for patients and dialysis facilities," *Clinical Journal of the American Society of Nephrology*, vol. 2, no. 4, pp. 825–838, 2007.

[28] M. Tracy, F. H. Norris, and S. Galea, "Differences in the determinants of posttraumatic stress disorder and depression after a mass traumatic event," *Depression and Anxiety*, vol. 28, no. 8, pp. 666–675, 2011.

[29] R. C. Kessler, A. Sonnega, E. Bromet, M. Hughes, and C. B. Nelson, "Posttraumatic stress disorder in the national comorbidity survey," *Archives of General Psychiatry*, vol. 52, no. 12, pp. 1048–1060, 1995.

[30] M.-L. Meewisse, M. Olff, R. Kleber, N. J. Kitchiner, and B. P. R. Gersons, "The course of mental health disorders after a disaster: predictors and comorbidity," *Journal of Traumatic Stress*, vol. 24, no. 4, pp. 405–413, 2011.

[31] E. Önder, Ü. Tural, T. Aker, C. Kiliç, and S. Erdoğan, "Prevalence of psychiatric disorders three years after the 1999 earthquake in Turkey: Marmara Earthquake Survey (MES)," *Social Psychiatry and Psychiatric Epidemiology*, vol. 41, no. 11, pp. 868–874, 2006.

[32] E. B. Foa, D. J. Stein, and A. C. McFarlane, "Symptomatology and psychopathology of mental health problems after disaster," *Journal of Clinical Psychiatry*, vol. 67, supplement 2, pp. 15–25, 2006.

[33] R. Shah, A. Shah, and P. Links, "Post-traumatic stress disorder and depression comorbidity: severity across different populations," *Neuropsychiatry*, vol. 2, no. 6, pp. 521–529, 2012.

[34] Ü. Tural, E. Önder, and T. Aker, "Effect of depression on recovery from PTSD," *Community Mental Health Journal*, vol. 48, no. 2, pp. 161–166, 2012.

[35] The Committee of Statistical Survey-the Japanese Society for Dialysis Therapy, An Overview of Regular Dialysis Treatment in Japan, 2012, http://docs.jsdt.or.jp/overview/pdf2013/p008.pdf.

[36] T. Tohyama, "Stressors associated with the subsequent mental conditions of the outpatients exposed to the Great Hanshin Earthquake," *Journal of Nara Medical Association*, vol. 49, no. 5, pp. 295–311, 1998 (Japanese).

[37] A. Roussos, A. K. Goenjian, A. M. Steinberg et al., "Post-traumatic stress and depressive reactions among children and adolescents after the 1999 earthquake in Ano Liosia, Greece," *The American Journal of Psychiatry*, vol. 162, no. 3, pp. 530–537, 2005.

[38] S. Galea, M. Tracy, F. Norris, and S. F. Coffey, "Financial and social circumstances and the incidence and course of PTSD in Mississippi during the first two years after Hurricane Katrina," *Journal of Traumatic Stress*, vol. 21, no. 4, pp. 357–368, 2008.

[39] F. M. Shrive, H. Stuart, H. Quan, and W. A. Ghali, "Dealing with missing data in a multi-question depression scale: a comparison of imputation methods," *BMC Medical Research Methodology*, vol. 6, article 57, 2006.

[40] C. Bono, L. D. Ried, C. Kimberlin, and B. Vogel, "Missing data on the Center for Epidemiologic Studies Depression Scale: a comparison of 4 imputation techniques," *Research in Social and Administrative Pharmacy*, vol. 3, no. 1, pp. 1–27, 2007.

[41] K. B. Johannesson, T. Lundin, T. Fröjd, C. M. Hultman, and P.-O. Michel, "Tsunami-exposed tourist survivors: signs of recovery in a 3-year perspective," *Journal of Nervous & Mental Disease*, vol. 199, no. 3, pp. 162–169, 2011.

[42] Hurricane Katrina Community Advisory Group, *Baseline Interview for the Hurricane Katrina Community Advisory Group*, Hurricane Katrina Community Advisory Group, 2006, http://www.hurricanekatrina.med.harvard.edu/pdf/baseline_overview_1-06.pdf.

[43] Department of Social Welfare. Tokyo Metropolitan Institute of Gerontology, Ed., *Family Caregiving for the Elderly and Service Needs for Caregiving*, Koseikan, Tokyo, Japan, 1996, (Japanese).

[44] J. S. House, *Americans' Changing Lives: Waves I and II, 1986 and 1989. ICPSR Version*, Survey Research Center, University of Michigan, Ann Arbor, Mich, USA, 1997.

[45] H. Sugisawa, J. Liang, and X. Liu, "Social networks, social support, and mortality among older people in Japan," *Journals of Gerontology*, vol. 49, no. 1, pp. S3–S13, 1994.

[46] E. M. Ginexi, K. Weihs, S. J. Simmens, and D. R. Hoyt, "Natural disaster and depression: a prospective investigation of reactions to the 1993 Midwest Floods," *American Journal of Community Psychology*, vol. 28, no. 4, pp. 495–518, 2000.

[47] D. S. Weiss and C. R. Marmer, "The impact of event scale-revised," in *Assessing Psychological Trauma and PTSD*, J. P. Wilson and T. M. Keane, Eds., pp. 399–411, Guilford Press, New York, NY, USA, 1997.

[48] N. Asukai, H. Kato, N. Kawamura et al., "Reliability and validity of the Japanese-language version of the impact of event scale-revised (IES-R-J): four studies of different traumatic events," *Journal of Nervous and Mental Disease*, vol. 190, no. 3, pp. 175–182, 2002.

[49] R. C. Kessler, G. Andrews, L. J. Colpe et al., "Short screening scales to monitor population prevalences and trends in non-specific psychological distress," *Psychological Medicine*, vol. 32, no. 6, pp. 959–976, 2002.

[50] T. A. Furukawa, N. Kawakami, M. Saitoh et al., "The performance of the Japanese version of the K6 and K10 in the World Mental Health Survey Japan," *International Journal of Methods in Psychiatric Research*, vol. 17, no. 3, pp. 152–158, 2008.

[51] P. Udomratn, "Mental health and the psychosocial consequences of natural disasters in Asia," *International Review of Psychiatry*, vol. 20, no. 5, pp. 441–444, 2008.

[52] Y. Neria, A. Nandi, and S. Galea, "Post-traumatic stress disorder following disasters: a systematic review," *Psychological Medicine*, vol. 38, no. 4, pp. 467–480, 2008.

[53] S. Kuriyama, N. Nakaya, K. Ohmori-Matsuda et al., "Factors associated with psychological distress in a community-dwelling Japanese population: the Ohsaki Cohort 2006 study," *Journal of Epidemiology*, vol. 19, no. 6, pp. 294–302, 2009.

[54] J. Chilcot, D. Wellsted, M. Da Silva-Gane, and K. Farrington, "Depression on dialysis," *Nephron—Clinical Practice*, vol. 108, no. 4, pp. c256–c264, 2008.

[55] M. Başoğlu, C. Kiliç, E. Şalcioğlu, and M. Livanou, "Prevalence of posttraumatic stress disorder and comorbid depression in earthquake survivors in Turkey: an epidemiological study," *Journal of Traumatic Stress*, vol. 17, no. 2, pp. 133–141, 2004.

[56] S. Priebe, F. Marchi, L. Bini, M. Flego, A. Costa, and G. Galeazzi, "Mental disorders, psychological symptoms and quality of life 8 years after an earthquake: findings from a community sample in Italy," *Social Psychiatry and Psychiatric Epidemiology*, vol. 46, no. 7, pp. 615–621, 2011.

[57] M. Fazel, J. Wheeler, and J. Danesh, "Prevalence of serious mental disorder in 7000 refugees resettled in western countries: a systematic review," *The Lancet*, vol. 365, no. 9467, pp. 1309–1314, 2005.

4

Self-Determination Theory and First-Episode Psychosis: A Replication

Nicholas J. K. Breitborde,[1] Cindy Woolverton,[1] R. Brock Frost,[2] and Nicole A. Kiewel[3]

[1] *Department of Psychiatry, The University of Arizona, Tucson, AZ 85713, USA*
[2] *Department of Psychiatry, University of New Mexico, Albuquerque, NM 87131, USA*
[3] *Department of Psychiatry, Cleveland Clinic, Cleveland, OH 44195, USA*

Correspondence should be addressed to Nicholas J. K. Breitborde; breitbor@email.arizona.edu

Academic Editor: Takahiro Nemoto

Self-determination theory (SDT) posits that human well-being depends on the satisfaction of three basic psychological needs: autonomy, competence, and relatedness. Although many scholars have suggested that SDT may be relevant to psychotic disorders, only one empirical study of SDT in individuals with psychosis has been completed to date by Breitborde and colleagues (2012). This study revealed that individuals with first-episode psychosis reported lower satisfaction of the three basic psychological needs as compared to individuals without psychosis. Moreover, greater satisfaction of basic psychological needs was modestly associated with lower general symptoms (e.g., anxiety and depression), greater social functioning, and better quality of life. Thus, the goal of this project was to replicate Breitborde et al.'s (2012) investigation of basic psychological need satisfaction among individuals with first-episode psychosis. Our results supported the conclusion that individuals with first-episode psychosis report lower autonomy, competence, and relatedness than individuals without psychosis. Moreover, our results comport with the finding that greater need satisfaction was associated with less severe symptomatology and better social functioning and quality of life. In total, the findings lend further credence to the hypothesis that SDT may help to inform the development of improved clinical services for individuals with psychotic disorders.

1. Introduction

Self-determination theory (SDT: [1]) posits that human well-being and motivation are dependent on the satisfaction of three basic psychological needs: autonomy (i.e., viewing oneself as the volitional source of one's actions), competence (i.e., perceiving one's self as effective in interactions in one's local world), and relatedness (i.e., feeling a sense of connectedness and belongingness with others in one's local world). Recently, several scholars have suggested that SDT theory may be relevant to psychotic disorders [2, 3]. For example, Choi and colleagues [4] have shown that greater intrinsic motivation—a construct underpinned by the three basic psychological needs [1]—is associated with greater participation in and response to cognitive remediation among individuals with schizophrenia.

Yet, despite this potential utility of SDT, only one study to date has examined basic psychological need satisfaction among individuals with psychosis. In this study, Breitborde and colleagues [5] found that individuals with first-episode psychosis reported lower feelings of autonomy, competence, and relatedness as compared to individuals without psychosis. Moreover, greater satisfaction of basic psychological needs was modestly associated with lower general symptoms (e.g., anxiety and depression), greater social functioning, and better quality of life. Among the three basic psychological needs, relatedness was found to be the most frequent correlate of clinical and functional status among individuals with first-episode psychosis.

With only one investigation of basic psychological need satisfaction among individuals with psychosis completed to date, the reliability of Breitborde and colleagues' [5] findings is unclear. This limitation is not unique to the Breitborde et al. study specifically; within psychiatric research, there is growing recognition of the limited reliability of findings from single studies [6, 7]. In response to this concern, scholars have advocated for the systematic replication of research findings prior to assuming that such findings are reliable [8, 9].

Thus, the goal of this project is to replicate Breitborde and colleagues' [5] investigation of basic psychological need satisfaction among individuals with first-episode psychosis. Consistent with the previous study, we first compared levels of basic psychological need satisfaction among individuals with first-episode psychosis to levels of need satisfaction among individuals without psychosis. Second, we investigated the association between need satisfaction and measures of symptomatology, social functioning, and quality of life among individuals with first-episode psychosis.

2. Methods

2.1. Participants. Forty-three individuals with first-episode psychosis were recruited from the Early Psychosis Intervention Center (EPICENTER: [10]). EPICENTER eligibility criteria include (i) diagnosis of a schizophrenia-spectrum or affective disorder with psychotic features as determined using the Structured Clinical Interview for the DSM-IV [11], (ii) less than 5 years of psychotic symptoms established using the Symptom Onset in Schizophrenia Inventory [12], (iii) ages 18–35, and (iv) no evidence of mental retardation or organic brain impairment. Participants in the study include 31 males and 12 females with an average age of 22.16 years (SD = 4.10). The median duration of psychotic symptoms was 13.94 months.

This project was completed in accordance with the Declaration of Helsinki. The study was approved by the University of Arizona Institutional Review Board, and all participants provided informed consent prior to enrolling in this study.

2.2. Procedures and Measures. Upon enrollment in EPICENTER and prior to the start of treatment, participants completed a series of assessments that were part of a larger research battery.

2.3. Basic Psychological Needs. Basic psychological need satisfaction was assessed using the Basic Psychological Needs Scale-General (BPNS: [13]). The BPNS is a 21-item self-report measure that assesses satisfaction of the need for autonomy, competence, and relatedness across life in general. All items are scored on seven-point Likert scale, with higher scores indicative of greater need satisfaction. Psychometric evaluations of the BPNS have revealed that this measure possesses good to excellent internal consistency [13, 14]. The BPNS also has demonstrated predictive validity with regard to differentiating between individuals with psychopathology versus those without [5, 14].

Normative data for the BPNS are lacking. However, in their previous study, Breitborde and colleagues [5] created pseudonormative data for the three BPNS subscales (i.e., autonomy, competence, and relatedness) from the 9145 individuals without a known psychotic disorders included in all previously published studies that used the 17-item BPNS and reported means and standard deviations. More specifically, they calculated means and standard deviations for each BPNS

subscale weighted by the number of subjects in each study. A list of these studies can be found in Breitborde et al. [5]. Among the 9145 individuals in these studies, the average age was 20.45 years (SD = 2.98) and 39% of the individuals were male.

2.4. Symptomatology. The Positive and Negative Syndrome Scale (PANSS: [15]) was used to assess symptomatology among study participants. The PANSS is a 30-item clinician-rated instrument that assesses three domains of symptomatology: positive symptoms (e.g., hallucinations and delusions), negative symptoms (e.g., blunted affect and social withdrawal), and general symptoms (e.g., anxiety and depression). Higher PANSS scores are indicative of worse symptomatology.

2.5. Social Functioning. Participants' level of social functioning was measured using the Social Functioning Scale (SFS: [16]). The SFS is a 79-item instrument that assesses seven areas of functioning: (i) social engagement/withdrawal, (ii) interpersonal behavior/communication, (iii) participation in prosocial activities, (iv) participation in recreational activities, (v) independence competence (i.e., ability to perform tasks of independent living), (vi) independence performance (i.e., completion of tasks of independent living), and (vii) educational/vocational functioning. Higher scores on the SFS are indicative of greater social functioning.

2.6. Quality of Life. The WHO Quality of Life Instrument-Brief (WHOQOL-BREF: [17]) was used to assess quality of life among study participants. The WHOQOL-BREF is a 26-item self-report scale that measures four domains of quality of life: (i) physical health, (ii) psychological health, (iii) social relationships, and (iv) quality of one's environment. Scores for each domain range from 0 to 100, with higher scores indicative of greater quality of life.

2.7. Analyses. Prior to the analyses, missing data points were replaced using multiple imputation (MI: [18]). This strategy comports with current guidelines for addressing missing data [19]. Comparison of BPNS scores between individuals with first-episode psychosis and individuals without a known psychotic disorder was completed using independent t-tests controlling for the additional variance created through the use of MI [20]. Evaluation of the association between BPNS subscales and measures of symptomatology, social functioning, and quality of life was completed using Pearson correlation coefficients controlling for the additional variance created through the use of MI [20].

3. Results

3.1. Satisfaction of Basic Psychological Needs. Among individuals with first-episode psychosis, there were no statistically significant differences between scores on the autonomy, competence, and relatedness subscales (all P values > 0.05). BPNS scores for individuals with first-episode psychosis versus those with no known psychotic disorder are shown

TABLE 1: Demographics and BPNS scores among individuals with first-episode psychosis versus individuals with no known psychotic disorder.

	Individuals with first-episode psychosis	Individuals with no known psychotic disorder
N	43	9145
Age	M = 22.16	M = 20.45
Percent male—female	74%—26%	39%—61%
Autonomy	M = 4.26	M = 5.00
Competence	M = 4.04	M = 5.07
Relatedness	M = 4.18	M = 5.33

in Table 1. Compared to individuals without psychosis, individuals with first-episode psychosis reported lower autonomy [$t(7622) = 5.43; P < 0.01$], competence [$t(7924) = 7.15; P < 0.01$], and relatedness [$t(7945) = 8.26; P < 0.01$].

Of note, there were a number of demographic variables that differed between the individuals with first-episode psychosis and the participants from the comparison studies (see Table 1). Specifically, individuals with first-episode psychosis were more likely to be men [$\chi^2(1) = 19.93; P < 0.01$] and were older [$t(8320) = 3.74; P < 0.01$] than the individuals without psychosis. Available research suggests that there is no association between gender and psychological need satisfaction [21]. Moreover, although need satisfaction has been shown to increase with age [22], our sample of individuals with first-episode psychosis reported lower need satisfaction than the younger cohort of individuals without a known psychotic disorder.

3.2. Symptomatology. Correlations between BPNS and PANSS are shown in Table 2. There were no statistically significant associations between severity of positive or negative symptoms and levels of autonomy, competence, or relatedness. Higher levels of general symptoms were associated with lower levels of autonomy and competence.

3.3. Social Functioning. Correlations between BPNS and SFS are shown in Table 2. Better interpersonal communication was associated with greater autonomy, competence, and relatedness. Higher levels of competence were also associated with greater success in the performance of independent living skills (i.e., Independence-Performance subscale). Greater perceived competence with regard to the performance of independent living skills (i.e., Independence-Competence subscale) was associated with higher autonomy and competence.

3.4. Quality of Life. Correlations between BPNS and WHO-QOL-BREF are shown in Table 2. Better physical health was associated with higher levels of autonomy. Greater psychological health was associated with higher levels of autonomy, competence, and relatedness. Better social relationships were associated with greater autonomy and relatedness. There were no statistically significant associations between quality of one's environment and BPNS subscales.

4. Discussion

Consistent with the results from Breitborde et al. [5], individuals with first-episode psychosis in our study reported lower autonomy, competence, and relatedness than individuals without psychosis. Similar reports of reduced need satisfaction have also been noted in studies of individuals with other forms of psychopathology (e.g., posttraumatic stress disorder [14] and major depressive disorder [23]). Our finding likely cannot be accounted for due to demographic differences between the two groups (i.e., gender and age). Available research suggests that there is no association between gender and psychological need satisfaction [21]. Moreover, although need satisfaction has been shown to increase with age [22], our sample of individuals with first-episode psychosis reported lower need satisfaction than the younger cohort of individuals without a known psychotic disorder. Additionally, our results further comport with findings by Breitborde et al. in that we found modest associations between basic psychological need satisfaction and symptomatology, social functioning, and quality of life among individuals with first-episode psychosis.

Of note, there is a key difference between our results and those reported by Breitborde and colleagues [5]. Specifically, whereas Breitborde et al. found that relatedness was the psychological need most frequently associated with clinical/functional status, among our sample, no single psychological need stood out as the best predictor of clinical/functional status. Important differences among the participants in these two studies may have contributed to this finding. For example, compared to participants in the Breitborde et al. study, our subjects had a longer duration of psychotic symptoms (Median = 13.94 versus 3.46 months, Wilcoxon rank-sum $z = -3.71$; $P < 0.01$) but a shorter duration of participation in specialized treatment for first-episode psychosis (Mean = 0 versus 9.91 months, Wilcoxon rank-sum $z = 5.22$; $P < 0.01$). This raises the possibility that satisfaction of the needs for autonomy and competence may be more important later in the early course of psychotic disorders and/or earlier during individuals' participation in specialized clinical services for first-episode psychosis. Relatedness, on the other hand, may be important throughout the early course of psychotic disorders as well as throughout participation in care for first-episode psychosis.

Our study did suffer from a number of limitations. The sample size was small and comprised predominantly of men. Likewise, our results may not generalize to individuals with longstanding psychotic illnesses. Finally, given our cross-sectional study design, the direction of the relationship between psychological need satisfaction and clinical/functional status is unclear.

In conclusion, the results of our replication study support the hypothesis that deficits in satisfaction of basic psychological needs are present early in the course of psychotic disorders and are associated with measures of clinical/functional status.

TABLE 2: Symptomatology, social functioning, and quality of life: descriptive statistics and correlations with BPNS scores.

	M (SD)	Autonomy	Competence	Relatedness
Symptomatology				
Positive symptoms	15.30 (2.41)	−0.16	−0.22	−0.09
Negative symptoms	13.71 (2.33)	0.12	0.13	−0.02
General symptoms	30.95 (2.66)	−0.41*	−0.36*	−0.25
Social functioning				
Social engagement/withdrawal	10.24 (1.74)	0.15	0.29	0.20
Interpersonal communication	6.86 (1.55)	0.42*	0.50*	0.44*
Independence performance	23.60 (2.77)	0.27	0.42*	0.18
Recreation	17.72 (2.58)	0.19	0.12	−0.03
Prosocial activities	14.35 (2.95)	0.13	0.24	0.06
Independence competence	34.13 (2.35)	0.36*	0.35*	0.20
Educational/occupational functioning	6.45 (1.90)	0.13	0.10	0.06
Quality of life				
Physical health	53.16 (5.43)	0.40*	0.19	0.16
Psychological health	39.65 (5.48)	0.48*	0.40*	0.36*
Social relationships	34.31 (5.21)	0.43*	0.18	0.35*
Environment	52.63 (5.44)	0.29	0.21	0.10

*$P < 0.05$.

Ultimately, developing clinical environments designed to address these deficits may facilitate greater motivation among individuals with first-episode psychosis to participate in treatment activities [2, 3].

Conflict of Interests

The authors declare that there is no conflict of interests regarding the publication of this paper.

Acknowledgments

This work was supported by funds from the University of Arizona and grant from the Institute for Mental Health Research to Nicholas J. K. Breitborde.

References

[1] R. M. Ryan and E. L. Deci, "Self-determination theory and the facilitation of intrinsic motivation, social development, and well-being," *The American Psychologist*, vol. 55, no. 1, pp. 68–78, 2000.

[2] A. D. Mancini, "Self-determination theory: a framework for the recovery paradigm," *Advances in Psychiatric Treatment*, vol. 14, no. 5, pp. 358–365, 2008.

[3] A. Medalia and J. Brekke, "In search of a theoretical structure for understanding motivation in schizophrenia," *Schizophrenia Bulletin*, vol. 36, no. 5, pp. 912–918, 2010.

[4] J. Choi, T. Mogami, and A. Medalia, "Intrinsic motivation inventory: an adapted measure for schizophrenia research," *Schizophrenia Bulletin*, vol. 36, no. 5, pp. 966–976, 2010.

[5] N. J. K. Breitborde, P. Kleinlein, and V. H. Srihari, "Self-determination and first-episode psychosis: associations with symptomatology, social and vocational functioning, and quality of life," *Schizophrenia Research*, vol. 137, no. 1–3, pp. 132–136, 2012.

[6] J. P. Ioannidis, "Why most published research findings are false," *PLoS Medicine*, vol. 2, no. 8, p. e124, 2005.

[7] Y. Amir and I. Sharon, "Replication research: a " must" for the scientific advancement of psychology," *Journal of Social Behavior & Personality*, vol. 5, no. 4, pp. 51–69, 1990.

[8] R. Moonesinghe, M. J. Khoury, and A. C. J. W. Janssens, "Most published research findings are false—but a little replication goes a long way," *PLoS Medicine*, vol. 4, no. 2, p. e28, 2007.

[9] J. Cohen, "The earth is round (p < 0.05)," *The American Psychologist*, vol. 49, no. 12, pp. 997–1003, 1994.

[10] N. J. K. Breitborde et al., "The Early Psychosis Intervention Center: exploring the mechanisms of change for psychosocial interventions for first-episode psychosis," *Early Intervention in Psychiatry*, vol. 4, supplement 1, p. 56, 2010.

[11] M. B. First, R. L. Spitzer, M. Gibbon, and J. B. W. Williams, *Structured Clinical Interview for DSM-IV-TR Axis I Disorders*, Research Version, Patient Edition (SCID-I/P), Biometrics Research, New York State Psychiatric Institute, New York, NY, USA, 2002.

[12] D. O. Perkins, J. Leserman, L. F. Jarskog, K. Graham, J. Kazmer, and J. A. Lieberman, "Characterizing and dating the onset of symptoms in psychotic illness: the Symptom Onset in Schizophrenia (SOS) inventory," *Schizophrenia Research*, vol. 44, no. 1, pp. 1–10, 2000.

[13] M. Gagné, "The role of autonomy support and autonomy orientation in prosocial behavior engagement," *Motivation and Emotion*, vol. 27, no. 3, pp. 199–223, 2003.

[14] T. B. Kashdan, T. Julian, K. Merritt, and G. Uswatte, "Social anxiety and posttraumatic stress in combat veterans: relations to well-being and character strengths," *Behaviour Research and Therapy*, vol. 44, no. 4, pp. 561–583, 2006.

[15] S. R. Kay, A. Fiszbein, and L. A. Opler, "The positive and negative syndrome scale (PANSS) for schizophrenia," *Schizophrenia Bulletin*, vol. 13, no. 2, pp. 261–276, 1987.

[16] M. Birchwood, J. Smith, R. Cochrane, S. Wetton, and S. Copestake, "The Social Functioning Scale. The development and validation of a new scale of social adjustment for use in family intervention programmes with schizophrenic patients," *The British Journal of Psychiatry*, vol. 157, pp. 853–859, 1990.

[17] The WHOQOL Group, "Development of the World Health Organization WHOQOL-BREF quality of life assessment," *Psychological Medicine*, vol. 28, no. 3, pp. 551–558, 1998.

[18] D. B. Rubin, *Multiple Imputation for Non-Response in Surveys*, John Wiley & Sons, New York, NY, USA, 1987.

[19] J. W. Graham, "Missing data analysis: making it work in the real world," *Annual Review of Psychology*, vol. 60, pp. 549–576, 2009.

[20] P. Royston, "Multiple imputation of missing values: update of ice," *Stata Journal*, vol. 5, no. 4, pp. 527–536, 2005.

[21] T. B. Kashdan, A. Mishra, W. E. Breen, and J. J. Froh, "Gender differences in gratitude: examining appraisals, narratives, the willingness to express emotions, and changes in psychological needs," *Journal of Personality*, vol. 77, no. 3, pp. 691–730, 2009.

[22] J. A. Hicks, J. Trent, W. E. Davis, and L. A. King, "Positive affect, meaning in life, and future time perspective: an application of socioemotional selectivity theory," *Psychology and Aging*, vol. 27, no. 1, pp. 181–189, 2012.

[23] M. S. Ibarra-Rovillard and N. A. Kuiper, "Social support and social negativity findings in depression: perceived responsiveness to basic psychological needs," *Clinical Psychology Review*, vol. 31, no. 3, pp. 342–352, 2011.

5

Rate of Nonadherence to Antipsychotic Medications and Factors Leading to Nonadherence among Psychiatric Patients in Gondar University Hospital, Northwest Ethiopia

Abyot Endale Gurmu, Esileman Abdela, Bashir Allele, Ermias Cheru, and Bemnet Amogne

School of Pharmacy, College of Medicine and Health Sciences, University of Gondar, P.O. Box 196, Gondar, Ethiopia

Correspondence should be addressed to Abyot Endale Gurmu; abiymille99@yahoo.com

Academic Editor: Xingguang Luo

Objective. The main aim of this study was to assess the rate of medication nonadherence among psychiatry patients at University of Gondar Hospital. *Materials and Methods.* Cross-sectional, descriptive method was conducted over a period of one month in May, 2013, at University of Gondar Hospital. Rate of nonadherence was computed using Medication Adherence Rating Scale questionnaire and self-reporting via a structured patient interview. Chi-square was used to determine the statistical significance of the association of variables with adherence. *Result.* Out of 209 respondents, 105 (50.2%) were found to be nonadherent. Patients who were forced to take their medication against their will ($P < 0.001$), those who did not believe they require medication ($P = 0.026$), and those who discontinued their medication without consulting their prescriber ($P < 0.001$) had significant association with nonadherence. Adherence among schizophrenia was 75.7%; psychotic was 46.7%; bipolar disorder was 37.5%; and psychosis with depression was 52.6%. Reasons for nonadherence included recovery from the illness (26.7%), seeking alternative therapy and unavailability of drugs (18.1% each), adverse drug reaction (12.7%), forgetfulness (10.6%), and being busy (8.6%). *Conclusion.* The observed rate of antipsychotic medication nonadherence in this study was high. Interventions to increase adherence are therefore crucial.

1. Introduction

Adherence to medication regimens has been monitored since the time of Hippocrates [1]. Adherence to a medication regimen is generally defined as the extent to which patients take medications as prescribed by their health care providers. It is clear that the full benefit of the many effective medications that are available will be achieved only if patients follow prescribed treatment regimens reasonably [2]. Because of the difficulties in measuring adherence, no estimate of adherence or nonadherence can be generalized, but poor adherence is to be expected in 30–50% of all patients, irrespective of disease, prognosis, or setting [3]. Study done in Washington showed that 74% of outpatients with schizophrenia stop taking neuroleptics or antipsychotics within two years of leaving a hospital and 20 to 57% patients with bipolar affective disorder are nonadherent [4].

Nonadherence to medication is known to be associated with poorer treatment outcomes, particularly in the management of chronic disease. In the treatment and management of psychotic disorders, the maximum benefit that a patient derives from these medications is highly dependent on their adherence to treatment. Although nonadherence is a ubiquitous problem in medicine, the nature of psychotic disorders makes it especially difficult for patients to adhere to treatment [1–5]. The consequences of nonadherence have been studied extensively and are significant, especially lack of disease control and hospital admissions or readmissions [6]. The impact of nonadherence on antipsychotic medication leads to diseases relapse, increased clinical and emergency room visit, and hospitalization. Nonadherent patients are over 10 times more likely to have a psychotic relapse and four times more likely to be hospitalized than adherent patients [7].

In Ethiopia, due to the underresourced health care system, medication nonadherence rates are potentially much higher thereby contributing to substantial worsening of disease, increased mortality, and increased health care cost [5]. Assessing medication adherence might lead to a better understanding of reasons for nonadherence in psychiatric patients and lay the groundwork for interventions aimed at increasing adherence [8]. In addition, understanding the extent of the problem is half of the solution and the result of study can help as a baseline for further study on psychiatric patient's adherence and open the door to determining various adherence and nonadherence issues.

The objective of this study was, first, to evaluate adherence rates and, second, to identify possible reasons for nonadherence to antipsychotic medications, among patients with psychiatric disorders at University of Gondar Hospital.

2. Materials and Methods

2.1. Study Design. A cross-sectional study design was conducted over a month period in 2013 (May 01 to May 30, 2013), on psychiatric clinic, University of Gondar Hospital (UoGH). UoGH is located 727 km Northwest of Addis Ababa, Ethiopia. It is one of the largest teaching institutions among federally established teaching hospitals and serving about five million populations in and around Gondar town [9].

2.2. Patient Selection Criteria. Convenience sampling was used to select patients. All patients who visited psychiatric clinic during the study period and fulfilled the inclusion criteria were recruited. Patients whose age was greater than or equal to eighteen years, who were diagnosed with psychiatric illness, who took antipsychotic medication for at least three months, who were conscious, and who volunteered to give consent were included.

2.3. Data Collection Tool. Data were collected using a structured and pretested questionnaire. The questionnaire was adapted from Medication Adherence Rating Scale (MARS) which was developed by Thompson et al., 2000 [10], for assessment of adherence in psychiatric patients and translated to local language (Amharic). It examines adherence behaviour and attitude towards medication with relatively simple scoring and includes 10 items. If the patient scored greater than or equal to six, he/she will be considered adherent and if the patient scored less than six, he/she was considered nonadherent. The questionnaire was pretested to identify potential problem of the questionnaires, unanticipated interpretations, and cultural objections to any of the questions on 11 (5%) respondents having similar characteristics to the study subjects on nonparticipants. Apart from MARS questionnaire, there was also section regarding sociodemographic characteristics, treatment duration, and insight about their medication/illness. Considering those respondents who were illiterate (cannot write and read), the questionnaire was read out to them by data collectors. The diagnosis on psychiatric disorder was done as per Diagnostic and Statistical Manual of Mental disorder (http://www.dsm.org/).

2.4. Data Analysis. Data were coded, checked for completeness and consistency, and analyzed using SPSS version 20.0. Descriptive statistics were used to determine patient demographics, medication information, and adherence rates. The association between variables was calculated with chi-square test of association. Frequency tables, graphs, percentages, and means were used to display results.

2.5. Ethical Approval. The study was conducted after getting letter of permission from School of Pharmacy, University of Gondar. Confidentiality of respondents was granted by keeping the privacy while filling the questionnaire.

3. Results

Among two hundred and eighty patients who were approached for the study, 63 did not fulfil the inclusion criteria and 8 either did not complete interview or were not willing to be included in the study. Finally 209 were included, resulting in a response rate of 96.3%. Male to female ratio was approximately 1 : 1 (50.2% to 49.8%) (Table 1).

3.1. Clinical Characteristics of the Study Participants. Regarding the insight about their mental illness, majority 162 (77.5%) had good understanding (59.9% were from rural) while the rest 47 (22.5%) feel they did have mental illness (55.5% were from rural) and even did not know why they came to hospital. Of patients who reportedly had good insight into their illness, 90% believed they require medication 46.8% of patients who do not think they are ill reported that they require medication. Ninety percent of respondents have had good relationship with their mental health care provider and replied that they got sufficient information concerning their medication (Table 2).

3.2. Nonadherence Level of Respondents. Based on MARS (Medication Adherence Rating Scale), out of total respondents, half of them (50.2%) were found nonadherent to their medication. The relative risk of residence on adherence odd ratio equals 0.962 (95% CI; 0.766–0.206) for rural area and odd ratio equals 1.058 (95% CI; 0.765–1.463) for urban. This implies that being from rural area had slight risk to be nonadherent even though being urban resident had no association with adherence. With regard to age, patients between 18 and 49 years old had adherence rate below 50% whereas those above 49 years had adherence rate of 65%. Correlating adherence with psychiatric disorders, schizophrenic patients were found to be the most nonadherent (75.7%) whereas bipolar disorder accounts for the least (37.5%) (Table 3).

Based on the association of different variables and rate of adherence, there was no statistically significant association between age, medication regimen, income, educational status, marital status, and occupational status of the respondents ($P > 0.05$).

TABLE 1: Sociodemographic characteristics of respondents, University of Gondar Hospital, Psychiatric Clinic, May, 2013.

Sociodemographics	Characteristics	Frequency (%)
Gender	Male	105 (50.2)
	Female	104 (49.8)
Age (years)	18–24	26 (12.4)
	25–30	94 (45.0)
	31–40	42 (20.1)
	41–50	24 (11.5)
	>50	23 (11.0)
Religion	Orthodox	182 (87.1)
	Islam	25 (12.0)
	Protestant	2 (1.0)
Education level	Illiterate	77 (33.6)
	Read and write	11 (5.3)
	Grades 1–6	24 (11.5)
	Grades 7–10	46 (22.0)
	Grades 11 and 12	14 (6.7)
	>Grade 12	37 (17.7)
Residence	Urban	86 (41.1)
	Rural	123 (58.9)
Marital status	Married	67 (32.1)
	Single	95 (45.5)
	Divorced	35 (16.7)
	Widowed	12 (5.7)

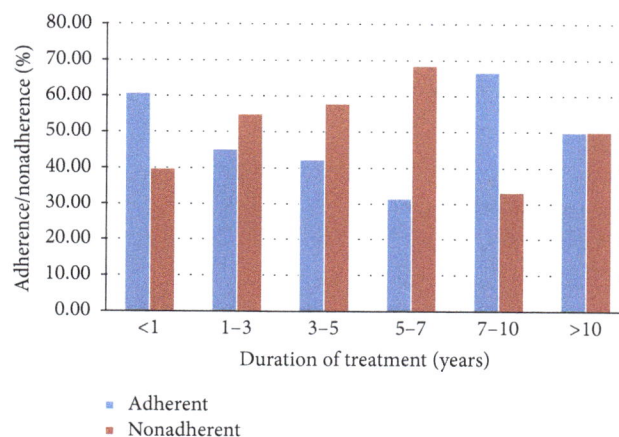

FIGURE 1: Duration on drug treatment and nonadherence rate of respondents, University of Gondar Hospital, Psychiatric Clinic, May, 2013.

TABLE 2: Clinical characteristics of respondents, Gondar University Hospital, May, 2013.

Psychiatry disorder	Number (%)
Psychosis	75 (35.9%)
Major depression disorder	60 (28.7%)
Schizophrenia	37 (17.7%)
Depression with psychotic feature	19 (9.1%)
Bipolar disorder	8 (3.8%)
Others (like sleep disorder, anxiety delusional)	10 (4.8%)

As shown in Table 4, majority of psychiatric patients ranges in the age group of 21–30 years, of which psychosis was the Major Psychiatric disorder (39.4%) followed by depression and schizophrenia with 23.4% each. Depression was found to be the major psychiatric illness (38.4%) within the age group of 10–20 years, whereas psychosis was found to be the major psychiatric illness in the elderly (39.1%).

Approximately, 90% of participants took medication from 3 months to seven years. It was found that as treatment duration increases, nonadherence rate also increases from 39.7% to 68.4% till year 7 (Figure 1).

3.3. Factors Leading to Nonadherence. Of all, 94 participants discontinued medication without consulting their prescribers for various reasons. Recovery from their illness (26%), unavailability of drugs (18.1%), adverse drug reactions (12.7%), forgetfulness (10.6%), being busy (8.6%), and seeking alternative therapy (5.3%) were found to be the reasons for nonadherence among respondents. With regard to those patient who had good insight into their illness, recovery from their illness (10.7%), unavailability of drugs (10.1%) and adverse drug reactions (6.7%), and forgetfulness (5.6%) were found to be the major factors for the nonadherence whereas other factors (19.1%) and recovery from their illness (14.7%) were the major factors for those ones who do not think they are ill (Table 5).

4. Discussion

This study showed that 105 (50.2%) of respondents were nonadherent using MARS. Accessing medication adherence might lead to a better understanding level of adherence and lays groundwork for interventions and aimed at increasing adherence. Previously reported rate of adherence to antipsychotic medication in USA was ranging from 25 to 75% [11]. This was consistent with the current study.

In this study, being from rural area was found to have slight association with nonadherence rate. Another study also showed that nonadherence among rural population was more common in 1 in 5 individuals [12].

Patients who believed that they required medication were approximately 1.6 times more adherent than those who did not (OR = 1.56, 95%). This was consistent with a study conducted by Adams, 2000, which predicted that the association between adherence and perceived benefits of treatment is logical and may reflect the reported relationship between insight and adherence in people with mental disorders [13]. In this study, schizophrenic patients were the most nonadherent (75.7%) compared to other psychiatry disorders while patients with bipolar disorder were the least (37.5%). In another study rates of adherence among patients with schizophrenia were reported between 50 and 60 percent, and among those with bipolar affective disorder the rates were as low as 35 percent [1]. In a systematic review by Cramer and Rosenheck, the mean rate of medication adherence with

TABLE 3: Nonadherence and psychotic illness among respondents, in University of Gondar Hospital, May, 2013.

Diagnosis	Adherent (number, %)	Nonadherent (number, %)	Total	
Psychosis	40 (53.3)	35 (46.7)	75 (100.0%)	
Depression	35 (58.5)	25 (41.7)	60 (100.0%)	
Schizophrenia	9 (24.3)	28 (75.7)	37 (100.0%)	$P = 0.026$
Psychosis with depression	9 (47.4)	10 (52.6)	19 (100.0%)	
Bipolar disorder	5 (62.5)	3 (37.5)	8 (100%)	
Other	6 (60)	4 (40)	10 (100.0%)	
Total	104 (49.8)	105 (50.2)	209 (100.0%)	

TABLE 4: Psychiatric illness in age distribution among respondents, in University of Gondar Hospital, May, 2013.

Age	Diagnosis						Total
	Psychosis	Depression	Schizophrenia	Psychosis with depression	Bipolar disorder	Others	
10–20	9	10	3	0	2	2	26
21–30	37	22	22	7	3	3	94
31–40	16	11	6	6	1	2	42
41–50	4	11	2	4	1	2	24
>50	9	6	4	2	1	1	23
Total	75	60	37	19	8	10	209

TABLE 5: Factors leading to nonadherence among respondents, University of Gondar Hospital, May, 2013.

Reasons for nonadherence	Adherent	Nonadherent	Total	
Get improved	5 (18.5%)	20 (29.8%)	25 (26.6%)	
Alternative therapy	0 (0%)	5 (7.4%)	5 (5.3%)	
Due to ADR	5 (18.5%)	7 (10.44%)	12 (12.7%)	
Due to unavailability of drugs	7 (25.9%)	10 (14.9%)	17 (18%)	$P = 0.00$
Forgetfulness	3 (11.1%)	7 (10.4%)	10 (10.6%)	
Being busy	4 (14.8%)	4 (5.9%)	8 (8.5%)	
Others	3 (11.1%)	14 (20.8%)	17 (18%)	
Total	27	67	94	

psychoses was 58 percent (range: 24 to 90 percent) and among those with depression the mean rate was 65 percent (range: 58 to 90 percent) [14].

In the present study, patients above 49 years old were more adherent (65.2%) than those under 49 years old (adherence rates range from 37.5% to 51.1%). This is consistent with expert consensus guideline and Oslin et al. studies which reported that patients who are younger were more likely to have adherence problems than older patients [15, 16].

Among participants, 94 (45%) discontinued medication without mental health care provider. Given the consequences of antipsychotic discontinuation and haphazard antipsychotic use, the poor adherence rates demonstrated in this study and other studies are troubling. Fenton et al., 1997, reported that patients who discontinued antipsychotics may be two to five times more likely to relapse than other patients, leading to unnecessary suffering [17]. Robinson and colleagues reported that 82% of first-episode patients experienced at least one relapse within 5 years of follow-up and that patients who discontinued medication were five times more likely to relapse. It might be speculated that, after

experiencing one relapse, patients would be substantially less likely to discontinue medication, so our study was particularly noteworthy in suggesting factors that might contribute to nonadherence [18].

Common barriers to adherence are under the patient's control, so attention to them is a necessary and important step in improving adherence [19, 20]. In the current study, recovery from the illness (26.6%) was found to be the most reason for drug discontinuation. Study done in Jimma University, Ethiopia, reported the following reasons for nonadherence among psychiatry patients: forgetfulness (36.2%), being busy (21.0%), and lack of sufficient information about the medication (10.0%) [5]. In other studies typical reasons cited by patients for not taking their medications included forgetfulness (30%), other priorities (16%), decision to omit doses (11%), lack of information (9%), and emotional factors (7%) [2]. In a study conducted by Taj et al. reasons for nonadherence included sedation (30%), medication cost (22%), forgetting to take medication (36%), and inability of the physicians to explain timing and dose (92%) or benefit of medication (76%) [1].

5. Limitation

Being a cross-sectional design conducted at a single university hospital, our study findings cannot be generalized to all areas of the country. The self-report method used in this study to measure treatment adherence might substantially overestimate medication adherence, as it relies on patient recall.

6. Conclusion

This study found that nonadherence to psychiatric medication was high in the study area. Forcing patients to take their medication against their will, recovery from first episodes of their illness, and discontinuation of medication without consulting their prescribers were found to be the main contributing factors to nonadherence. Nonadherence must therefore be considered when planning treatment strategies among psychiatric patients.

Conflict of Interests

The authors declare that they have no conflict of interests.

Acknowledgment

The authors are grateful to Mr. Niguse Yigzaw, Head of Department of Psychiatry, University of Gondar, for his help during data collection.

References

[1] F. Taj, M. Tanwir, Z. Aly et al., "Factors associated with non-adherence among psychiatric patients at a tertiary care hospital, Karachi, Pakistan: a questionnaire based cross-sectional study," *Journal of the Pakistan Medical Association*, vol. 58, no. 8, pp. 432–436, 2008.

[2] L. Osterberg and T. Blaschke, "Adherence to medication," *The New England Journal of Medicine*, vol. 353, no. 5, pp. 487–497, 2005.

[3] E. Vermeire, H. Hearnshaw, P. van Royen, and J. Denekens, "Patient adherence to treatment: three decades of research. A comprehensive review," *Journal of Clinical Pharmacy and Therapeutics*, vol. 26, no. 5, pp. 331–342, 2001.

[4] A. Elixhauser, S. A. Eisen, J. C. Romeis, and S. M. Homan, "The effects of monitoring and feedback on compliance.," *Medical care*, vol. 28, no. 10, pp. 882–893, 1990.

[5] M. Alene, M. D. Wiese, M. T. Angamo, B. V. Bajorek, E. A. Yesuf, and N. T. Wabe, "Adherence to medication for the treatment of psychosis: rates and risk factors in an Ethiopian population," *BMC Clinical Pharmacology*, vol. 12, article 10, 2012.

[6] R. Taj and S. Khan, "A study of reasons of non-compliance to psychiatric treatment," *Journal of Ayub Medical College*, vol. 17, no. 2, pp. 26–28, 2005.

[7] G. Morken, J. H. Widen, and R. W. Grawe, "Non-adherence to antipsychotic medication, relapse and rehospitalisation in recent-onset schizophrenia," *BMC Psychiatry*, vol. 8, article 32, 2008.

[8] S. Mahaye, T. Mayime, S. S. Nkosi et al., "Medication adherence of psychiatric patients in an outpatient setting," *African Journal of Pharmacy & Pharmacology*, vol. 6, pp. 608–612, 2012.

[9] WHO, "Patient safety 2013," 2013, http://www.who.int/patient-safety/implementation/apps/first_wave/ethiopia_leicester/en.

[10] K. Thompson, J. Kulkarni, and A. A. Sergejew, "Reliability and validity of a new medication adherence rating scale (MARS) for the psychoses," *Schizophrenia Research*, vol. 42, no. 3, pp. 241–247, 2000.

[11] C. R. Dolder, J. P. Lacro, L. B. Dunn, and D. V. Jeste, "Antipsychotic medication adherence: Is there a difference between typical and atypical agents?" *The American Journal of Psychiatry*, vol. 159, no. 1, pp. 103–108, 2002.

[12] H. Thomas and E. Donald, "Primary medication adherence in rural population," *The Journal of American Family Medicine*, vol. 12, pp. 27–59, 2006.

[13] J. Adams and J. Scott, "Predicting medication adherence in severe mental disorders," *Acta Psychiatrica Scandinavica*, vol. 101, no. 2, pp. 119–124, 2000.

[14] J. A. Cramer and R. Rosenheck, "Compliance with medication regimens for mental and physical disorders," *Psychiatric Services*, vol. 49, no. 2, pp. 196–201, 1998.

[15] D. I. Velligan, P. J. Weiden, M. Sajatovic et al., "The expert consensus guideline series: adherence problems in patients with serious and persistent mental illness," *The Journal of Clinical Psychiatry*, vol. 70, supplement 4, pp. 1–48, 2009.

[16] D. W. Oslin, H. Pettinati, and J. R. Volpicelli, "Alcoholism treatment adherence: older age predicts better adherence and drinking outcomes," *American Journal of Geriatric Psychiatry*, vol. 10, no. 6, pp. 740–747, 2002.

[17] W. S. Fenton, C. R. Blyler, and R. K. Heinssen, "Determinants of medication compliance in schizophrenia: empirical and clinical findings," *Schizophrenia Bulletin*, vol. 23, no. 4, pp. 637–651, 1997.

[18] D. Robinson, M. G. Woerner, J. M. J. Alvir et al., "Predictors of relapse following response from a first episode of schizophrenia or schizoaffective disorder," *Archives of General Psychiatry*, vol. 56, no. 3, pp. 241–247, 1999.

[19] S. Magura, A. Roseblum, and C. Fong, "Factor associated with medication adherence among psychiatric outpatients at substance abuse risk," *The Open Addiction Journal*, vol. 4, pp. 58–64, 2011.

[20] K. S. Latha, "The noncompliant patient in psychiatry: the case for and against covert/surreptitious medication," *Mens Sana Monographs*, vol. 8, no. 1, pp. 96–121, 2010.

6

Cytokine Serum Levels as Potential Biological Markers for the Psychopathology in Schizophrenia

Dimitre H. Dimitrov, Shuko Lee, Jesse Yantis, Craig Honaker, and Nicole Braida

South Texas Veterans Health Care Systems, San Antonio, TX 78229-4404, USA

Correspondence should be addressed to Dimitre H. Dimitrov; dimitre.dimitrov@va.gov

Academic Editor: Livia Carvalho

We discuss the role of immune system disturbance in schizophrenia and especially changes of serum levels of cytokines in patients with schizophrenia. The cytokines are essential to wide range of functions related to the defense of the organisms from infectious and environmental dangers. However it is not known whether cytokines influence the presentation of psychotic symptoms. Identification of changes in the serum level of certain cytokines and their correlation with distinct psychopathological symptoms may facilitate the identification of subgroups of patients who are likely to benefit from immunotherapy or anti-inflammatory therapy. Such patients may benefit from tailored immunotherapy designed for modulation of abnormal cytokine levels related to specific positive or negative symptoms of schizophrenia.

1. Introduction

Accumulating evidence supports the view that immunological dysfunction may have a role in the etiology of psychotic disorders. In a recent publication in Nature by the Schizophrenia Working Group of the Psychiatric Genomic Consortium were identified 108 schizophrenia associated loci [1]. Notable associations with the dopaminergic and glutaminergic neurotransmitters as well as associations with voltage gated calcium channels subunits were found. The most significant association was with the major histocompatibility complex and with a region involved in acquired immunity. A recent study provides encouraging evidence that biological signatures for schizophrenia can be identified in blood serum [2]. The role of the immune system disturbance was recently reviewed [3]. An important role leading to these changes is played by the cytokines [4, 5].

Cytokines are low-molecular weight proteins secreted by immune cells and other cell types in response to a number of environmental stimuli, particularly infections. They have wide-ranging roles in the innate and adaptive immune systems, where they help regulate the recruitment and activation of lymphocytes as well as immune cell differentiation and homeostasis. In addition, some cytokines possess direct effector mechanisms, including induction of cell apoptosis and inhibition of protein synthesis. Previously we described dysregulated production of cytokines and their association with psychopathology of schizophrenia as well as the possible involvement of the Th17/IL-17 pathway [6, 7]. We found significantly increased levels of GRO, MCP-1, MDC, and sCD40L and significantly decreased levels of IFN-γ, IL-2, IL12-p70, and IL-17. In addition, we observed positive correlations between levels of cytokines and the Positive and Negative Symptom scale (PANSS) scores in subjects with schizophrenia for G-CSF, IL-1β, IL-1ra, IL-3, IL-6, IL-9, IL-10, sCD40L, and TNFβ. The main objective of this review is to provide further evidence of cytokines linked to severity and duration of schizophrenia as well as with distinct symptoms of psychopathology based on the obtained PANSS scores. Such approach may lead to the discovery of reliable biomarkers for schizophrenia and new immunological therapy designed to control different distinct symptoms of schizophrenia.

2. Evidence Obtained on the Basis of the Classical Th1/Th2 Model

The importance of macrophages and T lymphocytes and the cytokines produced by them has been highlighted in the macrophage—T cell theory of bipolar disorder and schizophrenia [8]. T cells are divided into Th8—cytotoxic cells and CD4 cells—T helper cells (Th). According to a model proposed by Mosmann and Coffman [9] the Th cells were divided into Th1 and Th2. Currently two new subtypes of T cells, Th17 and T regulatory cells (Tregs), are emerging as important factors in the etiology of schizophrenia [10].

According to the classical model Th1 cells support cell-mediated immune responses and activate macrophages via IFN-γ. Th2 cells support humoral and allergic responses and play a major role in the transformation of B cells into plasma cells which secrete IL-4, IL-5, IL-9, and IL-13 [11]. By analyzing the type 1 and type 2 responses a decreased production of IFN-γ and IL-2 in schizophrenia was reported in vitro reflecting a blunted production of type 1 cytokines [12, 13]. An activation of the type 2 immune response is also described in schizophrenia including increased levels of IL-4 and IL-10.

The IFN-γ is essential for Th1 cellular response. High levels of IFN-γ may lead to CNS inflammation and damage to oligodendrocytes, and this may be one of the reasons why in patients with schizophrenia there is a switch from cellular to humoral Th2 immunity. IFN-γ is found in neuronal synapses and it may act at the level of the synapse to influence brain function [14]. Alterations in the levels of cytokines and combinations of cytokines can act synergistically or antagonistically. This depends upon the state of the target cells and the combination of doses and temporal sequence of cytokine secretion. Chronic exposure to proinflammatory cytokines may cause premature maturation and stabilization of these synapses. Thus, alterations in the levels of cytokines can profoundly change synaptic efficiency and changes of synaptic efficiency may lead to changes of cytokine level. For example, it was described that IL-6 and IL-2 inhibit the long-term plasticity and the short-term potentiation of neuronal circuits [14]. IL-6 is viewed as a key danger signal initiating the inflammatory cascade. This cytokine together with IFN-γ and IL-12 control the Th17 response [15, 16]. Overproduction of IL-17 may aggravate inflammatory reactions and contribute to tissue damage. We observed lower levels of IL-17 in veterans with schizophrenia who were treated with different antipsychotics. This may be a compensatory mechanism to lessen the extent of injury due to inflammation [7].

In patients with schizophrenia there is also activation of the type 2 immune response with increased production of Ig E and IL-10 [17]. In CSF, IL-10 levels were found to be related to the severity of psychosis [18]. IL-4, the key cytokine of type 2 immune response, is increased in the CSF of juvenile schizophrenic patients [19]. In a recent meta-analysis, 40 studies of the acute phase of schizophrenia were reviewed. High levels of IL-1β, IL-6, and TGF-β were observed, which were considered to be state markers for schizophrenia. Elevated levels of IFN-γ, TNF-α, and soluble IL-2 receptor (sIL-2R) were considered to be trait markers of schizophrenia [20]. Results reported in another meta-analysis suggested that in vivo there are increased peripheral levels of IL-1ra, sIL-2R, and IL-6 [4].

Additionally, the type 1/type 2 imbalance is associated with an activation of astrocytes and an imbalance in the activation of astrocytes/microglial cells [21]. Microglial cells, deriving from peripheral macrophages, secrete preferably type 1 cytokines such as IL-12, while astrocytes inhibit the production of IL-12 and secrete IL-10 [21]. The view of an overactivation of astrocytes in schizophrenia is supported by the findings of increased levels of the calcium binding protein S100B which is considered a marker of astrocyte overactivation [22].

3. Cytokines Involved in Regulation of Calcium Channels and Formation of Synapses

Increased serum levels of eotaxin/CCL-11 were described in patients with schizophrenia [23]. The protein sequence of eotaxin is 66% similar to human MCP-1 and acts on the chemokine receptor CCR3 which is expressed on eosinophils and mast cells. This data is consistent with the idea that preferential activation of Th2 lymphocytes plays a role in the pathogenesis of schizophrenia. Eotaxin is involved in the regulation of the calcium binding proteins such as calcineurin. Calcineurin is linked to receptors for several brain chemicals including NMDA, dopamine, and GABA. Conditioned calcineurin knockout mice exhibit multiple abnormal behaviors related to schizophrenia [24]. Calcineurin in reactive astrocytes plays a key role in the interaction between proinflammatory and anti-inflammatory signals. In quiescent astrocytes inflammatory mediators such as TNFα recruit calcineurin to stimulate canonical inflammatory pathway involving NF-κB. However in reactive astrocytes calcineurin involves anti-inflammatory mediators that inhibit NF-κB. These results suggest that calcineurin forms a molecular pathway whereby reactive astrocytes determine the outcome of the neuron inflammatory process by directing it towards either its resolution or its progression [25]. The recent genome-wide study describing associations of schizophrenia with voltage gated calcium channels may outline the possibility that levels of eotaxin and calcium binding proteins could be used as potential markers for schizophrenia [1].

During the neuroinflammatory process of schizophrenia, cytokines like eotaxin appear to facilitate calcium waves. According to this concept if calcium levels are tweaked different neurotransmitters would be expressed. In depression there would be too few calcium waves and in mania and psychosis calcium waves would be fluid and intense. Cannabis may cause ripples of calcium waves and dreamlike states.

Increased eotaxin/CCL11 levels in blood plasma are associated with ageing in mice and humans [26]. Exposing young mice to CCL11 or the blood plasma of older mice decreases their neurogenesis and cognitive performance [26].

Fractalkine is a transmembrane chemokine and is expressed only by neurons, while the fractalkine receptor

CX3CR1 is exclusively present on microglial cells. Fractalkine (CX3CL1) and its receptor are also involved in immune cell trafficking to the CNS. Mice that lack the receptor for fractalkine have impaired cognitive function and synaptic plasticity. Microglial cells which have receptor for fractalkine are also required to support hippocampal neurogenesis [27]. Fractalkine is recently described as neuronal "off signal" that keeps microglia in resting states. The chemokine CX3CL1 induced chemokine release of CXCL16-CCL2. This interaction involves neurons, microglia, and astrocytes and that represents an endogenous self-protecting mechanism. It was reported that in this way cell damage due to brain ischemia may be limited by counteracting neuronal death due to glutamate excitotoxicity [28, 29]. The release of CCL2/MCP-1 by astrocytes involves synergistic activity of adenosine and adenosine type 3 receptor on astrocytes.

Fractalkine on one hand appears to prevent excess microglial activation in the absence of injury while promoting activation of microglia and astrocytes during inflammatory episodes [30]. Expression levels of fractalkine and its receptor have been found to change in and around the demyelinating lesions that accompany experimental autoimmune encephalomyelitis (EAE) disease progression. In Alzheimer's disease there is increased activation of microglia around amyloid beta plaques. There are data that fractalkine is increased in patients with mild cognitive impairment as compared to healthy controls and the levels of fractalkine were decreased in severe forms of Alzheimer's disease [31].

The fractalkine receptor is synthesized exclusively by microglia and is essential for their survival and migration. Neurons in the brain increase fractalkine production when they are forming synapses. A very interesting observation was that microglia actively engulf synaptic material and play a major role in synaptic pruning during postnatal development in mice [32]. The authors used mutant mice lacking the gene encoding the fractalkine receptor. The mice lacking the fractalkine receptor had significantly greater numbers of synapses leading to increases in the frequency of spontaneous electrical impulses. According to the authors it appears that the developing brain treats unwanted synapses as if they are invading microorganisms and dispatches the microglial cells to survey the state of the synapses and dispose those deemed unwanted and superfluous [32].

4. Cytokines in the CNS

Increased inflammatory markers were found in the dorsolateral prefrontal cortex by using SOLiD next generation sequencing to quantify neuroimmune inflammatory transcripts in postmortem brain samples from patients with schizophrenia [33]. By using a two-step factor analysis in this cluster a high mRNA expression of IL-1β, IL-6, and IL-8 was reported in 18 individuals and it was concluded that IL-1β is linked to MHC-II-expressing cells in the white matter and that the disease duration had a positive correlation with IL-6 and IL-1β [33]. Elevated IL-1β expression is known to cause increased secretion of IL-6 from microglia, astrocytes, and neurons and IL-6 may lead to problems of cell migration,

which may be one of the reasons for greater density of inhibitory neurons in the white matter of patients with schizophrenia [34]. In a review of the fetal brain cytokine imbalance of schizophrenia it was report that IL-1β is most capable in inducing the conversion of rat mesencephalic progenitor cells into a dopaminergic phenotype and that IL-6 is highly efficacious in decreasing the survival of fetal brain serotonin neurons [35]. It is interesting that enhanced levels of IL-10 during prenatal development are sufficient to prevent the emergence of multiple behavior abnormalities [35].

Neuroinflammation is characterized by the activation of the microglial cells which exhibit an increase in the expression of the peripheral benzodiazepine receptor. An 11C radiolabeled isoquinoline is a peripheral receptor ligand and PET imaging was used for the detection of the activated microglial cells [36].

In this report it was demonstrated that there is an increase in the expression of the peripheral benzodiazepine receptor indicative of neuroinflammation and that focal neuroinflammation is a feature of psychosis and not necessarily present in stable schizophrenic patients. The calcium binding protein S100B expressed in activated astrocytes is increased in the serum and plasma of schizophrenia patients and there is a higher binding potential of the radioactive ligand in the hippocampus of schizophrenic patients [36]. Th17 response could be significantly amplified by dopamine. For example, the stimulation of dopamine receptor D5 expressed on dendritic cells can potentiate Th17 immunity [37]. Dopamine receptors expressed on immune cells modulate Th17-mediated inflammation [37] and the Th17-mediated immune response can be attenuated by D1-like receptor antagonists [38].

The inflammatory cytokines may influence tryptophan degradation, leading to elevated levels of the kynurenine metabolites, and as endogenous kynurenic acid modulates the extracellular levels of glutamate and acetylcholine such increases may be of pathophysiologic significance [12].

5. Autoimmune Diseases and Psychosis

A range of psychiatric disorders including psychosis have been observed to occur more frequently in some autoimmune diseases such as systemic lupus erythematosus and multiple sclerosis. There is a similarity in the immune pathogenic principles involved in autoimmunity, chronic inflammation, and psychosis [39]. A 30-year population-based register study has shown that having a prior autoimmune disease and a history of hospitalization with infection increased the risk of schizophrenia by 29% and 60%, respectively [40].

The Th17 lineage is now implicated in a number of autoinflammatory disorders such as rheumatoid arthritis, multiple sclerosis, and psoriasis [41]. It is also implicated in the autoimmune encephalitis and its role in the neuroinflammatory process in multiple sclerosis [42]. Interestingly an IL-17 producing CD8+ T cells (termed Tc17) was discovered in mice and humans. These Tc17 cells can initiate Th17 autoimmunity by supporting Th17 pathogenicity [43].

In a subgroup of psychotic patients the high comorbidity with autoimmune and chronic inflammatory conditions suggests a common underlying immune abnormality underlying both conditions. Immune biomarkers might be found in raised monocyte and microglia inflammatory activation patterns together with reduced numbers and reduced proliferation activity of T cells. In such case high number of T reg cells may predominate leading to high serum level of sIL2R and inflammatory skewing of T cells in direction of Th1/Th17 with high levels of IL-12 and IFN-γ [44].

6. Review of the IL-17/Th17

Previously we reported positive correlation between the levels of cytokines and PANSS scores in patients with schizophrenia. Pathway analyses showed these cytokines to be part of the IL-17 pathway [7]. IL-17 has a remarkable homology with herpes virus saimiri and this led to the hypothesis that during evolution the virus captures a portion of the human gene in order to gain survival advantage during infection [45, 46]. The Th17 responses are very important in host defense but also in promoting chronic inflammation and autoimmunity [16]. Th17 cells appear to have evolved as cells bridging the innate and the adaptive immunity and are specialized for enhanced cell protection from microorganisms that are not well guarded by the Th1 and Th2 immunity. Th17 cells an IL-17 contribute to host defense against bacterial and fungal infections [15, 16]. Human Th17 cells remain in the body as a long-lived proliferating effector memory T cells with unique genetic and functional characteristic [47]. It was reported that inflammation in the brain parenchyma occurs only when Th17 cells outnumber Th1 cells [48]. IL-17 increases the level of GRO and MCP-1 [49, 50]. On the other hand the IL-17 mediated monocyte migration occurs partially through MCP-1 induction [51].

IL-17 has been shown to induce expression of several cytokines known to contain nuclear factor kappa (NF-κB) binding sites in their promoters. NF-κB is the principal transcription factor in the initiation of the inflammatory response. The precise mechanism by which cell generates IL-17 is not fully elucidated but it probably involves calcineurin and cyclic AMP. In response to IL-17 neutrophil specific chemokines such as IL-8 and GRO are generated as well as granulopoietic cytokines such as G-CSF and GM-CSF. By acting on macrophages IL-17 stimulates the release of TNF-α [46].

In patients with schizophrenia increased levels of sCD40L are associated with endothelial damage and this event triggers the release of inflammatory mediators [52]. In studies of EAE in mice IL-17 disrupts the blood brain barrier tight junctions [53]. In order for the Th17 cells to enter the CNS CCR6 expression on Th17 cells was required in the first wave of Th17 cells that enter the CNS through the epithelial cells of the choroid plexus. After that IL-17 induces inflammatory gene expression in the astrocytes which triggers a second wave of Th-17 cells. Th17 cells then enter the inflamed brain in a CCR6 independent manner leading to explosive inflammatory cascade with the onset of EAE [54]. The low levels of IL-17 in the veterans observed by us could be due

to low levels of IFN-γ and IL-12 which do not exert enough inhibitory effect on Th17 cells [7]. The inflammatory changes in astrocytes lead to increased levels of IL-10 and decreased levels of IL-12. The decreased levels of IL-12 lead to decreased IL-17 [21, 22]. Recent study described a subpopulation of Th17 cells that are highly pathogenic and can induce EAE in mice [55]. Generation of the pathogenic cells requires IL-23 stimulation following IL-6 and TGFβ stimulation [15].

Not all Th17 cells are involved in autoimmune processes. In contrast to the autoimmunity-promoting Th17 cells, thymus derived natural regulatory cells (nTreg) represent a unique population of cells that inhibits T cell proliferation and autoimmune processes [56]. T regulatory cells are a component of the immune system that suppresses immune responses of other T cells. This is an important "self-check" built into the immune system to prevent excessive reactions. These cells are involved in shutting down immune responses after they have successfully eliminated invading organisms and also in preventing autoimmunity. Low levels of IL-2 may impair the proliferation of Treg cells and ultimately result in autoimmunity. The low serum levels of IL-2 could lead to proliferation of Th2 response in the presence of IL-4. This would lead to an allergic response with increased levels of IL-4 and IL-13 which leads to isotype switching to IgE [11]. The eosinophilia may lead to lower levels of IL-17.

The expansion and proliferation of Treg cells is dependent on the activity of IL-2. IL-2 activates Treg cells to proliferate and differentiate via the IL-2 receptor. Activated Treg cells shed the IL-2 receptors and the shed receptor (sIL-2R) binds IL-2, inactivates it, and so fine-tunes the immune response. Th17 cells and regulatory T (Treg) cells play opposite roles in autoimmune disease. The Treg cells use Foxp3 transcription factor. The process of differentiation of Th17 requires STAT3 transcription factor. At the same time both cell subsets require TGF-β for their development but there is reciprocal regulation in the generation of these cells. While TGF-β induces Foxp3 expression, in the absence of IL-6 and IL-21, TGF-β will instead induce Th17 differentiation [56].

Tregs were found to have neuroprotective effect, attenuating microglia-mediated inflammation [57]. Microglia can adopt a neuroprotective phenotype upon activation by cytokines such as IL-4. On the other hand activated microglia produce high level of MCP-1 which triggers microglia proliferation and also serves as a microglia-induced neurodegeneration [57].

7. Emerging Theories for the Etiology of Psychopathology

By using convergent functional genomics it was proposed that fibronectin is decreased in high hallucination states and high delusional states and also in fibroblasts from schizophrenic patients [58]. In the above report the authors concluded that a decreased fibronectin and increased neuregulin are involved in high delusional states and decreased fibronectin and increased calcyclin S100A6 in high hallucination states. Of interest is the fact that fibronectin is also a top gene for alcoholism. The authors also propose that genes involved in cancer, plasticity, and connectivity (cell morphology, cell to cell signaling, and interaction) are prominent players in psychotic disorders. This hypothesis provides encouraging evidence that there may be different biological markers involved in delusions and hallucinations [58].

If the developing brain treats imperfect synapses as if they were invading microorganisms and dispatches the microglial cells to survey the state of the synapses and dispose of those that are unwanted and superfluous, this may suggest a speculative conclusion that an evolutionary process in nature may have selected primitive cellular mechanisms. These mechanisms are involved in the response to damage, insults, and stressors for analogous higher organism level functions (i.e., increased neuregulin and decreased fibronectin and increased S100A6 and decreased APOE). In this view, psychosis becomes the higher organism brain equivalent of cellular dedifferentiation and disconnection, such as occurring in early stages of inflammation, tissue remodeling, and cancer metastasis.

The evolutionary process has also changed the ratio of astrocytes per neuron. In mice the ratio is 0.3 astrocytes per neuron and in humans this ratio is 1.4 astrocytes per neuron [59]. The dramatic increase of astrocytes in the human brain could be a reason for the occurrence of imbalance between astrocytes and microglia. The overactivation of the astrocytes in schizophrenia is supported by the findings of increased levels of S100B [22].

8. Prospective Immunological Therapy of Schizophrenia

According to the cytokine model of schizophrenia it is considered that elevated levels of IL-6 and other proinflammatory cytokines play a key role and cause a wide adverse effect on the brain including facilitation of the dopaminergic sensitization, diminished hippocampal volumes, and impaired glutamatergic functions [5]. According to this model aberrant fetal programming results in elevation of IL-6 level around puberty and when this is reinforced by peripubertal stress they interact with one another leading to emergence of positive and negative symptoms and cognitive deficits. This model leads to the conclusions that immunological immunotherapy leading to opposing the effect of IL-6 may represent a useful strategy for treatment and that the IL-17 pathway is emerging as a major target in autoimmune disease. For example, Tocilizumab is an anti-IL-6 receptor antibody that is approved by the FDA for treatment of rheumatoid arthritis in individuals who have not responded to anti-TNF alpha therapy [5]. On the other hand a recent study has demonstrated that inhibition of STAT3 blocks Th17 development and inhibits experimental uveitis [60]. Inhibition of the STSAT3 pathway offers an additional approach to immunotherapy of schizophrenia.

Conflict of Interests

The authors declare that there is no conflict of interests regarding the publication of this paper.

Acknowledgment

The authors would like to thank Dr. Kelly Arneman, Ph.D., for editorial assistance.

References

[1] Schizophrenia Working Group of the Psychiatric Genome Consortium, "Biological insights from 108 schizophrenia-associated genetic loci," Nature, vol. 511, pp. 421–427, 2014.

[2] E. Schwarz, P. C. Guest, H. Rahmoune et al., "Identification of a biological signature for schizophrenia in serum," Molecular Psychiatry, vol. 17, no. 5, pp. 494–502, 2012.

[3] S. Horváth and K. Mirnics, "Immune system disturbances in schizophrenia," Biological Psychiatry, vol. 75, no. 4, pp. 316–323, 2014.

[4] S. Potvin, E. Stip, A. A. Sepehry, A. Gendron, R. Bah, and E. Kouassi, "Inflammatory cytokine alterations in schizophrenia: a systematic quantitative review," Biological Psychiatry, vol. 63, no. 8, pp. 801–808, 2008.

[5] R. R. Girgis, S. S. Kumar, and A. S. Brown, "The cytokine model of schizophrenia: emerging therapeutic strategies," Biological Psychiatry, vol. 75, no. 4, pp. 292–299, 2014.

[6] D. H. Dimitrov, "Correlation or coincidence between monocytosis and worsening of psychotic symptoms in veterans with schizophrenia?" Schizophrenia Research, vol. 126, no. 1–3, pp. 306–307, 2011.

[7] D. H. Dimitrov, S. Lee, J. Yantis et al., "Differential correlations between inflammatory cytokines and psychopathology in veterans with schizophrenia: potential role for IL-17 pathway," Schizophrenia Research, vol. 151, no. 1–3, pp. 29–35, 2013.

[8] R. C. Drexhage, E. M. Knijff, R. C. Padmos et al., "The mononuclear phagocyte system and its cytokine inflammatory networks in schizophrenia and bipolar disorder," Expert Review of Neurotherapeutics, vol. 10, no. 1, pp. 59–76, 2010.

[9] T. R. Mosmann and R. L. Coffman, "TH1 and TH2 cells: different patterns of lymphokine secretion lead to different functional properties," Annual Review of Immunology, vol. 7, pp. 145–173, 1989.

[10] M. Debnath and M. Berk, "Th17 pathway–mediated immunopathogenesis of schizophrenia: mechanisms and implications," Schizophrenia Bulletin, vol. 40, no. 6, pp. 1412–1421, 2014.

[11] D. D. Chaplin, "Overview of the immune response," Journal of Allergy and Clinical Immunology, vol. 125, no. 2, pp. S3–S23, 2010.

[12] N. Muller and M. J. Schwarz, "Immune system in schizophrenia," Current Immunology Reviews, vol. 6, pp. 213–220, 2010.

[13] V. Arolt, M. Rothermundt, K.-P. Wandinger, and H. Kirchner, "Decreased in vitro production of interferon-gamma and interleukin-2 in whole blood of patients with schizophrenia during treatment," Molecular Psychiatry, vol. 5, no. 2, pp. 150–158, 2000.

[14] P. A. Garay and A. K. McAllister, "Novel roles for immune molecules in neural development: implications for neurodevelopmental disorders," Frontiers in Synaptic Neuroscience, vol. 2, pp. 136–162, 2010.

[15] C. T. Weaver, R. D. Hatton, P. R. Mangan, and L. E. Harrington, "IL-17 family cytokines and the expanding diversity of effector T cell lineages," Annual Review of Immunology, vol. 25, pp. 821–852, 2007.

[16] T. Korn, E. Bettelli, M. Oukka, and V. K. Kuchroo, "IL-17 and Th17 cells," *Annual Review of Immunology*, vol. 27, pp. 485–517, 2009.

[17] M. J. Schwarz, S. Chiang, N. Müller, and M. Ackenheil, "T-helper-1 and T-helper-2 responses in psychiatric disorders," *Brain, Behavior, and Immunity*, vol. 15, no. 4, pp. 340–370, 2001.

[18] D. P. van Kammen, C. G. McAllister-Sistilli, and M. E. Kelly, "Relationship between immune and behavioral measures in schizophrenia," in *Current Update in Psychoimmunology*, G. Wiesselmann, Ed., New York, NY, USA, pp. 51–55, Springer, 1997.

[19] B. B. Mittleman, F. X. Castellanos, L. K. Jacobsen, J. L. Rapoport, S. E. Swedo, and G. M. Shearer, "Cerebrospinal fluid cytokines in pediatric neuropsychiatric disease," *The Journal of Immunology*, vol. 159, no. 6, pp. 2994–2999, 1997.

[20] B. J. Miller, P. Buckley, W. Seabolt, A. Mellor, and B. Kirkpatrick, "Meta-analysis of cytokine alterations in schizophrenia: clinical status and antipsychotic effects," *Biological Psychiatry*, vol. 70, no. 7, pp. 663–671, 2011.

[21] F. Aloisi, G. Penna, J. Cerase, B. M. Iglesias, and L. Adorini, "IL-12 production by the central nervous system microglia is inhibited by astrocytes," *Journal of Immunology*, vol. 159, no. 4, pp. 1604–1612, 1997.

[22] M. Rothermundt, P. Falkai, G. Ponath et al., "Glial cell dysfunction in schizophrenia indicated by increased S100B in the CSF," *Molecular Psychiatry*, vol. 9, no. 10, pp. 897–899, 2004.

[23] A. L. Teixeira, H. J. Reis, R. Nicolato et al., "Increased serum levels of CCL11/eotaxin in schizophrenia," *Progress in Neuropsychopharmacology and Biological Psychiatry*, vol. 32, no. 3, pp. 710–714, 2008.

[24] T. Miyakawa, L. M. Leiter, D. J. Gerber et al., "Conditional calcineurin knockout mice exhibit multiple abnormal behaviors related to schizophrenia," *Proceedings of the National Academy of Sciences of the United States of America*, vol. 100, no. 15, pp. 8987–8992, 2003.

[25] A. M. Fernandez, S. Fernandez, P. Carrero, M. Garcia-Garcia, and I. Torres-Aleman, "Calcineurin in reactive astrocytes plays a key role in the interplay between proinflammatory and anti-inflammatory signals," *The Journal of Neuroscience*, vol. 27, no. 33, pp. 8745–8756, 2007.

[26] S. A. Villeda, J. Luo, K. I. Mosher et al., "The ageing systemic milieu negatively regulates neurogenesis and cognitive function," *Nature*, vol. 477, pp. 90–94, 2011.

[27] A. D. Bachstetter, J. M. Morganti, J. Jernberg et al., "Fractalkine and CX$_3$CR1 regulate hippocampal neurogenesis in adult and aged rats," *Neurobiology of Aging*, vol. 32, no. 11, pp. 2030–2044, 2011.

[28] K. Biber, H. Neumann, K. Inoue, and H. W. G. M. Boddeke, "Neuronal "on" and "off" signals control microglia," *Trends in Neurosciences*, vol. 30, no. 11, pp. 596–602, 2007.

[29] M. Rosito, C. Lauro, G. Chece et al., "Trasmembrane chemokines CX3CL1 and CXCL16 drive interplay between neurons, microglia and astrocytes to counteract pMCAO and excitotoxic neuronal death," *Frontiers in Cellular Neuroscience*, vol. 8, article 193, 2014.

[30] G. K. Sheridan and K. J. Murphy, "Neuron-glia crosstalk in health and disease: fractalkine and CX3CR1 take centre stage," *Open Biology*, vol. 3, no. 1, Article ID 130181, 2013.

[31] T.-S. Kim, H.-K. Lim, J. Y. Lee et al., "Changes in the levels of plasma soluble fractalkine in patients with mild cognitive impairment and Alzheimer's disease," *Neuroscience Letters*, vol. 436, no. 2, pp. 196–200, 2008.

[32] R. C. Paolicelli, G. Bolasco, F. Pagani et al., "Synaptic pruning by microglia is necessary for normal brain development," *Science*, vol. 333, no. 6048, pp. 1456–1458, 2011.

[33] S. G. Fillman, N. Cloonan, V. S. Catts et al., "Increased inflammatory markers identified in the dorsolateral prefrontal cortex of individuals with schizophrenia," *Molecular Psychiatry*, vol. 18, no. 2, pp. 206–214, 2013.

[34] Y. Yang, S. J. Fung, A. Rothwell, S. Tianmei, and C. S. Weickert, "Increased interstitial white matter neuron density in the dorsolateral prefrontal cortex of people with schizophrenia," *Biological Psychiatry*, vol. 69, no. 1, pp. 63–70, 2011.

[35] U. Meyer, J. Feldon, and B. K. Yee, "A review of the fetal brain cytokine imbalance hypothesis of schizophrenia," *Schizophrenia Bulletin*, vol. 35, no. 5, pp. 959–972, 2009.

[36] J. Doorduin, E. F. J. de Vries, A. T. M. Willemsen, J. C. de Groot, R. A. Dierckx, and H. C. Klein, "Neuroinflammation in schizophrenia-related psychosis: a PET study," *Journal of Nuclear Medicine*, vol. 50, no. 11, pp. 1801–1807, 2009.

[37] C. Prado, F. Contreras, H. González et al., "Stimulation of dopamine receptor D5 expressed on dendritic cells potentiates Th17-mediated immunity," *Journal of Immunology*, vol. 188, no. 7, pp. 3062–3070, 2012.

[38] K. Nakagome, M. Imamura, H. Okada et al., "Dopamine D1-like receptor antagonist attenuates Th17-mediated immune response and ovalbumin antigen-induced neutrophilic airway inflammation," *The Journal of Immunology*, vol. 186, no. 10, pp. 5975–5982, 2011.

[39] M. E. Benros, P. R. Nielsen, M. Nordentoft, W. W. Eaton, S. O. Dalton, and P. B. Mortensen, "Autoimmune diseases and severe infections as risk factors for schizophrenia: a 30-year population-based register study," *The American Journal of Psychiatry*, vol. 168, no. 12, pp. 1303–1310, 2011.

[40] M. E. Benros, W. W. Eaton, and P. B. Mortensen, "The epidemiologic evidence linking autoimmune diseases and psychosis," *Biological Psychiatry*, vol. 75, no. 4, pp. 300–306, 2014.

[41] T. A. Moseley, D. R. Haudenschild, L. Rose, and A. H. Reddi, "Interleukin-17 family and IL-17 receptors," *Cytokine and Growth Factor Reviews*, vol. 14, no. 2, pp. 155–174, 2003.

[42] F. Jadidi-Niaragh and A. Mirshafiey, "Th17 Cell, the new player of neuroinflammatory process in multiple sclerosis," *Scandinavian Journal of Immunology*, vol. 74, no. 1, pp. 1–13, 2011.

[43] M. Huber, S. Heink, A. Pagenstecher et al., "IL-17A secretion by CD8+ T cells supports Th17-mediated autoimmune encephalomyelitis," *Journal of Clinical Investigation*, vol. 123, no. 1, pp. 247–260, 2013.

[44] V. Bergink, S. M. Gibney, and H. A. Drexhage, "Autoimmunity, inflammation, and psychosis: a search for peripheral markers," *Biological Psychiatry*, vol. 75, no. 4, pp. 324–331, 2014.

[45] Z. Yao, W. C. Fanslow, M. F. Seldin et al., "Herpesvirus Saimiri encodes a new cytokine, IL-17, which binds to a novel cytokine receptor," *Immunity*, vol. 3, no. 6, pp. 811–821, 1995.

[46] J. Witowski, K. Książek, and A. Jörres, "Interleukin-17: a mediator of inflammatory responses," *Cellular and Molecular Life Sciences*, vol. 61, no. 5, pp. 567–579, 2004.

[47] I. Kryczek, E. Zhao, Y. Liu et al., "Human TH17 cells are long-lived effector memory cells," *Science Translational Medicine*, vol. 3, no. 104, pp. 104–ra100, 2011.

[48] I. M. Stromnes, L. M. Cerretti, D. Liggitt, R. A. Harris, and J. M. Goverman, "Differential regulation of central nervous system autoimmunity by TH1 and TH17 cells," *Nature Medicine*, vol. 14, no. 3, pp. 337–342, 2008.

[49] Y. Hu, F. Shen, N. K. Crellin, and W. Ouyang, "The IL-17 pathway as a major therapeutic target in autoimmune diseases," *Annals of the New York Academy of Sciences*, vol. 1217, no. 1, pp. 60–76, 2011.

[50] F. J. Dumont, "IL-17 cytokine/receptor families: emerging targets for the modulation of inflammatory responses," *Expert Opinion on Therapeutic Patents*, vol. 13, no. 3, pp. 287–303, 2003.

[51] S. Shahrara, S. R. Pickens, A. M. Mandelin II et al., "IL-17-mediated monocyte migration occurs partially through CC chemokine ligand 2/monocyte chemoattractant protein-1 induction," *The Journal of Immunology*, vol. 184, no. 8, pp. 4479–4487, 2010.

[52] P. I. Johansson, A. M. Sørensen, A. Perner et al., "High sCD40L levels early after trauma are associated with enhanced shock, sympathoadrenal activation, tissue and endothelial damage, coagulopathy and mortality," *Journal of Thrombosis and Haemostasis*, vol. 10, no. 2, pp. 207–216, 2012.

[53] H. Kebir, K. Kreymborg, I. Ifergan et al., "Human TH17 lymphocytes promote blood-brain barrier disruption and central nervous system inflammation," *Nature Medicine*, vol. 13, no. 10, pp. 1173–1175, 2007.

[54] A. Reboldi, C. Coisne, D. Baumjohann et al., "C-C chemokine receptor 6-regulated entry of TH-17 cells into the CNS through the choroid plexus is required for the initiation of EAE," *Nature Immunology*, vol. 10, no. 5, pp. 514–523, 2009.

[55] Y. Lee, A. Awasthi, N. Yosef et al., "Induction and molecular signature of pathogenic T_H17 cells," *Nature Immunology*, vol. 13, no. 10, pp. 991–999, 2012.

[56] T. Yamazaki, X. O. Yang, Y. Chung et al., "CCR6 regulates the migration of inflammatory and regulatory T cells," *Journal of Immunology*, vol. 181, no. 12, pp. 8391–8401, 2008.

[57] L. R. Frick, K. Williams, and C. Pittenger, "Microglial dysregulation in psychiatric disease," *Clinical and Developmental Immunology*, vol. 2013, Article ID 608654, 10 pages, 2013.

[58] S. M. Kurian, H. Le-Niculescu, S. D. Patel et al., "Identification of blood biomarkers for psychosis using convergent functional genomics," *Molecular Psychiatry*, vol. 16, no. 1, pp. 37–58, 2011.

[59] M. Nedergaard, B. Ransom, and S. A. Goldman, "New roles for astrocytes: redefining the functional architecture of the brain," *Trends in Neurosciences*, vol. 26, no. 10, pp. 523–530, 2003.

[60] C.-R. Yu, Y. S. Lee, R. M. Mahdi, N. Surendran, and C. E. Egwuagu, "Therapeutic targeting of STAT3 (signal transducers and activators of transcription 3) pathway inhibits experimental autoimmune uveitis," *PLoS ONE*, vol. 7, no. 1, Article ID e29742, 2012.

7

Early Detection and Treatment of Psychosis: The Bern Child and Adolescent Psychiatric Perspective

Frauke Schultze-Lutter and Benno G. Schimmelmann

University Hospital of Child and Adolescent Psychiatry and Psychotherapy, University of Bern, Bolligenstrasse 111, Haus A, 3000 Bern 60, Switzerland

Correspondence should be addressed to Frauke Schultze-Lutter; frauke.schultze-lutter@kjp.unibe.ch

Academic Editor: Jane E. Boydell

Commonly conceptualized as neurodevelopmental disorders of yet poorly understood aetiology, schizophrenia and other nonorganic psychoses remain one of the most debilitating illnesses with often poor outcome despite all progress in treatment of the manifest disorder. Drawing on the frequent poor outcome of psychosis and its association with the frequently extended periods of untreated first-episode psychosis (FEP) including its prodrome, an early detection and treatment of both the FEP and the preceding at-risk mental state (ARMS) have been increasingly studied. Thereby both approaches are confronted with different problems, for example, treatment engagement in FEP and predictive accuracy in ARMS. They share, however, the problems related to the lack of understanding of developmental, that is, age-related, peculiarities and of the presentation and natural course of their cardinal symptoms in the community. Most research on early detection and intervention in FEP and ARMS is still related to clinical psychiatric samples, and little is known about symptom presentation and burden and help-seeking in the general population related to these experiences. Furthermore, in particular in the early detection of an ARMS, studies often address adolescents and young adults alike without consideration of developmental characteristics, thereby applying risk criteria that have been developed predominately in adults. Combining our earlier experiences described in this paper in child and adolescent, and general psychiatry as well as in both lines of research, that is, on early psychosis and its treatment and on the early detection of psychosis, in particular in its very early states by subjective disturbances in terms of basic symptoms, age-related developmental and epidemiological aspects have therefore been made the focus of our current studies in Bern, thus making our line of research unique.

1. Introduction

Schizophrenia and other nonorganic psychoses remain one of the most debilitating illnesses [1, 2], despite all the progress in treatment that has been made since the introduction of antipsychotics in the 1960s. Though generally conceptualized as a neurodevelopmental disorder, their aetiology is still only poorly understood. Psychotic disorders have a life-time prevalence of approximately 3.5% [3] and a 12-month incidence rate of about 0.035% [4]. They usually first strike early in life, between the ages of 20 and 25 [4, 5]; approximately 10–15% are early-onset psychoses (EOP) manifesting themselves before the age of 18, and approximately 1–3% are very-early-onset psychoses (VEOP) with an onset before the age of 13 [6]. Despite their relatively low prevalence, psychoses are

one of the top-ten diseases with regard to disability-adjusted life years (DALYs) [7–9]. Furthermore, the immense indirect costs of these disorders, for example, caused by early and lasting loss of productivity on the part of both patients and their carers, make them one of the most costly disorders for society [8, 9].

The high societal and personal cost are driven in part by the poor course that psychoses tend to take after their initial manifestation. A poor course however is, among others, a consequence of the frequently long duration of unrecognized and untreated psychosis (DUP) and illness, including the prodrome (DUI) [10–13] even in persons seeking help early [14, 15]. An extended prodrome of more than three years precedes the majority of first-episode psychoses (FEP) [13, 16, 17]; however, the gradual progression characteristic of

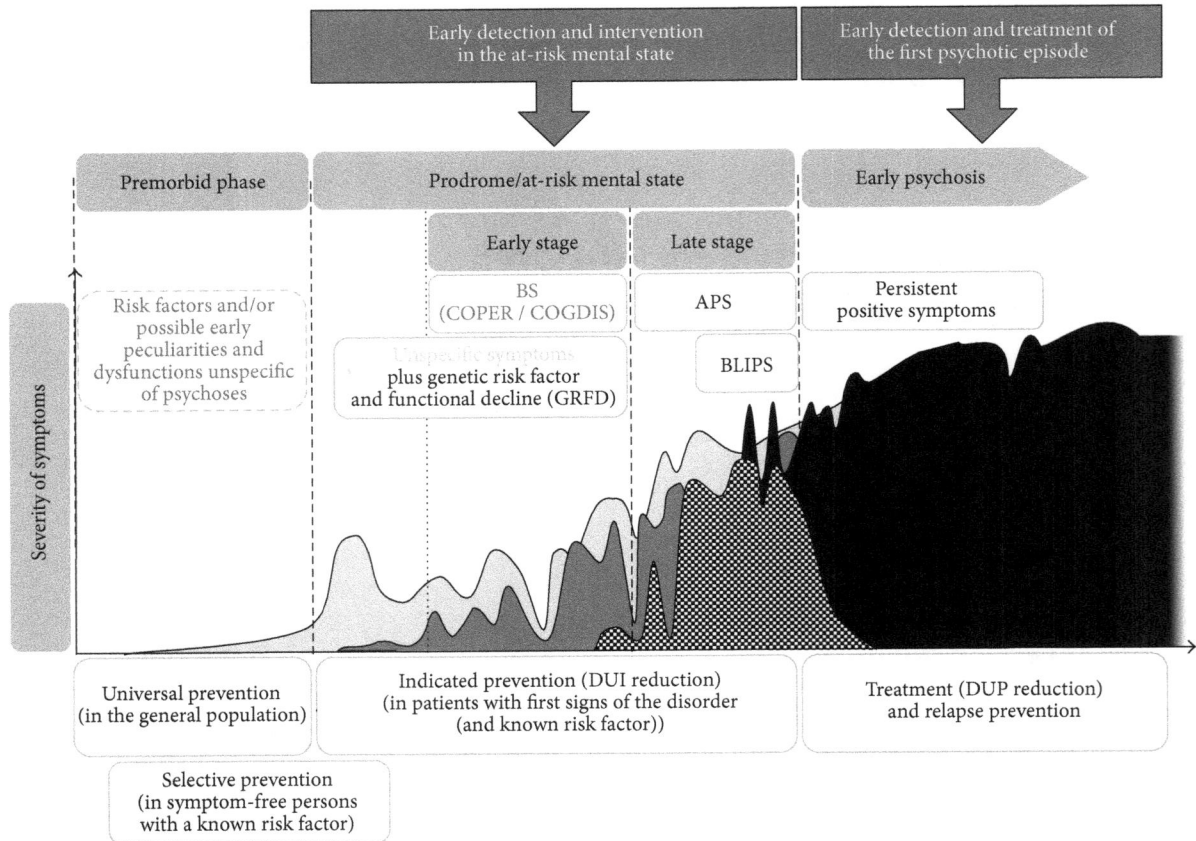

FIGURE 1: Hypothetical early course of psychosis in relation to primary and secondary preventive approaches (according to [164]). Annotations: BS: basic symptoms; COPER: cognitive-perceptive basic symptoms; COGDIS: cognitive disturbances; APS: attenuated psychotic symptoms; BLIPS: brief limited intermittent psychotic symptoms; DUP: duration of untreated psychosis; DUI: duration of untreated illness.

psychoses impedes the identification of a disorder by patients and healthcare professionals. Thus, since the 1990s, efforts have increasingly focused on detecting and treating FEP early, preferably, in terms of indicated prevention, while the patient is still within the prodromal state and before the onset of persisting positive psychotic symptoms (Figure 1) [18–20].

As an example of these efforts, the present outlook paper will summarize the research conducted by the two authors, both being experts in this area of research, and their perspectives on it and conclude with an outlook on future questions that will have to be addressed.

2. The First Episode of Psychoses

2.1. The Melbourne Early Psychosis Prevention and Intervention Centre (EPPIC). The Early Psychosis Prevention and Intervention Centre (EPPIC) in Melbourne has been one of the first programmes with a mandate to detect and treat all patients with FEP of both early and young adult onset (mid-teens to midtwenties) [21]. Gradually developing between 1984 and 1992, EPPIC services a sector with a population of about 800,000 people. Working within a national mental health system, it receives all referrals with suspicion of a FEP. Thus, its database provides a unique and, in terms of sampling, unbiased opportunity to analyse the characteristics

and treatment outcomes of all types of FEP [22–30] and has a special focus on bipolar psychoses [23, 31, 32]. Such detailed knowledge is important for identifying obstacles to care and for detecting starting-points for early detection and intervention in FEP and has therefore been in the special focus of the work of Benno Schimmelmann.

2.1.1. The Early Course of First-Episode Psychosis. One important finding of the EPPIC data was that diagnostic stability over 18 months is high for first episodes of schizophrenic psychoses with few shifts from schizophrenia to other diagnoses. On the other hand, patients with a FEP diagnosis of schizophreniform or bipolar disorder were diagnostically unstable, with frequent shifts to other psychotic disorders, mainly schizophrenia, necessitating longitudinal reassessment of their diagnoses [33]. Thus, after their first episode, most psychoses had a poor outcome within the first 18 months with the frequency of the diagnosis of its most severe type, schizophrenia, increasing. Thereby, persistent substance use over the treatment period but not baseline substance use was associated with nonremission of psychotic symptoms after 18 months, even after controlling for many relevant predictors of outcome [34]. Similarly, persistent cannabis use but not cannabis use at baseline was a significant predictor of worse outcome in early-onset psychosis [35]. Additionally cannabis use disorders starting before age 14 seem to predict an earlier onset of psychosis [36]; an earlier onset, in turn, had been associated with a poorer outcome [16]. Thus, substance and in particular cannabis use seem to have differential and age-related effects on the course of psychosis: accelerating the onset of psychosis in young psychosis-prone adolescents and corrupting the outcome of FEP in general, that is, across all age groups.

2.1.2. Treatment Compliance in First-Episode Psychosis. Adherence to treatment and medication is a significant problem in early psychosis. In the FEP cohort of EPPIC (N = 661), 19% never took the prescribed medication and 23% disengaged from the program despite significant efforts to keep patients engaged in treatment (such as assertive community treatment, specific crisis teams, and highly specialized case managers). Predictors of service disengagement and medication nonadherence or refusal were persistent substance use over the treatment period, a forensic history, and lack of family support [37, 38]. Those consistently refusing all medications from the outset were more likely to have a forensic history compared to those who became nonadherent later on [38]. Service disengagement was further predicted by moderate illness severity and a lack of significant treatment success until disengagement from both the entire sample and the adolescent subsample [37, 39].

2.1.3. Early-Onset and Adult Onset Psychosis. With regard to developmental peculiarities, the EPPIC cohort has provided a unique opportunity to assess differences between EOP and young adult onset psychosis (AOP; starting between ages 18 and 28). Due to EPPIC's focus on a young age range, about 19% of the sample was EOP patients (onset between 8.2 and 17.9 years). Compared to AOP patients, EOP had a slightly lower premorbid functioning and considerably longer duration of untreated psychosis (median 26.3 weeks in EOP compared to 8.7 weeks in AOP). Notably, the significantly longer DUP in EOP accounted for their worse course after controlling for type of psychosis, level of premorbid functioning, family support, and psychiatric history. No significant outcome differences including illness severity, global functioning, remission of positive symptoms, or employment status were detected between EOP and AOP [40, 41]. Hence the negative effects of DUI and DUP may be exacerbated in EOP. The treatment delay observed in EOP may be due to several factors, including the more pronounced neurodevelopmental and cognitive deficits, the insidious onset of less pronounced positive symptoms, and/or the atypical clinical picture of the beginning EOP—potentially misinterpreted as "adolescent crisis" [40]. Furthermore, as the age of onset of symptoms seems to be earlier in adolescent cannabis users [42], early symptoms might also be mistaken as substance-induced. Thus, early detection and treatment of persons with the first signs of the disorder, which is currently regarded as a promising strategy in fighting the consequences of psychosis, may face different or additional challenges in EOP as compared to AOP.

2.2. The Hamburg Psychosis Early Detection and Intervention Project (PEDIC). Based on the EPPIC experience, the Psychosis Early Detection and Intervention Project (PEDIC) was implemented in Hamburg in 2003. One early research focus of PEDIC was on remission and recovery of symptoms, functioning, and subjective well-being in adults with FEP [43–45].

2.2.1. Remission and Recovery in First-Episode Schizophrenia. In a 3-year follow-up study of 392 never-treated patients with schizophrenia cared for within PEDIC, remission rates were 60% for symptoms, 45% for functional deficits, and 57% for subjective well-being; corresponding recovery rates were 52%, 35%, and 44%; 28% were in combined remission and 17% in combined recovery (fulfilling all remission or recovery criteria, resp.). Studies examining predictors of remission and functional outcome have shown that premorbid and baseline psychosocial functioning and good treatment response with symptom remission within the first 3 months are the best predictors of both [45–51]. These findings have important clinical implications whereby the low proportion of patients who met remission or recovery criteria clearly highlights the importance of making adaptations to treatment early on [45]. Furthermore, our studies suggested that measures of quality of life and subjective well-being should be assessed when measuring the outcome of psychotic disorders [52–54]. The patient's perspective and experience might be particularly important when it comes to assessment of the side effects of antipsychotics. Because objective and subjective side effects often differ and subjective impairment may be a stronger predictor of nonadherence than objective measures of the severity of side effects, assessing both objective and subjective side effects has been strongly recommended [54].

2.2.2. Assertive Community Treatment in Schizophrenia-Spectrum Disorders: The Access Trial. Despite all of the knowledge gained about moderators of outcome in FEP, a crucial, yet unresolved, question is how patients with psychotic disorders are optimally treated. In Hamburg, we constructed a comprehensive treatment model for patients with both first- and multiple-episode schizophrenia-spectrum disorders, the ACCESS model, which included assertive community treatment, specialized personnel, integration of specific treatment options for psychotic patients such as cognitive-behavioural psychotherapy, metacognitive training, and a general psychotherapeutic approach including techniques of open dialogue [55–57]. At 12 months, patients treated in the ACCESS program had better outcomes than those treated as usual in an integrated care setting without assertive community treatment, case management, or specialized personnel in terms of service engagement, symptoms, functioning, quality of life, and satisfaction with care. The additional treatment effect of the ACCESS program was clearly significant, and the costs of ACCESS were similar to treatment as usual; therefore inpatient days were significantly decreased while outpatient contacts were increased [58, 59]. ACCESS was then translated into clinical practice and extended to bipolar psychotic disorders. The benefits of the ACCESS treatment model, particularly in terms of high service engagement and low hospitalization rates, remained stable over a 2-year period [60], yet their longer-term effects remain to be studied.

2.3. Getting There Even Earlier: Lessons from First-Episode Psychosis Research. Despite a broad range of efforts to improve the outcome of FEP but also of multiepisode psychosis, many patients continue to suffer from symptoms as well as poor functioning and quality of life. Thus, not only is the early identification of patients with manifest psychotic disorders important in order to reduce the DUP [41], but also the early detection of at-risk mental states (ARMS) is mandatory for the reduction of DUI and the burden of psychotic disorders in both adults [61] and children and adolescents [62–65].

3. The At-Risk Mental State

Since Kraepelin's description of dementia praecox more than a century ago [66], diagnosis, treatment, and studies of psychosis have focused mainly on its cardinal positive and negative symptoms. In the last two decades, however, the growing interest in prodromal or risk states of the illness has generated renewed interest in the early subclinical expressions and subtle, self-experienced changes in mentation that had already been observed by Kraepelin [66, 67].

Until the 1980s, scattered and mainly retrospective reports of the psychotic prodrome prevailed that led to the formulation of early developmental models of schizophrenia such as Conrad's [68] and Docherty's [69] staging models, both assuming a unidirectional mandatory pattern of symptom manifestation. These invariant models, however, could not be confirmed by retrospective data on the early course assessed on FEP patients in the Age, Beginning, Course (ABC) study [16, 70], suggesting that the road to psychosis might not be a straight one but rather twisted with stops and returns being possible at any stage [71, 72]. Thus, not knowing where the road is leading when looking at it prospectively, there is common agreement in prospective research nowadays not to use the retrospectively defined term "prodrome" that would indicate that a certain outcome is inevitable but to emphasise the risk along with the only more or less probable outcome. To this end, several terms have been proposed that are often used and considered interchangeable, even if they originally related to distinct concepts or assessments. This fact has unfortunately created Babylonian speech confusion as well as heterogeneity and variance of findings [73, 74]. In the following, the term "at-risk mental state" (ARMS) that is not linked to a specific operationalization or assessment is used when prospectively relating to a state which may be the prodrome of a FEP.

3.1. Symptomatic Risk Criteria for First-Episode Psychosis. For the indicated prevention of psychosis in help-seeking persons already suffering from first signs and symptoms of the emerging disorder, two approaches were developed in parallel [75]. Both approaches distinguish between affective and nonaffective psychotic disorders and nonpsychotic affective disorders [76, 77]: the basic symptom (BS) approach

targeting the earliest possible specific risk symptoms by our Cologne group and the ultrahigh risk (UHR) approach targeting an imminent risk of psychosis with a conversion within the next 12 months by the Melbourne and New Haven groups of Patrick McGorry and Thomas McGlashan (Figure 1).

3.1.1. Basic Symptom Criteria

(1) The Basic Symptom Concept. Relating to early descriptions of prodromal changes by Mayer-Gross [78], the most thorough early description of subtle early symptoms has been provided within the framework of the BS concept [20, 71, 79]. BS are subtle, subjectively experienced subclinical disturbances in drive, stress tolerance, affect, thinking, speech, attention, body and sensory perception, and motor action [71]. These subjective symptoms were regarded as the earliest perceivable signs of the developing psychotic disorder and its neurobiological correlates—hence the term "basic" [20]. Although BS vary in their specificity for psychoses and can occur in nonpsychotic disorders to various degrees [76, 80, 81], they are recognized nowadays mainly for their occurrence in initial prodromal states of psychoses including potential outpost syndromes (i.e., spontaneously remitting "prodrome-like" phases preceding the prodrome leading to frank psychosis; Figure 2). Yet, they are not restricted to the early states but are an integral part of the disorder and can occur in all states [80–82], that is, within the prodrome of FEP, within prodromal states of relapse, within residual states, and even within acute psychotic episodes; consequently, the assessment of BS can serve several clinical and scientific purposes (Figure 2).

By definition, BS are not evoked by substance misuse or somatic illness and differ from what is considered to be one's "normal" mental self [71]. Being subjective, they remain predominately private and apparent only to the affected person and are rarely directly observable to others but might be indirectly observed by a patient's self-initiated coping strategies in response to BS such as social withdrawal or other avoidance strategies. It is this emphasis on the subjective, self-experienced character that distinguishes BS from (i) negative symptoms in terms of functional deficits observable to others and (ii) frank psychotic symptoms which are experienced by the patient as real and normal thoughts and feelings. The ability to experience BS with insight, however, often attenuates with progressive illness and emerging (attenuated) psychotic symptoms but is commonly restored upon remission [71].

(2) Assessment Instruments of Basic Symptoms. Two instruments for the binary assessment of presence or absence of BS were initially developed in concerted action [83]: a semistructured clinical interview, the Bonn Scale for the Assessment of Basic Symptoms (BSABS) [84, 85], and a self-report questionnaire, the Frankfurt Complaint Questionnaire (FCQ) [86]. Nevertheless, the correspondence between BSABS and FCQ subscales was poor, indicating that the mode of assessment is a crucial factor in the evaluation of BS [67, 87].

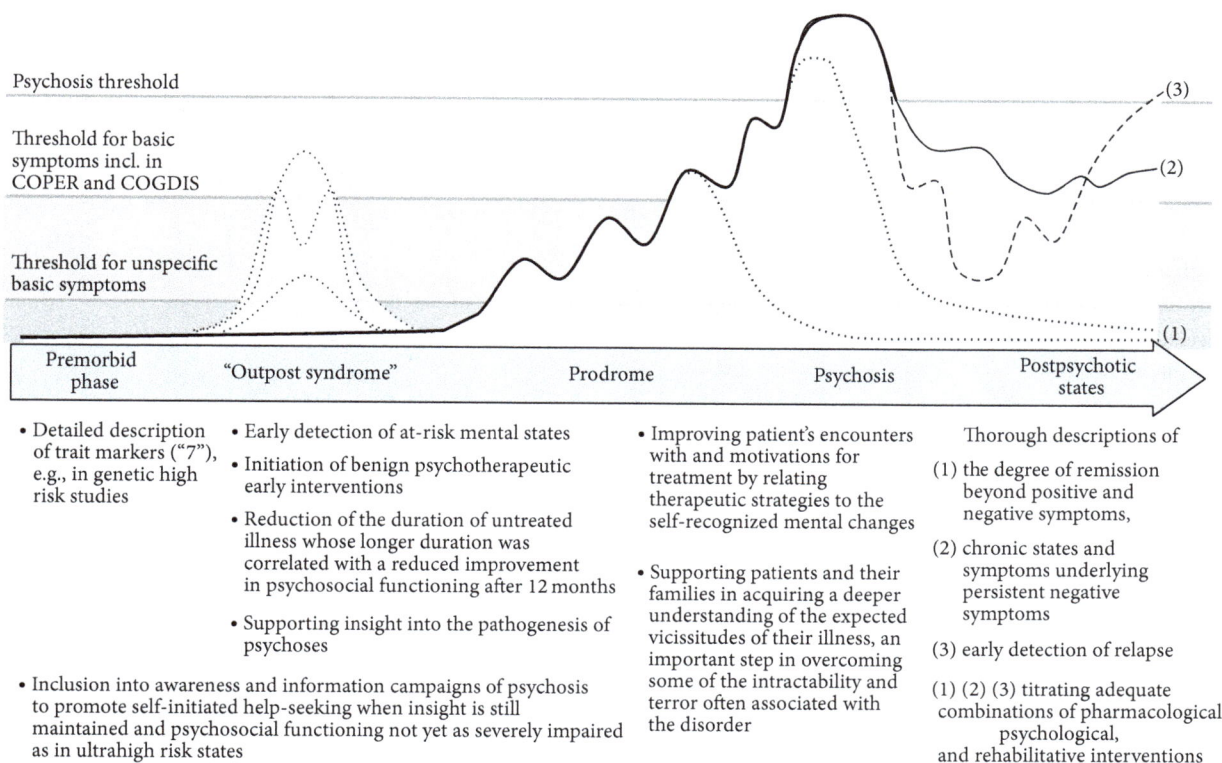

FIGURE 2: Range of possible applications of basic symptom assessment (according to [71, 91]). Annotation: ("7"): SPI-A/SPI-CY rating for basic symptom-like phenomena that are reported as having always been present in the current frequency in a trait-like manner.

Based on the BSABS, we developed an instrument for the quantitative clinical assessment of BS [67, 88], that is, the Schizophrenia Proneness Instrument, in two versions, that is, an Adult (SPI-A; [89]) and a Child and Youth version (SPI-CY; [90, 91]). With regard to the development of the SPI-A, the six BS dimensions in adult samples exhibited a robust structure across samples in different stages of the illness [88]. This structure even remained largely unchanged when BS assessment turned from the binary assessment of presence in the BSABS to an ordinal assessment of frequency-guided severity in the SPI-A. Yet, the structure could not be replicated in a sample of patients with nonpsychotic depressive disorders. Thus, it was concluded that these dimensions might be inherent and unique to schizophrenia and other psychoses and, therefore, can serve as valid and reliable subscales of an instrument for the assessment of BS [88]. Building on this, the final version of the SPI-A was developed after validation on a second prospectively assessed truly prodromal sample [67, 89]. The SPI-A has shown good interrater reliability with an increase of the overall concordance rate with an expert rating from 60% to 89% across five training sessions [67, 89].

Though very consistent in adult samples, the six-dimensional structure of BS was absent in an EOP sample [62, 67]. Rather, a four-dimensional structure was revealed that formed the basis for the subscales of the SPI-CY—thus far the only early detection instrument especially designed for use in children and adolescents aged 8 and older [62, 67, 91].

A striking structural difference between the SPI-A and SPI-CY was that adynamic BS (e.g., lack of energy, motivation, drive, or (positive) feelings including sudden depressive mood, decreased stress tolerance, increased emotional responsiveness, and general cognitive impediments such as concentration, memory, and attention problems or reports of a "blank mind") appeared to play a central role in children and adolescents; this central position was held in adults by mainly cognitive BS, including those included in BS risk criteria described below [67]. The discriminative validity of the SPI-CY was preliminarily confirmed on three groups of children and adolescents: risk patients meeting UHR and/or BS criteria (AtRisk), clinical inpatient controls not suspected to be at risk for developing psychosis (ClinS), and children and adolescents from the general population (GPS) [92]. As expected, the groups differed significantly on all four SPI-CY subscales with the AtRisk sample scoring highest and the GPS lowest and at least moderate between-group effects that were largest for the subscale "Adynamia." However, these results require validation in a larger sample, and longitudinal studies should examine the psychosis-predictive ability of the subscales in different young age groups, especially the role of Adynamia. In cooperation with the Cologne and Zurich University Hospitals for Child and Adolescent Psychiatry, we are currently addressing these questions in a prospective study, the Binational Evaluation of At-Risk Symptoms in Children and Adolescents (BEARS-Kid) study,

TABLE 1: At-risk criterion cognitive-perceptive basic symptoms (COPER) [89, 97].

Presence of at least any one of the following ten basic symptoms with at least weekly occurrence (i.e., a SPI-A/SPI-CY score of ≥3) within the last three months *and* first occurrence at least 12 months ago (irrespective of frequency and persistence during this time):

(i) thought interference (C2)[a]

(ii) thought perseveration (O1)

(iii) thought pressure (D3)

(iv) thought blockages (C3)

(v) disturbance of receptive speech (C4)

(vi) decreased ability to discriminate between ideas and perception, fantasy and true memories (O2)

(vii) unstable ideas of reference (D4)

(viii) derealisation (O8)

(ix) visual perception disturbances, excl. blurred vision and hypersensitivity to light (D5, F2, F3, and O4)

(x) acoustic perception disturbances, excl. hypersensitivity to sounds (F5, O5)

[a] Item numbers refer to the SPI-A.

TABLE 2: High risk criterion cognitive disturbances (COGDIS) [89, 97].

Presence of at least any two of the following nine basic symptoms with at least weekly occurrence (i.e., a SPI-A/SPI-CY score of ≥3) within the last three months:

(i) inability to divide attention (B1)[a]

(ii) thought interference (C2)

(iii) thought pressure (D3)

(iv) thought blockages (C3)

(v) disturbance of receptive speech (C4)

(vi) disturbance of expressive speech (C5)

(vii) unstable ideas of reference (D4)

(viii) disturbances of abstract thinking (O3)

(ix) captivation of attention by details of the visual field (O7)

[a] Item numbers refer to the SPI-A.

which is funded by a common grant of the Swiss National Science Foundation and the German Research Foundation and examines four groups of altogether 800 children and adolescents (e.g., patients meeting ARMS criteria, inpatients with no clinical suspicion of an ARMS, patients with an EOP, and children and adolescents of the general population) for three years [http://p3.snf.ch/project-144100].

(3) The Basic Symptom Criteria for an At-Risk Mental State. The Cologne Early Recognition (CER) study [67, 85, 93–95] was the first ever long-term naturalistic prospective early detection study with a mean follow-up period of 9.6 years and investigated the psychosis-predictive accuracy of BS assessed with the BSABS in 160 adult patients clinically suspected to be at risk for schizophrenia. Based on different types of analyses, two BS criteria that share some of the included BS were developed from its data [67, 85, 93–95]: "cognitive-perceptive basic symptoms" (COPER; Table 1) and "cognitive disturbances" (COGDIS; Table 2).

Compared to COPER, COGDIS seem to have a higher specificity, that is, are associated with higher conversion rates (Table 3), yet this might be at the cost of sensitivity, that is, related to missing more patients who are in fact about to develop a FEP [67]. In other words, COGDIS performed better in ruling in conversion to psychosis (moderate positive diagnostic likelihood ratio of 3.9), while COPER performed better in ruling it out (moderate negative diagnostic likelihood ratio of 0.23) [93, 96]. Thus, in terms of a clinical staging, these BS criteria were thought to be possibly able to serve different clinical purposes in adult samples, that is, broad risk detection and symptom monitoring based on COPER versus risk detection with the intention to initiate specific psychosis-preventive treatment by COGDIS [93].

Subsequent studies by our group [97–100] and others [101, 102] confirmed the psychosis-predictive ability of both COPER and COGDIS, although conversion rates were somewhat lower at comparable follow-ups (Table 3). This decline might be caused by conservatively accounting for drop-outs as nonconverters [97–100], exclusion of symptomatic UHR criteria [98], age-related peculiarities [102], or other factors related to changes in referral and treatment practice that had been discussed in relation to the much more severe decline in conversion rates observed in UHR samples [103]. In addition, differences in conversion rates might also be related to differences in the BS composition of samples. Analyses of converters of the CER study with different duration of the prodrome defined as short (<1 year), medium (1–6 years), and long (>6 years) revealed group differences particularly in

TABLE 3: Conversion rates for COPER and COGDIS in (sub)samples not systematically treated for psychosis-risk.

Study	BS criterion, N (N criterion positive), predominant age group, n (%) lost-to-last-follow-up of total sample	Conversion rate at month				
		12	18	24	36	>36
[93, 95]	COPER, 160 (106), adults, n.a.	20%		37%	50%	65%[c]
	COGDIS, 160 (67), adults, n.a.	24%		46%	61%	79%[c]
[97]	COPER, 146 (146), adults, 60 (41%)[b]	25%		33%		
	COGDIS, 146 (124), adults, 60 (41%)[b]	25%		33%		
[98][a]	COPER, 128 (64), adults, 23 (36%)[b]	17%		20%		
[99, 114]	COGDIS, 245 (171), adults, 62 (25%)[b]	14%	19%			
[101]	COGDIS, 73 (48), adults, n.a.			25%		
[102]	COGDIS, 72 (39), adolescents, 15 (21%)[b]			18%		
[100]	COGDIS, 246 (158), adults, 56 (23%)[b]	23%		34%	40%	42%[d]

[a]Supportive counselling control condition only; conversion rate includes conversion to a late state, that is, development of APS or BLIPS.
[b]Those lost-to-follow-up were conservatively regarded as nonconverters, symptomatic UHR criteria excluded.
[c]Minimum of 60 months, maximum of 359 months.
[d]Months 36 to 48.
n.a.: not applicable; only patients with complete follow-up data were included.

cognitive BS constellations that could be interpreted in terms of differences in underlying deficits in information processes, that is, in bottom-up, top-down, or central integrative processes [104]. Because of the current lack of sufficiently long follow-up data, these etiological considerations still await confirmation in independent samples as well as examination in neurocognitive studies.

3.1.2. Combining Basic Symptom and Ultrahigh Risk Criteria. Initially developed independently of each other, BS and UHR criteria (Table 4) frequently cooccur and are increasingly applied together—first within our Cologne Early Recognition and Intervention Centre (FETZ), Europe's pioneer early detection service for adults in an ARMS [97, 100, 105, 106]. A combined approach was adopted and first operationalized within the German Research Network on Schizophrenia (GRNS) [107] as a clinical staging model [108, 109] distinguishing an early from a late risk state [110] (Figure 1): an early risk state was alternatively defined by COPER and the UHR state-trait criterion, and a late risk state was alternatively defined by attenuated psychotic symptoms (APS) and brief limited intermittent psychotic symptoms (BLIPS).

The sequence by which symptoms progress according to the clinical staging model for ARMS [107–111]—from unspecific mental problems via first BS of COPER and second APS to psychotic symptoms (Figure 1)—was supported on retrospective data of FEP inpatients [17]. Furthermore, both approaches exhibited good sensitivity in this sample: 79% of the sample reported COPER and 71% APS, whereby 63% reported both APS and COPER [17]. A rather large but not complete overlap between BS and UHR criteria was also apparent in other ARMS studies [97, 99–102, 105].

Moreover, the highest 18-month and 48-month conversion rates showed for the combination of COGDIS and UHR criteria (mainly APS) compared to either COGDIS or UHR criteria alone [67, 99, 100]. For example, within a 48-month follow-up [100], COPER and UHR criteria exclusive of each other revealed hazard rates of 0.23 and 0.28. In line with the GRNS staging model, in the "only UHR" group, conversions occurred between months 1 and 8, while in the "only COGDIS" group, conversions occurred after month 5 but continued throughout the follow-up thereafter. The combined group "COGDIS plus UHR" showed conversions throughout the 48 months at a hazard rate of 0.66. Notably, irrespective of each other both COGDIS and UHR showed an equal but lower hazard rate of 0.56 [100].

These findings support the merits of considering both COGDIS and UHR criteria in the early detection of persons who are at high clinical risk of developing a FEP; the combination with COPER has not yet been explicitly studied. Applying both sets of criteria improves the sensitivity of risk detection and the individual risk estimation; it may thereby support the development of stage-targeted interventions. Moreover, since the combination of COGDIS and UHR criteria enables the identification of considerably more homogeneous ARMS samples, it should support both preventive and basic research [100]. However, for the still considerable number of false-positive predictions, potential additional predictors enhancing the overall predictive accuracy—ideally without simultaneously reducing sensitivity—continue to be studied at all levels.

3.2. Searching for Additional Predictors to Enhance Predictive Accuracy. Across early detection studies, the addition of predictors frequently raised specificity at the cost of sensitivity, that is, frequently leading to a higher rate of exclusion of truly prodromal patients from preventive measures [112]. A possible solution to this dilemma, well-established in somatic medicine, is risk stratification [112, 113]. Risk stratification was first introduced in psychiatric prevention research within the European Prediction of Psychosis Study (EPOS) [99, 114], which used COGDIS and UHR criteria as assessed with the Structured Interview for Psychosis-Risk Syndromes (SIPS; [115]) to detect mainly adult ARMS patients. Examining additional psychopathological predictors, four risk classes for the 18-month conversion risk were identified based on a prognostic index calculated from APS severity, sleep disturbances, schizotypal personality disorder, and functioning and educational level [28]. Notably, the highest risk class contained a much higher percentage (83%) of persons reporting both

TABLE 4: Ultrahigh risk criteria according to the Structured Interview for Psychosis-Risk Syndromes (SIPS) [115].

"Brief limited intermittent psychotic symptom" (BLIPS) syndrome
(i) At least any 1 of the following SIPS P-items scored 6 "severe and psychotic":
(a) P1 unusual thought content/delusional ideas[a]
(b) P2 suspiciousness/persecutory ideas
(c) P3 grandiose ideas
(d) P4 perceptual abnormalities/hallucinations
(e) P5 disorganized communication
(ii) First appearance in the past three months
(iii) Present for at least several minutes per day at a frequency of at least once per month but less than 7 days
"Attenuated psychotic symptom" (APS) syndrome[b]
(i) At least any 1 of the following SIPS P-items scored 3 "moderate" to 5 "severe but not psychotic":
(a) P1 unusual thought content/delusional ideas
(b) P2 suspiciousness/persecutory ideas
(c) P3 grandiose ideas
(d) P4 perceptual abnormalities/hallucinations
(e) P5 disorganized communication
(ii) First appearance within the past year or current rating one or more scale points higher compared to 12 months ago
(iii) Symptoms have occurred at an average frequency of at least once per week in the past month
"Genetic risk and functional deterioration" (GRFD) syndrome
(1) Patient meets criteria for schizotypal personality disorder according to SIPS
(2) Patient has 1st degree relative with a psychotic disorder
(3) Patient has experienced at least 30% drop in the global assessment of functioning (GAF) score over the last month compared to 12 months ago
[1 and 3] or [2 and 3] or all are met

[a] Item numbers refer to the SIPS.
[b] In the definition of the Attenuated Psychosis Syndrome of DSM-5, requirements (i) to (iii) are complimented a fourth requirement; that is, significant disability or distress is caused by APS.

COGDIS and UHR criteria than all other risk classes (55–57%).

Other possible psychopathological predictors in adult samples were bipolar, somatoform, and unipolar depressive disorders at baseline, while anxiety disorders at baseline were negatively associated with conversion [116], the Strauss and Carpenter Prognostic Scale items assessing quality of useful work and social relations, positive symptoms and subjective distress [117], presence of ideas of reference and lack of close interpersonal relations as assessed with the Schizotypal Personality Questionnaire [118], and schizoid personality traits but neither schizotypal personality traits [119] nor dimensions of normal personality [120]. Together, these results point to an important role of functional deficits, especially in social contexts, high emotional responsiveness, and severity and persistence of APS in the development of psychosis in adult ARMS patients.

Another line of research on predictors has focussed on deficits in information processing that are common in FEP and have also been observed in ARMS patients, albeit to a lesser degree [121–124]. Objectively assessed neurocognitive deficits were widely independent of the subjectively reported cognitive disturbances included in COPER and COGDIS, thus offering the possibility to explain additional variance between ARMS patients who do or do not convert to psychosis [125]. Conversion was repeatedly related to processing speed deficits and lower premorbid verbal IQ, while results on the additional value of verbal memory deficits were conflicting [126, 127].

Similar to neurocognitive deficits, also electrophysiological abnormalities have been reported in both psychosis and adult ARMS patients with only slight differences [128, 129]. Abnormalities in mismatch negativity and quantitative EEG parameters have been associated with conversion [130, 131]. Another line of research, which evaluated biochemical abnormalities as potentially valuable predictors, found that anandamidergic upregulation might be a protector against conversion in ARMS patients [132, 133].

As many of these results have been generated independently of one another, future research should use large samples to ensure a sufficient number of converters so that simultaneous analyses of potential predictors and their interactions can be performed. In this way, nonredundant predictors that are most useful for a risk stratification of ARMS patients can be identified. Furthermore, while some of the potential predictors such as functional deficits, greater symptom severity, abnormalities in mismatch negativity, and processing speed deficits have already been replicated by other work groups (see [75] for overview), other results such as the protective role of an anandamidergic upregulation are still in need for replication in independent samples. And last but not least, all potential predictors still need to be studied for developmental differences in children and adolescent samples.

3.3. Clinical Significance of the At-Risk Mental State. ARMS patients, however, not only are at risk for future psychosis but also are already suffering from a wide range of mental problems. In addition to the neurocognitive and electrophysiological abnormalities described above, they exhibit poor premorbid adjustment and deficits in psychosocial functioning and subjective quality of life that tend to worsen from the early to the late risk state [134–137]. Notably, a considerable number experience improvement in psychosocial outcome following the detection of an ARMS [138]. Furthermore, many ARMS patients suffer from other nonpsychotic mental disorders, frequently depression and anxiety [105, 116, 139]. Thus it was not surprising that the pattern of coping, self-efficacy, and control beliefs of ARMS patients closely resembled that of depressive patients in its frequent lack of positive coping strategies, low self-efficacy, and a fatalistic externalizing bias [140].

As we and others [75, 141] have shown that help-seeking ARMS samples are clinically significant, in 2008, we raised the question of whether current early detection approaches really target the "prodrome" of psychosis or rather a psychosis-spectrum disorder with a high risk for psychotic symptoms as one of the key questions in early detection research [142]. This issue became widely discussed a year later with the suggestion of including a psychosis-risk syndrome based on APS in DSM-5 [143]. In line with our rationale for a self-contained disorder [112, 144], this proposal was later revised to an APS-based self-contained disorder, the Attenuated Psychosis Syndrome [145]. As such, it was finally included in Section III of DSM-5 as a condition for future studies [146, 147]. Besides questions related to reliability, this decision was made for the unknown prevalence and clinical significance of such a syndrome outside help-seeking samples in the community [147].

3.4. Risk Criteria and Symptoms in the Community. The clinical significance of risk symptoms, in particular APS, outside help-seeking samples in the community had been called into question by the high prevalence rates reported for subclinical psychotic symptoms or psychotic-like experiences (PLEs) in the community. PLEs, however, have commonly been assessed by self-report questionnaires or layperson fully structured interviews and thus provide no valid measure of clinician-assessed APS or psychotic symptoms but significantly overestimate their prevalence [148]. Thus it was concluded that dedicated studies are warranted, in which APS—and other risk criteria—are assessed in a way that equates to their clinical evaluation. Supported by a grant from the Swiss National Science Foundation and following confirmation of the reliability of telephone assessments of risk symptoms [149], we started such a study, the Bern Epidemiological At-Risk (BEAR) study, in 2011 (http://p3.snf.ch/project-135381). Both an interim analysis of the BEAR study and results from a proof-of-concept study [150, 151]confirmed our expectation that APS criteria and Attenuated Psychosis Syndrome are infrequent: they were met by less than 0.5% of the 1229 mainly adult interviewees that entered the interim analyses of the BEAR study. At symptom level, APS were reported by 13% of the sample and, indicating a clinical significance of APS in the

community, were associated with functional impairments, current mental disorders, and help-seeking although they were not a reason for help-seeking [150]. Future analyses of the full sample of 16–40-year-olds after conclusion of the BEAR study in July 2014 will show if these results are maintained in a larger sample, while comparison with data with the 8–17-year-old community sample of the BEARS-Kid study will help to identify age-related peculiarities that were suggested by Kelleher et al. in their adolescent samples [152]. Furthermore, the aspired follow-up of the BEAR sample will reveal the course and impact of risk symptoms and criteria over time.

As regards BS criteria, COPER and COGDIS and their included BS were as equally rare as APS in the small proof-of-concept study [151], though further confirmation is needed from the larger sample queried in the BEAR study [150]. Furthermore, irrespective of their frequency, any one COPER-BS and any two COGDIS-BS were reported by only 8% and 3% of adolescents in the general population [153].

4. Conclusion and Outlook

For the lack of a significant breakthrough in the treatment of psychotic disorders after the onset of the first episode and due to the negative impact of the frequent and often years-long delays in the initiation of an adequate treatment on outcome, hopes are that indicated prevention of psychotic disorders in persons with first signs of the developing disorder will provide such a breakthrough [61, 75, 109, 154, 155]. To this end, an accurate and reliable early detection, that is, the development of exact, broadly applicable, and economic risk criteria, is a prerequisite.

Thus, the accuracy of prediction along with the safety of treatment has been in the main focus of critics and of, sometimes heated, ethical debates [156]. While further research is certainly needed, it is confronted with a dilemma of preventive research: with the growing awareness of the need for treatment in help-seeking ARMS patients and, consequently, its provision, the observation of the long-term natural course of potential risk symptoms that is necessary to develop accurate prediction models is increasingly impossible in clinical samples. The consideration of treatment effects as confounders in prediction analyses however not only raises the need for ever larger samples but also is hindered by the lack of knowledge about their long-term effectiveness [157, 158]. Yet a recent review reported a rather robust overall risk reduction across ten pharmacological and psychological early intervention studies at 12 months of 54% with a number-needed-to-treat of nine [159]. For this reason, *longitudinal epidemiological studies* that reliably and validly assess clinical risk criteria and symptoms in the general population become increasingly important, such as our BEAR study, the first epidemiological study on a large random representative sample of a broad age range and with a sufficient response rate of nearly 70% [150]. Such studies in unselected community samples might also help to alleviate fears about pathologising "normal" experiences that have been raised by reports on frequent and mostly benign PLEs in the community [147]. However, the benign PLEs measured by self-report in community samples may not be a valid measure of clinician-assessed symptoms [148]. Furthermore, community studies should increase knowledge about help-seeking to detect starting-points for increasing early help-seeking, because, at the currently low rate of only about 30% of FEP patients seeking help prior to the onset of frank psychotic symptoms [13, 14], a significant reduction of the incidence of psychosis—the ultimate target of prevention—will not be in sight. Another question that epidemiological research will help to address is whether to continue to regard current criteria as risk criteria with the main outcome being progression to psychosis and the main treatment target being its prevention or to rather perceive them as a self-contained syndrome in that remission, persistence, and progression, for example, to psychosis, are equally possible outcomes and in that the main treatment targets are current symptoms [112, 144]. In both cases, however, the search for additional predictors of psychosis will continue.

Today, this search mainly relies on group differences that greatly depend on the studied sample and, consequently, are hard to *transfer into clinical practice*, that is, on the risk estimation of an individual patient [127, 140]. Thus, where available such as for neurocognitive or psychological tests, deficits should be defined according to independent test norms, and risk stratification approaches should be presented in a way acceptable to clinicians, that is, not as scores of a complex regression equation but as clear decision rules relying on certain patterns of aberrations [127, 160]. Such a presentation would also facilitate the validation of prediction rules in other samples. The *use of norms* that are generally already gender- and age-adjusted might also help to avoid heterogeneity in data related to gender and, more importantly, *age effects* that have just been started to be addressed in this line of research [62–65, 67, 92, 161, 162], for example, by our multicentre BEARS-Kid study.

Age effects and needs of young age will also have to be considered in *early intervention research* in both ARMS and FEP patients, in particular with regard to more benign psychotherapeutic interventions [161]. Early interventions in an ARMS that have so far mainly focussed on risk symptoms and comorbidities [155, 157] might thereby broaden their focus to enhancing general *resilience factors* such as adequate coping strategies, metacognitive beliefs, or sleep [140, 163].

In summary, while exciting process has already been made in the field of early psychosis—both ARMS and FEP—much remains to be done. And while psychosis research has traditionally been mainly carried out in general psychiatry and adult samples, research on early psychosis and, consequently, rather young patients calls for a stronger involvement of child and adolescent psychiatry and reconsideration of the often strict age-related separation of fields of responsibility of the two professions. A successful example is the FETZ Bern (http://www.fetz.gef.be.ch/fetz_gef/de/index/navi/index.html), an early detection and intervention service that serves patients between the ages of 8 and 40—and, at this, the worldwide largest age range—and is run as a cooperation of the Bern University Hospitals for Child and Adolescent Psychiatry, and Psychiatry, and the Soteria Bern.

Conflict of Interests

Frauke Schultze-Lutter declares that there is no conflict of interests in relation to any subject of this paper. Benno G. Schimmelmann has been a consultant and/or advisor for or has received honoraria from Eli Lilly and Shire.

Acknowledgments

Studies presented in this paper were funded by the German Research Foundation, the Koeln Fortune Program/Faculty of Medicine (University of Cologne), the German Federal Ministry of Education and Health, the Swiss National Science Foundation, AstraZeneca (investigator initiated), Eli Lilly, Sanofi-Aventis, the Werner-Otto-Stiftung, and the National Health and Medical Research Council, Australia. Furthermore, many of the works presented in this paper would not have been possible without the support of the authors' respective earlier work groups and the cooperation of colleagues, of whom the authors would like to name Philippe Conus (Lausanne), Joachim Klosterkötter (Cologne), Martin Lambert (Hamburg), Patrick McGorry (Melbourne), Chantal Michel (Bern), and Stephan Ruhrmann (Cologne). SPI-A and SPI-CY are available in English and other languages at http://www.fioriti.it/.

References

[1] F. M. Gore, P. J. N. Bloem, G. C. Patton et al., "Global burden of disease in young people aged 10-24 years: a systematic analysis," *The Lancet*, vol. 377, no. 9783, pp. 2093–2102, 2011.

[2] J. Olesen and M. Leonardi, "The burden of brain diseases in Europe," *European Journal of Neurology*, vol. 10, no. 5, pp. 471–477, 2003.

[3] J. Perälä, J. Suvisaari, S. I. Saarni et al., "Lifetime prevalence of psychotic and bipolar I disorders in a general population," *Archives of General Psychiatry*, vol. 64, no. 1, pp. 19–28, 2007.

[4] J. B. Kirkbride, P. Fearon, C. Morgan et al., "Heterogeneity in incidence rates of schizophrenia and other psychotic syndromes: findings from the 3-center ÆSOP study," *Archives of General Psychiatry*, vol. 63, no. 3, pp. 250–258, 2006.

[5] J. B. Kirkbride, C. Stubbins, and P. B. Jones, "Psychosis incidence through the prism of early intervention services," *The British Journal of Psychiatry*, vol. 200, no. 2, pp. 156–157, 2012.

[6] B. G. Schimmelmann, S. J. Schmidt, M. Carbon, and C. U. Correll, "Treatment of adolescents with early-onset schizophrenia spectrum disorders: in search of a rational, evidence-informed approach," *Current Opinion in Psychiatry*, vol. 26, no. 2, pp. 219–230, 2013.

[7] H. U. Wittchen, F. Jacobi, J. Rehm et al., "The size and burden of mental disorders and other disorders of the brain in Europe 2010," *European Neuropsychopharmacology*, vol. 21, no. 9, pp. 655–679, 2011.

[8] A. Gustavsson, M. Svensson, F. Jacobi et al., "Cost of disorders of the brain in Europe 2010," *European Neuropsychopharmacology*, vol. 21, no. 10, pp. 718–779, 2011.

[9] N. Charrier, K. Chevreul, and I. Durand-Zaleski, "The cost of schizophrenia: a literature review," *Encephale*, vol. 39, supplement 1, pp. S49–S56, 2013.

[10] M. Marshall, S. Lewis, A. Lockwood, R. Drake, P. Jones, and T. Croudace, "Association between duration of untreated psychosis and outcome in cohorts of first-episode patients: a systematic review," *Archives of General Psychiatry*, vol. 62, no. 9, pp. 975–983, 2005.

[11] M. S. Keshavan, G. Haas, J. Miewald et al., "Prolonged untreated illness duration from prodromal onset predicts outcome in first episode psychoses," *Schizophrenia Bulletin*, vol. 29, no. 4, pp. 757–769, 2003.

[12] D. Köhn, A. Niedersteberg, A. Wieneke et al., "Frühverlauf schizophrener Ersterkrankungen mit langer Dauer der unbehandelten Erkrankung—eine vergleichende Studie," *Fortschr Neurol Psychiatr*, vol. 72, no. 2, pp. 88–92, 2004.

[13] N. Schaffner, B. G. Schimmelmann, A. Niedersteberg, and F. Schultze-Lutter, "Versorgungswege von erstmanifesten psychotischen Patienten—eine Übersicht internationaler Studien," *Fortschr Neurol Psychiatr*, vol. 80, no. 2, pp. 72–78, 2012.

[14] D. Köhn, R. Pukrop, A. Niedersteberg et al., "Wege in die Behandlung: Hilfesuchverhalten schizophrener Ersterkrankter," *Fortschr Neurol Psychiatr*, vol. 72, no. 11, pp. 635–642, 2004.

[15] H. G. von Reventlow, S. Krüger-Özgürdal, S. Ruhrmann et al., "Pathways to care in subjects at high risk for psychotic disorders—a European perspective," *Schizophrenia Research*, vol. 152, no. 2-3, pp. 400–407, 2014.

[16] H. Hafner, B. Nowotny, W. Löffler, W. an der Heiden, and K. Maurer, "When and how does schizophrenia produce social deficits?" *European Archives of Psychiatry and Clinical Neuroscience*, vol. 246, no. 1, pp. 17–28, 1995.

[17] F. Schultze-Lutter, S. Ruhrmann, J. Berning, W. Maier, and J. Klosterkötter, "Basic symptoms and ultrahigh risk criteria: symptom development in the initial prodromal state," *Schizophrenia Bulletin*, vol. 36, no. 1, pp. 182–191, 2010.

[18] T. H. McGlashan and J. O. Johannessen, "Early detection and intervention with schizophrenia: rationale," *Schizophrenia Bulletin*, vol. 22, no. 2, pp. 201–222, 1996.

[19] P. D. McGorry, "'A stitch in time'... the scope for preventive strategies in early psychosis," *European Archives of Psychiatry and Clinical Neuroscience*, vol. 248, no. 1, pp. 22–31, 1998.

[20] G. Huber and G. Gross, "The concept of basic symptoms in schizophrenic and schizoaffective psychoses," *Recenti Progressi in Medicina*, vol. 80, no. 12, pp. 646–652, 1989.

[21] P. D. McGorry, J. Edwards, C. Mihalopoulos, S. M. Harrigan, and H. J. Jackson, "EPPIC: an evolving system of early detection and optimal management," *Schizophrenia Bulletin*, vol. 22, no. 2, pp. 305–326, 1996.

[22] P. Conus, S. Cotton, B. G. Schimmelmann, P. McGorry, and M. Lambert, "The First-episode Psychosis Outcome Study (FEPOS): pre-morbid and baseline characteristics of an epidemiological cohort of 661 first-episode psychosis patients," *Early Intervention in Psychiatry*, vol. 1, no. 2, pp. 191–200, 2007.

[23] P. Conus, S. Cotton, B. G. Schimmelmann, P. D. McGorry, and M. Lambert, "Pretreatment and outcome correlates of sexual and physical trauma in an epidemiological cohort of first-episode psychosis patients," *Schizophrenia Bulletin*, vol. 36, no. 6, pp. 1105–1114, 2010.

[24] S. M. Cotton, M. Lambert, B. G. Schimmelmann et al., "Differences between first episode schizophrenia and schizoaffective disorder," *Schizophrenia Research*, vol. 147, no. 1, pp. 169–174, 2013.

[25] S. M. Cotton, M. Lambert, B. G. Schimmelmann et al., "Gender differences in premorbid, entry, treatment, and outcome characteristics in a treated epidemiological sample of 661 patients with first episode psychosis," *Schizophrenia Research*, vol. 114, no. 1–3, pp. 17–24, 2009.

[26] S. M. Cotton, M. Lambert, B. G. Schimmelmann et al., "Depressive symptoms in first episode schizophrenia spectrum disorder," *Schizophrenia Research*, vol. 134, no. 1, pp. 20–26, 2012.

[27] M. Lambert, P. Conus, B. G. Schimmelmann et al., "Comparison of olanzapine and risperidone in 367 first-episode patients with non-affective or affective psychosis: results of an open retrospective medical record study," *Pharmacopsychiatry*, vol. 38, no. 5, pp. 206–213, 2005.

[28] K. K. Morley, S. M. Cotton, P. Conus et al., "Familial psychopathology in the first episode psychosis outcome study," *Australian and New Zealand Journal of Psychiatry*, vol. 42, no. 7, pp. 617–626, 2008.

[29] S. Rebgetz, P. Conus, L. Hides et al., "Predictors of substance use reduction in an epidemiological first-episode psychosis cohort," *Early Intervention in Psychiatry*, vol. 24, pp. 1–24, 2013.

[30] J. Robinson, S. Cotton, P. Conus, B. G. Schimmelmann, P. McGorry, and M. Lambert, "Prevalence and predictors of suicide attempt in an incidence cohort of 661 young people with first-episode psychosis," *Australian and New Zealand Journal of Psychiatry*, vol. 43, no. 2, pp. 149–157, 2009.

[31] S. M. Cotton, M. Lambert, M. Berk et al., "Gender differences in first episode psychotic mania," *BMC Psychiatry*, vol. 13, no. 1, article 82, 2013.

[32] D. Schöttle, B. G. Schimmelmann, P. Conus et al., "Differentiating schizoaffective and bipolar I disorder in first-episode psychotic mania," *Schizophrenia Research*, vol. 140, no. 1–3, pp. 31–36, 2012.

[33] B. G. Schimmelmann, P. Conus, J. Edwards, P. D. McGorry, and M. Lambert, "Diagnostic stability 18 months after treatment initiation for first-episode psychosis," *Journal of Clinical Psychiatry*, vol. 66, no. 10, pp. 1239–1246, 2005.

[34] M. Lambert, P. Conus, D. I. Lubman et al., "The impact of substance use disorders on clinical outcome in 643 patients with first-episode psychosis," *Acta Psychiatrica Scandinavica*, vol. 112, no. 2, pp. 141–148, 2005.

[35] B. G. Schimmelmann, P. Conus, S. Cotton, S. Kupferschmid, P. D. McGorry, and M. Lambert, "Prevalence and impact of cannabis use disorders in adolescents with early onset first episode psychosis," *European Psychiatry*, vol. 27, no. 6, pp. 463–469, 2012.

[36] B. G. Schimmelmann, P. Conus, S. M. Cotton et al., "Cannabis use disorder and age at onset of psychosis—a study in first-episode patients," *Schizophrenia Research*, vol. 129, no. 1, pp. 52–56, 2011.

[37] P. Conus, M. Lambert, S. Cotton, C. Bonsack, P. D. McGorry, and B. G. Schimmelmann, "Rate and predictors of service disengagement in an epidemiological first-episode psychosis cohort," *Schizophrenia Research*, vol. 118, no. 1–3, pp. 256–263, 2010.

[38] M. Lambert, P. Conus, S. Cotton, J. Robinson, P. D. McGorry, and B. G. Schimmelmann, "Prevalence, predictors, and consequences of long-term refusal of antipsychotic treatment in first-episode psychosis," *Journal of Clinical Psychopharmacology*, vol. 30, no. 5, pp. 565–572, 2010.

[39] B. G. Schimmelmann, P. Conus, M. Schacht, P. McGorry, and M. Lambert, "Predictors of service disengagement in first-admitted adolescents with psychosis," *Journal of the American Academy of Child and Adolescent Psychiatry*, vol. 45, no. 8, pp. 990–999, 2006.

[40] B. G. Schimmelmann, P. Conus, S. Cotton, P. D. McGorry, and M. Lambert, "Pre-treatment, baseline, and outcome differences between early-onset and adult-onset psychosis in an epidemiological cohort of 636 first-episode patients," *Schizophrenia Research*, vol. 95, no. 1–3, pp. 1–8, 2007.

[41] B. G. Schimmelmann, C. G. Huber, M. Lambert, S. Cotton, P. D. McGorry, and P. Conus, "Impact of duration of untreated psychosis on pre-treatment, baseline, and outcome characteristics in an epidemiological first-episode psychosis cohort," *Journal of Psychiatric Research*, vol. 42, no. 12, pp. 982–990, 2008.

[42] S. Dragt, D. H. Nieman, F. Schultze-Lutter et al., "Cannabis use and age at onset of symptoms in subjects at clinical high risk for psychosis," *Acta Psychiatrica Scandinavica*, vol. 125, no. 1, pp. 45–53, 2012.

[43] M. Lambert, A. Karow, S. Leucht, B. G. Schimmelmann, and D. Naber, "Remission in schizophrenia: validity, frequency, predictors, and patients' perspective 5 years later," *Dialogues in Clinical Neuroscience*, vol. 12, no. 3, pp. 393–407, 2010.

[44] M. Lambert, D. Naber, A. Karow et al., "Subjective wellbeing under quetiapine treatment: Effect of diagnosis, mood state, and anxiety," *Schizophrenia Research*, vol. 110, no. 1–3, pp. 72–79, 2009.

[45] M. Lambert, D. Naber, A. Schacht et al., "Rates and predictors of remission and recovery during 3 years in 392 never-treated patients with schizophrenia," *Acta Psychiatrica Scandinavica*, vol. 118, no. 3, pp. 220–229, 2008.

[46] M. Lambert, B. G. Schimmelmann, D. Naber et al., "Early- and delayed antipsychotic response and prediction of outcome in 528 severely impaired patients with schizophrenia treated with amisulpride," *Pharmacopsychiatry*, vol. 42, no. 6, pp. 277–283, 2009.

[47] M. Lambert, B. G. Schimmelmann, A. Schacht et al., "Long-term patterns of subjective wellbeing in schizophrenia: Cluster, predictors of cluster affiliation, and their relation to recovery criteria in 2842 patients followed over 3 years," *Schizophrenia Research*, vol. 107, no. 2-3, pp. 165–172, 2009.

[48] M. Lambert, D. Naber, F. X. Eich, M. Schacht, M. Linden, and B. G. Schimmelmann, "Remission of severely impaired subjective wellbeing in 727 patients with schizophrenia treated with amisulpride," *Acta Psychiatrica Scandinavica*, vol. 115, no. 2, pp. 106–113, 2007.

[49] M. Lambert, B. G. Schimmelmann, D. Naber et al., "Prediction of remission as a combination of symptomatic and functional remission and adequate subjective well-being in 2960 patients with schizophrenia," *The Journal of Clinical Psychiatry*, vol. 67, no. 11, pp. 1690–1697, 2006.

[50] H. Meng, B. G. Schimmelmann, B. Mohler et al., "Pretreatment social functioning predicts 1-year outcome in early onset psychosis," *Acta Psychiatrica Scandinavica*, vol. 114, no. 4, pp. 249–256, 2006.

[51] P. M. Wehmeier, M. Kluge, A. Schacht et al., "Patterns of physician and patient rated quality of life during antipsychotic treatment in outpatients with schizophrenia," *Journal of Psychiatric Research*, vol. 42, no. 8, pp. 676–683, 2008.

[52] B. G. Schimmelmann, C. Mehler-Wex, M. Lambert et al., "A prospective 12-week study of quetiapine in adolescents with schizophrenia spectrum disorders," *Journal of Child and Adolescent Psychopharmacology*, vol. 17, no. 6, pp. 768–778, 2007.

[53] A. Karow, J. Czekalla, R. W. Dittmann et al., "Association of subjective well-being, symptoms, and side effects with compliance after 12 months of treatment in schizophrenia," *The Journal of Clinical Psychiatry*, vol. 68, no. 1, pp. 75–80, 2007.

[54] B. G. Schimmelmann, S. Paulus, M. Schacht, C. Tilgner, M. Schulte-Markwort, and M. Lambert, "Subjective distress related to side effects and subjective well-being in first admitted adolescents with early-onset psychosis treated with atypical antipsychotics," *Journal of Child and Adolescent Psychopharmacology*, vol. 15, no. 2, pp. 249–258, 2005.

[55] M. Lambert, T. Bock, A. Daubmann et al., "Integrierte Versorgung von Patienten mit psychotischen Erkrankungen nach dem Hamburger Modell: Teil 1," *Psychiatrische Praxis*, vol. 41, no. 5, pp. 257–265, 2014.

[56] A. Karow, T. Bock, A. Daubmann et al., "Integrierte Versorgung von Patienten mit psychotischen Erkrankungen nach dem Hamburger Modell: Teil 2," *Psychiatrische Praxis*, vol. 41, no. 5, pp. 266–273, 2014.

[57] D. Schöttle, A. Karow, B. G. Schimmelmann, and M. Lambert, "Integrated care in patients with schizophrenia: results of trials published between 2011 and 2013 focusing on effectiveness and efficiency," *Current Opinion in Psychiatry*, vol. 26, no. 4, pp. 384–408, 2013.

[58] M. Lambert, T. Bock, D. Schöttle et al., "Assertive community treatment as part of integrated care versus standard care: A 12-month trial in patients with first- and multiple-episode schizophrenia spectrum disorders treated with quetiapine immediate release (ACCESS trial)," *Journal of Clinical Psychiatry*, vol. 71, no. 10, pp. 1313–1323, 2010.

[59] A. Karow, J. Reimer, H. H. König et al., "Cost-effectiveness of 12-month therapeutic assertive community treatment as part of integrated care versus standard care in patients with schizophrenia treated with quetiapine immediate release (ACCESS trial)," *Journal of Clinical Psychiatry*, vol. 73, no. 3, pp. e402–e408, 2012.

[60] D. Schöttle, B. G. Schimmelmann, and A. Karow, "Translating Research into clinical practice: effectiveness of integrated care including therapeutic assertive community treatment in severe schizophrenia-spectrum and bipolar I disorders—a 24-month follow-up study (ACCESS-II study)," *Journal of Clinical Psychiatry*. In press.

[61] F. Schultze-Lutter, "Prediction of psychosis is necessary and possible," in *Schizophrenia: Challenging the Orthodox*, C. McDonald, K. Schultz, R. Murray, and P. Wright, Eds., pp. 81–90, Taylor & Francis, London, UK, 2004.

[62] E. Koch, F. Schultze-Lutter, B. G. Schimmelmann, and F. Resch, "On the importance and detection of prodromal symptoms from the perspective of child and adolescent psychiatry," *Clinical Neuropsychiatry*, vol. 7, no. 2, pp. 38–48, 2010.

[63] B. G. Schimmelmann, P. Walger, and F. Schultze-Lutter, "The significance of at-risk symptoms for psychosis in children and adolescents," *Canadian Journal of Psychiatry*, vol. 58, no. 1, pp. 32–40, 2013.

[64] B. G. Schimmelmann and F. Schultze-Lutter, "Early detection and intervention of psychosis in children and adolescents: urgent need for studies," *European Child and Adolescent Psychiatry*, vol. 21, no. 5, pp. 239–241, 2012.

[65] F. Schultze-Lutter, F. Resch, E. Koch, and B. G. Schimmelmann, "Früherkennung von Psychosen bei Kindern und Adoleszenten—sind entwicklungsbezogene Besonderheiten ausreichend berücksichtigt?" *Zeitschrift für Kinder- und Jugendpsychiatrie und Psychotherapie*, vol. 39, no. 5, pp. 301–311, 2011.

[66] E. Kraepelin, *Psychiatrie. Ein Lehrbuch für Studierende und Ärzte. 8. vollständig umgearbeitete Auflage*, Johann Ambrosius Barth, Leipzig, Germany, 1909.

[67] F. Schultze-Lutter, S. Ruhrmann, P. Fusar-Poli, A. Bechdolf, B. G. Schimmelmann, and J. Klosterkötter, "Basic symptoms and the prediction of first-episode psychosis," *Current Pharmaceutical Design*, vol. 18, no. 4, pp. 351–357, 2012.

[68] K. Conrad, *Die beginnende Schizophrenie. Versuch einer Gestalt-analyse des Wahns*, Thieme, Stuttgart, Germany, 1958.

[69] J. P. Docherty, D. P. Van Kammen, S. G. Siris, and S. R. Marder, "Stages of onset of schizophrenic psychosis," *The American Journal of Psychiatry*, vol. 135, no. 4, pp. 420–426, 1978.

[70] H. Häfner, K. Maurer, W. Löffler, W. An der Heiden, M. Hambrecht, and F. Schultze-Lutter, "Modeling the early course of schizophrenia," *Schizophrenia Bulletin*, vol. 29, no. 2, pp. 325–340, 2003.

[71] F. Schultze-Lutter, "Subjective symptoms of schizophrenia in research and the clinic: the basic symptom concept," *Schizophrenia Bulletin*, vol. 35, no. 1, pp. 5–8, 2009.

[72] A. R. Yung and P. O. McGorry, "The prodromal phase of first-episode psychosis: Past and current conceptualizations," *Schizophrenia Bulletin*, vol. 22, no. 2, pp. 353–370, 1996.

[73] F. Schultze-Lutter, B. G. Schimmelmann, and S. Ruhrmann, "The near babylonian speech confusion in early detection of psychosis," *Schizophrenia Bulletin*, vol. 37, no. 4, pp. 653–655, 2011.

[74] F. Schultze-Lutter, B. G. Schimmelmann, S. Ruhrmann, and C. Michel, "'A rose is a rose is a rose', but at-risk criteria differ," *Psychopathology*, vol. 46, no. 2, pp. 75–87, 2013.

[75] P. Fusar-Poli, S. Borgwardt, A. Bechdolf et al., "The psychosis high-risk state: a comprehensive state-of-the-art review," *JAMA Psychiatry*, vol. 70, no. 1, pp. 107–120, 2013.

[76] F. Schultze-Lutter, S. Ruhrmann, H. Picker, H. G. von Reventlow, A. Brockhaus-Dumke, and J. Klosterkötter, "Basic symptoms in early psychotic and depressive disorders," *British Journal of Psychiatry*, vol. 191, supplement 51, pp. S31–S37, 2007.

[77] F. Schultze-Lutter, B. G. Schimmelmann, J. Klosterkötter, and S. Ruhrmann, "Comparing the prodrome of schizophrenia-spectrum psychoses and affective disorders with and without psychotic features," *Schizophrenia Research*, vol. 138, no. 2-3, pp. 218–222, 2012.

[78] W. Mayer-Gross, "Die klinik," in *Handbuch der Geisteskrankheiten—Spezieller Teil V: Die Schizophrenie*, O. Bumke, Ed., Julius Springer, Berlin, Germany, 1932.

[79] G. Huber, "Reine Defektsyndrome und Basisstadien endogener Psychosen," *Fortschritte der Neurologie-Psychiatrie*, vol. 34, pp. 409–426, 1966.

[80] J. Klosterkotter, H. Ebel, F. Schultze-Lutter, and E. M. Steinmeyer, "Diagnostic validity of basic symptoms," *European Archives of Psychiatry and Clinical Neuroscience*, vol. 246, no. 3, pp. 147–154, 1996.

[81] F. Schultze-Lutter and J. Klosterkotter, "Do basic symptoms provide a possible explanation for the elevated risk for schizophrenia among mentally retarded?" *Neurology Psychiatry and Brain Research*, vol. 3, no. 1, pp. 29–34, 1995.

[82] A. Bechdolf, F. Schultze-Lutter, and J. Klosterkötter, "Self-experienced vulnerability, prodromal symptoms and coping strategies preceding schizophrenic and depressive relapses," *European Psychiatry*, vol. 17, no. 7, pp. 384–393, 2002.

[83] L. Süllwold and G. Huber, *Schizophrene Basisstörungen*, Springer, Berlin, Germany, 1986.

[84] G. Gross, G. Huber, J. Klosterkötter, and M. Linz, *Bonner Skala für die Beurteilung von Basissymptomen (BSABS; Bonn Scale for the Assessment of Basic Symptoms)*, Springer, Berlin, Germany, 1987.

[85] J. Klosterkötter, G. Gross, G. Huber, A. Wieneke, E. M. Steinmeyer, and F. Schultze-Lutter, "Evaluation of the "bonn scale for the assessment of basic symptoms—BSABS" as an instrument for the assessment of schizophrenia proneness: a review of recent findings," *Neurology, Psychiatry and Brain Research*, vol. 5, no. 3, pp. 137–150, 1997.

[86] L. Süllwold, *Manual Zum Frankfurter Beschwerde-Fragebogen (FBF)*, Springer, Berlin, Germany, 1991.

[87] R. Mass, K. Hitschfeld, E. Wall, and H. B. Wagner, "Validität der Erfassung schizophrener Basissymptome," *Nervenarzt*, vol. 68, no. 3, pp. 205–211, 1997.

[88] F. Schultze-Lutter, E. M. Steinmeyer, S. Ruhrmann, and J. Klosterkötter, "The dimensional structure of self-reported prodromal disturbances in schizophrenia," *Clinical Neuropsychiatry*, vol. 5, no. 3, pp. 140–150, 2008.

[89] F. Schultze-Lutter, J. Addington, S. Ruhrmann, and J. Klosterkötter, *Schizophrenia Proneness Instrument-Adult Version (SPI-A)*, Giovanni Fioriti Editore, Rome, Italy, 2007.

[90] F. Schultze-Lutter and E. Koch, *Schizophrenia Proneness Instrument—Child and Youth Version (SPI-CY)*, Giovanni Fioriti Editore, Rome, Italy, 2010.

[91] F. Schultze-Lutter, M. Marshall, and E. Koch, *Schizophrenia Proneness Instrument, Child and Youth Version*, Extended English Translation (SPI-CY EET), Giovanni Fioriti Editore, Rome, Italy, 2012.

[92] L. Fux, P. Walger, B. G. Schimmelmann, and F. Schultze-Lutter, "The schizophrenia proneness instrument, child and youth version (SPI-CY): practicability and discriminative validity," *Schizophrenia Research*, vol. 146, no. 1–3, pp. 69–78, 2013.

[93] F. Schultze-Lutter, S. Ruhrmann, and J. Klosterkötter, "Can schizophrenia be predicted phenomenologically?" in *Evolving Psychosis. Different Stages, Different Treatments*, J. O. Johannessen, B. Martindale, and J. Cullberg, Eds., pp. 104–123, Routledge, London, UK, 2010.

[94] M. Albers, F. Schultze-Lutter, E. M. Steinmeyer, and J. Klosterkötter, "Can self-experienced neuropsychological deficits indicate propensity to schizophrenic psychosis? Results of an 8-year prospective follow-up study," *International Clinical Psychopharmacology*, vol. 13, supplement 1, pp. S75–S80, 1998.

[95] J. Klosterkötter, M. Hellmich, E. M. Steinmeyer, and F. Schultze-Lutter, "Diagnosing schizophrenia in the initial prodromal phase," *Archives of General Psychiatry*, vol. 58, no. 2, pp. 158–164, 2001.

[96] F. Schultze-Lutter, "Ruling in or ruling out the schizophrenic prodrome: what criteria for symptom selection should be used?" *Schizophrenia Research*, vol. 41, no. 1, p. 179, 2000.

[97] F. Schultze-Lutter, J. Klosterkötter, H. Picker, E.-M. Steinmeyer, and S. Ruhrmann, "Predicting first-episode psychosis by basic symptom criteria," *Clinical Neuropsychiatry*, vol. 4, no. 1, pp. 11–22, 2007.

[98] A. Bechdolf, M. Wagner, S. Ruhrmann et al., "Preventing progression to first-episode psychosis in early initial prodromal states," *The British Journal of Psychiatry*, vol. 200, no. 1, pp. 22–29, 2012.

[99] S. Ruhrmann, F. Schultze-Lutter, R. K. R. Salokangas et al., "Prediction of psychosis in adolescents and young adults at high risk: results from the prospective European prediction of psychosis study," *Archives of General Psychiatry*, vol. 67, no. 3, pp. 241–251, 2010.

[100] F. Schultze-Lutter, J. Klosterkötter, and S. Ruhrmann, "Improving the clinical prediction of psychosis by combining ultra-high risk criteria and cognitive basic symptoms," *Schizophrenia Researc*, vol. 154, no. 1–3, pp. 100–106, 2014.

[101] E. Velthorst, D. H. Nieman, H. E. Becker et al., "Baseline differences in clinical symptomatology between ultra high risk subjects with and without a transition to psychosis," *Schizophrenia Research*, vol. 109, no. 1–3, pp. 60–65, 2009.

[102] T. B. Ziermans, P. F. Schothorst, M. Sprong, and H. van Engeland, "Transition and remission in adolescents at ultra-high risk for psychosis," *Schizophrenia Research*, vol. 126, no. 1–3, pp. 58–64, 2011.

[103] A. R. Yung, H. P. Yuen, G. Berger et al., "Declining transition rate in ultra high risk (prodromal) services: dilution or reduction of risk?" *Schizophrenia Bulletin*, vol. 33, no. 3, pp. 673–681, 2007.

[104] F. Schultze-Lutter, S. Ruhrmann, C. Hoyer, J. Klosterkötter, and F. M. Leweke, "The initial prodrome of schizophrenia: different duration, different underlying deficits?" *Comprehensive Psychiatry*, vol. 48, no. 5, pp. 479–488, 2007.

[105] F. Schultze-Lutter, S. Ruhrmann, and J. Klosterkötter, "Early detection of psychosis—establishing a service for persons at risk," *European Psychiatry*, vol. 24, no. 1, pp. 1–10, 2009.

[106] F. Schultze-Lutter, S. Ruhrmann, and J. Klosterkötter, "Early detection and early intervention in psychosis in Western Europe," *Clinical Neuropsychiatry*, vol. 5, no. 6, pp. 303–315, 2008.

[107] H. Häfner, K. Maurer, S. Ruhrmann et al., "Early detection and secondary prevention of psychosis: facts and visions," *European Archives of Psychiatry and Clinical Neuroscience*, vol. 254, no. 2, pp. 117–128, 2004.

[108] J. Klosterkötter, "The clinical staging and the endophenotype approach as an integrative future perspective for psychiatry," *World Psychiatry*, vol. 7, no. 3, pp. 159–160, 2008.

[109] J. Klosterkötter, F. Schultze-Lutter, and S. Ruhrmann, "Prediction and prevention of schizophrenia: what has been achieved and where to go next?" *World Psychiatry*, vol. 10, no. 3, pp. 165–174, 2011.

[110] S. Ruhrmann, F. Schultze-Lutter, and J. Klosterkötter, "Early detection and intervention in the initial prodromal phase of schizophrenia," *Pharmacopsychiatry*, vol. 36, supplement 3, pp. S162–S167, 2003.

[111] J. Klosterkötter, F. Schultze-Lutter, and S. Ruhrmann, "Kraepelin and psychotic prodromal conditions," *European Archives of Psychiatry and Clinical Neuroscience*, vol. 258, no. 2, pp. 74–84, 2008.

[112] S. Ruhrann, F. Schultze-Lutter, and J. Klosterkötter, "Subthreshold states of psychosis—a challenge to diagnosis and treatment," *Clinical Neuropsychiatry*, vol. 7, no. 2, pp. 72–87, 2010.

[113] J. T. Bigger Jr., C. A. Heller, T. L. Wenger, and F. M. Weld, "Risk stratification after acute myocardial infarction," *The American Journal of Cardiology*, vol. 42, no. 2, pp. 202–210, 1978.

[114] J. Klosterkötter, S. Ruhrmann, F. Schultze-Lutter et al., " The European prediction of psychosis study (EPOS): integrating early recognition and intervention in Europe," *World Psychiatry*, vol. 4, no. 3, pp. 161–167, 2005.

[115] T. H. McGlashan, B. C. Walsh, and S. W. Woods, *The Psychosis-Risk Syndrome*, Oxford University Press, New York, NY, USA, 2010.

[116] R. K. R. Salokangas, S. Ruhrmann, H. G. von Reventlow et al., "Axis I diagnoses and transition to psychosis in clinical high-risk patients EPOS project: Prospective follow-up of 245 clinical high-risk outpatients in four countries," *Schizophrenia Research*, vol. 138, no. 2-3, pp. 192–197, 2012.

[117] D. H. Nieman, E. Velthorst, H. E. Becker et al., "The Strauss and Carpenter Prognostic Scale in subjects clinically at high risk of psychosis," *Acta Psychiatrica Scandinavica*, vol. 127, no. 1, pp. 53–61, 2013.

[118] R. K. R. Salokangas, P. Dingemans, M. Heinimaa et al., "Prediction of psychosis in clinical high-risk patients by the Schizotypal Personality Questionnaire. Results of the EPOS project," *European Psychiatry*, vol. 28, no. 8, pp. 469–475, 2013.

[119] F. Schultze-Lutter, J. Klosterkötter, C. Michel, K. Winkler, and S. Ruhrmann, "Personality disorders and accentuations in at-risk persons with and without conversion to first-episode psychosis," *Early Intervention in Psychiatry*, vol. 6, no. 4, pp. 389–398, 2012.

[120] F. Schultze-Lutter, J. Klosterkötter, A. Nikolaides, and S. Ruhrmann, "Personality dimensions in subjects symptomatically at-risk of psychosis: pronounced but lacking a characteristic profile," *Early Intervention in Psychiatry*, 2014.

[121] R. Pukrop, F. Schultze-Lutter, S. Ruhrmann et al., "Neurocognitive functioning in subjects at risk for a first episode of psychosis compared with first- and multiple-episode schizophrenia," *Journal of Clinical and Experimental Neuropsychology*, vol. 28, no. 8, pp. 1388–1407, 2006.

[122] E. Gouzoulis-Mayfrank, M. Balke, S. Hajsamou et al., "Orienting of attention in unmedicated patients with schizophrenia, prodromal subjects and healthy relatives," *Schizophrenia Research*, vol. 97, no. 1–3, pp. 35–42, 2007.

[123] D. Koethe, C. W. Gerth, M. A. Neatby et al., "Disturbances of visual information processing in early states of psychosis and experimental delta-9-tetrahydrocannabinol altered states of consciousness," *Schizophrenia Research*, vol. 88, no. 1–3, pp. 142–150, 2006.

[124] D. Koethe, L. Kranaster, C. Hoyer et al., "Binocular depth inversion as a paradigm of reduced visual information processing in prodromal state, antipsychotic-naïve and treated schizophrenia," *European Archives of Psychiatry and Clinical Neuroscience*, vol. 259, no. 4, pp. 195–202, 2009.

[125] F. Schultze-Lutter, S. Ruhrmann, H. Picker et al., "Relationship between subjective and objective cognitive function in the early and late prodrome," *The British Journal of Psychiatry*, vol. 191, supplement 51, pp. s43–s51, 2007.

[126] R. Pukrop, S. Ruhrmann, F. Schultze-Lutter, A. Bechdolf, A. Brockhaus-Dumke, and J. Klosterkötter, "Neurocognitive indicators for a conversion to psychosis: comparison of patients in a potentially initial prodromal state who did or did not convert to a psychosis," *Schizophrenia Research*, vol. 92, no. 1–3, pp. 116–125, 2007.

[127] C. Michel, S. Ruhrmann, B. G. Schimmelmann, J. Klosterkötter, and F. Schultze-Lutter, "A stratified model for psychosis prediction in clinical practice," *Schizophrenia Bulletin*, 2014.

[128] A. Brockhaus-Dumke, I. Tendolkar, R. Pukrop, F. Schultze-Lutter, J. Klosterkötter, and S. Ruhrmann, "Impaired mismatch negativity generation in prodromal subjects and patients with schizophrenia," *Schizophrenia Research*, vol. 73, no. 2-3, pp. 297–310, 2005.

[129] A. Brockhaus-Dumke, F. Schultze-Lutter, R. Mueller et al., "Sensory gating in schizophrenia: P50 and N100 gating in antipsychotic-free subjects at risk, first-episode and chronic patients," *Biological Psychiatry*, vol. 64, no. 5, pp. 376–384, 2008.

[130] M. J. van Tricht, S. Ruhrmann, M. Arns et al., "Can quantitative EEG measures predict clinical outcome in subjects at clinical high risk for psychosis? A prospective multicenter study," *Schizophrenia Research*, vol. 153, no. 1–3, pp. 42–47, 2014.

[131] M. Bodatsch, S. Ruhrmann, M. Wagner et al., "Prediction of psychosis by mismatch negativity," *Biological Psychiatry*, vol. 69, no. 10, pp. 959–966, 2011.

[132] J. T. Huang, F. M. Leweke, T. M. Tsang et al., "CSF metabolic and proteomic profiles in patients prodromal for psychosis," *PLoS ONE*, vol. 2, no. 8, article e756, 2007.

[133] D. Koethe, A. Giuffrida, D. Schreiber et al., "Anandamide elevation in cerebrospinal fluid in initial prodromal states of psychosis," *British Journal of Psychiatry*, vol. 194, no. 4, pp. 371–372, 2009.

[134] A. Bechdolf, R. Pukrop, D. Köhn et al., "Subjective quality of life in subjects at risk for a first episode of psychosis: a comparison with first episode schizophrenia patients and healthy controls," *Schizophrenia Research*, vol. 79, no. 1, pp. 137–143, 2005.

[135] S. Ruhrmann, J. Paruch, A. Bechdolf et al., "Reduced subjective quality of life in persons at risk for psychosis," *Acta Psychiatrica Scandinavica*, vol. 117, no. 5, pp. 357–368, 2008.

[136] E. Velthorst, D. H. Nieman, D. Linszen et al., "Disability in people clinically at high risk of psychosis," *The British Journal of Psychiatry*, vol. 197, no. 4, pp. 278–284, 2010.

[137] R. K. R. Salokangas, M. Heinimaa, T. From et al., "Short-term functional outcome and premorbid adjustment in clinical high-risk patients. Results of the EPOS project," *European Psychiatry*, vol. 29, no. 6, pp. 371–380, 2014.

[138] R. K. R. Salokangas, D. H. Nieman, M. Heinimaa et al., "Psychosocial outcome in patients at clinical high risk of psychosis: a prospective follow-up," *Social Psychiatry and Psychiatric Epidemiology*, vol. 48, no. 2, pp. 303–311, 2013.

[139] F. Schultze-Lutter, H. Picker, S. Ruhrmann, and J. Klosterkötter, "Das Kölner Früh-Erkennungs- & Therapie-Zentrum für psychische Krisen (FETZ)," *Medizinische Klinik*, vol. 103, no. 2, pp. 81–89, 2008.

[140] S. J. Schmidt, V. M. Grunert, B. G. Schimmelmann, F. Schultze-Lutter, and C. Michel, "Differences in coping, self-efficacy, and external control beliefs between patients at-risk for psychosis and patients with first-episode psychosis," *Psychiatry Research*, vol. 219, no. 1, pp. 95–102, 2014.

[141] F. Schultze-Lutter and S. Ruhrmann, *Früherkennung und Frühbehandlung von Psychosen*, Uni-Med, Bremen, Germany, 2008.

[142] A. Grispini and F. Schultze-Lutter, "Introductory remarks to special issue: early detection and intervention in psychosis around the world," *Clinical Neuropsychiatry*, vol. 5, no. 5, article 261, 2008.

[143] S. W. Woods, J. Addington, K. S. Cadenhead et al., "Validity of the prodromal risk syndrome for first psychosis: findings from the north american prodrome longitudinal study," *Schizophrenia Bulletin*, vol. 35, no. 5, pp. 894–908, 2009.

[144] S. Ruhrmann, F. Schultze-Lutter, and J. Klosterkötter, "Probably at-risk, but certainly ill—advocating the introduction of a psychosis spectrum disorder in DSM-V," *Schizophrenia Research*, vol. 120, no. 1–3, pp. 23–37, 2010.

[145] W. T. Carpenter Jr., "Criticism of the DSM-V risk syndrome: a rebuttal," *Cognitive Neuropsychiatry*, vol. 16, no. 2, pp. 101–106, 2011.

[146] F. Schultze-Lutter and B. G. Schimmelmann, "Psychotische Störungen im DSM-5," *Zeitschrift für Kinder- und Jugendpsychiatrie und Psychotherapie*, vol. 42, no. 3, pp. 193–202, 2014.

[147] A. R. Yung, S. W. Woods, S. Ruhrmann et al., "Whither the attenuated psychosis syndrome?" *Schizophrenia Bulletin*, vol. 38, no. 6, pp. 1130–1134, 2012.

[148] F. Schultze-Lutter, F. Renner, J. Paruch, D. Julkowski, J. Klosterkötter, and S. Ruhrmann, "Self-reported psychotic-like experiences are a poor estimate of clinician-rated attenuated and frank delusions and hallucinations," *Psychopathology*, vol. 47, no. 3, pp. 194–201, 2014.

[149] C. Michel, B. G. Schimmelmann, S. Kupferschmid, M. Siegwart, and F. Schultze-Lutter, "Reliability of telephone assessments of at-risk criteria of psychosis: a comparison to face-to-face interviews," *Schizophrenia Research*, vol. 153, no. 1–3, pp. 251–253, 2014.

[150] F. Schultze-Lutter, C. Michel, S. Ruhrmann, and B. G. Schimmelmann, "Prevalence and clinical significance of DSM-5-attenuated psychosis syndrome in adolescents and young adults in the general population: the bern epidemiological at-risk (BEAR) study," *Schizophr Bull*, 2013.

[151] B. G. Schimmelmann, C. Michel, N. Schaffner, and F. Schultze-Lutter, "What percentage of people in the general population satisfies the current clinical at-risk criteria of psychosis?" *Schizophrenia Research*, vol. 125, no. 1, pp. 99–100, 2011.

[152] I. Kelleher, H. Keeley, P. Corcoran et al., "Clinicopathological significance of psychotic experiences in non-psychotic young people: evidence from four population-based studies," *The British Journal of Psychiatry*, vol. 201, no. 1, pp. 26–32, 2012.

[153] H. Meng, B. G. Schimmelmann, E. Koch et al., "Basic symptoms in the general population and in psychotic and non-psychotic psychiatric adolescents," *Schizophrenia Research*, vol. 111, no. 1–3, pp. 32–38, 2009.

[154] A. R. Yung, E. Killackey, S. E. Hetrick et al., "The prevention of schizophrenia," *International Review of Psychiatry*, vol. 19, no. 6, pp. 633–646, 2007.

[155] S. Ruhrmann, J. Klosterkötter, M. Bodatsch et al., "Chances and risks of predicting psychosis," *European Archives of Psychiatry and Clinical Neuroscience*, vol. 262, supplement 2, pp. 85–90, 2012.

[156] J. Klosterkötter and F. Schultze-Lutter, "Prevention and early treatment," in *Ethics in Psychiatry—European Contributions*, H. Helmchen and N. Sartorius, Eds., pp. 235–262, Springer Science+Business Media B.V., Heidelberg, The Netherlands, 2010.

[157] S. Ruhrmann, F. Schultze-Lutter, and J. Klosterkötter, "Intervention in the at-risk state to prevent transition to psychosis," *Current Opinion in Psychiatry*, vol. 22, no. 2, pp. 177–183, 2009.

[158] S. Ruhrmann, J. Klosterkötter, M. Bodatsch et al., "Pharmacological prevention and treatment in clinical at-risk states for psychosis," *Current Pharmaceutical Design*, vol. 18, no. 4, pp. 550–557, 2012.

[159] M. van der Gaag, F. Smit, A. Bechdolf et al., "Preventing a first episode of psychosis: meta-analysis of randomized controlled prevention trials of 12month and longer-term follow-ups," *Schizophrenia Research*, vol. 149, no. 1–3, pp. 56–62, 2013.

[160] F. Schultze-Lutter, *Früherkennung der Schizophrenie anhand subjektiver Beschwerdeschilderungen: ein methodenkritischer Vergleich der Vorhersageleistung nonparametrischer statistischer und alternativer Verfahren zur Generierung von Vorhersagemodelle [dissertation]*, Philosophical Faculty of the University of Cologne, 2001.

[161] S. J. Schmidt and B. G. Schimmelmann, "Evidence-based psychotherapy in children and adolescents: advances, methodological and conceptual limitations, and perspectives," *European Child & Adolescent Psychiatry*, vol. 22, no. 5, pp. 265–268, 2013.

[162] B. G. Schimmelmann, "Früherkennung von Psychosen Risiken und Nutzen bei Kindern und Jugendlichen abwägen," *Zeitschrift für Kinder und Jugendpsychiatrie und Psychotherapie*, vol. 39, no. 5, pp. 297–299, 2011.

[163] L. Tarokh, C. Hamann, and B. G. Schimmelmann, "Sleep in child and adolescent psychiatry: overlooked and underappreciated," *European Child & Adolescent Psychiatry*, vol. 23, no. 6, pp. 369–372, 2014.

[164] F. Schultze-Lutter, "Früherkennung von psychosen vor deren erstmanifestation: chance oder sackgasse? Die kerbe," *Forum für Sozialpsychiatrie*, vol. 3, pp. 36–39, 2014.

8

The Cloninger Type I/Type II Typology: Configurations and Personality Profiles in Socially Stable Alcohol Dependent Patients

Peter Wennberg,[1] Kristina Berglund,[2] Ulf Berggren,[3] Jan Balldin,[3] and Claudia Fahlke[2]

[1]Centre for Social Research on Alcohol and Drugs, Stockholm University, 10691 Stockholm, Sweden
[2]Department of Psychology, University of Gothenburg, 405 30 Gothenburg, Sweden
[3]Department of Psychiatry and Neurochemistry, Institute of Neuroscience and Physiology, University of Gothenburg, 413 45 Gothenburg, Sweden

Correspondence should be addressed to Peter Wennberg; peter.wennberg@ki.se

Academic Editor: Georges Brousse

Many attempts have been made to derive alcohol use typologies or subtypes of alcohol dependence and this study aimed at validating the type I/type II typology in a treatment sample of socially stable alcohol dependent males and females. A second aim was to compare the two types with respect to their temperament profiles. Data was part of a larger ongoing longitudinal study, the Gothenburg Alcohol Research Project, and included 269 alcohol dependent males and females recruited from three treatment centers. The results showed that type II alcoholism occurred as a more homogenous type than type I alcoholism, and type I alcoholism seemed too heterogeneous to be summarized into one single type. When adapting a strict classification, less than a third of the study population could be classified in accordance with the typology, suggesting that the typology is not applicable, at least in socially stable individuals with alcohol dependence. The results also showed that type II alcoholics showed higher levels of novelty seeking than did the individuals that were classified as type I alcoholics. Quite surprisingly, the individuals classified as type II alcoholics also showed higher levels of harm avoidance than did the individuals that were classified as type I alcoholics.

1. Background

As a means of understanding the high level of heterogeneity among individuals with alcohol use disorders (AUD) in terms of etiology and manifestations, many attempts have been made to derive alcohol use typologies or alcoholic subtypes. Although a great deal of effort has been put into this area of research, no generally accepted typology has yet been presented. As the concept is employed here, a typology refers to a set of fairly homogenous classes with respect to some specified characteristics. Belonging to any of these classes does not have to be a fixed and unchangeable feature but might be seen as a more or less temporary state in the context of a dynamic process (see a discussion in [1]). We believe that a good typology includes three basic features: (1) some form of face validity or heuristic power, (2) the types occur more frequently than would be expected if the criteria were randomly distributed across the subjects (i.e., the types form natural clusters), and (3) a majority (read more than 50 percent) of the subjects could be classified according to the typology in question.

In a study by Cloninger and colleagues [2] a population of 862 male adoptees was described in detail including data from temperance registers, child welfare agencies records, criminal records, and medical diagnoses. All in the study population were sons of single mothers and were adopted at an early age. The circumstance that the project had extensive information on the biological as well as the adoptive parents made it possible to single out the contribution of genetic from social heritage in the etiology of alcoholism. Furthermore, two quite different forms of alcoholism were also described as type I and type II alcoholism. While this study was based exclusively on males, another study by the same researchers [3] later added a female study population of adoptees. In summary, type I alcoholism includes influence of a childhood family environment, late-onset of alcohol-related problems (after age 25), men and women being affected equally, ability to abstain from drinking (at least temporarily), using alcohol as self-medication, and responding better to treatment. In summary, type II includes inheritance of the disease from the father, onset of alcohol-related problems before the age of 25 years, primarily males, inability to abstain from alcohol, history of antisocial acts, and poor response to treatment. In the present study we have focused on four key features to distinguish these types: gender, age of debut of alcohol-related problems, antisocial behavior, and paternal alcoholism. In addition to these features, the two types of alcoholism are also suggested to have different temperament profiles (Cloninger, 1987). [4] with higher levels of novelty seeking (NS) among type II alcoholics and higher levels of harm avoidance (HA) and reward dependence (RD) in type I alcoholics.

According to Cloninger et al. [4] the temperament traits are highly inherited personality traits that are underlined by specific neurotransmitters in the brain. The temperament traits are stable over time in contrary to the character traits, which are more determined by environmental factors and therefore less stable. In addition, the temperament traits are independently inherited of each other and therefore there are several combinations of them, which interact with several character profiles.

A study by Wills et al. [5] gave some support for the temperament profiles for type II alcoholics (high NS, low HA, and low RD). However, a review by Howard et al. [6] showed that NS was consistently associated with early onset alcohol abuse and antisocial behavior while the results regarding HA and RD were more inconsistent.

1.1. Aims. This study aimed at validating the Cloninger type I/type II typology (as described in [2, 3]) in a treatment sample of socially stable (for definition, see Berglund 2009) alcohol dependent males and females. More specifically we aimed at (1) testing to what extent the most important characteristics were grouped together relative to chance in the two types and (2) how the two types differ with respect to their personality profiles.

2. Methods

This study was part of a larger ongoing longitudinal study (Gothenburg Alcohol Research Project—GARP) which aims to investigate the interaction between psychological, psychiatric, as well as neurobiological, and genetic characteristics in alcohol dependent individuals and also to evaluate whether these variables influence treatment outcome. The project has earlier been described in more detail [7–9].

2.1. Subjects. In this study, 269 individuals participated (61 females and 208 males), consecutively recruited from three different treatment centers in the western part of Sweden (two of which used 12-step programs (n = 192) and one of which used a psychosocial relapse prevention program

(n = 77)). Before inclusion in the study a psychiatric assessment was conducted and patients with severe psychiatric comorbidity were excluded. Participants included in the study met the diagnostic criteria for alcohol dependence as classified by DSM-IV [10]. In addition, three percent of the participants also met the DSM-IV criteria for other drug abuse/dependencies. The mean age of the subjects was 47.9 ± 10.3 years (ranging from 21 to 71 years). Ninety-one percent had a permanent residence and 83% were employed for which reasons this group can be described as socially stable.

The recruitment procedure for inpatients and outpatients was somewhat different. Patients at an inpatient care unit were asked about participation in the project during the first week in treatment and if accepting interviewed 4-5 days later. In all, 65% of the inpatients agreed to participate. Outpatients were asked about participation during weeks 1–3 in treatment and if accepting interviewed one week later.

2.2. Procedure and Instruments. When arriving to treatment, the individuals were informed about the longitudinal study. Short thereafter they were interviewed by a trained interviewer from the research group. In addition, they also completed a number of psychological self-rating scales. As an interview instrument, the Addiction Severity Index (ASI [11]) was used. This interview assesses the following, on the basis of self-report, life-time, and recent severity of different life-domains: family and social relationships, work and education, somatic symptoms, psychiatric symptoms, alcohol use, use of other drugs, and legal problems. ASI has acceptable reliability and validity [12, 13]. Data on early debut, antisocial behavior, and paternal alcoholism was derived from the ASI. The indicator of debut before the age of 25 was defined as drinking until intoxication three times or more per week before that age. The indicator of antisocial behavior included prosecution for any of the following offences: violent crimes (robbery, assault, murder, or manslaughter), drug-related criminality, or drunken driving. The indicator of paternal alcoholism included answering yes to a question of whether the father had serious alcohol-related problems.

Personality was assessed by the Temperament and Character Inventory (TCI), a 238-item true-false self-rating questionnaire [14]. The TCI assesses four basic dimensions of temperament (novelty seeking (NS), harm avoidance (HA), reward dependence (RD), and persistence (PS)) and three dimensions of character (self-directedness (SD), cooperativeness (CO), and self-transcendence (ST)). The Swedish version of the TCI has earlier showed satisfactory psychometric properties for adults [15].

2.3. Data Processing and Analysis. A Configural Frequency Analysis [16, 17] was conducted with the purpose of finding specific configurations that were more frequent ("types") or less frequent ("antitypes") than expected by chance. We hypothesized that two specific configurations would come up as typical for type I: being a man or woman with late debut of alcohol problems and without signs of antisocial behavior or paternal alcoholism. Further, we hypothesized that one specific configuration would come up as typical for type II: being a man with early debut of alcohol problems, debut with signs of antisocial behavior, and paternal alcoholism.

Next, a crude classification was made to group the individuals in the sample into the two types. This was done by counting criteria (gender, age of debut, antisocial behavior, and paternal alcoholism). Subjects with equal number of type I/II criteria were defined as type I. A more strict classification was also done which only included subjects that fulfilled all the criteria for the respective type. Thereafter the personality profiles according to the TCI were compared between the classified types. Since the results include multiple statistical tests, significant results on the 5% level should be interpreted with caution.

3. Results

The first analysis of the 269 subjects included a test of whether the indicators of type I and type II, respectively, form naturally occurring configurations. This was done by including four important features of the types into a Configural Frequency Analysis. We hypothesized that three configurations would come out as more frequent than expected by chance: male gender, early debut of alcohol problems, antisocial behavior, and paternal alcoholism (type II); male gender, late debut of alcohol problems, no antisocial behavior, and no paternal alcoholism (type I); and female gender, late debut of alcohol problems, no antisocial behavior, and no paternal alcoholism (type I). While the configuration that indicates type II alcoholism came out as a significant type ($P = 0.007$), neither of the two configurations that would constitute type I alcoholism occurred more frequently than expected by chance. One configuration also came out as antitypical (i.e., occurring less frequently than expected by chance), namely, being male, with late debut of alcohol problems, antisocial behavior, and paternal alcoholism ($P = 0.02$). However, one configuration that resembled type I came out as statistically significant (female, late debut of alcohol problems, no antisocial behavior, and paternal alcoholism; $P = 0.008$). In all, 85 subjects out of 269 (i.e., 31.6 percent) could be defined as either type I or type II by the definitions used in this study. See Table 1.

Next, a crude classification was made of the two types, contingent of the number of criteria each subject fulfilled. Based on this classification 192 subjects (or 71.4 percent) were classified as type I and 77 subjects were classified as type II (or 28.6 percent). These two types were thereafter compared with respect to their temperament and character profile on the TCI. While there were no statistically significant differences between the two types with regard to their temperament profile, there were several differences in their character profile. While type I group had higher levels of self-directedness ($F_{(1,216)} = 7.1$; $P = 0.008$) and cooperativeness ($F_{(1,216)} = 4.1$; $P = 0.043$), type II group showed higher levels of self-transcendence ($F_{(1,216)} = 5.6$; $P = 0.019$). When including all temperament and character traits as independent continuous variables and type (I or II)

as dependent one in a logistic regression (Nagelkerke $R^2 = .087$), only self-transcendence remains statistically significant ($P = 0.046$). See Figures 1(a) and 1(b).

While this classification above forced all subjects into any of the two types only a minority could be classified as more strictly defined type I's or more strictly defined type II's. More specifically, 62 subjects fulfilled all the criteria for type I and 23 subjects fulfilled all criteria for type II. When the temperament and character profiles were compared between these two more strictly defined types, type II group came out as more prone to novelty seeking ($F_{(1,73)} = 6.5$; $P = 0.013$) and, quite surprisingly, *more* harm avoidant ($F_{(1,73)} = 6.1$; $P = 0.016$). Furthermore, the pattern regarding character differences was similar to that in the previous analysis.

4. Discussion

This study aimed at examining to what extent type I and type II alcoholism exists as natural clusters and the personality profiles associated with these types. In our results, type II alcoholism occur as a more homogenous type than type I alcoholism and type I alcoholism was too heterogeneous as a phenomenon to be summarized into one single type. Furthermore, it should be noted that less than a third of the study population could be classified in accordance with the typology. This latter finding raises the possibility that this typology is not applicable to socially stable or socially well-preserved alcoholics. If so, this hampers the use of this typology since this group may comprise the majority of alcohol dependent individuals (see Berglund 2009 and references therein).

Our results give support to other typologies that distinguish between different forms of late onset alcoholism. One such example is the typology suggested by Zucker [18, 19] including four types and distinguishing between two late onset types (negative effect alcoholism that includes depression or anxiety) and developmentally cumulative (also labeled "primary alcoholism" without severe comorbidity other than the consequences of the alcohol disorder).

Quite according to theory, individuals that fulfilled the criteria for type II showed higher levels of novelty seeking than did the individuals that were classified as type I alcoholics. However, quite surprisingly, the individuals classified as type II alcoholics also showed higher levels of harm avoidance than did the individuals that were classified as type I alcoholics. This is in line with the overview by Howard et al. [6] stating that the results linking high levels of novelty to type II alcoholism are more consistent than results linking low levels of harm avoidance and reward dependence to type II. Furthermore, not to our surprise, type I alcoholics showed higher levels of self-directedness and cooperativeness and lower levels of self-transcendence than type II alcoholic.

While we believe that this study is relevant and employs a novel methodological approach, it also has some limitations. The main limitation concerns the representativeness of our sample of treatment seeking and, to some degree, socially well-adjusted alcohol dependent individuals. Although treatment seeking individuals often display severe psychiatric

Table 1: Prevalence of different configurations and their relative probability ($n = 269$).

Gender	Early debut (<25 yrs)	Antisocial behavior	Paternal alcoholism	Obs. freq.	Exp. freq.	P (bin. prob.)	Sign type/antitype
Male	Yes	Yes	Yes	23	13.1	0.007	Type
Female	Yes	Yes	Yes	4	3.8	Ns	
Male	No	Yes	Yes	11	20.1	0.02	Antitype
Female	No	Yes	Yes	2	5.9	Ns	
Male	Yes	No	Yes	22	24.4	Ns	
Female	Yes	No	Yes	8	7.2	Ns	
Male	No	No	Yes	33	37.5	Ns	
Female	No	No	Yes	20	11.0	0.008	Type
Male	Yes	Yes	No	17	15.6	Ns	
Female	Yes	Yes	No	2	4.6	Ns	
Male	No	Yes	No	31	23.9	Ns	
Female	No	Yes	No	4	7.0	Ns	
Male	Yes	No	No	23	28.9	Ns	
Female	Yes	No	No	7	8.5	Ns	
Male	No	No	No	48	44.5	Ns	
Female	No	No	No	14	13.1	Ns	

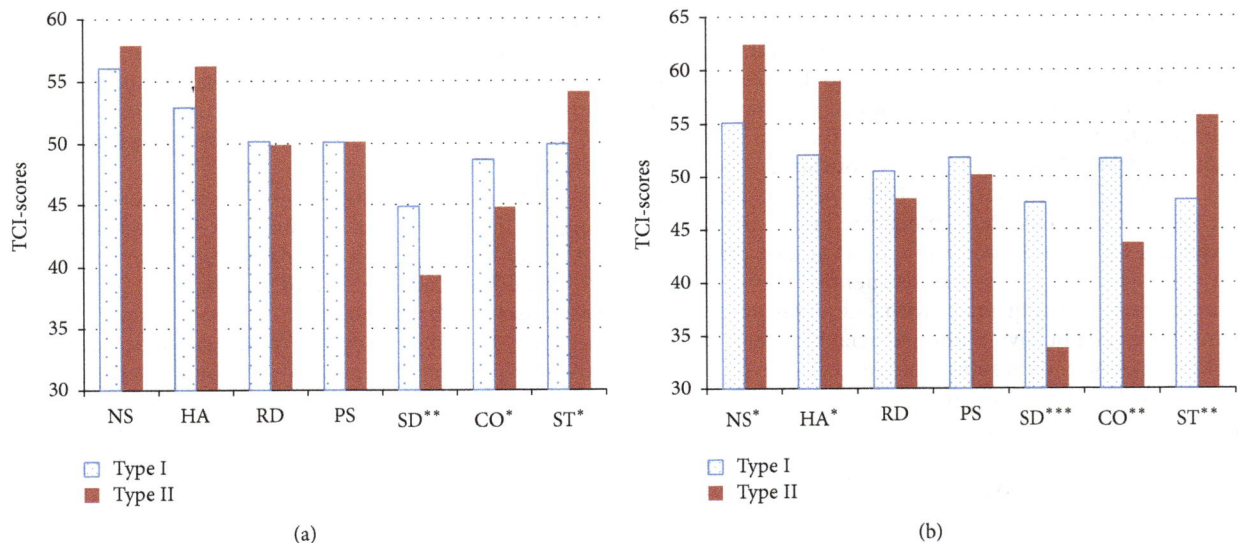

Figure 1: (a) Temperament and character profiles for the type I and type II alcoholics ($n = 218$). $^*P < 0.05$; $^{**}P < 0.01$; NS = novelty seeking, HA = harm avoidance, RD = reward dependence, PS = persistence, SD = self-directedness, CO = cooperativeness, and ST = self-transcendence. (b) Temperament and character profiles for the strictly defined type I and type II alcoholics ($n = 75$). $^*P < 0.05$; $^{**}P < 0.01$; $^{***}P < 0.001$; NS = novelty seeking, HA = harm avoidance, RD = reward dependence, PS = persistence, SD = self-directedness, CO = cooperativeness, ST = self-transcendence.

comorbidity, we have in the present study excluded patients with severe psychiatric comorbidity and therefore the level of comorbidity in this sample is lower than in the general alcohol dependent population. Further, while we have extensive data for every individual in the study, the sample size is relatively small.

Studies on alcohol typologies call for an integration of finding from genetics, personality, and social psychology into a developmental model. To be valuable as an intellectual tool, typologies should also be clinically relevant. Future research within this project will focus on the validity of other common alcohol typologies and an examination of the clinical relevance of these typologies in terms of treatment outcome.

Conflict of Interests

The authors declare that there is no conflict of interests regarding the publication of this paper.

References

[1] L. R. Bergman, "The application of a person oriented approach: types and clusters," in *Developmental Science and the Holistic Approach*, L. R. Bergman, R. B. Cairns, L.-G. Nilsson, and L. Nystedt, Eds., pp. 137–154, Lawrence Erlbaum Associates, Mahwah, NJ, USA, 2000.

[2] C. R. Cloninger, M. Bohman, and S. Sigvardsson, "Inheritance of alcohol abuse. Cross-fostering analysis of adopted men," *Archives of General Psychiatry*, vol. 38, no. 8, pp. 861–868, 1981.

[3] M. Bohman, S. Sigvardsson, and C. R. Cloninger, "Maternal inheritance of alcohol abuse: cross-fostering analysis of adopted women," *Archives of General Psychiatry*, vol. 38, no. 9, pp. 965–969, 1981.

[4] C. R. Cloninger, S. Sigvardsson, and M. Bohman, "Type I and type II alcoholism: an update," *Alcohol Health & Research World*, vol. 20, pp. 18–23, 1996.

[5] T. A. Wills, D. Vaccaro, and G. McNamara, "Novelty seeking, risk taking, and related constructs as predictors of adolescent substance use: an application of Cloninger's theory," *Journal of Substance Abuse*, vol. 6, no. 1, pp. 1–20, 1994.

[6] M. O. Howard, D. Kivlahan, and R. D. Walker, "Cloninger's tridimensional theory of personality and psychopathology: applications to substance use disorders," *Journal of Studies on Alcohol*, vol. 58, no. 1, pp. 48–66, 1997.

[7] K. Berglund, U. Berggren, C. Fahlke, and J. Balldin, "Self-reported health functioning in Swedish alcohol-dependent individuals: age and gender perspectives," *Nordic Journal of Psychiatry*, vol. 62, no. 5, pp. 405–412, 2008.

[8] K. J. Berglund, J. Balldin, U. Berggren, A. Gerdner, and C. Fahlke, "Childhood maltreatment affects the serotonergic system in male alcohol-dependent individuals," *Alcoholism: Clinical and Experimental Research*, vol. 37, no. 5, pp. 757–762, 2013.

[9] C. Fahlke, U. Berggren, K. J. Berglund et al., "Neuroendocrine assessment of serotonergic, dopaminergic, and noradrenergic functions in alcohol-dependent individuals," *Alcoholism: Clinical and Experimental Research*, vol. 36, no. 1, pp. 97–103, 2012.

[10] American Psychiatric Association, *Diagnostic and Statistical Manual of Mental Disorders*, American Psychiatric Association, Washington, DC, USA, 1st edition, 994.

[11] A. T. McLellan, H. Kushner, D. Metzger et al., "The fifth edition of the addiction severity index," *Journal of Substance Abuse Treatment*, vol. 9, pp. 199–213, 1992.

[12] C. Leonhard, K. Mulvey, D. R. Gastfriend, and M. Shwartz, "The Addiction Severity Index: a field study of internal consistency and validity," *Journal of Substance Abuse Treatment*, vol. 18, no. 2, pp. 129–135, 2000.

[13] B. E. Stöffelmayr, B. E. Mavis, and R. M. Kasim, "The longitudinal stability of the addiction severity index," *Journal of Substance Abuse Treatment*, vol. 11, no. 4, pp. 373–378, 1994.

[14] C. R. Cloninger, T. R. Przybeck, D. M. Svrakic, and R. D. Wetzel, *The Temperament and Character Inventory (TCI): A Guide to Its Development and Use*, Center for Psychobiology of Personality, Washington University, St. Louis, Mo, USA, 1994.

[15] S. Brändström, S. Sigvardsson, P.-O. Nylander, and J. Richter, "The Swedish version of the Temperament and Character Inventory (TCI): a cross-validation of age and gender influences," *European Journal of Psychological Assessment*, vol. 24, no. 1, pp. 14–21, 2008.

[16] A. von Eye, *Configural frequency analysis-Methods, models, and applications*, Lawrence Erlbaum, Mahwah, NJ, USA, 2001.

[17] A. von Eye, C. Spiel, and P. K. Wood, "CFA models, tests, interpretation, and alternatives: a rejoinder," *Applied Psychology: An International Review*, vol. 45, no. 4, pp. 345–352, 1996.

[18] R. A. Zucker, "The four alcoholisms: a developmental account of the etiologic process," in *Proceedings of the Nebraska Symposium on Motivation. Alcohol and Addictive Behaviors*, P. C. Rivers, Ed., vol. 34, pp. 27–83, University of Nebraska Press, Lincoln, Neb, USA, 1987.

[19] R. A. Zucker, "Pathways to alcohol problems and alcoholism: A developmental account of the evidence for multiple alcoholisms and for contextual contributions to risk," in *The Development of Alcohol Problems: Exploring the Biopsychosocial Matrix of Risk*, R. Zucker, G. Boyd, and J. Howard, Eds., NIAAA Research Monograph No. 26, pp. 255–289, NIAAA, Rockville, Md, USA, 1994.

9

The Effectiveness and Applicability of Compensatory Cognitive Training for Japanese Patients with Schizophrenia: A Pilot Study

Sadao Otsuka,[1] **Mie Matsui,**[1] **Takatoshi Hoshino,**[1] **Kayoko Miura,**[1] **Yuko Higuchi,**[2] **and Michio Suzuki**[2]

[1]*Department of Psychology, Graduate School of Medicine and Pharmaceutical Sciences, University of Toyama, Toyama 930-0194, Japan*
[2]*Department of Neuropsychiatry, Graduate School of Medicine and Pharmaceutical Sciences, University of Toyama, Toyama 930-0194, Japan*

Correspondence should be addressed to Mie Matsui; mmatsui@las.u-toyama.ac.jp

Academic Editor: Raphael J. Braga

Although cognitive remediation or training for schizophrenia has been developed, few studies on the subject have focused on Japanese patients. The aim of the present study was to examine the effectiveness and applicability of compensatory cognitive training (CCT) in Japanese patients with schizophrenia. Twenty-six participants diagnosed with schizophrenia were assigned to either the CCT plus treatment as usual group ($n = 13$) or the treatment as usual alone group ($n = 13$). CCT is a 12-session, manualized, group-based training that coaches compensatory strategies in four cognitive domains (prospective memory, attention, verbal memory, and executive functions). Cognitive, functional, and clinical symptom measures were implemented at baseline, after treatment, and at 3-month follow-up. Mixed design analyses of variance with group and time for each measure demonstrated that effects of CCT on verbal memory, processing speed, and social functioning at postintervention were significant, and the effects on processing speed were maintained at follow-up. Our study suggests that CCT has beneficial effects on cognitive performance, improving functional outcomes in Japanese patients with schizophrenia. Additionally, the high degrees of attendance rates and level of satisfaction rated by the CCT participants ensure the applicability of this methodology to this population.

1. Introduction

Cognitive impairment is broadly considered as one of the core components of schizophrenia, along with well-known psychotic symptoms such as positive and negative symptoms [1]. Previous studies have reported that the severity of cognitive impairments in individuals with schizophrenia is related to difficulties in social participation and could predict later functional outcomes including employment and independence in everyday living, though the explained variance in functional outcomes was modest [2–6]. While the progress of antipsychotic medications can serve to reduce positive symptoms dramatically, improvements in everyday functioning and the promotion of social participation remain as issues to be solved. Consequently, there is strong interest in advancing interventions aimed at improving cognitive performance, leading to the enhancement of everyday and social functioning in individuals with schizophrenia.

Cognitive impairments in schizophrenia are evident in a wide range of domains, including attention, memory, and executive functions [7–10]. The psychotic symptoms in schizophrenia are manifested more commonly in adolescents and young adults and require lifelong treatment to stabilize. In contrast, cognitive impairments are known to appear before the symptomatic manifestation of the illness [11–14] and are relatively stable over time after the onset of the illness [15]. Importantly, performance on the cognitive tasks shows the weakest or no relationship with positive symptoms, though a significant relationship with negative symptoms is reported [16–20]. These findings support the idea that cognitive impairments in schizophrenia are relatively independent of psychotic symptoms, or at least of positive symptoms [1].

The treatment of schizophrenia predominantly relies on pharmaceutical drugs. Thus, there are a number of studies examining the improvement effects of antipsychotic drugs on cognitive impairments in schizophrenia. Specifically, studies report that significant effects of antipsychotic drugs on cognitive functions were observed when comparing cognitive performance before and after treatment, but no differences were observed when comparing the effects of atypical and typical drugs on cognitive performance [21, 22]. In addition, the magnitude of cognitive improvements associated with atypical drugs is relatively small and in fact is similar to practice effects in healthy controls [23]. Thus, the effects of antipsychotic medications on cognitive functions are far from satisfactory, and little is known about the improvement effects of antipsychotic drugs on everyday and social functioning in patients with schizophrenia.

Against this background, cognitive remediation or training for schizophrenia has been developed as a psychosocial therapeutic approach to directly address cognitive impairments. Cognitive remediation is defined as "a behavioral training-based intervention that aims to improve cognitive processes (attention, memory, executive function, social cognition, or metacognition) with the goal of durability and generalization" [24]. The effectiveness of cognitive remediation has been repeatedly demonstrated through randomized controlled trials and meta-analyses. For example, Wykes et al. [24] conducted a meta-analysis and showed that the improvement effect of cognitive remediation on global cognition was medium (Cohen's $d = 0.45$, group comparison after treatment). This study also showed that the effects of cognitive remediation on global cognition were durable after the completion of the intervention ($d = 0.43$, a comparison between pretreatment and follow-up evaluations within the cognitive remediation group). The effect sizes reported in their meta-analytic study on the respective cognitive domains were small to medium ($d = 0.25$ on attention, $d = 0.26$ on processing speed, $d = 0.35$ on verbal working memory, $d = 0.41$ on verbal learning/memory, $d = 0.57$ on reasoning/problem solving, and $d = 0.65$ on social cognition). The effect sizes did not differ according to the type of intervention approach, duration of treatment, or use of computers. In addition, the authors found that cognitive remediation had a small-to-medium effect (0.42) on functional outcomes. Regarding the effectiveness of cognitive remediation on psychosocial functioning, McGurk et al. [25] conducted a meta-analysis and demonstrated that cognitive remediation programs that used strategy coaching in addition to the drill-and-practice method had greater effects ($d = 0.62$) when compared to programs using the drill-and-practice method alone ($d = 0.24$). Wykes et al. [24] also confirmed this finding.

These findings suggest that we could expect to obtain equivalent effects of cognitive remediation in Japanese individuals with schizophrenia. However, to date, only four studies have reported the effectiveness and validity of cognitive remediation for schizophrenia in Japan, all without

referring to strategy coaching [26–29]. Therefore, in this study, we focused on a compensatory cognitive training (CCT) that includes strategy coaching developed by Twamley and colleagues, the effectiveness of which has been sufficiently demonstrated in the US [30, 31]. Although the term "strategy coaching" is not well defined, it commonly includes instructions on using cognitive or behavioral strategies to cope with cognitive activities effectively, to avoid overloading one's cognitive capability. The characteristic feature of CCT is that the approach focuses on compensatory strategies that the participants can use on their own in real-world conditions. Compensatory approach, in contrast to restorative approaches such as utilizing repetitive drill practices [32, 33], is intended for the participants to acquire new ways to apply their capability in order to compensate for the cognitive impairments and interact with the world suitably. The compensatory strategies coached in the CCT intervention include not only the use of external or environmental aids (e.g., writing down the things to do later) but also internal or psychological attempts (using categorization or visual imagery to retain information). Specifically, acquisition of these internal strategies would improve cognitive performance evaluated using neuropsychological tests, without the use of any external tools during a test circumstance and any drill in the CCT intervention, as reported in previous studies [30, 31]. We translated the therapist's manual and the participant's workbook of CCT [30, 31] into Japanese and partially modified them while considering the cultural backgrounds of the Japanese participants. The following modifications were made. First, changes to the scenarios used for role-play training were made and some scenarios were added. Second, the commonly used "Goroawase" method was added, in which the participants create a meaningful sentence by utilizing the phonological aspects of a series of digits (like a wordplay), when memorizing digits such as a phone number or a year in which a historical event occurred. As a preliminary step of effect research on CCT for Japanese patients with schizophrenia, we need to confirm that the Japanese version has not lost the advantages of CCT during the translation process and after the modifications mentioned above.

The aim of this pilot study was to examine the effectiveness and applicability of CCT for Japanese patients with schizophrenia. We predicted that the application of CCT in Japanese patients with schizophrenia would benefit cognitive and functional outcomes, as was noted in previous studies [30, 31]. The improvement effects of CCT on cognitive performance combined with antipsychotic medication would be greater than the effectiveness of antipsychotic medication alone. In addition, CCT should positively operate upon the everyday and social functioning of patients with improvements in cognitive performance. We expected these improvement effects to be durable at follow-up evaluations implemented several months after the completion of the CCT intervention. We also expected that the CCT intervention would be feasible with Japanese individuals with schizophrenia, as reflected in high attendance rates and high satisfaction reported by participants.

2. Method

2.1. Protocol. The study protocol is presented in Figure 1. Our trial compared CCT plus treatment as usual (CCT group) with treatment as usual alone (TAU group). The CCT intervention was delivered over 12 weeks in weekly 2-hour group sessions for the CCT group. Cognitive measures (neuropsychological tests), functional measures (questionnaires asking participants and their families about everyday and social functioning), and clinical symptom measures were implemented at preintervention (baseline, T1), immediately following the completion of CCT (postintervention, T2), and three months following the completion of CCT (follow-up, T3), to evaluate the efficacy of CCT. It was explained to the participants in both groups that the tests would assess their current status, and they were encouraged to perform well to the extent that they could at the three time points. Clinical symptoms were assessed by the Scale for the Assessment of Positive Symptoms [34] and the Scale for the Assessment of Negative Symptoms [35]. The study was approved by the Committee on Medical Ethics of the University of Toyama, and all participants provided written informed consent prior to participating in the study.

2.2. Participants. Participants included inpatients and outpatients recruited from the same hospital. All participants were diagnosed with schizophrenia or schizoaffective disorder according to DSM-IV-TR criteria [36]. The participants were aged 18 years or older and showed evidence of cognitive difficulties (i.e., scored more than 1 SD below average on at least one of the neuropsychological tests at baseline). They maintained a stable dose of medication for at least 1 month prior to inclusion in the study. The following exclusion criteria were applied: neurological illness, traumatic head injury, current substance or alcohol abuse, and an estimate of premorbid IQ > 90 as assessed by the Japanese Adult Reading Test (JART) [37]. The demographic and clinical characteristics of the participants are presented in Table 1.

Twenty-six participants were enrolled in the study. We used posters and brochures to recruit patients for the study. All participants were recommended for the study by their attending psychiatrist. Thirteen participants were assigned to the CCT group and the other 13 to the TAU group. The CCT and TAU groups did not differ statistically on age, gender, years of education, duration of illness, age at onset, antipsychotic dose (risperidone equivalents) [38], symptom severity, or any of the neuropsychological tests at the beginning of the CCT intervention (i.e., baseline). More than half the participants were living with their families (65%), about one-third were in the hospital (31%), and only one participant was living alone (4%). Some participants worked part-time (12%) and the others were unemployed (88%). In the CCT group, 12 participants completed the postintervention evaluations and 11 completed the follow-up evaluations; in the TAU group, 11 completed the postintervention evaluations and 8 completed the follow-up evaluations.

2.3. CCT Intervention. The CCT intervention delivered in the study was a 12-session, manualized, group-based training

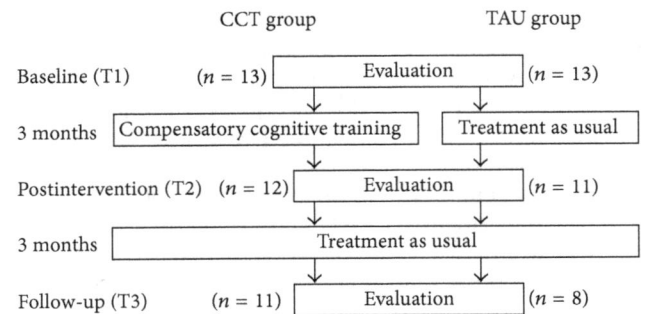

FIGURE 1: Flowchart of the study design. CCT: compensatory cognitive training. TAU: treatment as usual. n: number of patients who finished evaluations at each time point. The CCT group received the CCT intervention plus treatment as usual for 3 months after baseline evaluations. The TAU group received treatment as usual for 3 months after baseline evaluations. After that, both groups underwent postintervention assessment and follow-up evaluations after 3 months of treatment as usual.

focusing on the 4 cognitive domains presented in Table 2. The CCT groups consisted of fewer than 6 participants and more than 2 therapists who were certified clinical psychologists and a doctoral-level clinical neuropsychologist. Before starting the study, we role-played all 12 sessions with members of our laboratory as staff training in order to enhance the fidelity of the treatment procedure and refine the Japanese manual.

In this approach, homework assignments are important. Homework is assigned at the end of each session and enables participants to identify situations in which they would use a given strategy. In addition, participants are provided with an opportunity to troubleshoot any difficulties concerning the homework at the beginning of each session. These procedures encourage participants to develop learned strategies into new habits in their real-world circumstances. The learning of habits has been shown to be intact in individuals with schizophrenia [39, 40], and habits are particularly resistant to forgetting [41]. Thus, the effects of the compensatory approach based on habit learning are expected to endure for a longer period of time and be generalized to everyday living and social activities.

CCT covers prospective memory, attention/vigilance, verbal learning/memory, and executive functions, in that order. These four cognitive domains were selected based on their degree of impairment in schizophrenia spectrum disorders, relevance for psychosocial functioning, and potential modifiability [4, 42, 43]. In addition, CCT has the following features: no use of computer and being delivered anywhere, interactive, game-like format as much as possible to maintain the interest and attention of participants, and a workbook whereby participants could review the things they had worked on anywhere and anytime. A short break between the first and second hours of each session is given to reduce fatigue (see [30, 31] for more details).

2.4. Measures

2.4.1. Cognitive Measures. The neuropsychological tests were implemented as cognitive measures in the following cognitive

TABLE 1: Baseline group comparison of participants ($n = 26$).

	CCT ($n = 13$) Mean (SD)	TAU ($n = 13$) Mean (SD)	t or χ^2	p value	d
Demographics					
Age (years)	34.6 (10.2)	39.5 (8.9)	1.31	0.20	0.51
Gender (% male)	61.5%	46.2%	0.62	0.43	
Education (years)	14.7 (1.5)	14.0 (1.8)	1.06	0.30	0.42
Illness burden					
Illness duration (years)	11.8 (6.8)	16.5 (9.4)	1.61	0.16	0.57
Age at onset (years)	22.8 (6.6)	22.9 (7.5)	0.01	0.94	0.02
Antipsychotic dose (mg/day, RPD equivalent)	5.5 (3.6)	5.7 (3.6)	0.11	0.91	0.06
SAPS positive symptoms	19.5 (14.3)	29.4 (21.8)	1.36	0.19	0.54
SANS negative symptoms	43.3 (17.4)	43.5 (20.0)	0.12	0.98	0.01
Cognitive functions					
Verbal memory					
JVLT total score	29.5 (6.9)	28.1 (7.7)	0.74	0.62	0.19
RBMT immediate recall	13.2 (4.9)	13.0 (4.7)	0.10	0.92	0.04
Processing speed					
Digit symbol raw score	70.5 (16.0)	76.2 (21.2)	0.77	0.45	0.30
TMT-A time	40.0 (13.2)	35.9 (11.4)	0.84	0.41	0.33
Executive functioning					
WCST completed category	5.5 (1.7)	5.2 (2.1)	0.42	0.68	0.16
TMT-B time	77.6 (34.7)	75.8 (24.3)	0.15	0.88	0.06

RPD = risperidone, SAPS = Scale for Positive Symptoms, SANS = Scale for Negative Symptoms, JVLT = Japanese Verbal Learning Test, RBMT = Rivermead Behavioral Memory Test, TMT-A = Trail Making Test-A, WCST = Wisconsin Card Sorting Test, and TMT-B = Trail Making Test-B.

TABLE 2: Domains and strategies included in compensatory cognitive training [31].

Targeted domain	Importance for everyday functioning	Compensatory strategies
Prospective memory	(i) Remembering to go to work or school (ii) Remembering to take medications (iii) Remembering to turn in school assignments (iv) Remembering to do assigned tasks at work in response to cues	(1) Daily calendar use (2) To-do lists and prioritizing tasks (3) Linking tasks by using reminders or using routines to automate tasks (4) Automatic place
Attention and vigilance	(i) Paying attention to communications from supervisors and coworkers (ii) Maintaining attention in class or while studying (iii) Maintaining attention for work tasks or household projects without getting distracted	(1) Conversational vigilance skills (reduce distractions, eye contact, paraphrasing, and asking questions) (2) Task vigilance skills (use self-talk during tasks to maintain focus, taking breaks to refocus)
Learning and memory	(i) Learning and remembering work tasks (ii) Learning novel information in school or vocational training (iii) Learning and remembering names of supervisors and coworkers	(1) Encoding strategies (taking notes, paraphrasing, association, chunking, categorizing, acronyms, rhymes, visual imagery, and overlearning) (2) Retrieval strategies (3) Name-learning strategies
Executive functioning	(i) Problem solving and coping with unexpected situations on the job or in vocational training, or at home (ii) Being able to balance demands of work/school with home/family needs (iii) Thinking flexibly and self-monitoring performance at work	(1) 6-step problem solving method (define problem, brainstorm solutions, evaluate solutions systematically, select a solution, try it, and evaluate how it worked) (2) Self-talk while solving problems (3) Hypothesis testing (4) Self-monitoring

domains. All measures were administered by experienced psychologists trained in standardized testing procedures.

(1) Verbal learning/memory: the Japanese Verbal Learning Test (JVLT) [44, 45] based on Gold et al. [46], in which scores are given for the number of words recalled immediately (0–48) and after a delay (0–16, see [44, 45] for more details), and the story subtest of the Japanese version of the Rivermead Behavioral Memory Test (RBMT) [47, 48], where scores are given for the number of sentences recalled immediately (0–25) and after a delay (0–25).

(2) Processing speed: digit symbols subtest of the Japanese version of the Wechsler Adult Intelligence Scale, third edition (WAIS-III) [49, 50], in which scores (0–133) are given for the number of symbols copied within 120 s, and the Trail Making Test part A (TMT-A) [51], in which the time taken to complete the test was scored.

(3) Executive function: Wisconsin Card Sorting Test (WCST) [52, 53], where the number of categories completed was scored (0–6), and the Japanese version of the Trail Making Test part B (TMT-B) [10, 51], in which the time taken to complete the task was scored.

These cognitive measures, including some measures which were different from those used in previous studies [30, 31], were selected according to the content in the training (e.g., the RBMT story test for conversational attention, processing speed tests for task attention) and the possibility of improved performance in the tasks by applying the coached strategies. Prospective memory performance could be inferred from the attendance rate of the participants to some extent, although there was no standardized test with which to measure this domain in Japanese.

2.4.2. Functional Measures. The Social Functioning Scale Japanese version (SFS-J) [54, 55] was implemented as functional measures. SFS-J evaluates the functioning in everyday and social living, reported by participants and their families (score range: 0–226).

2.5. Data Analyses. The statistical analyses were administered based on the intent-to-treat principle and therefore included all available data from the 26 participants completing the baseline evaluations regardless of whether they adhered to treatment (see Table 1). In order to compare the results of each measure on cognitive functions, everyday/social functioning, and clinical symptoms at three time points (baseline, T1; postintervention, T2; follow-up, T3), we performed two-way mixed factor analyses of variance (ANOVAs) with group (CCT versus TAU) as a between-subject factor and time points (T1 versus T2 versus T3) as a within-subject factor. In these analyses, we adjusted the significance level (alpha) for the ANOVAs with Bonferroni correction. In the study, we focused on group-by-time interactions because the CCT intervention was considered effective when the improvement effects in the CCT group were beyond the

effects of medication or natural course of time seen in the TAU group. Furthermore, we performed follow-up t-tests with Bonferroni correction (T2 versus T1, T3 versus T1) to examine changes from the baseline of each measure when the significant interactions were detected. In addition, we calculated Cohen's d [56] using the change scores from baseline (T2-T1, T3-T1) of each measure to evaluate the magnitude of improvement effects with or without the CCT intervention.

3. Results

Table 3 presents the results of the mixed ANOVAs in terms of group-by-time interactions for all measures. The patterns of the significant interaction are seen in Figure 2. Two of the 11 participants in the CCT group who completed follow-up evaluations did not answer the questionnaires, so we analyzed data from 9 participants in the CCT group and 8 in the TAU group regarding functional measures.

3.1. Effects on Cognitive Functions. Regarding verbal memory, significant group-by-time interactions were found for JVLT total recall ($F = 5.25$, $p = 0.018$, and $\eta_p^2 = 0.479$). A series of Bonferroni-corrected paired comparisons revealed that the CCT group showed significant improvements in JVLT total recall at postintervention compared to baseline ($t = 2.80$, $p = 0.027$, and $d = 1.26$). In contrast, the TAU group did not show any changes from baseline on this measure ($t = 1.21$, $p = 0.839$, and $d = -0.47$). Additionally, a similar trend was found on RBMT story immediate recall. The interaction was close to significance ($F = 3.65$, $p = 0.049$, and $\eta_p^2 = 0.313$), and paired comparisons indicated that the CCT group but not the TAU group showed significant improvements from baseline at postintervention ($t = 3.28$, $p = 0.021$, and $d = 0.81$, Bonferroni-corrected). As for the follow-up period, there were no significant differences from baseline on all measures of verbal memory ($ts \leq 2.47$, $ps \geq 0.080$, and $ds \leq 0.61$). That is, the improvement effects seen in the CCT group at postintervention were not maintained several months after the completion of CCT.

As shown in Table 3, significant interactions were found in processing speeds for both WAIS-III digit symbol and TMT-A ($Fs \geq 5.09$, $ps \leq 0.020$, and $\eta_p^2 \geq 0.389$). A series of paired comparisons indicated that the CCT group showed significant improvements from baseline on both digit symbol ($t = 6.09$, $p = 0.002$, and $d = 0.66$) and TMT-A ($t = 5.36$, $p = 0.000$, and $d = 1.01$) at the postintervention period. Furthermore, the CCT group performed better at follow-up on both digit symbol ($t = 3.66$, $p = 0.002$, and $d = 0.57$) and TMT-A ($t = 2.66$, $p = 0.030$, and $d = 0.59$) compared to baseline, suggesting that the improvements seen in the CCT group on these cognitive measures were maintained for several months. The TAU group did not show significant changes on these measures at postintervention or follow-up compared to baseline ($ts \leq 2.25$, $ps \geq 0.214$, and $d \leq 0.70$).

Regarding executive function, no significant interactions were found on WCST or TMT-B, as shown in Table 3 ($Fs \leq 1.12$, $ps \geq 0.350$, and $\eta_p^2 \leq 0.123$).

TABLE 3: Means and standard deviations of evaluation time by group and group-by-time interaction effects.

	CCT group T1 Mean (SD)	CCT group T2 Mean (SD)	CCT group T3 Mean (SD)	TAU group T1 Mean (SD)	TAU group T2 Mean (SD)	TAU group T3 Mean (SD)	Interaction F	Interaction p value	η_p^2
Neuropsychological scores									
Verbal memory			($n = 11$)			($n = 8$)			
JVLT recall total	28.9 (6.1)	35.9 (5.0)	31.1 (7.0)	26.5 (6.5)	23.8 (4.9)	24.4 (7.5)	5.25	**0.018**	**0.396**
RBMT immediate recall	13.1 (4.2)	16.1 (3.1)	15.0 (5.2)	12.6 (5.4)	11.4 (5.8)	12.9 (5.5)	3.65	0.049	0.313
JVLT delayed recall	11.4 (2.9)	13.1 (2.7)	12.2 (2.8)	10.5 (2.3)	8.6 (3.1)	8.5 (3.4)	2.77	0.093	0.257
RBMT delayed recall	11.6 (4.0)	14.4 (4.0)	14.6 (5.7)	11.4 (5.2)	10.9 (6.2)	10.9 (4.8)	3.03	0.077	0.274
Processing speed									
Digit symbol raw score	70.6 (14.8)	80.7 (15.7)	79.5 (16.2)	76.3 (18.0)	78.0 (16.9)	76.3 (16.7)	7.37	**0.005**	**0.479**
TMT-A time	39.8 (14.4)	27.2 (10.3)	31.0 (15.3)	38.0 (11.1)	34.5 (11.1)	31.1 (8.51)	5.09	**0.020**	**0.389**
Executive functioning			($n = 9$)			($n = 8$)			
WCST completed categories	5.4 (1.8)	6.0 (0.0)	6.0 (0.0)	5.3 (2.1)	5.0 (2.1)	4.5 (2.8)	1.12	0.350	0.123
TMT-B time	75.6 (36.2)	65.9 (35.1)	68.0 (29.3)	74.3 (27.4)	69.4 (18.5)	66.5 (31.2)	0.23	0.796	0.028
Functional outcomes			($n = 11$)			($n = 8$)			
Social functioning, SFS-J	93.7 (25.4)	109.2 (17.8)	105.3 (23.3)	109.5 (20.5)	108.9 (24.4)	119.1 (21.3)	2.16	0.152	0.244
SFS-J for family	94.8 (27.5)	120.6 (28.6)	105.4 (25.4)	102.0 (21.9)	96.8 (25.1)	102.0 (32.8)	6.91	**0.008**	**0.483**
Clinical symptoms									
SAPS positive symptoms	15.7 (11.8)	9.1 (12.8)	8.4 (10.4)	33.9 (26.1)	31.0 (26.0)	32.4 (35.1)	1.15	0.341	0.126
SANS negative symptoms	42.5 (17.2)	38.2 (9.9)	37.1 (9.5)	51.5 (13.2)	46.8 (11.7)	44.9 (11.7)	0.03	0.972	0.004

T1 = baseline evaluation time, T2 = postintervention evaluation time, T3 = follow-up evaluation time, JVLT = Japanese Verbal Learning Test, RBMT = Rivermead Behavioral Memory Test, TMT-A = Trail Making Test-A, WCST = Wisconsin Card Sorting Test, TMT-B = Trail Making Test-B, SFS-J = Social Functioning Scale, Japanese version, SAPS = Scale for Positive Symptoms, and SANS = Scale for Negative Symptoms.

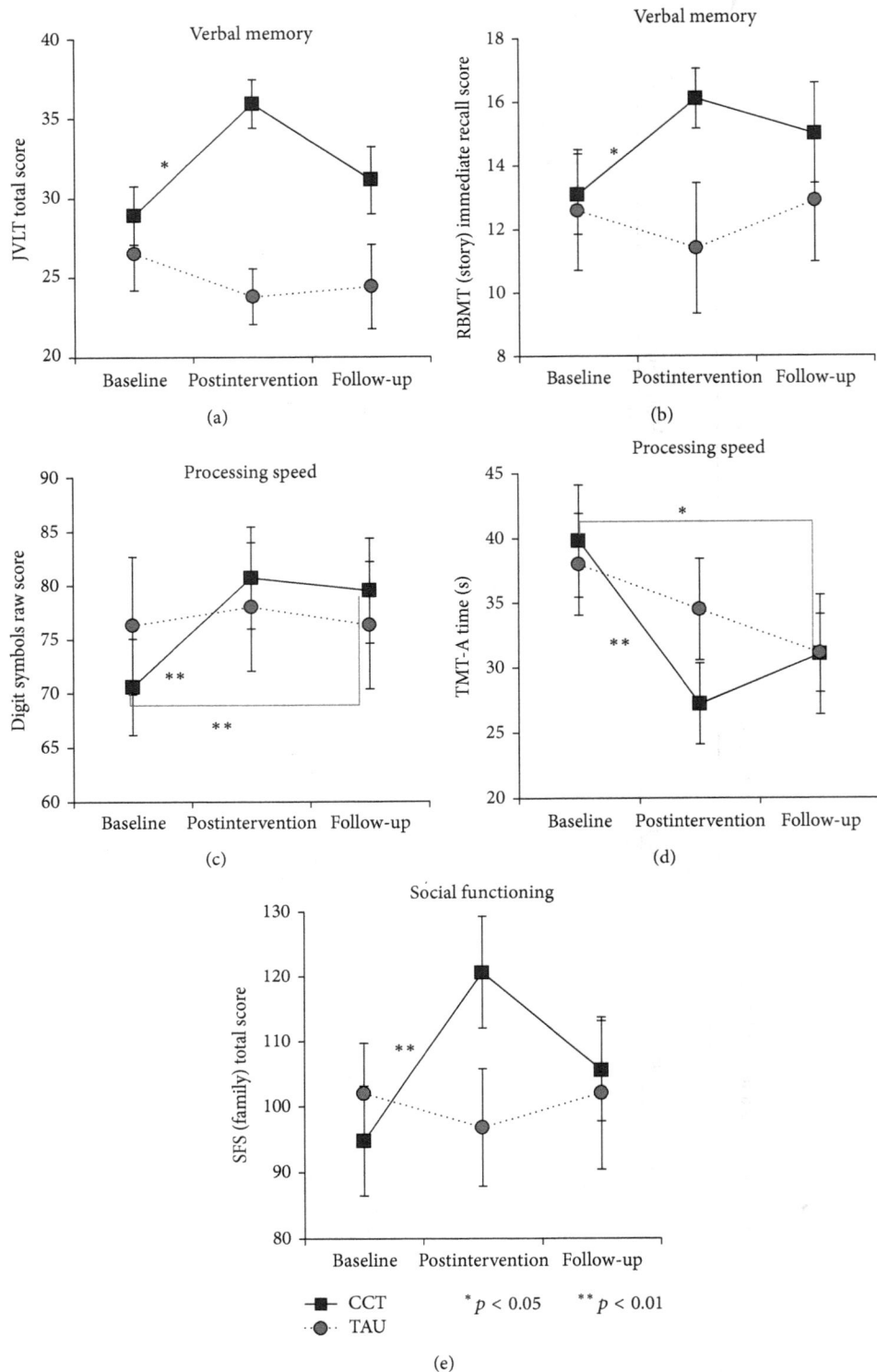

FIGURE 2: Means and standard deviations by evaluation times and outcome scores for each group. Square: compensatory cognitive training group; Circle: treatment as usual group. ((a), (b)) For verbal memory, ((c), (d)) for processing speed, and (e) for social functioning. The horizontal axis indicates evaluation times. Baseline: before CCT intervention, postintervention: after 3-month CCT intervention, and follow-up: 3 months after postintervention. The vertical axis indicates outcome scores. (a) Total score (0–48) of the Japanese Verbal Learning Test, (b) immediate recall score (0–25) of the story subtest from the Rivermead Behavioural Memory Test, (c) raw score (0–133) of the digit symbol subtest from the Wechsler Adult Intelligence Scale—Third Edition, (d) time required to finish the Trail Making Test part A in seconds, and (e) total score (0–226) of Social Functioning Scale, Japanese version, rated by participants' family members. Error bars denote ±1 SD.

3.2. Effects on Everyday and Social Functioning. Of two measures, only the interaction on SFS-J score rated by participants' family members was significant ($F = 6.91$, $p = 0.008$, and $\eta_p^2 = 0.483$). A series of paired comparisons revealed that the CCT group showed significant improvements on social functioning at the postintervention period compared to baseline ($t = 3.44$, $p = 0.004$, and $d = 0.92$) but that the TAU group showed no change ($t = -0.95$, $p = 1.000$, and $d = 0.22$). At the follow-up period, both groups did not show any significant changes compared to baseline ($ts \leq 2.07$, $ps \geq 0.250$, and $d \leq 0.40$), suggesting that the improvement effects seen in the CCT group on the SFS-J for families at postintervention were not maintained for several months.

3.3. Effects on Clinical Symptoms. As for clinical symptoms, no significant interactions were observed for both positive and negative symptoms, as seen in Table 3 ($Fs \leq 1.15$, $ps \geq 0.341$, and $\eta_p^2 \leq 0.126$).

3.4. Effect Sizes. The effect sizes of the CCT intervention were calculated using the change scores from baseline for all measures to contrast the magnitude of the improvement effects between the groups. Table 4 presents the effect sizes of the CCT intervention. Regarding verbal memory, CCT had medium-to-large effect sizes on JVLT immediate recall, delayed recall ($d = 0.95, 0.69$), and RBMT story immediate recall and delayed recall ($d = 1.00, 0.88$) at postintervention. Furthermore, the equivalent effect sizes of CCT were maintained at follow-up (JVLT, $d = 0.55, 0.75$; RBMT, $d = 0.50, 0.85$, resp.).

Large effect sizes of CCT were found in processing speed in both WAIS-III digit symbol ($d = 0.97$) and TMT-A ($d = 1.22$) at postintervention. The equivalent effect size of CCT on digit symbol was maintained at follow-up ($d = 1.29$), but not the effect size on TMT-A ($d = 0.19$). Regarding executive functions, there were small-to-large effect sizes on WCST ($d = 0.58$) and TMT-B ($d = 0.33$) at postintervention. The effect sizes on WCST were maintained at follow-up ($d = 0.71$). On the other hand, the effect size on TMT-B ($d = -0.01$) was not maintained.

With regard to functional measures, the CCT intervention had medium-to-large effect sizes on the SFS-J rated by the participants themselves and their families at postintervention ($d = 0.47$ and 1.56, resp.). The effect size of the self-rating was not maintained ($d = 0.011$) while that of family rating decreased ($d = 0.049$). Regarding the measures on clinical symptoms, a small-to-medium effect ($d = 0.52$) was found on positive symptoms at postintervention, and the effect was maintained at follow-up ($d = 0.48$); however, there were no effects on negative symptoms at both times ($d = 0.02$ and 0.08, resp.).

4. Discussion

The study examined the effectiveness and applicability of CCT for Japanese patients with schizophrenia. Compared to participants receiving treatment consisting mainly of medication as usual (i.e., the TAU group), those receiving

TABLE 4: Effect sizes for group differences in change scores.

	Postintervention T2-T1	Follow-up T3-T1
Neuropsychological scores		
Verbal memory		
JVLT recall total	0.95	0.55
RBMT immediate recall	1.00	0.50
JVLT delayed recall	0.69	0.75
RBMT delayed recall	0.88	0.85
Processing speed		
Digit symbols raw score	0.97	1.29
TMT-A time	1.22	0.19
Executive functioning		
WCST completed categories	0.58	0.71
TMT-B time	0.33	-0.01
Functional outcomes		
Social functioning (SFS-J)	0.47	0.11
(SFS-J for family)	1.56	0.49
Clinical symptoms		
SAPS positive symptoms	0.52	0.48
SANS negative symptoms	0.02	0.08

T1 = baseline evaluation time, T2 = postintervention evaluation time, T3 = follow-up evaluation time, JVLT = Japanese Verbal Learning Test, RBMT = Rivermead Behavioral Memory Test, TMT-A = Trail Making Test-A, WCST = Wisconsin Card Sorting Test, TMT-B = Trail Making Test-B, SFS-J = Social Functioning Scale, Japanese version, SAPS = Scale for Positive Symptoms, and SANS = Scale for Negative Symptoms.

the CCT intervention along with treatment as usual (i.e., the CCT group) showed greater improvements on measures of cognitive functions such as verbal memory, or processing speed, and social functioning. Our results demonstrate that CCT benefits Japanese individuals with schizophrenia. In addition, the high attendance and level of satisfaction rated by the participants in the CCT group indirectly support the notion that this intervention could be effectively applied on Japanese individuals with schizophrenia. The high attendance rate in the CCT group could also imply that they took advantage of the strategies for prospective memory such as the use of calendar for scheduling. They are expected to acquire this new habit through homework exercises. The participants in the CCT group who completed the intervention ($n = 11$) attended 84.9% of the sessions. Although this percentage decreased to 78.9% after considering the two participants who dropped out, overall attendance was still high. Participants also reported that the sessions were well conducted (mean rating = 76.6 on a 0–100 visual analogue scale). Although definite judgment on whether some of the homework assignments were completed or not was difficult, all participants executed an assignment to call a therapist and leave a message on Saturday using their calendar, once or more in two sessions, for example. Few participants missed all of their homework assignments at each session.

Since impairments on verbal memory in individuals with schizophrenia have been demonstrated to be particularly severe relative to other cognitive domains [9, 10, 57], it is one of the main targets of CCT. Therefore, the successful replication of improvements on verbal memory performance observed in a previous study [31] is a clear indicator of the methodological validity and effectiveness of the Japanese version we administered in this study. JVLT has three or more versions of parallel tests, which we administered randomly to each participant at the three time points. Influences of repetition are considered to be modest, as seen in the performance of the TAU group on these measures. The participants learned a number of memory strategies in the verbal memory sessions and practiced choosing adequate strategies depending on the circumstances. For example, the encoding strategies, such as the use of categorization or visual imagery, are useful for remembering a list for shopping, people's names, and important information in each participant's real-world circumstances. These strategies are considered relevant in performing the JVLT.

As for the other cognitive domains targeted in the CCT intervention, the participants in the CCT group showed greater improvements on measures of processing speed such as the WAIS-III digit symbol or TMT-A compared to those in the TAU group. Since the participants in both groups showed trends in improvement on these measures to some degree, it is plausible that these measures were subjected to the effect of repetition. Nevertheless, the significant group-by-time interactions indicate that the effect of the CCT intervention should be detected beyond that of repetition seen in the TAU group. Indeed, participants in the CCT group showed improvements in processing speed or sustained the level of attention necessary to perform these tasks quickly. Task attention strategies, such as paraphrasing and self-talk, were practiced in the letter cancellation tasks and card games with the goal of utilizing these strategies in everyday activities under real-world circumstances. These strategies are considered relevant for performance on both tests of processing speed (the TMT and WAIS-III digit symbol task). The previous studies [30, 31] reported inconsistent effects of CCT on processing speed, showing that CCT led to improvement on the attention measure (digit span) but no improvement on the WAIS-III digit symbol task. Further studies are needed to investigate the effects of CCT on processing speed.

On the other hand, the CCT group did not show significant changes on measures of executive function, which is consistent with previous studies [30, 31]. The ceiling effects observed in WCST could make it difficult to examine the effectiveness of the intervention on executive functions in this study and possibly in previous studies [30, 31]. Careful selection of additional assessment tools, along with some revisions in the CCT program, might be necessary for examining executive function in future studies.

The effect sizes associated with CCT on cognitive measures at postintervention were as follows: medium-to-large (0.69–1.00) on verbal memory, large (0.97–1.22) on processing speed, and small-to-medium (0.33–0.58) on executive function. Additionally, the effect sizes on social functioning were much larger (0.47–1.56). These results suggest that CCT has promising effects on cognitive performance and that improvements in social functioning occur as well when CCT is applied to Japanese individuals with schizophrenia. These effect sizes were somewhat larger than those in a recent report [31] but are generally similar to those in the first report by Twamley et al. [30]. The results of the previous studies [30, 31] showed that effect sizes for functional measures such as subjective quality of life and functional capacity were larger than those for cognitive measures. Consistent with these findings, we observed the same tendencies in this study. Conversational attention strategies, including paraphrasing and asking questions, were practiced by discussing daily topics and sample scenarios with other participants in the sessions. Somewhat larger effect sizes seen in the functional measures suggest that these strategies might encourage patients to take part in social interactions in everyday life and that these strategies possibly had an effect on social functioning independent of the cognitive aspects.

Although effect sizes on cognitive measures were smaller than those on functional measures, significant improvement effects of this compensatory approach on cognitive performance, which has been reported previously [30, 31], were replicated in this study. As Twamley et al. [30] pointed, it is difficult to know whether these effects of CCT represent an attenuation of cognitive deficits or an increase in the ability to compensate for them. Nevertheless, we believe it is unlikely that the intervention is correcting underlying cognitive deficits, because the CCT intervention does not use any drills to improve the cognitive capability itself. Similarly, the improvements on neuropsychological tests seen in the CCT group may reflect the utilization of the strategies participants acquired in the CCT, because none of the neuropsychological tests implemented as cognitive measures was referred to in the sessions. This also implies that the cognitive strategies coached can easily be generalized in various situations, as long as the strategies are applicable. For clarification of the mechanism of action in this compensatory intervention, in future studies, we should include a variety of measures on which the compensatory strategies show improvements or no effects.

In light of the aim of cognitive training, it is worth noting that the improvements on cognitive measures such as verbal memory or processing speed were maintained over a three-month follow-up period. Medium-to-large effects on verbal memory and those on measures of processing speed (WAIS-III digit symbol) and executive function (WCST) were maintained. These results are roughly consistent with those in previous studies [30, 31]. Although we did not collect data on the frequency and way in which the strategy was used by CCT participants in everyday living, we could expect, from the above, that the participants made the strategies their new habits and generalized them to everyday tasks. Further studies are required to examine the generalization and availability of the strategies in real-world circumstances.

The impressive improvements on social functioning were moderately maintained (0.49) at follow-up. However, the effect size decreased compared to that of the postintervention period. These results suggest that social interactions or instructions encouraging interpersonal behaviors or prosocial activities provided by the CCT intervention contribute to improvements on social functioning immediately after

CCT. It is reported that the cognitive remediation provided in conjunction with adjunctive psychiatric rehabilitations has significantly stronger effects compared to cognitive remediation alone [24, 25]. However, in this study, we did not control for psychosocial intervention (excluding the CCT sessions) in keeping with previous work [31]. Conjunction with periodical psychosocial intervention may be effective in maintaining the improvement effects on social functioning for a longer period of time.

Regarding clinical symptoms, although significant group differences were not observed, CCT had small-to-medium effects (0.47–0.51) on positive symptoms. This result raises questions on whether the improvement effects of CCT on cognitive performance are associated with symptomatology. Therefore, we also conducted correlational analyses on positive symptoms and cognitive function measures. The results showed that positive symptoms were negatively correlated with WCST ($r = -0.91$, $p = 0.000$), but not with any other cognitive measures ($rs \leq |0.38|$, $p \geq 0.070$), suggesting that the observed effects of CCT on measures of verbal memory and processing speed have little association with the severity of positive symptoms. Nevertheless, significant correlations between positive symptoms and executive functions represent the possibility that a certain type of cognition is not independent of positive symptoms. The relationship between clinical symptoms and cognitive abilities should be examined in future studies in order to investigate the effectiveness of CCT on cognitive functions more optimally. On the other hand, the previous study [30] showed significant effects on negative symptoms but not positive symptoms. This issue should be carefully examined using larger sample sizes.

Although our results are potentially fruitful, this pilot study has several limitations. The small sample size limits the generalizability of our findings. Regarding the study protocol, we did not employ a rigorous randomization procedure, assessment of treatment fidelity, active control group, or group allocation masking. Although the previous meta-analyses showed that variation in methodological quality (such as lacking these procedures) in cognitive remediation intervention studies had no effect on most cognitive and functioning outcomes [24], these limitations would need to be addressed in future studies. In our results, the effect size of social functioning rated by the participants' families was larger than those rated by participants themselves, suggesting that the expectation of the participants' families biased their evaluations. The result of larger effects in functional outcomes than for cognitive functions is consistent with previous studies [30, 31]. However, it is possible that nonspecific factors including social contact in weekly group sessions could enhance arousal and affect social functioning as well as some of the cognitive measures, in which the effects were attenuated during the follow-up period. Additionally, we could not exclude the interpretation that the CCT participants might be motivated to put more effort into the neuropsychological tests at postintervention and follow-up than that by the TAU participants, with expectation for positive effects of the CCT intervention. In order to clarify these issues, a study of CCT using an active control group to control therapist-time and attention is needed. Finally, Twamley et al. [31] reported

a high rate of dropout, but only two participants dropped out during the CCT intervention in our study. To enhance the applicability of this approach, strategies for maintaining participation in CCT sessions are worth investigating in the future.

In conclusion, this pilot study provides the first piece of preliminary evidence on the effectiveness and applicability of CCT for Japanese individuals with schizophrenia. The results suggest that the CCT intervention substantially benefits not only cognitive performance but also functional outcomes in this population. The results of the previous studies were generally replicated, ensuring that the advantages of CCT were not lost in the Japanese version. On the other hand, some different patterns of results were observed in this study, which provides us with new insights relevant to CCT itself and to issues specific to the Japanese version. The promising results observed in this pilot study would encourage further research on CCT in Japan. Investigation into the biological basis of the effects of cognitive remediation is a key challenge. As several studies using cognitive remediation programs based on restorative approaches have shown that cognitive remediation has positive effects on brain structure, brain function, and biomarkers such as brain-derived neurotrophic factors [58–60], studies on CCT are expected to lead to further investigations into its effectiveness from multiple viewpoints, including its neural basis or functional mechanism.

Conflict of Interests

The authors declare that there is no conflict of interests regarding the publication of this paper.

Acknowledgments

This study was supported by a Grant-in-Aid for Scientific Research (B) 20330141, 26285155 and Grant-in-Aid for Scientific Research on Innovative Areas 26118707 from the Japan Society for the Promotion of Science (JSPS). The authors thank Dr. Twamley for providing them with the CCT manual and allowing them to use it.

References

[1] J. M. Gold, "Cognitive deficits as treatment targets in schizophrenia," *Schizophrenia Research*, vol. 72, no. 1, pp. 21–28, 2004.

[2] A.-K. J. Fett, W. Viechtbauer, M.-D. Dominguez, D. L. Penn, J. van Os, and L. Krabbendam, "The relationship between neurocognition and social cognition with functional outcomes in schizophrenia: a meta-analysis," *Neuroscience and Biobehavioral Reviews*, vol. 35, no. 3, pp. 573–588, 2011.

[3] M. F. Green, "What are the functional consequences of neurocognitive deficits in schizophrenia?" *American Journal of Psychiatry*, vol. 153, no. 3, pp. 321–330, 1996.

[4] M. F. Green, R. S. Kern, D. L. Braff, and J. Mintz, "Neurocognitive deficits and functional outcome in schizophrenia: are we measuring the 'right stuff'?" *Schizophrenia Bulletin*, vol. 26, no. 1, pp. 119–136, 2000.

[5] M. F. Green, R. S. Kern, and R. K. Heaton, "Longitudinal studies of cognition and functional outcome in schizophrenia: implications for MATRICS," *Schizophrenia Research*, vol. 72, no. 1, pp. 41–51, 2004.

[6] K. H. Nuechterlein, K. L. Subotnik, M. F. Green et al., "Neurocognitive predictors of work outcome in recent-onset schizophrenia," *Schizophrenia Bulletin*, vol. 37, supplement 2, pp. S33–S40, 2011.

[7] R. M. Bilder, R. S. Goldman, D. Robinson et al., "Neuropsychology of first-episode schizophrenia: initial characterization and clinical correlates," *American Journal of Psychiatry*, vol. 157, no. 4, pp. 549–559, 2000.

[8] R. W. Heinrichs and K. K. Zakzanis, "Neurocognitive deficit in schizophrenia: a quantitative review of the evidence," *Neuropsychology*, vol. 12, no. 3, pp. 426–445, 1998.

[9] R. I. Mesholam-Gately, A. J. Giuliano, K. P. Goff, S. V. Faraone, and L. J. Seidman, "Neurocognition in first-episode schizophrenia: a meta-analytic review," *Neuropsychology*, vol. 23, no. 3, pp. 315–336, 2009.

[10] M. Matsui, H. Yuuki, K. de Kato et al., "Schizotypal disorder and schizophrenia: a profile analysis of neuropsychological functioning in Japanese patients," *Journal of the International Neuropsychological Society*, vol. 13, no. 4, pp. 672–682, 2007.

[11] W. J. Brewer, S. M. Francey, S. J. Wood et al., "Memory impairments identified in people at ultra-high risk for psychosis who later develop first-episode psychosis," *The American Journal of Psychiatry*, vol. 162, no. 1, pp. 71–78, 2005.

[12] R. E. Carrión, T. E. Goldberg, D. McLaughlin, A. M. Auther, C. U. Correll, and B. A. Cornblatt, "Impact of neurocognition on social and role functioning in individuals at clinical high risk for psychosis," *American Journal of Psychiatry*, vol. 168, no. 8, pp. 806–813, 2011.

[13] P. Jones, B. Rodgers, R. Murray, and M. Marmot, "Child developmental risk factors for adult schizophrenia in the British 1946 birth cohort," *The Lancet*, vol. 344, no. 8934, pp. 1398–1402, 1994.

[14] T. A. Niendam, C. E. Bearden, I. M. Rosso et al., "A prospective study of childhood neurocognitive functioning in schizophrenic patients and their siblings," *The American Journal of Psychiatry*, vol. 160, no. 11, pp. 2060–2062, 2003.

[15] A. L. Hoff, C. Svetina, G. Shields, J. Stewart, and L. E. DeLisi, "Ten-year longitudinal study of neuropsychological functioning subsequent to a first episode of schizophrenia," *Schizophrenia Research*, vol. 78, no. 1, pp. 27–34, 2005.

[16] C.-H. Lin, C.-L. Huang, Y.-C. Chang et al., "Clinical symptoms, mainly negative symptoms, mediate the influence of neurocognition and social cognition on functional outcome of schizophrenia," *Schizophrenia Research*, vol. 146, no. 1–3, pp. 231–237, 2013.

[17] G. Heydebrand, M. Weiser, J. Rabinowitz, A. L. Hoff, L. E. DeLisi, and J. G. Csernansky, "Correlates of cognitive deficits in first episode schizophrenia," *Schizophrenia Research*, vol. 68, no. 1, pp. 1–9, 2004.

[18] D. S. O'Leary, M. Flaum, M. L. Kesler, L. A. Flashman, S. Arndt, and N. C. Andreasen, "Cognitive correlates of the negative, disorganized, and psychotic symptom dimensions of schizophrenia," *Journal of Neuropsychiatry and Clinical Neurosciences*, vol. 12, no. 1, pp. 4–15, 2000.

[19] J. Ventura, G. S. Hellemann, A. D. Thames, V. Koellner, and K. H. Nuechterlein, "Symptoms as mediators of the relationship between neurocognition and functional outcome in

schizophrenia: a meta-analysis," *Schizophrenia Research*, vol. 113, no. 2-3, pp. 189–199, 2009.

[20] J. Ventura, K. L. Subotnik, A. Ered et al., "The relationship of attitudinal beliefs to negative symptoms, neurocognition, and daily functioning in recent-onset schizophrenia," *Schizophrenia Bulletin*, vol. 40, no. 6, pp. 1308–1318, 2014.

[21] M. Davidson, S. Galderisi, M. Weiser et al., "Cognitive effects of antipsychotic drugs in first-episode schizophrenia and schizophreniform disorder: a randomized, open-label clinical trial (EUFEST)," *American Journal of Psychiatry*, vol. 166, no. 6, pp. 675–682, 2009.

[22] R. S. E. Keefe, R. M. Bilder, S. M. Davis et al., "Neurocognitive effects of antipsychotic medications in patients with chronic schizophrenia in the CATIE trial," *Archives of General Psychiatry*, vol. 64, no. 6, pp. 633–647, 2007.

[23] T. E. Goldberg, R. S. Goldman, K. E. Burdick et al., "Cognitive improvement after treatment with second-generation antipsychotic medications in first-episode schizophrenia: is it a practice effect?" *Archives of General Psychiatry*, vol. 64, no. 10, pp. 1115–1122, 2007.

[24] T. Wykes, V. Huddy, C. Cellard, S. R. McGurk, and P. Czobor, "A meta-analysis of cognitive remediation for schizophrenia: methodology and effect sizes," *American Journal of Psychiatry*, vol. 168, no. 5, pp. 472–485, 2011.

[25] S. R. McGurk, E. W. Twamley, D. I. Sitzer, G. J. McHugo, and K. T. Mueser, "A meta-analysis of cognitive remediation in schizophrenia," *The American Journal of Psychiatry*, vol. 164, no. 12, pp. 1791–1802, 2007.

[26] S. Ikezawa, T. Mogami, Y. Hayami et al., "The pilot study of a Neuropsychological Educational Approach to Cognitive Remediation for patients with schizophrenia in Japan," *Psychiatry Research*, vol. 195, no. 3, pp. 107–110, 2012.

[27] M. Matsui, H. Arai, M. Yonezawa, T. Sumiyoshi, M. Suzuki, and M. Kurachi, "The effects of cognitive rehabilitation on social knowledge in patients with schizophrenia," *Applied Neuropsychology*, vol. 16, no. 3, pp. 158–164, 2009.

[28] S. Pu, K. Nakagome, T. Yamada et al., "A pilot study on the effects of cognitive remediation on hemodynamic responses in the prefrontal cortices of patients with schizophrenia: a multi-channel near-infrared spectroscopy study," *Schizophrenia Research*, vol. 153, no. 1–3, pp. 87–95, 2014.

[29] S. Sato, K. Iwata, S.-I. Furukawa, Y. Matsuda, N. Hatsuse, and E. Ikebuchi, "The effects of the combination of cognitive training and supported employment on improving clinical and working outcomes for people with Schizophrenia in Japan," *Clinical Practice & Epidemiology in Mental Health*, vol. 10, pp. 18–27, 2014.

[30] E. W. Twamley, G. N. Savla, C. H. Zurhellen, R. K. Heaton, and D. V. Jeste, "Development and pilot testing of a novel compensatory cognitive training intervention for people with psychosis," *The American Journal of Psychiatric Rehabilitation*, vol. 11, no. 2, pp. 144–163, 2008.

[31] E. W. Twamley, L. Vella, C. Z. Burton, R. K. Heaton, and D. V. Jeste, "Compensatory cognitive training for psychosis: effects in a randomized controlled trial," *Journal of Clinical Psychiatry*, vol. 73, no. 9, pp. 1212–1219, 2012.

[32] S. Barlati, G. Deste, L. de Peri, C. Ariu, and A. Vita, "Cognitive remediation in schizophrenia: current status and future perspectives," *Schizophrenia Research and Treatment*, vol. 2013, Article ID 156084, 12 pages, 2013.

[33] A. Medalia and A. M. Saperstein, "Does cognitive remediation for schizophrenia improve functional outcomes?" *Current Opinion in Psychiatry*, vol. 26, no. 2, pp. 151–157, 2013.

[34] N. C. Andreasen, *The Scale for the Assessment of Positive Symptoms (SAPS)*, The University of Iowa, Iowa City, Iowa, USA, 1984.

[35] N. C. Andreasen, *The Scale for the Assessment of Negative Symptoms (SANS)*, The University of Iowa, Iowa City, Iowa, USA, 1983.

[36] American Psychiatric Association, *Diagnostic and Statistical Manual of Mental Disorders, Text Revision (DSM-4-TR)*, American Psychiatric Association, Washington, DC, USA, 2000.

[37] K. Matsuoka and Y. Kim, *Japanese Adult Reading Test: JART*, Shinkou Igaku Shuppan, Tokyo, Japan, 2006.

[38] A. Inagaki and T. Inada, "Dose equivalence of new psychotropic drugs—version 6: risperidone extended-release tablets," *Rinsyou Seishin Yakuri*, vol. 15, no. 3, pp. 397–404, 2012 (Japanese).

[39] L. Clare, P. J. McKenna, A. M. Mortimer, and A. D. Baddeley, "Memory in schizophrenia: what is impaired and what is preserved?" *Neuropsychologia*, vol. 31, no. 11, pp. 1224–1241, 1993.

[40] S. Kéri, A. Juhász, Á. Rimanóczy et al., "Habit learning and the genetics of the dopamine D3 receptor: evidence from patients with schizophrenia and healthy controls," *Behavioral Neuroscience*, vol. 119, no. 3, pp. 687–693, 2005.

[41] P. J. Bayley, J. C. Frascino, and L. R. Squire, "Robust habit learning in the absence of awareness and independent of the medial temporal lobe," *Nature*, vol. 436, no. 7050, pp. 550–553, 2005.

[42] S. R. McGurk and H. Y. Meltzer, "The role of cognition in vocational functioning in schizophrenia," *Schizophrenia Research*, vol. 45, no. 3, pp. 175–184, 2000.

[43] W. Spaulding, D. Reed, D. Storzbach, M. Sullivan, M. Weiler, and C. Richardson, "The effects of a remediational approach to cognitive therapy for schizophrenia," in *Outcome and Innovation in Psychological Treatment of Schizophrenia*, T. Wykes, N. Tarrier, and S. Lewis, Eds., pp. 145–160, John Wiley & Sons, London, UK, 1998.

[44] M. Matsui, H. Yuuki, K. Kato, and M. Kurachi, "Impairment of memory-organization in patients with schizophrenia or schizotypal disorder," *Journal of the International Neuropsychological Society*, vol. 12, no. 5, pp. 750–754, 2006.

[45] M. Matsui, T. Sumiyoshi, K. Kato, and M. Kurachi, "Development of alternate forms of Japanese verbal learning test," *Seishin Igaku*, vol. 49, no. 1, pp. 31–34, 2007 (Japanese).

[46] J. M. Gold, C. Randolph, C. J. Carpenter, T. E. Goldberg, and D. R. Weinberger, "Forms of memory failure in schizophrenia," *Journal of Abnormal Psychology*, vol. 101, no. 3, pp. 487–494, 1992.

[47] S. Watamori, H. Hara, T. Miyamori, and F. Eto, *The Rivermead Behavioral Memory Test (RMBT)*, Japanese Version, Chiba Test Center, Tokyo, Japan, 2002.

[48] B. A. Wilson, J. Cockburn, and A. Baddeley, *The Rivermead Behavioral Memory Test (RMBT)*, Thames Valley Test Company, Bury St Edmunds, UK, 1986.

[49] K. Fujita, H. Maekawa, H. Dairoku, and K. Yamanaka, *Wechsler Adult Intelligence Scale*, Nihon Bunka Kagakusha, Tokyo, Japan, 3rd edition, 2006, (Japanese).

[50] D. Wechsler, *Wechsler Adult Intelligence Scale—Third Edition (WAIS-III)*, The Psychological Corporation, San Antonio, Tex, USA, 1997.

[51] R. M. Reitan and D. Wolfson, *The Halstead-Reitan Neuropsychological Test Battery*, Neuropsychology Press, Tucson, Ariz, USA, 1985.

[52] R. K. Heaton, G. J. Chelune, J. K. Talley, G. G. Kay, and G. Curtiss, *Wisconsin Card Sorting Test Manual: Revised and Expanded*, Psychological Assessment Resources, Odessa, Tex, USA, 1993.

[53] T. Nemoto, C. Fujii, Y. Miura et al., "Reliability and validity of the Social Functioning Scale Japanese version (SFS-J)," *Japanese Bulletin of Social Psychiatry*, vol. 17, pp. 188–195, 2008 (Japanese).

[54] M. Birchwood, J. Smith, R. Cochrane, S. Wetton, S. Copestake, and M. Birchwood, "The social functioning scale. The development and validation of a new scale of social adjustment for use in family intervention programmes with schizophrenic patients," *The British Journal of Psychiatry*, vol. 157, no. 6, pp. 853–859, 1990.

[55] H. E. Nelson, "A modified card sorting test sensitive to frontal lobe defects," *Cortex*, vol. 12, no. 4, pp. 313–324, 1976.

[56] J. Cohen, *Statistical Power Analysis for the Behavioral Sciences*, Lawrence Erlbaum Associates, Hillsdale, NJ, USA, 2nd edition, 1988.

[57] A. Aleman, R. Hijman, E. H. F. de Haan, and R. S. Kahn, "Memory impairment in schizophrenia: a meta-analysis," *The American Journal of Psychiatry*, vol. 156, no. 9, pp. 1358–1366, 1999.

[58] S. M. Eack, G. E. Hogarty, R. Y. Cho et al., "Neuroprotective effects of cognitive enhancement therapy against gray matter loss in early schizophrenia: results from a 2-year randomized controlled trial," *Archives of General Psychiatry*, vol. 67, no. 7, pp. 674–682, 2010.

[59] S. Vinogradov, M. Fisher, C. Holland, W. Shelly, O. Wolkowitz, and S. H. Mellon, "Is serum brain-derived neurotrophic factor a biomarker for cognitive enhancement in schizophrenia?" *Biological Psychiatry*, vol. 66, no. 6, pp. 549–553, 2009.

[60] B. E. Wexler, M. Anderson, R. K. Fulbright, and J. C. Gore, "Preliminary evidence of improved verbal working memory performance and normalization of task-related frontal lobe activation in schizophrenia following cognitive exercises," *American Journal of Psychiatry*, vol. 157, no. 10, pp. 1694–1697, 2000.

10

Occupational Performance and Affective Symptoms for Patients with Depression Disorder

Åsa Daremo,[1,2] **Anette Kjellberg,**[2] **and Lena Haglund**[2]

[1]*Department of Psychiatry, University Hospital, 581 85 Linköping, Sweden*
[2]*Department of Social and Welfare Studies, Faculty of Health Sciences, Linköping University, Linköping, Sweden*

Correspondence should be addressed to Åsa Daremo; asa.daremo@regionostergotland.se

Academic Editor: Raphael J. Braga

The aim of this study was to describe recovering over time in occupational performance and in affective symptoms for patients with depression disorder by using different assessments and methods for collecting data. A longitudinal design with data collections on repeated occasions was used. The Occupational Circumstances Assessment Interview and Rating Scale and Occupational Self-Assessment were used for measuring occupational performance, and for affective symptoms, a Comprehensive Psychopathological Rating Scale Self-Assessment was used. Fourteen patients with depression disorder were included in the study. The result indicates that affective symptoms improve earlier than occupational performance. Furthermore, self-assessment seems to reflect more improvement to the patient than interview-based assessment. Different kinds of assessment and different kinds of data collection methods seem to facilitate the understanding of the patients recovering. In addition habituation was the most important item for the patients to manage. One implication for practice is that patients may need an extended period of treatment supporting occupational performance.

1. Introduction

Depression is a common mental disorder and affects people of all ages. The disorder is so common that most people have either experienced it themselves or have a near relative who has suffered from it [1]. Depression is the most common reason for ill health, lost productivity, and work disability in the world. It is the leading cause of disability as measured by Years Lived with Disability (YLD) and was the fourth leading contributor to the global burden of disease by Disability Adjusted Life Years (DALY) in 2000. By the year 2020, depression is projected to reach second place in the ranking of DALYs calculated for all ages and for both sexes, and about 121 million people worldwide are affected today [2]. The picture in Sweden does not differ from the global perspective [3].

DSM-V states that at least two of the symptoms of depression, lack of energy, and reduced activity must have been experienced for at least two weeks in order for a diagnosis of depression to be given. When suffering depression,

the patient lacks self-esteem, has feelings of guilt, and experiences hopelessness and meaninglessness. Self-confidence is reduced and the low self-esteem is like a loss of inner certainty and power [4]. All these symptoms have an impact on occupational performance. Since the cognitive, the behavioural, social, and physiological areas are affected, most patients have difficulties performing daily activities. Daily routine activities such as home care, meal preparation, and self-care are often affected, as well as the ability to interact with others [5]. Furthermore, the area of work often presents many problems for adults with depression [6].

The Model of Human Occupation (MOHO) attempts to explain how humans are motivated toward and choose to do things in their patterns of everyday life and in their individual capacities. There is evidence that MOHO has become the most widely used occupation-focused model; about 80% of occupational therapists worldwide have indicated that they use MOHO in everyday practice [7, 8]. In the model, interrelated components such as volition, habituation, and performance capacity are understood in relation to the

TABLE 1: Demographic data for the patients and the number of assessments.

Patient $n = 14$	Sex	Age	Treatment period	OCAIRS-S $n = 46$	OSA $n = 75$	CPRS-S-A $n = 73$	Total assessments $n = 194$
1	Woman	29	4 months and 3 weeks	5	8	8	21
2	Man	47	2 months and 1 week	3	2	2	7
3	Woman	49	8 months and 2 weeks	7	12	12	31
4	Woman	49	7 months	4	12	12	28
5	Man	59	2 months	3	5	4	12
6	Man	24	26 days	2	2	1	5
7	Woman	18	5 months and 2 weeks	4	8	8	20
8	Man	45	1 month	2			2
9	Man	48	5 months	3	6	6	15
10	Man	58	2 months and 1 week	3			3
11	Man	27	25 days	1	2	2	5
12	Woman	63	7 months and 3 weeks	2	8	8	18
13	Woman	62	3 months	4	5	5	14
14	Woman	28	2 months and 1 week	3	5	5	13

influence of the physical and social environments on the occupation. Volition refers to the motivation for occupation and it reflects, for example, the individual's interest and values. Habituation refers to the process by which occupation is organized into routine behaviour in daily life, and performance capacity refers to the ability to do things. As a function of the interaction between the personal components (volition, habituation, and performance capacity) and the environment, skills are used; these skills are observable and goal-directed actions. Several structured assessments have been developed for use with MOHO. They all reflect years of development and have been studied and worked up to enhance their psychometric status and practical usefulness [9].

Furthermore, it is important to clarify what the patient wants and needs to do and measure the actual performance. This can be done with different data collection methods such as self-assessment, interviews, or observation. To our knowledge no other studies have been performed using a longitudinal design in combination with using evidence based measures including self-assessment and interviewing patients with depressions. In addition comparing occupational performance and affective symptoms has not been investigated. Therefore the aim is to describe recovering over time in occupational performance and affective symptoms for patients with depression by using different methods for collecting data and assessments.

2. Method

The study attempted to gain a longitudinal perspective [10], with data collections on repeated occasions. To investigate change over time in occupational performance, the Occupational Circumstances Assessment Interview and Rating Scale (OCAIRS) [11] and Occupational Self-Assessment (OSA) [12] were used, and for affective symptoms, the Comprehensive

Psychopathological Rating Scale Self-Assessment (CPRS-S-A) [13] was used.

In total 45 patients were treated in psychiatric institutional care in two different hospitals, located in the southern part of Sweden. Both hospitals are located in rural areas. All patients were diagnosed by the medical doctor at the ward. The inclusion criteria for the study were depression with suicidal behaviour according to DSM-V [4]. An inquiry about participation in the study was consecutively asked, the first week at the psychiatric ward, by the occupational therapist or the occupational therapist assistant belonging to the ward.

Eighteen patients gave informed consent to participate and 14 patients completed the study.

The 14 patients included seven women and seven men. The ages ranged between 18 and 63 years, with an average age of 39 years. The treatment periods varied from 25 days to eight and a half months (mode = two months and one week) and during this period the patients could be treated in both institutional care and noninstitutional care (Table 1). The Regional Ethical Review Board in Linköping, Sweden, approved the study.

2.1. Data Collection

2.1.1. Assessments. The OCAIRS, which is a MOHO-based assessment, was originally developed for use in acute psychiatric settings [9]. It is often used as an initial interview and it collects information about the patient's participation and ability to manage daily activities. OCAIRS is a semistructured interview. There is a structure to the type of information that is gathered and how it is interpreted. The OCAIRS uses a 4-point rating scale (Table 2) [11, 14]. The development of the OCAIRS started in 1989 and several studies examining the quality of the assessment have been completed. These studies provide evidence of reliability and concurrent validity [14–16]. The Swedish version of the assessment which is used in this study is designated OCAIRS-S.

TABLE 2: Grades in the rating scales.

Grades		Number of items	Score interval
OCAIRS-S	0 = "Competent" 1 = "Some difficulties/challenges" 2 = "Explicit difficulties/challenges" 3 = "Problems in highly restrictive"	12	0–36
OSA	0 = "I do it well" 1 = "I manage it" 2 = "I have a problem with it"	29	0–58
CPRS-S-A	0 = "I often feel calm" 2 = "Sometimes I have unpleasant feelings of anxiety" 4 = "I often have feelings of anxiety, which sometimes can be very strong, and which I make an effort to master" 6 = "I have terrible, protracted or unbearable anxiety feelings"	19	0–114

The OSA, which also is a MOHO-based assessment, is an evaluation tool and an outcome measurement. The OSA is a two-part self-rating form. It is designed to capture patients' perceptions of their own occupational competence and of the occupations they consider important. In this study, version 1 was used, and this has a two-part rating form, with a 3-point rating scale in each part (Table 2). First, the patient responds to items about his occupational competence and then indicates the importance of each of these items. When the patient has responded to the questions about competence and values he can go on to choose the areas he would most like to change. In this study the patients did not carry out this last step.

Several international studies have been conducted on the OSA, confirming that the OSA items and ratings (competence and value) can be used as valid and reliable measures of a patient's occupational competence and the value of occupation [12, 17]. In this study, a Swedish version of the OSA is used that is called "Min Mening."

CPRS-S-A is a self-rating scale for affective syndromes. The assessment was developed on the basis of the original CPRS from 1978 [18]. The resulting subscale, for affective syndromes (CPRS-A), was then revised to a self-rating format (CPRS-S-A) [19]. CPRS-S-A covers depression, anxiety, and obsessional symptoms. The purpose of the assessment is to give a detailed picture of the patient's present sense of his condition. The patient grades how he has felt over the previous three days. CPRS-S-A has a 7-point rating scale (Table 2). The assessment has been used frequently since the end of 1970 in different studies and has shown good values concerning reliability and clinical usefulness [19, 20].

2.2. Procedure. The patients were initially interviewed with the OCAIRS-S and the patients also filled in the self-rating

assessments, OSA and CPRS-S-A. Occupational therapists performed the interviews with OCAIRS-S; they had several years of experience in the area of psychiatric care.

After the first occasion the patient filled in these two self-rating assessments every fortnight and the interview using the OCAIRS-S was repeated every month until the patient was discharged.

The interviews were conducted at the hospital or in the patient's home or, in exceptional cases, by telephone. The interviews lasted from 30 to 60 minutes. The self-rating assessments (OSA, CPRS-S-A) were given to the patient at the hospital or sent by post if the patient was treated as an outpatient. The total number of assessments for each patient is presented in Table 1. In total, 194 assessments—on average 14 (range 3–31) assessments per patient—were performed during the period.

2.3. Data Analysis. For identifying intraindividual differences for each patient the sum scores from each occasion from OCAIRS-S, OSA, and CPRS-S-A were compared. The differences for each patient over time are based on a period of four months since most of the patients were discharged after that time (Table 3). In addition an investigation was also made of whether or not there were changes over time regarding occupational performance measured by OCAIRS-S and OSA and symptoms measured by CPRS-S-A. These changes were investigated for each patient.

3. Results

Nine of the 14 patients (9/14) showed a positive trend during the treatment period (Table 3). For some of these nine patients, their score constantly changed in a positive way and for some patients the scores varied during the treatment period. However, all of these nine patients (patients 1, 4, 5, 6, 7, 9, 11, 13, and 14) changed in a positive way, both in occupational performance and in affective symptoms, when the first and the last occasions were compared.

No clear trend could be seen for two of the 14 patients (patients 2 and 12) since the scores shifted and there was no homogenous pattern between the three assessments. Patient number 3 had a negative development during the treatment period related to occupational performance. Furthermore, missing data was frequent for two of the patients (patients 8 and 10).

Occupational performance was measured with OCAIRS-S and OSA. In total, the results showed that the patients still had problems in occupational performance after discharge. Comparing between the first and the last occasion the patients improved more when measuring with the self-assessment OSA (8 of 14 patients) than when the occupational therapist interviewed the patient with OCAIRS-S (6 of 14 patients) (Table 3).

The study indicates that patients can have low scores measured with the CPRS-S-A, that is, few symptoms, but still have problems with their occupational performance. The sum score of CPRS-S-A indicates an earlier improvement than the sum score based on OCAIRS-S and OSA. Less affective

TABLE 3: Sum scores of the different assessments for each patient ($n = 14$).

Patient	Occasion 1			Occasion 2			Occasion 3			Occasion 4		
	OCAIRS	OSA	CPRS	OCAIRS	OSA	CPRS	OCAIRS	OSA	CPRS	OCAIRS	OSA	CPRS
1	16	39	53	12 (I)	37 (I)	46 (I)	11 (S)	29 (I)	27 (I)	9 (I)	38 (R)	36 (R)
2	6	12	18	12 (R)	15 (R)	25 (R)	11 (S)	—	—	d	d	d
3	12	24	61	17 (R)	29 (R)	44 (I)	10 (I)	30 (R)	66 (R)	15 (R)	26 (I)	46 (I)
4	14	53	54	10 (I)	41 (I)	37 (I)	16 (R)	49 (R)	39 (R)	13 (I)	49 (I)	30 (I)
5	16	32	35	4 (I)	19 (I)	17 (I)	5 (S)	7 (I)	14 (I)	—	—	14 (S)
6	11	38	43	11 (S)	36 (I)	27 (I)	d	d	d	d	d	d
7	10	49	51	10 (S)	30 (I)	27 (I)	0 (I)	29 (I)	8 (I)	—	25 (I)	6 (I)
8	1	—	—	3 (R)	—	—	d	d	d	d	d	d
9	13	31	80	16 (R)	38 (R)	81 (S)	—	34 (I)	69 (I)	10 (I)	29 (I)	43 (I)
10	9	—	—	5 (I)	—	—	7 (R)	—	—	d	d	d
11	6	39	24	—	37 (I)	22 (I)	d	d	d	d	d	d
12	x	34	43	—	28 (I)	46 (R)	5	51 (R)	45 (S)	0 (I)	33 (I)	43 (I)
13	22	37	60	19 (I)	42 (R)	34 (I)	15 (I)	35 (I)	18 (I)	14 (I)	33 (I)	19 (S)
14	24	54	43	16 (I)	37 (I)	28 (I)	13 (I)	37 (S)	35 (R)	d	d	d

I = improved score (lower score than the occasion before).
S = stable score (same score or only one point difference).
R = reduced score (higher score than the occasion before).
— = drop out.
d = discharged.

symptoms and fewer difficulties in occupational performance do not seem to arise at the same time.

When analysing each assessment separately at item level some homogeneous trends could be seen, based on CPRS-S-A. Symptoms of depression related to mood, feelings of unease, sleep, appetite, ability to concentrate, initiative, emotional involvement, pessimism, and zest for life all showed a positive trend during the treatment period. The same trend could not be seen for anxiety and obsession symptoms.

The occupational therapist rated most improvements for patients regarding the items of "Habituation" when using OCAIRS-S. The items "Skills" and "Environment" were mostly rated as stable. The items in OSA "Habituation" and "Volition" were the items that the patients themselves rated as giving them the most problems and also considered as most important for them to manage at the first occasion. However, "Habituation" was the item that had the most improvement during the treatment period referring to the patients' own ratings.

4. Discussion

The aim of the study was to describe recovering over time in occupational performance and affective symptoms for patients with depression. The sum score of CPRS-S-A reflected an earlier improvement than the sum score of OCAIRS-S and OSA. The items in CPRS-S-A that describe depressive symptoms had a positive trend during the treatment period. However, this study indicates that even if the patients' affective symptoms improved after a while compared to the acute phase, it took time for the patients to resume their earlier occupational performance. This result adds a new perspective for patients with depression disorders, showing that occupational performance needs to be considered when discharge. Maybe the patient will need an extended period

of occupational focused treatment. To support and enable occupational performance in order to manage activities of everyday life are important. There is, for example, evidence for that treatment for patients with mood disorders should include promotion of regularity in everyday activities as Grandin et al. stated in 2006 [21].

By the end of the treatment period this study showed more improvements with OSA, the self-rating assessment (8 of 14 patients), than by interviewing the patients with the OCAIRS-S (6 of 14 patients). This indicates that it is important to use more than one type of data collection method, such as interviewing and self-rating. This is in line with what Möller [22] argues regarding the multimethod data-collection approach in the treatment of patients with affective disorders. Möller also points out that different areas, such as medical symptoms and social functioning, should be measured. We argue that occupational performance must also be measured in order to understand patients with depressive disorders since occupational performance is affected.

The longitudinal design with repeated measures [10] applied in this study shows that it is necessary to gather data in clinical practice several times during a treatment period, since both occupational performance and affective symptoms varied during the period of four months for the patients in this study. For some of the patients, the variation showed a negative pattern. This should be considered since it will influence the content of the short-term goals and the offered interventions.

In the interview with OCAIRS-S and in the self-rating with OSA, habituation was the item most frequently rated as a problem and at the same time was considered as important to manage. At the end of the treatment, habituation was the item that had the most improvement but still problems existed. This also indicates the need for occupational focused treatment. Habituation influences significantly performance of activities in everyday life. Habituation forming the structure and routine of daily life, gives patterns for activities that influence the life style. Habituation holds together the patterns of occupations that give life its effectiveness and familiar character [9]. When there are difficulties in habits and routines for patients with psychiatric diagnoses they often need occupational therapy [23].

There were too few patients in the study to make any statistical calculations. The explorative nature of the study also confirmed that statistical tests were not suitable. There were variations in the investigated group concerning gender, age, and variation of sick leave. Even if 194 assessments were included in the study, no generalizing to larger or other populations should be made. The longitudinal design [10] gave a description of change in occupational performance and affective syndromes within each patient. The data collection at multiple time points gave a valuable understanding of each patient but also across patients. One limitation when using time series studies can be missing data. In the present study this occurred relatively few times and mainly for just two of the patients (patients 8 and 10).

This study is based on patients who received inpatient care in the beginning of their illness. This will influence the generalization of the result. People who received inpatient care have met the criteria for admission to a department; that is, the severity was of such a degree that outpatient treatment was judged not to be successful by the medical doctor. The degree of the severity may have influenced the time for improving on symptoms. In addition the small study group weakens generalization of the result.

A period of four months with data from four occasions was considered reasonable to analyse since eight of fourteen patients were discharged during a four-month period. Nevertheless a longer period would be of interest for future studies. In addition future studies including greater number of subjects and using a mixed methods design with quantitative and qualitative data will improve and deepen the knowledge in the area.

In conclusion this study indicates that reduced affective symptoms and fewer problems in occupational performance do not seem to arise at the same time. Consequently, occupational performance needs to be noticed when discharged from treatment caused by depression.

The result also suggests the importance of measuring on repeated occasions during the treatment period since this allows identification of the changes in occupational performance and affective symptoms for the patient and how these vary over time. The most affected item related to occupational performance was habituation, both in the interviews with OCAIRS-S and in the self-ratings with OSA. Habituation was the item that the patients themselves rated as giving the most problems and was also determined as most important for them to manage.

Conflict of Interests

The authors declare that there is no conflict of interests regarding the publication of this paper.

References

[1] Socialstyrelsen, October 2013, http://www.socialstyrelsen.se/.

[2] World Health Organization, 2013, http://www.who.int/en/.

[3] J.-O. Ottosson, *Psykiatri*, Liber AB, Stockholm, Sweden, 7th edition, 2009 (Swedish).

[4] American Psychiatric Association, *Diagnostic and Statistical Manual of Mental Disorders 5 (DSM-5)*, American Psychiatric Association, Washington, DC, USA, 2013.

[5] D. Bilsker, M. Gilbert, T. Myette, and C. Stewart-Patteson, "Depression and work funktion: bridging the gap between mental health care and the workplace," in *Occupational Therapy in Mental Health. A Vision for Participation*, C. Brown and V. Stoffel, Eds., F.A. Davis Company, Philadelphia, Pa, USA, 2011.

[6] N. Spangler, "Mood disorders," in *Occupational Therapy in Mental Health. A Vision for Participation*, C. Brown and V. Stoffel, Eds., Davis Company, Philadelphia, Pa, USA, 2011.

[7] L. Haglund, E. Ekbladh, L.-H. Thorell, and I. R. Hallberg, "Practice models in Swedish psychiatric occupational therapy," *Scandinavian Journal of Occupational Therapy*, vol. 7, no. 3, pp. 107–113, 2000.

[8] S. W. Lee, R. Taylor, G. Kielhofner, and G. Fisher, "Theory use in practice: a national survey of therapists who use the model of human occupation," *The American Journal of Occupational Therapy*, vol. 62, no. 1, pp. 106–117, 2008.

[9] G. Kielhofner, *Model of Human Occupation*, Lippincott: Williams & Wilkins, Baltimore, Md, USA, 4th edition, 2008.

[10] D. F. Polit and C. T. Beck, *Nursing Research: Generating and Assessing Evidence for Nursing Practice*, Lippincott Williams & Wilkins, Philadelphia, Pa, USA, 8th edition, 2008.

[11] S. Deshpande, G. Kielhofner, C. Henriksson et al., *A User's Manual for The Occupational Circumstances Assessment Interview and Rating Scale, Version 2.0*, University of Illinois at Chicago, Chicago, Ill, USA, 2002.

[12] K. Baron, G. Kielhofner, A. Iyenger, V. Goldhammer, and J. Wolenski, *A User's Manual for the Occupational Self Assessment (OSA)*, Version 2.2, University of Illinois at Chicago, 2006.

[13] P. Svanborg and M. Åsberg, "A new self-rating scale for depression and anxiety states based on the comprehensive psychopathological rating scale," *Acta Psychiatrica Scandinavica*, vol. 89, no. 1, pp. 21–28, 1994.

[14] C. Henriksson and L. Haglund, *Occupational Circumstance Assessment Interview and Rating Scale*, Swedish Version 4.0, Department of Occupational Therapy, Faculty of Health Science, Linköping University, 2005.

[15] L. Haglund and C. Henriksson, "Testing a Swedish version of OCAIRS on two different patient groups," *Scandinavian Journal of Caring Sciences*, vol. 8, no. 4, pp. 223–230, 1994.

[16] J.-S. Lai, L. Haglund, and G. Kielhofner, "Occupational case analysis interview and rating scale—an examination of construct validity," *Scandinavian Journal of Caring Sciences*, vol. 13, no. 4, pp. 267–273, 1999.

[17] E. M. Hellsvik, *Min Mening. Version 1.0. Swedish version of Occupational Self Assessment by Baron K, Kielhofner G, Iyenger A, Goldhammer V & Wolenski J. Stockholm*, Förbundet Sveriges Arbetsterapeuter, 2000.

[18] M. Åsberg, S. A. Montgomery, C. Perris, D. Schalling, and G. Sedvall, "CPRS: development and applications of a psychiatric rating scale," *Acta Psychiatrica Scandinavica*, supplement 271, pp. 5–32, 1978.

[19] C. Holmstrand, G. Engström, and L. Träskman-Bendz, "Disentangling dysthymia from major depressive disorder in suicide attempters' suicidality, comorbidity and symptomatology," *Nordic Journal of Psychiatry*, vol. 62, no. 1, pp. 25–31, 2008.

[20] M. Mattila-Evenden, P. Svanborg, P. Gustavsson, and M. Åsberg, "Determinants of self-rating and expert rating concordance in psychiatric out-patients, using the affective subscales of the CPRS," *Acta Psychiatrica Scandinavica*, vol. 94, no. 6, pp. 386–396, 1996.

[21] L. D. Grandin, L. B. Alloy, and L. Y. Abramson, "The social zeitgeber theory, circadian rhythms, and mood disorders: review and evaluation," *Clinical Psychology Review*, vol. 26, no. 6, pp. 679–694, 2006.

[22] H. J. Möller, "Rating depressed patients: observer- vs self-assessment," *European Psychiatry*, vol. 15, no. 3, pp. 160–172, 2000.

[23] L. Haglund, L.-H. Thorell, and J. Wålinder, "Occupational functioning in relation to psychiatric diagnoses: schizophrenia and mood disorders," *Nordic Journal of Psychiatry*, vol. 52, no. 3, pp. 223–229, 1998.

11

The Psychosocial Consequences of Sports Participation for Individuals with Severe Mental Illness: A Metasynthesis Review

Andrew Soundy,[1] Paul Freeman,[2] Brendon Stubbs,[3] Michel Probst,[4,5] Carolyn Roskell,[1] and Davy Vancampfort[4,5]

[1]School of Sport, Exercise and Rehabilitation Sciences, University of Birmingham, Birmingham B15 2TT, UK
[2]School of Biological Sciences, University of Essex, Essex CO4 3SQ, UK
[3]School of Health and Social Care, University of Greenwich, London SE10 9LS, UK
[4]Department of Neurosciences, University Psychiatric Centre, KU Leuven, Leuvensesteenweg 517, 3070 Kortenberg, Belgium
[5]Department of Rehabilitation Sciences, KU Leuven, Tervuursevest 101, 3001 Leuven, Belgium

Correspondence should be addressed to Andrew Soundy; a.a.soundy@bham.ac.uk

Academic Editor: Takahiro Nemoto

The purpose of the current metasynthesis review was to explore the psychosocial benefits of sport and psychosocial factors which impact on sports participation for individuals with severe mental illness. AMED, CINAHL Plus, Medline, EMBASE, ProQuest Nursing & Allied Health Source, and Science Citation Index were searched from inception until January 2014. Articles included use qualitative methods to examine the psychosocial effects of sports participation in people with severe mental illness. Methodological quality was assessed using the Consolidated Criteria for Reporting Qualitative Studies and a case study tool. Included studies were analysed within a metasynthesis approach. Eight articles involving 56 patients met the inclusion criteria. The results identified the broader and direct psychosocial benefits of sport. Sport provided a "normal" environment and interactions that were not associated with an individual's mental illness. Sport provided individuals with a sense of meaning, purpose, belonging, identity, and achievement. Other findings are discussed. Direct psychosocial benefits are a consequence of sports participation for the vast majority of individuals with severe mental illness. Further to this, sports participation was associated with a reduction in social isolation and an increase in social confidence, autonomy, and independence.

1. Introduction

The Council of Europe [1] defines the term sports participation as all forms of physical activity which, through casual or organised participation, aim at expressing or improving physical fitness and mental wellbeing, forming social relationships or obtaining results in competitions at all levels. Within the context of physical activity, sport is considered a particular type of leisure time physical activity [2]. Sports participation may be one way in which individuals with severe mental illness can achieve the current physical activity recommendations [3] and it is very likely, based on literature from other populations, that the participation itself has biopsychosocial benefits [4–6]. These benefits are important when considering the physical [7] and social [8] health

disparity between individuals with severe mental illness and the general population.

It is important to recognise that the benefits of physical activity are most often derived from research that has focused on the effects of exercise therapy. In contrast to sport, exercise therapy is physical activity that is repetitive, structured, and planned and is able to improve or maintain one or more components of physical fitness [9]. Thus, understanding the direct benefits of sports participation would be extremely useful. A previous review [10] has suggested that sports participation can have a positive effect on several psychosocial domains that relate to an individuals mental health, including self-esteem, body awareness, social interaction, and ability to organise time and undertake physical activity. A recent qualitative metaethnographic review [11] has highlighted the postive impact exercise therapy has on several important psychosocial domains, including, but not limited to, an individual's autonomy and athletic identity; however, this research did not establish the broader direct benefits (benefits that were generic and could assist social engagement, interaction, or behaviour in other settings and contexts) on other aspects of the individuals life. Recently, research [12] coindering the views of indivduals with schizophrenia has identified broader psychosocial benefits of undertaking phyical activity. These include self-initiated positive changes in behaviour and increased confidence in other settings, having a sense of purpose and meaning and providing a sense of achievement, pride, and confidence. Further direct benefits included a sense of belonging, cohesion, and support from similar others. These findings require further consideration. Within previous sports reviews, the potential social value of sport has been considered by Langle et al. [10] who identified that sports participation can benefit self-esteem and social interactions. Given the above findings, it is reasonable to assume that sports participation may have a direct and broader social benefit for individuals with severe mental illness. For instance, it may be that sports participation can increase self- and social-confidence, which are both important factors that are assoicated with improvements in an individual's mental health [13]. However, further research is required to establish this.

Aims of the Study. The aim of the present study is to conduct a metasynthesis review to explore the broader psychosocial benefits of sport particpation for individuals with severe mental illness.

2. Methods

A metasynthesis [14] (a particular review technique, which was used in order to synthesise qualitative data) was undertaken and is reported in 3 phases [12]: (1) a systematic search of the literature, (2) a critical appraisal of identified studies, and (3) a synthesis of research to reveal overarching and emerging themes regarding the broader psychosocial value of sport for individuals with severe mental illness.

2.1. Phase 1: Systematic Search. A systematic search of major electronic databases was conducted from inception until January 2014 including AMED, CINAHL Plus, Medline EMBASE, ProQuest Nursing & Allied Health Source, and Science Citation Index. The key search terms included sport OR exercise OR physical activity OR training AND schizophrenia OR severe mental illness OR bipolar disorder OR schizoaffective disorder AND qualitative OR ethnography OR phenomenology OR grounded theory OR case study OR case series. In addition, we conducted hand searching of the included articles' reference lists.

2.1.1. Eligibility Criteria. Articles were eligible if (1) they included individuals with a diagnosis that fell within the range of severe and enduring mental health problems including individuals with schizophrenia, bipolar disorder, and schizo-affective disorder (DSM-V, ICD-10). The classification

of severe mental illness is defined by other features in addition to the diagnosis [15, 16], these include the need for formal and informal care, the impaired ability to cope on a daily basis, an extended period of time with the illness (>6 months), and finally the need to consider safety for the individual (intentional/unintentional self-harm, abuse from others, and safety for others), (2) the research utilised qualitative methods, (3) the study reported the views, perceptions, or experiences of sports participation, and (4) the research was published in English. Articles were excluded if (1) they were presented as stories or (2) if they were presented commentaries which did not provide any analysis or did not consider taking part in sport.

2.1.2. Study Selection Process and Data Extraction. Two authors (AS/DV) screened the titles and abstracts of all identified articles. A paper was included when it was considered that it satisfied all eligibility criteria.

2.2. Phase 2: Critical Appraisal of the Included Studies. In order to assess the quality of included qualitative articles, we used the Consolidated Criteria for Reporting Qualitative Studies (COREQ) [17]. The COREQ provides clear guidelines to enable a gold standard approach in reporting qualitative studies. We report a summary score from each of the three COREQ domains, as well as a total score. The score is based on each question either being reported correctly (scoring a point) or not (scoring no point), with a maximum possible score of 32. Domain 1 entitled "the research team and reflexivity" is split into two areas of assessment, first, the personal characteristics of the research team which may impact on the researchers observations and interpretations, and second, the relationship established, or the interactions with the participants under investigation. Domain 2 entitled "study design" is split into four areas of assessment and includes the theoretical framework used, how the participants were selected, the chosen setting with contextual details, and how the data was collected, recorded, and transcribed. Domain 3 entitled "study design, and analysis and findings" considers two areas of assessment including identifying the process undertaken for data analysis, method of triangulation, and validation processes. Second, this domain considers how the reporting is undertaken, considering the consistency in reporting findings, consideration to major and minor themes.

In order to assess the quality of nonqualitative articles we used criteria established by Crombie [18]. We created a 10-question assessment tool which was based on questions proposed by the author. The tick box scoring system for this tool was utilised as answers to the proposed questions, the answers included "yes," "no," or unsure. For example "Is the researcher's perspective clearly described and taken into account?" When an answer of no was recorded, a comments box was provided to detail why.

2.3. Phase 3: The Synthesis. Thematic line-by-line coding was undertaken using participants' quotes and authors' comments [14]. Themes were then rearranged and streamlined.

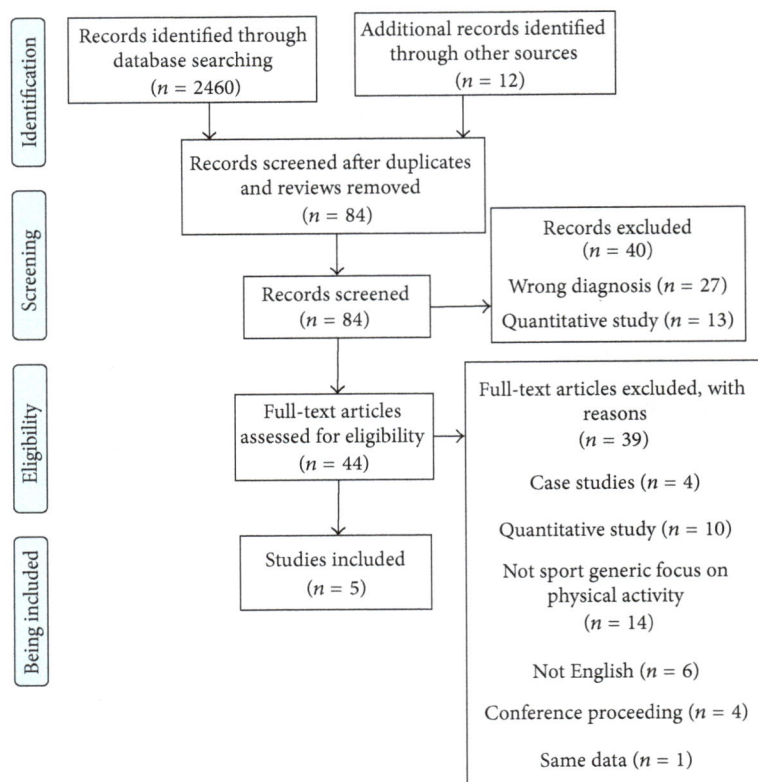

FIGURE 1: A PRISMA diagram for the study. Adapted from Moher et al. [27]. For more information, visit http://www.prisma-statement.org/.

An audit trail of the thematic development is available from the primary author.

3. Results

3.1. The Systematic Search. Eight articles [19–26] met the inclusion criteria. Figure 1 provides the results of the search using a traditional review flow diagram [27]. The eight articles included 56 individuals (39 male, 2 female, and 15 not identified). Table 1 provides the summary characteristics of the included studies.

3.2. Critical Appraisal of the Studies. No studies that were assessed using the COREQ ($n = 5$) had data that was considered as flawed for the purposes of the metasynthesis analysis [28]. Thus, all five studies were included in the synthesis. Across studies the weakest of the three domains assessed was details regarding the study designs. The study by Iancu et al. [23] had the lowest score. However, the available data was considered to be authentic and usable within the synthesis. Table 2 provides a summary of COREQ scores. Three studies [24–26] were assessed using the alternative appraisal form. Only one study [23] was considered unclear in some several domains, including the researcher's perspective, the methods for data collection and analysis, and if more than one researcher took part in this analysis.

3.3. The Synthesis. Four themes and 18 subthemes were identified. The themes were (1) the social meaning of sport in the lives of patients and what it represents in participants' lives, (2) the direct benefits of sport, (3) the organisation, processes, and challenges of the sports activity, and (4) the use of functional social support. Indicative quotes from first order and second order interpretations are available from the primary author. Supplementary File A (see Supplementary Material available online at http://dx.doi.org/10.1155/2015/261642) provides a full thematic breakdown and Supplementary File B provides the translational benefits of sports model.

3.3.1. The Social Meaning of Sport in the Lives of Patients. Three subthemes were generated from this theme: (1) a positive social experience to look forward to, be part of, and reflect about, (2) feeling part of a community and creating a positive identity, and (3) an activity that promoted autonomous behaviour and social engagement.

The sporting activities seemed to generate enthusiasm among the patients before and after the activity [19, 21, 23]. This could represent a positive topic of conversation and through this means served to promote sport to peers within the mental health setting. In contrast to this, one study [22] identified that users could find difficulty in the effort required to undertake the activity and be tired following the activity. The second theme detailed the social aspects of the sporting experience. These included that sport meant

TABLE 1: The study characteristics of the included studies.

Study	Design	Participants	Assessment, Intervention and setting	Outcome measures	Main results
Carless and Douglas (2004) [19]	Case study design within an ideographic approach	9 ♂ with severe and enduring mental illness	9-week Golf Project. Mental health staff was involved in recruiting and publicising the group before study starting. Tangible support was provided including; free transport, entry, equipment and tea, coffee, and biscuits. Also "some" were telephoned before session as a reminder. The golf project was planned by the second author (a PGA golf coach). A staged approach across 9 weeks was undertaken: (1) social meeting in the café centre with indoor putting instruction and a game, (2) two introductory sessions within the driving range, (3) a supported par 3 course session, (4) a third driving range session, (5) two supported sessions on the par 3 course, (6) two free play sessions on the par 3 course.	Focused themes around attendance considering factors that threatened attendance (competition, crossing the bridge, Texas scramble, and time to move on) and factors which encouraged attendance (doing something normal, a safety net, bubbling about golf, a relaxing sport, and caring golf).	Money and transport barriers to autonomous play. A transfer of responsibility occurred and autonomy increased across time. Enthusiasm was demonstrated about golf. The low intensity nature of the sport was valuable. A caring environment and atmosphere was valued. It was important to do something normal.
Clark et al. (1991) [20]	Phenomenological approach	8 ♂ patients with schizophrenia Age range 19–42	5-day white water canoe trip in Northern Ontario. Support team included occupational therapist, nurse, and 5 skilled canoe instructors. Days 1-2 2 days for training canoeing strokes, river morphology, camping skills, and safety way to fall into the rapids. Days 2-5 Canoeing down river, camping, and working as a group Semi-interviews were 1-hour long >6 months after experience.	Questions from interviews on critical incidents, interactions with others, emotional experiences, and self-perceptions.	Benefits in three broad categories: the experience of pleasure, belonging, and ability to talk. Challenging activity provided accomplishment and pride. Positive emotions, fun excitement, and fear also. Normalising activity for interactions between staff and patients.
Carter-Morris and Faulkner (2003) [21]	Phenomenological approach	5 (♂ = 4) 3 individuals with schizophrenia. 1 with manic depression and 1 with chronic anxiety.	Interviewing participants who had become part of a football team for individuals with severe and enduring mental illness. Team trained "regularly." Involved in national tournaments and took part in "Pallastrad" in Italy = team travelled to Italy and participated in football and other sporting events with mental health services users across Europe.	Questions from interview schedule not identified.	Project as a normalising activity and meaningful experience. Importance of accessing a positive identity. Activity benefited positive symptoms. Barriers to participation associated with medication.
Crone and Guy (2008) [22]	Grounded theory approach Using focus groups	11 individuals (♂ = 10) with severe mental health problems	Sports therapy that was undertaken within an NHS trust for a period between 2 months and 4 years. Twice weekly sessions were available including outpatient and inpatient. Sessions included mainly badminton and the fitness gym.	Topics in focus groups included motivations for participation, experiences, perceptions on the role of sports therapy, and their perceived benefits from participation.	Themes included Taking part in that there was value in doing something rather than nothing. Reasons for participation: biopsychosocial reasons were given. Attitudes and opinions: the term therapy was not well liked. Perceived role of sports therapy: it was considered as beneficial on mental health symptoms. Factors affecting participation: classic motivation barriers are noted. Perceived benefits are noted on self-esteem, accomplishment, feeling positive, and being more mentally alert. Improvements for the future: participants identified changes to the program that may be beneficial.
Iancu et al. (2004) [23]	Case studies	8 ♂ with schizophrenia	Inpatient table tennis tournament was organised with tangible rewards including trophies, sport shirts and two hats. 4 therapists assisted in the doubles tournaments. Matches were 1 set up to 21 points.	Vignettes of the experience of three patients considered.	When enjoyed and successful, provides a sense of achievement and focus. Potential to cause negative emotions because of losing or being fearful of the experience.

TABLE 2: The summary of correctly scored domains of the COREQ (Tong et al., 2007 [17]) appraisal for the 4 included studies.

Author/year of publication	Domain 1 (/8) Research team and reflexivity	Domain 2 (/15) Study design	Domain 3 (9) Analysis and findings	Total (/32)
Clark et al. (1991) [20]	3	8	4	15/32
Carter-Morris and Faulkner (2003) [21]	7	9	6	24/32
Carless and Douglas (2004) [19]	7	11	6	24/32
Crone and Guy (2008) [22]	7	10	8	25/32
Iancu et al. (2004) [23]	4	6	2	12/32
Mean	5.6	8.8	5.2	20
Median	7	9	6	24

being part of a group and receiving an identity from that [20, 21, 24, 25], having a social interest which gave meaning [19–22], providing a topic of conversation which was different and interesting, for instance, being able to reflect on a task that was overcome, failed, or was achieved. More generally sport required individuals to undertake a social learning experience [20], which extended and enhanced their social network. Individuals demonstrated increases in social confidence [19–22], greater social skills [23], and a decrease in social withdrawal from experiencing a new social world [21]. This particular subtheme also represents a direct benefit of sport; however, it should be noted that one patient [25] stated it had not changed them as a person or impacted on their identity. The final subtheme identified that, through engaging in sport, individuals became more autonomous and had developed or enhanced their ability for social engagement. The development of autonomy was, in part, due to sport representing a challenge [20] that was overcome, by participants just by undertaking and enjoying the experience [22], and providing individuals with a sense of belief in themselves.

3.3.2. The Direct Benefits of Sport. Five subthemes are reported within this theme: (1) an activity that provided meaning and purpose, (2) undertaking a normalised activity, (3) the benefit of sport serving as a distraction, (4) achievement accomplishment and pride, and (5) feelings and emotions generated by the sports.

The first benefit identified by patients was that sport provided individuals with somewhere to go and something to do [19, 22]. This in essence means patients can feel they have a sense of purpose and have access to meaningful and valuable social experiences [24]; this is because sports can be highly valued by patients [25].

The second subtheme, undertaking a normalised activity, was represented by four major reasons. First, sport provided an opportunity to be someone within a positive group and provided a positive sense of identity [19, 21]. Second, interactions within the sporting environment were often different as conversation was represented by what the participants were doing rather than focusing on their mental illness or problems [21]. Third, sport was often associated with a normal trip with excitement and pleasure [22] or getting back to what was perceived as normal for the patient [25, 26]. It should be noted that patients in one study empathised

the detachment from the medical system within this as a benefit [19]. Finally, it represented a social learning opportunity as it could help break down perceptual biases. As one patient from the study by Carter-Morris and Faulkner [21] stated "it breaks down barriers and builds bridges."

The third subtheme identified that sport served as a distraction from individuals' typical worries, anxieties, or mental health symptoms [21, 22, 24]. The fourth subtheme illustrated the importance of accomplishing a task, which acted as a source of pride for individuals and the social network within the activity acted to support that achievement [19, 20, 22]. This included the ability to successfully complete the activity [25, 26]. The fifth subtheme highlighted the different emotions evoked by sports participation. Often this was centred on positive feelings such as fun [26], but also other feelings like being more positive or having more positive thoughts after the activity, for example, running [24]. However, emotions such as fear or apprehension were also reported. These were observed in different ways and were in a response to competitive situation [19]. For instance, Iancu et al. [23] noted an apprehension of the ability of others, whilst Clark et al. [20] identified the fear as well as excitement about the danger level of the activity. Finally, some participants noted that sport could be a way of releasing negative emotions such as anger or frustration.

3.3.3. The Organisation, Process, and Challenges of the Sports Programme. Three subthemes were identified within this theme: (1) the organisation and content of the sports programme, (2) the supported environment and atmosphere, and (3) challenges presented by the sport.

The first subtheme regarding the organisation of the sport identified the importance of how the sport was marketed and promoted by the researchers and health care professionals before the activity began [19, 22, 23]. Further to this, Carless and Douglas [19] highlighted the importance of progression of the task difficulty and the use of supported competition as an important aid to the initial experience. The second subtheme identified the importance of the environment and the need to use the sport to foster a sense of belonging, identity, and interaction [19, 21, 22, 24–26]. The final subtheme included the importance of individual considerations around sport which need to be known in order to foster participation. These included the importance of a holistic approach by staff [22], understanding the effects medication can have on individuals [21], being aware of incidences (perceptual and interactional) during the sport that may prevent further attendance [19], and finally responding to needs in order to help a situation [23].

3.3.4. The Use of Functional Social Support.

This theme was organised into four preexisting dimensions of social support [29]: (1) esteem, (2), emotional, (3) informational, and (4) tangible.

The importance of esteem support was recognised across all studies as a valuable facilitator of engagement, particularly when provided by the staff involved with sport. This included encouragement, as well as positive feedback about performance and accomplishments. In turn, participants learnt to provide each other with esteem support as well. Emotional support was the most specifically mentioned theme with specific techniques employed in order to help participants. Staff were required to be empathic towards the barriers faced by users [21]; this required individuals to be sensitive towards users in how they spoke to them and to take a real interest in their lives and be known by them [22]. Where a spirit of camaraderie between all could be generated, it provided positive effects for the users [20]. A further aspect of emotional support came from peers; in that it was positive for users to feel related to others [20, 22] and want others to do well [19], being willing to contact peers in order to support them to attend [22] or having a place where the patient felt being able to talk about worries in their life [25]. There was less evidence regarding informational support, but it was considered important for technical skills in golf and canoeing [19, 20] and it was clearly apparent in the strategies used within all studies to promote initial participation in sport. In one study, a patient cites a primary reason for undertaking the activity was due to a physiotherapist recommending that he should get fitter [25]. Finally, tangible support was dominated by the importance of cost, including cost of travel and participation in the activity [19, 22]. Tangible rewards were also utilised by Iancu et al. [23] in the form of prizes.

4. Discussion

The current results illustrate that sport can play a valuable role in helping individuals overcome the debilitating effects of social isolation. Participation in sport can assist individuals with severe mental illness in gaining social confidence by providing individuals with positive experiences and enabling them to become more independent and autonomous. Importantly, participation in sport provides individuals with access to an activity which provides a sense of meaning, purpose, and achievement in their lives, it gives access to more "normal" interactions, and it distracts from more negative thoughts and can create positive emotions and feelings. To generate a positive experience it is important that the sport is promoted before it starts and provides an environment which fosters support and an activity that has a progression in difficulty to enable positive experiences, assisted by their peers. Further, it is clear that the different dimensions of functional support are highly valuable and require consideration. A summary of the direct benefits of sports participation has

been included in a model generated from these results and can be obtained from the primary author.

4.1. The Importance of the Social Environment.

Sports and physical activity programmes for individuals with severe mental illness are frequently set up using social support as a core strategy to enhance engagement and adherence to physical activity. Key elements of support are recognised including the importance of the group leader [30] and supportive staff across the health care team [31] who are able to provide esteem and emotional support. The current study supports these positions but also identified the importance of the group dynamics and individuals feeling connected or a sense of belonging to a group, which was generated through peer support generated within the activity. Good examples of this can be seen in other physical activity interventions, for example, [32–34]. It is worth noting that peer led interventions are currently rarely used in individuals with severe mental illness [35]. Although it has been recognised, that act of support from peers and practitioners may be an essential part of promoting and sustaining the self-esteem of individuals, as well as creating a perception of control over their environment [13].

Different aspects of the environment and culture influenced the participants' physical activity behaviour. For instance, both a competitive and noncompetitive environment were reported as positive factors that could increase participant [19, 23]. By varying the competitive environments, it may be possible to influence attendance and enjoyment of the sport, although the reactions to this approach may be highly individual. An interesting finding from the study by Ginis and colleagues [35] was that the fear and excitement of activities with a danger element may distract individuals from negative thoughts and encourage a focus purely on the activity at hand. This in turn may have a positive influence on the experience of the sport and be positively identified in social discourse following the sport.

4.2. The Processes of Social Change Explored.

Mental health care programmes are needed which are designed to combat social isolation and develop social contact and community integration [8]. One reason for this is because establishing a good social network is an important aspect in recovery for mental illness [36]. The current results identify that sport can provide positive opportunities for social engagement. Perhaps the most central processes by which direct social benefits are gained is through social learning experiences, the opportunity to feel "normal," and access to new and different social discourses that have a "distance" from institutionalised settings and identities. Important aspects which make this possible are the physical location and environment where the activity takes place, the culture of that environment, and the unity and collective identity between different members who attend the sports activity [11]. Importantly, it is possible that the sport environment provided normative and behavioural guidance [13] by individuals within the sport setting by modelling values and beliefs which are positive regarding exercise, interactions, and behaviours.

It is evident from research literature that individuals with severe mental illness are vulnerable to social and cognitive biases [16]. One important role of sports may be to provide an environment where the effects of such perceptions are minimised and with further successful experiences individuals are able to engage in a greater range of activities. Once individuals are embedded within a sporting activity, it is possible that they can assume positive roles, for instance, organising the activity, which can facilitate autonomy and self-belief.

4.3. Limitations. Several limitations must be acknowledged; primarily, this research was restricted to a small number of sports activity and a small sample size. The analysis was focused on the social benefits and does not consider the physical benefits. Further, the primary author may have restricted the analysis by his theoretical position or limited understanding of previous literature.

Conflict of Interests

The authors declare that there is no conflict of interests regarding the publication of this paper.

Acknowledgment

Davy Vancampfort is funded by the Research Foundation-Flanders (FWO-Vlaanderen).

References

[1] Council of Europe, *The European Sports Charter*, Council of Europe, Brussels, Belgium, 2001.

[2] E. T. Howley, "Type of activity: resistance, aerobic and leisure versus occupational physical activity," *Medicine and Science in Sports and Exercise*, vol. 33, pp. S364–S369, 2001.

[3] D. Vancampfort, M. De Hert, L. H. Skjerven et al., "International Organization of Physical Therapy in Mental Health consensus on physical activity within multidisciplinary rehabilitation programmes for minimising cardio-metabolic risk in patients with schizophrenia," *Disability and Rehabilitation*, vol. 34, no. 1, pp. 1–12, 2012.

[4] M. Mountjoy, L. B. Andersen, N. Armstrong et al., "International Olympic Committee consensus statement on the health and fitness of young people through physical activity and sport," *British Journal of Sports Medicine*, vol. 45, no. 11, pp. 839–848, 2011.

[5] P. Krustrup, J. Dvorak, A. Junge, and J. Bangsbo, "Executive summary: the health and fitness benefits of regular participation in small-sided football games," *Scandinavian Journal of Medicine & Science in Sports*, vol. 20, pp. 132–135, 2010.

[6] P. Oja, S. Titze, A. Bauman et al., "Health benefits of cycling: a systematic review," *Scandinavian Journal of Medicine and Science in Sports*, vol. 21, no. 4, pp. 496–509, 2011.

[7] M. de Hert, J. M. Dekker, D. Wood, K. G. Kahl, R. I. G. Holt, and H.-J. Möller, "Cardiovascular disease and diabetes in people with severe mental illness position statement from the European Psychiatric Association (EPA), supported by the European Association for the Study of Diabetes (EASD) and the European Society of Cardiology (ESC)," *European Psychiatry*, vol. 24, no. 6, pp. 412–424, 2009.

[8] S. J. Linz and B. A. Sturm, "The phenomenon of social isolation in the severely mentally ill," *Perspectives in Psychiatric Care*, vol. 49, no. 4, pp. 243–254, 2013.

[9] C. J. Caspersen, K. E. Powell, and G. M. Christenson, "Physical activity, exercise and physical fitness: definitions and distinctions for health-related research," *Public Health Reports*, vol. 100, no. 2, pp. 126–131, 1985.

[10] G. Langle, G. Siemssen, and S. Hornberger, "The role of sports in the treatment and rehabilitation of schizophrenic patients," *Rehabilitation*, vol. 39, no. 5, pp. 276–282, 2000.

[11] A. Soundy, T. Kingstone, and P. Coffee, "Understanding the psychosocial process of physical activity for individuals with severe mental illness: a meta-ethnography," in *Mental Illness 2*, L. L'Abate, Ed., Intech, Vienna, Austria, 2012.

[12] A. Soundy, P. Freeman, B. Stubbs, M. Probst, P. Coffee, and D. Vancampfort, "The transcending benefits of physical activity for individuals with schizophrenia: a systematic review and meta-ethnography," *Psychiatry Research*, vol. 220, no. 1-2, pp. 11–19, 2014.

[13] P. A. Thoits, "Mechanisms linking social ties and support to physical and mental health," *Journal of Health and Social Behavior*, vol. 52, no. 2, pp. 145–161, 2011.

[14] J. Thomas and A. Harden, "Methods for the thematic synthesis of qualitative research in systematic reviews," *BMC Medical Research Methodology*, vol. 8, article 45, 2008.

[15] Department of Health, *Building Bridges: A Guide to Arrangements for Inter-Agency Working for the Care and Protection of Severely Mentally Ill People*, Department of Health, London, UK, 1995.

[16] A. Soundy, G. Faulkner, and A. Taylor, "Exploring variability and perceptions of lifestyle physical activity among individuals with severe and enduring mental health problems: a qualitative study," *Journal of Mental Health*, vol. 16, no. 4, pp. 493–503, 2007.

[17] A. Tong, P. Sainsbury, and J. Craig, "Consolidated criteria for reporting qualitative research (COREQ): a 32-item checklist for interviews and focus groups," *International Journal for Quality in Health Care*, vol. 19, no. 6, pp. 349–357, 2007.

[18] I. Crombie, *The Pocket Guide to Critical Apprasial*, BMJ Publishing Group, London, UK, 1996.

[19] D. Carless and K. Douglas, "A golf programme for people with severe and enduring mental health problems," *Journal of Public Mental Health*, vol. 3, no. 4, pp. 26–39, 2004.

[20] C. Clark, P. Goering, and G. Tomlinson, "Challenging expectations: client perceptions of white water canoeing," *Psychosocial Rehabilitation Journal*, vol. 14, no. 4, pp. 71–76, 1991.

[21] P. Carter-Morris and G. Faulkner, "A football project for service users: the role of football in educing social exclusion," *Journal of Mental Health Promotion*, vol. 2, pp. 24–30, 2003.

[22] D. Crone and H. Guy, "'I know it is only exercise, but to me it is something that keeps me going': a qualitative approach to understanding mental health service users' experiences of sports therapy: feature Article," *International Journal of Mental Health Nursing*, vol. 17, no. 3, pp. 197–207, 2008.

[23] I. Iancu, R. D. Strous, N. Nevo, and J. Chelben, "A Table Tennis Tournament in the Psychiatric Hospital: description and suggestion for salutogenic implications," *The International Journal of Psychosocial Rehabilitation*, vol. 9, article 11, 2004.

[24] D. Carless, "Narrative, identity, and recovery from serious mental illness: a life history of a runner," *Qualitative Research in Psychology*, vol. 5, no. 4, pp. 233–248, 2008.

[25] D. Carless and K. Douglas, "The role of sport and exercise in recovery from serious mental illness: two case studies," *International Journal of Men's Health*, vol. 7, no. 2, pp. 137–156, 2008.

[26] H. Leutwyler, E. M. Hubbard, S. Vinogradov, and G. A. Dowling, "Videogames to promote physical activity in older adults with schizophrenia," *Games for Health Journal: Research, Development, and Clinical Applications*, vol. 1, no. 5, pp. 381–383, 2012.

[27] D. Moher, A. Liberati, J. Tetzlaff, and D. G. Altman, "Preferred reporting items for systematic reviews and meta-analyses: the PRISMA statement," *British Medical Journal*, vol. 339, no. 7716, pp. 332–336, 2009.

[28] M. Dixon-Woods, A. Sutton, R. Shaw et al., "Appraising qualitative research for inclusion in systematic reviews: a quantitative and qualitative comparison of three methods," *Journal of Health Services Research and Policy*, vol. 12, no. 1, pp. 42–47, 2007.

[29] C. E. Cutrona and D. Russell, "Type of social support and specific stress: toward a theory of optimal matching," in *Social Support: An Interactional View*, B. R. Sarason, I. G. Sarason, and G. R. Pierce, Eds., Wiley, New York, NY, USA, 1990.

[30] C. R. Richardson, G. Faulkner, J. McDevitt, G. S. Skrinar, D. S. Hutchinson, and J. D. Piette, "Integrating physical activity into mental health services for persons with serious mental illness," *Psychiatric Services*, vol. 56, no. 3, pp. 324–331, 2005.

[31] A. Soundy, B. Stubbs, M. Probst, L. Hemmings, and D. Vancampfort, "Barriers to and facilitators of physical activity among persons with schizophrenia: a survey of physical therapists," *Psychiatric Services*, vol. 65, no. 5, pp. 693–696, 2014.

[32] L. H. Beebe and R. F. Harris, "Using pedometers to document physical activity in patients with schizophrenia spectrum disorders: a feasibility study," *Journal of Psychosocial Nursing and Mental Health Services*, vol. 50, no. 2, pp. 44–49, 2012.

[33] L. H. Beebe and K. Smith, "Feasibility of the Walk, Address, Learn and Cue (WALC) intervention for schizophrenia specturm disorders," *Archives of Psychiatric Nursing*, vol. 24, no. 1, pp. 54–62, 2010.

[34] L. H. Beebe, K. Smith, R. Burk et al., "Effect of a motivational intervention on exercise behavior in persons with schizophrenia spectrum disorders," *Community Mental Health Journal*, vol. 47, no. 6, pp. 628–636, 2011.

[35] K. A. M. Ginis, C. R. Nigg, and A. L. Smith, "Peer-delivered physical activity interventions: an overlooked opportunity for physical activity promotion," *Translational Behavioral Medicine*, vol. 3, no. 4, pp. 434–443, 2013.

[36] D. Elisha, D. Castle, and B. Hocking, "Reducing social isolation in people with mental illness: the role of the psychiatrist," *Australasian Psychiatry*, vol. 14, no. 3, pp. 281–284, 2006.

12

Limitations of Randomized Control Designs in Psychotherapy Research

Glenn Shean

College of William & Mary, P.O. Box 8795, Williamsburg, VA 23187-8795, USA

Correspondence should be addressed to Glenn Shean; gdshea@gmail.com

Academic Editor: Christine M. Blasey

Despite the growing influence of lists of empirically supported therapies (ESTs) there are concerns about the design and conduct of this body of research. These concerns include limitations inherent in the requirements of randomized control trials (RCTs) that favor those psychotherapies that define problems and outcome in terms of uncomplicated symptoms. Additional concerns have to do with criteria for patient selection, lack of integration with research on psychotherapy process and effectiveness studies, limited outcome criteria, and lack of controls for experimenter bias. RCT designs have an important place in outcome research; however it is important to recognize that these designs also place restrictions on what and how psychotherapy can be studied. There is a need for large scale psychotherapy outcome research based on designs that allow for inclusion of process variables and the study of the effects of those idiographic approaches to therapy that do not lend themselves to RCT designs. Interpretative phenomenological analysis may provide a useful method for the evaluation of the effectiveness of idiographic approaches to psychotherapy where outcome is not understood solely in terms of symptom reduction.

1. Introduction

There are several issues related to the external validity of lists of empirically supported psychotherapies (ESTs) that should be considered before broad policy changes are instituted based on this body of research. First, the design requirements of randomized control trial (RCT) studies do not allow for adequate understanding of the multifaceted nature of many mental health problems or the complex interplay of individual differences, interpersonal processes, and range of potential outcomes that are inherent in psychotherapy practice. Second, the EST literature is based on studies characterized by unacknowledged sampling issues, methodological constraints, researcher bias, and limited outcome criteria [1–3].

2. Background

A white paper issued by a Task Force of the American Psychological Association in 1995 stated that "in order to remain competitive in the mental health services marketplace psychologists must provide evidence of therapeutic efficacy in the form of lists of empirically supported psychotherapies (ESTs) for specific disorders" [4]. The APA paper specified RCTs as the ideal design for studies of psychotherapy efficacy, in which "a treatment is manualized and demonstrated to be more effective than other treatments or placebo..." [4]. A large number of efficacy studies have been published that are the basis for lists of ESTs [5]. These lists are the basis for proposals to differentiate between "psychological treatments" and "psychotherapy" [6]. As proposed by Barlow and Carl, for example, [6], the term "psychological treatment" would be restricted to ESTs designed to address specific diagnoses within a health-care context. "Psychotherapy" in turn would be limited to references to processes and procedures designed to resolve issues such as interpersonal and relationship problems and personal growth concerns and administered outside of the health-care system. Given the broad policy and social implications of this proposal, it is worthwhile to more closely examine the external validity of lists of ESTs.

2.1. RCT Designs. Double-blind randomized control trial designs are widely considered to be the "gold standard" for treatment efficacy studies [7]. RCTs are the most direct way of determining whether a cause-effect relation exists between treatment and outcome [8]. RCT designs include the following features [8]. (1) The first item is random allocation of participants to intervention and control groups, in order to minimize allocation bias and to balance known and unknown prognostic factors in the assignment of treatments. (2) Both patients and clinicians must remain unaware of which treatment (e.g., placebo control or a previously tested treatment positive control study) was given until the study is completed. (3) All intervention groups are treated identically except for the experimental treatment. (4) Patients are analyzed within the group to which they were allocated. (5) Analyses are designed to estimate the size of the difference in predicted outcomes between intervention and control groups. Valid studies using RCT designs also require representative samples of adequate size to support planned statistical analyses and close matching of treatment and control group patients based on defined criteria.

2.1.1. RCT Advantages and Limitations. The practice of patient selection based on uncomplicated DSM based symptoms, common to most RCT design EST studies, allows for enhanced matching of treatment and control groups and clarity of outcome criteria. On the other hand, this requirement restricts the population studied to a portion of the individuals who seek psychotherapy services, since many patients seek psychotherapy services for issues that transcend specific symptoms, and comorbidity of symptoms is common. The use of therapy manuals in RCT studies allows for enhanced control over the experimental treatment under study but restricts the types of psychotherapeutic interventions that can be studied. The requirements of RCT designs in effect help to ensure the reliability of reported effects but limit the manner in which problems, treatments, and outcome criteria are defined, understood, and assessed [3, 9–11]. The effects of therapy moderators are assumed to be randomized in RCT design studies based on the assumption that randomization of group assignment takes into account potential effects of known moderators of therapeutic effects such as level of distress, social impairment, comorbidity, self-reflectiveness, readiness for change, openness to experience, level of engagement, ability to verbalize feelings, social support, and coping [1–3, 7, 10, 11]. Differences in dispositional traits that are correlated with DSM diagnoses (e.g., negative affect, submissiveness, low affect tolerance, and introversion) are also assumed to be randomized in RCT designs [2, 3]. The assumption that randomization of patient assignment controls for the effects of therapy moderators and process variables is valid only if study sample sizes are large enough to allow for adequate levels of power for valid statistical comparisons. Many EST studies are based on relatively small sample sizes, justified by power estimates based on questionable effect sizes reported in previous non-double-blind psychotherapy efficacy studies. These estimates are likely to be inflated by the effects of "therapist allegiance."

In contrast to most manualized psychotherapies now listed as ESTs, idiographic psychotherapies emphasize the importance of process variables as moderators of therapeutic effectiveness and tailor the application of therapeutic strategies and techniques to the particular characteristics and circumstances of each individual patient. These approaches cannot be manualized in a manner that can be applied in the same manner across patients. The goals of idiographic therapies are typically described in terms of changes that are more in line with the concept of *recovery* than symptom reduction. Idiographic therapies emphasize the multifaceted origins and nature of mental disorders and understand recovery as an ongoing process that requires flexibility on the part of the therapists, as well as responsibility, commitment, and motivation to change on the part of the patient. The goals of idiographic therapies are not limited to symptom reduction and include enhanced connection of memories, emotions, changes in patterns of problematic experiences, and relating in ways that enable patients to live more satisfying and effective symptom-free lives, to have richer and more satisfying relationships, and to find new ways to become more effective agents in their lives [1, 7, 11, 12].

2.2. Issues Related to ESTs

2.2.1. Sampling Practices. The practice of limiting RCT psychotherapy studies to populations with a single diagnosis and few if any comorbid problems does not mirror the realities of most clinical practice. Individuals who meet single uncomplicated symptom criteria are estimated to represent no more than about 20% of the overall population seeking psychotherapy services [2, 3, 13]. Surveys indicate that at least one-third to one-half of people seeking mental health treatment do not meet criteria for any one diagnostic category [2, 14]. When specific symptoms are the initial focus of treatment about one-half of the patients add new target complaints or change their complaints over the course of treatment [10, 14]. It is estimated that between 40% and 70% of individuals who present for treatment in clinical practice settings are excluded from EST studies because they do not meet the restrictive criteria required by RCT designs [3, 14]. Finally, many EST studies are conducted in university affiliated related clinics [13]. Participants are often enrolled in studies of behavioral or cognitive-behavioral therapy (CBT). The individuals selected for the study are not likely to be blind to the treatment condition and likely were referred because of prior information about the lead therapist's reputation. In short, the patient samples in university affiliated studies are not representative of the population at large nor are they randomly selected.

2.2.2. Length of Therapy. The average number of sessions for published EST studies is sixteen [2, 3]. The assumption that mental health problems can be resolved in an average of 16 or fewer sessions is not consistent with evidence for a significant psychotherapy dose-response relationship [3, 9] or with field studies of CBT for depressed patients that report an average of 69 sessions [3]. In contrast to the EST literature on treatment for depression, the research team conducted by the National Institute of Mental Health Treatment of Depression Collaborative Research Program concluded that

16 weeks of cognitive-behavioral or interpersonal therapy is insufficient for most patients to achieve full recovery and lasting remission [15]. Follow-up assessments of participants in the NIMH study, conducted at 6, 12, and 18 months after treatment, indicated that the percent of patients who were rated as recovered following the end of treatment and remained well during follow-up did not differ between the four treatment groups: about 30% for cognitive-behavioral therapy, interpersonal therapy, imipramine plus clinical management, and placebo plus clinical management. Long-term studies of patients treated by ESTs indicate high rates of relapse and seeking of alternative therapies [3, 15]. Evidence indicates that short-term therapies produce benefits more quickly than more individually focused therapies but long-term therapy is superior to short-term therapies at three- and five-year follow-up [16, 17].

2.2.3. Therapy Manuals. The use of manuals in RCT outcome studies is based on the assumption that psychotherapy can be formulated as a standardized set of procedures that can be applied across matched individuals without significant variation related to differences between either therapists or patients. There is logic in attempting to describe as systematically as possible the various principles and strategies involved in each therapeutic approach but it is important to acknowledge that this requirement limits the scope and range of problems that can be treated as well as the therapies that can be studied. The use of therapy manuals biases psychotherapy outcome research in favor of those therapies that can be operationalized [13, 14, 18]. Idiographic therapies do not lend themselves to manualization or standardized application across patients [19].

Finally, evidence indicates therapists within treatments vary significantly in outcomes so that some people respond to certain types of psychotherapy provided by some practitioners and others do not, and moderators of treatment effectiveness for one outcome indicator may not be the same as moderators of treatment for another [7, 11]. A more fruitful direction for future research would be to design studies that seek to identify the characteristics of patients that are associated with positive responses to different approaches to psychotherapy, with adequate safeguards for researcher bias.

2.2.4. Therapist Allegiance. It is often not practical to conduct true double-blind RCT studies of psychotherapy since it is difficult for both researchers and patients to remain blind to the therapeutic approaches included in the study. Efforts have been made to control for this source of error variance in non-double-blind RCT psychotherapy studies but evidence consistently indicates that the "same" therapy performs better in studies conducted by researchers who are committed to the approach than it does in studies conducted by others [20, 21]. Therapist allegiance accounts for about 69% of the variance in psychotherapy outcome studies [21]. Double-blind studies of psychotherapy are admittedly difficult to conduct; however, controls for the effects of therapy allegiance are not that difficult to implement. Luborsky and colleagues have published guidelines for how to control

for the effects of therapist allegiance but these suggestions are ignored in the EST literature [20, 21]. The guidelines suggested by Luborsky et al. represent minimal standards for valid psychotherapy outcome research. (1) Comparative treatment studies should be conducted using raters of varied theoretical persuasion, and researchers who have minimal allegiances to the approaches studied should be involved in conducting the study. (2) Therapists for each treatment mode should be selected and supervised by those who represent the same treatment mode, and therapists should be assigned to each mode of treatment on the basis of ratings of their effectiveness. (3) Outcome criteria developed based on the input of the therapists of all persuasions under study and long-term functional follow-up evaluations should be conducted using consistent outcome criteria. (4) If all else fails efficacy studies include researcher/therapist allegiance as a variable in all analyses.

2.2.5. Idiographic Psychotherapy Effectiveness and Process. Numerous psychotherapy studies have been published that support the effectiveness of idiographic approaches but these studies are ignored in lists of ESTs [6, 22–24]. Meta-analytic analyses of comparative outcome studies also indicate that large differences in effectiveness are not observed among the major approaches to psychotherapy (e.g., cognitive-behavioral, interpersonal, behavioral activation, psycho-dynamic, problem solving, or social skills training) for many problems [25]. Researchers have identified practitioner related moderators that contribute to therapeutic outcome across approaches to therapy, including the quality of the therapeutic alliance, fostering a sense of hope and self-efficacy in the patient, and that encourage relevant emotional expression in combination with meaningful cognitive and emotional processing and integration [26–29]. Process variables, such as the quality of the therapeutic relationship estimated to account for between 15 and 30% of the variance in outcome; therapist techniques about 15%; expectancy (hope), therapist credibility about 15%; and environmental and patient characteristics (e.g., readiness for change, openness, engagement, active participation, and ability to verbalize feelings) about 40%, are ignored in RCT studies [12, 29].

3. Conclusion

The use of RCT designs for the evaluation of psychotherapy effectiveness works best for those symptom focused approaches to psychotherapy that can be manualized and applied in essentially the same manner across patients who share a certain uncomplicated diagnosis. RCT designs are ideal when cause and effect relationships can be clearly defined, interventions can be applied in a similar manner across patients, and outcome criteria are applicable across all study participants. RCT designed studies have resulted in useful lists of ESTs that can be applied effectively to address specific DSM symptoms. On the other hand the requirements of RCT designs limit how problems are understood, psychotherapy can be practiced, and outcome can be defined and assessed. These design requirements disadvantage idiographic approaches to psychotherapy. Research is needed on the effectiveness of idiographic approaches to psychotherapy that are characterized by broad descriptions of patients' problems and allow for flexibility in how therapeutic processes are described, applied, and assessed in individual cases and indicators of recovery are defined and measured over extended follow-up intervals [19]. Not everyone seeking psychotherapy services is interested to, able to, or motivated to commit to the demands and relative ambiguity of idiographic therapies, just as not everyone seeks targeted approaches to therapy for the resolution of specific uncomplicated symptoms. RCT design requirements do not allow for research on the effectiveness of idiographic psychotherapies, nor do they allow researchers to address the full range of problems for which people seek psychotherapy.

Advances in the application of phenomenological psychology appear to hold promise for the study of the effects of idiographic psychotherapies [30]. Phenomenological psychology is rooted in attempts to construct a philosophical science of consciousness that includes both hermeneutics (theory of interpretation) and symbolic interactionism (posits that individual meanings are of central concern and are only accessible through an interpretive process) [30, 31]. Methods have been developed that allow for reliable idiographic understandings of patients, their social realities, and what it means to live with symptoms in a particular situation. IPA allows us to situate and validate observations developed through discourse, subjective engagement, and careful and sympathetic attention to how another person cares for and about certain "things," how they are involved and/or distressed by them, and how they are involved and tied up with certain aspects of their lives [31]. These methods lack the potential for clear delineation of cause and effect relationships in outcome research but hold promise for research on the effects of idiographic therapies in particular because they allow for (1) descriptions of the patients' concerns and cares and their orientation to the world and (2) contextualization of phenomenological claims within the patient's social, cultural, and physical environments in ways that make sense of the mutually constitutive relationship between "person" and "world" within a psychological framework that describes what this means to this person in this context [31].

IPA, in combination with methodological safeguards against researcher bias, can allow for more appropriate ways of evaluating idiographic approaches to psychotherapy and broaden our understanding of psychotherapy process while minimizing the risks of ungrounded theoretical relativism and authoritarianism. RCT designs are the "gold standard" for determining cause and effect relationships in studies of treatment effectiveness but it is important to recognize that not all approaches to psychotherapy can be adequately described, understood, and evaluated within RCT design requirements. Alternative research approaches are necessary in order to evaluate the effectiveness of idiographic approaches to psychotherapy.

Conflict of Interests

The author declares that there is no conflict of interests regarding the publication of this paper.

References

[1] B. Wampold, "Do therapies designated as ESTs for specific disorders produce outcomes superior to non-EST therapies? Not a scintilla of evidence to support ESTs as more effective than other treatments," in *Evidence-Based Practices in Mental Health: Debate and Dialogue on the Fundamental Questions*, J. C. Norcross, L. E. Beutler, and R. F. Levant, Eds., pp. 299–308, American Psychological Association, Washington, DC, USA, 2005.

[2] D. Westen and K. Morrison, "A multidimensional meta-analysis of treatments for depression, panic, and generalized anxiety disorder: an empirical examination of the status of empirically supported therapies," *Journal of Consulting and Clinical Psychology*, vol. 69, no. 6, pp. 875–899, 2001.

[3] D. Westen, C. M. Novotny, and H. Thompson-Brenner, "The empirical status of empirically supported psychotherapies: assumptions, findings, and reporting in controlled clinical trials," *Psychological Bulletin*, vol. 130, no. 4, pp. 631–663, 2004.

[4] American Psychological Association Task Force on Psychological Intervention Guidelines, *Template for Developing Guidelines: Interventions for Mental Disorders and Psychosocial Aspects of Physical Disorders*, American Psychological Association, Washington, DC, USA, 1995.

[5] D. L. Chambless and T. H. Ollendick, "Empirically supported psychological interventions: controversies and evidence," *Annual Review of Psychology*, vol. 52, pp. 685–716, 2001.

[6] D. Barlow and J. Carl, "The future of clinical psychology: promises, perspectives, and predictions," in *The Oxford Handbook of Clinical Psychology*, D. H. Barlow and P. E. Nathan, Eds., pp. 891–911, Oxford University Press, New York, NY, USA, 2011.

[7] P. A. Arean and H. C. Kraemer, *High Duality Psychotherapy Research: From Conception to Piloting to National Trials*, Oxford University Press, New York, NY, USA, 2013.

[8] K. F. Schulz, L. Chalmers, R. J. Hayes, and D. G. Altman, "Empirical evidence of bias: dimensions of methodological quality associated with estimates of treatment effects in controlled trials," *The Journal of the American Medical Association*, vol. 273, no. 5, pp. 408–412, 1995.

[9] F. Richardson, B. Fowers, and C. Guignon, *Renewing Psychology: Beyond Scientisim and Constructivisim*, Jossey-Bass, San Francisco, Calif, USA, 1999.

[10] R. Frie, *Understanding Experience: Psychology and Postmodernism*, Routledge, New York, NY, USA, 2003.

[11] J. Martin and J. Thompson, "Psychotherapy as the interpretation of being: hermeneutic perspectives on psychotherapy," *Journal of Constructivist Psychology*, vol. 16, no. 1, pp. 1–16, 2003.

[12] E. Ansell, A. Pinto, M. O. Edelen et al., "The association of personality disorders with the prospective 7-year course of anxiety disorders," *Psychological Medicine*, vol. 41, no. 5, pp. 1019–1028, 2011.

[13] B. E. Wampold, "Psychotherapy: the Humanistic (and Effective) Treatment," *The American Psychologist*, vol. 62, no. 8, pp. 857–873, 2007.

[14] D. Westen, "Are research patients and clinical trials representative of clinical practice?" in *Evidence-Based Practices in Mental Health: Debate and Dialogue on the Fundamental Questions*, J. C. Norcross, L. E. Beutler, and R. F. Levant, Eds., pp. 161–171, 317–319, American Psychological Association, Washington, DC, USA, 2003.

[15] M. T. Shea, I. Elkin, S. D. Imber et al., "Course of depressive symptoms over follow-up: findings from the national institute

of mental health treatment of depression collaborative research program," *Archives of General Psychiatry*, vol. 49, no. 10, pp. 782–787, 1992.

[16] P. Knekt, O. Lindfors, T. Härkänen et al., "Randomized trial on the effectiveness of long-and short-term psychodynamic psychotherapy and solution-focused therapy on psychiatric symptoms during a 3-year follow-up," *Psychological Medicine*, vol. 38, no. 5, pp. 689–703, 2008.

[17] P. Knekt, O. Lindfors, M. A. Laaksonen, R. Raitasalo, P. Haaramo, and A. Järvikoski, "Effectiveness of short-term and long-term psychotherapy on work ability and functional capacity—a randomized clinical trial on depressive and anxiety disorders," *Journal of Affective Disorders*, vol. 107, no. 1–3, pp. 95–106, 2008.

[18] B. Wampold, *The Great Psychotherapy Debate: Models, Methods and Findings*, Erlbaum, Mahwah, NJ, USA, 2001.

[19] B. Wampold, S. Hollon, and C. Hill, "Unresolved questions and future directions in psychotherapy research," in *The Real Relationship in Psychotherapy: The Hidden Foundation of Change*, C. J. Gelso, Ed., chapter 11, pp. 333–355, American Psychological Association, Washington, DC, USA, 2011.

[20] L. Luborsky, L. Diguer, D. A. Seligman et al., "The researcher's own therapy allegiances: a "wild card" in comparisons of treatment efficacy," *Clinical Psychology: Science and Practice*, vol. 6, no. 1, pp. 95–106, 1999.

[21] L. Luborsky, M. Barrett, and D. Antonuccio, "What else materially influences what is represented and published as evidence?" in *Evidence-Based Practices in Mental Health: Debate and Dialogue on the Fundamental Questions*, J. C. Norcross, L. E. Beutler, and R. F. Levant, Eds., pp. 257–298, American Psychological Association, Washington, DC, USA, 2006.

[22] F. Leichsenring, "Are psychodynamic and psychoanalytic therapies effective? A review of empirical data," *International Journal of Psychoanalysis*, vol. 86, no. 3, pp. 841–868, 2005.

[23] J. Shedler, "The efficacy of psychodynamic psychotherapy," *American Psychologist*, vol. 65, no. 2, pp. 98–109, 2010.

[24] R. Levy and S. Ablon, *Handbook of Evidence-Based Psychodynamic Psychotherapy: Bridging the Gap Between Science and Practice*, Humana Press, New York, NY, USA, 2008.

[25] L. Luborsky, R. Rosenthal, and L. Diguer, "The dodo bird verdict is alive and well-mostly," *Clinical Psychology Science and Practice*, vol. 9, no. 1, pp. 2–12, 2002.

[26] M. Lambert, "The individual therapist's contribution to psychotherapy process and outcome," *Clinical Psychology Review*, vol. 9, no. 4, pp. 469–485, 1989.

[27] A. Horvath and R. Bedi, "The alliance," in *Psychotherapy Relationships That Work: Therapist Contributions and Responsiveness to Patients*, J. C. Norcross, Ed., pp. 37–70, Oxford University Press, New York, NY, USA, 2002.

[28] D.-M. Kim, B. E. Wampold, and D. M. Bolt, "Therapist effects in psychotherapy: a random-effects modeling of the national institute of mental health treatment of depression collaborative research program data," *Psychotherapy Research*, vol. 16, no. 2, pp. 161–172, 2006.

[29] E. Heinonen, O. Lindfors, M. A. Laaksonen, and P. Knekt, "Therapists' professional and personal characteristics as predictors of outcome in short- and long-term psychotherapy," *Journal of Affective Disorders*, vol. 138, no. 3, pp. 301–312, 2012.

[30] D. Biggerstaff and A. R. Thompson, "Interpretative Phenomenological Analysis (IPA): a qualitative methodology of choice in healthcare research," *Qualitative Research in Psychology*, vol. 5, no. 3, pp. 214–224, 2008.

[31] M. Larkin, S. Watts, and E. Clifton, "Giving voice and making sense in interpretative phenomenological analysis," *Qualitative Research in Psychology*, vol. 3, no. 2, pp. 102–120, 2006.

13

Valproate Prescribing in Women of Childbearing Age: An Audit of Clinical Practice

Harini Atturu[1] and Adedeji Odelola[2]

[1]Pennine Care NHS Foundation Trust, Royal Oldham Hospital, Oldham, Lancashire OL1 2JH, UK
[2]Pennine Care NHS Foundation Trust, Birch Hill Hospital, Rochdale OL12 9QB, UK

Correspondence should be addressed to Adedeji Odelola; deji.odelola@nhs.net

Academic Editor: Holly A. Garriock

Background. Evidence is accruing regarding the risks of valproate exposure in women of childbearing age. Recommendations have recently been made for a higher standard of prenatal counselling and prescribing practice in respect of valproate use in this patient group. *Aim and Method.* A reaudit was carried out to review the standard of clinical discussion around teratogenic risk and pregnancy planning offered to women of child-bearing age prescribed valproate. Case notes and prescription charts of women 45 years old or less were examined and compared with the results of a previous audit in 2005. *Results.* The use of valproate was increased overall by 64% and there was an 18% increase in off-label valproate use. The rate of clinical discussion carried out during commencement declined from 70% to 35% and at annual review from 50% to 22%. There was less clinical discussion in outpatients and in older patients. More than 40% of doctors surveyed were not confident about giving information to women. *Clinical Implication.* There is a need for a multidisciplinary approach and action at Healthcare Trust level, to increase awareness and reduce risks associated with valproate prescribing in childbearing women.

1. Introduction

The risks in women of childbearing age associated with prenatal valproate exposure are becoming established [1], and updated recommendations are being made nationally and internationally for restrictions to valproate use and enhanced preconceptual counselling in this patient group [2, 3]. Recent research has shown that in utero exposure to sodium valproate is associated with a range of neuropsychological, language, and developmental difficulties [4–9] and a higher incidence of autistic spectrum disorder compared to controls [10].

Valproate is now considered to be the most teratogenic of all the antiepileptics [11, 12]. Exposure to valproate doses greater than or equal to 1000 mgs is generally associated with a higher range of teratogenic risk (21.9%), compared to 2.5% with lower doses, and a fourfold increase in the rate of major anomalies is reported with antiepileptic polytherapy [1, 13]. Valproate is associated with a teratogenic risk of 6.3% compared to other medicines like carbamazepine (2.4%) and lamotrigine (2.7%). Lithium is associated specifically with a 0.1% risk of Ebstein's cardiacanomaly [14]. The least risk is attributed to antipsychotics [12, 15].

It is now not recommended that valproate should be prescribed routinely for women with child-bearing potential. If valproate use is inevitable, then recommendations are for a clinical discussion involving teratogenic risk, pregnancy planning, and contraception advice [1–3, 16].

In July 2005, a local audit showed inadequate clinical discussion associated with valproate prescribing, and specially designed "yellow monitoring forms" were developed to facilitate clinical discussion and documentation during initiation and follow-up of women prescribed valproate.

The current reaudit is to examine the extent to which clinical discussions regarding the teratogenic potential of valproate, contraceptive advice, and pregnancy planning are offered to women of child bearing age during commencement of valproate treatment and at review.

TABLE 1: Rates for clinical discussion in 2005 and 2012 audits.

Audit standard	Commencement 2005 (%)	Commencement 2012 (%)	Review 2005 (%)	Review 2012 (%)
Any clinical discussion documented	70%	35%	50%	22%
Discussion of teratogenicity	70%	35%	50%	22%
Discussion about contraception	70%	35%	50%	22%
Collaborative pregnancy planning discussed	70%	35%	50%	22%
Last menstrual period documented	70%	30%	—	13%
Communication with GP	70%	25%	50%	13%

2. Method

The current reaudit involved women between the ages of 18 to 45 years under the care of the Rochdale General Adult Psychiatric service from August 2005 till October 2012, receiving valproate preparations for psychiatric illness. Women taking valproate primarily for epilepsy were excluded as they are generally managed by primary care or epilepsy services. Using search terms "Valproate," "Depakote," or "Epilim" patients were identified from the department's electronic patient administration database.

Audit standards were set at a departmental meeting and were derived from a previous departmental audit done in 2005 and reflected guidance by NICE [16]. Agreed standards were the following. (1) For women of childbearing age, there should be evidence of a clinical discussion at initiation of valproate prescribing. (2) There should be a further discussion at subsequent clinical review for women prescribed valproate. (3) The clinical discussion should include the provision of contraceptive advice, discussion of the need for pregnancies to be planned collaboratively with the prescriber, a discussion of the risk of teratogenicity, and a record of the patient's last menstrual period (LMP). (4) Details of the clinical discussion should be communicated to the patient's General Practitioner. (5) Yellow monitoring forms developed after the previous audit (2005), specifically for the recording of information provided to patients, should be completed for each patient and filed in their case notes.

Consecutive patients who were under the care of either of two community sector teams were included in the study. One of the study authors (Harini Atturu) reviewed patient case notes and searched for the presence of the "yellow monitoring forms." In addition the same author examined handwritten case note entries and written correspondence for any other evidence of clinical discussion, contraceptive advice, or pregnancy planning contained within the records. Case notes were searched for evidence of adverse outcomes occurring in patients who received valproate during pregnancy and these were recorded as "near misses." Results were compared with those of the previous audit using basic statistics specifically prevalence rates expressed as percentages.

A separate survey was carried out prior to discussion of the audit findings, which included doctors within the department attending an educational meeting in January 2013. All doctors of various grades attending the meeting were invited to take part in the survey. Survey questions were agreed by consensus by both authors (Harini Atturu and Adedeji Odelola), based on the results of the previous

TABLE 2: Use of valproate for different psychiatric disorders.

Diagnosis	July 2005 ($n = 14$)	October 2012 ($n = 23$)
Bipolar disorder	78.7%	60.8%
Schizoaffective disorder	7.1%	17.4%
Paranoid schizophrenia	7.1%	8.7%
Psychotic depression	7.1%	4.3%
Personality disorder	0%	8.7%

audit (2005), and sought to uncover reasons for the poor practice identified in that audit. Questions were kept open-ended as much as possible, inviting a narrative response, and covered choice of medication, barriers to clinical discussion with women of childbearing age, and the scope of such discussions.

3. Results

In the 2012 audit, a total of 94 patients were identified from the database. Out of these 46 were male and 48 were female. 26 patients were women up to 45 years in age. Three women had a diagnosis of epilepsy and were excluded. 23 cases met the study criteria. The initial audit carried out in 2005 involved a sample of 14 women who received valproate.

The results in respect of clinical discussions carried out in 2005 are shown in Table 1 and are shown alongside findings in the current (2012) audit.

4. Diagnosis

Compared with the previous (2005) study, the present study found an increase in the use of valproate for psychiatric disorders other than bipolar disorders. The use of valproate for schizoaffective disorder and paranoid schizophrenia was increased. There were no cases of valproate use for personality disorder in 2005 but 8.7% of the 2012 sample received valproate for a personality disorder. The routine use of valproate for bipolar disorder and for depression with psychosis was found to be reduced (Table 2).

5. Age

The use of valproate in women less than or equal to 25 years of age had reduced from 50% to 4.3% when compared with the 2005 audit. The use of valproate had remained essentially

TABLE 3: Trends in the usage of valproate in different settings.

Different settings	% of patients on valproate in 2005 ($n = 14$)	% of patients on valproate in 2012 ($n = 23$)	Total change in usage of valproate between 2005 and 2012
Inpatient	35%	43.5%	8.5% increase
Outpatient	50%	43.5%	6.5% decrease
Other teams	14.3%	13%	1.3% decrease

TABLE 4: Clinical discussions in respect of valproate prescribing during 2012 audit.

Age group	Number of pts	Teratogenicity	Contraceptive advice	Pregnancy planning	LMP	GP advised
<25 y	1	100%	100%	100%	0%	100%
26–35 y	5	40%	40%	40%	40%	40%
36–45 y	14	29%	29%	29%	29%	14%
Commencement (all ages)	20	35%	35%	35%	30%	25%
Review (all ages)	23	22%	22%	22%	13%	13%

the same in the age group 26–35 years. However, in age group 36–45 years, the use of valproate had increased from 21.4% to 69.6%.

6. Use of Valproate in Inpatient and Outpatient Settings

There was an increased trend in the prescribing of valproate by 8.5% in inpatients and a decrease by 6.5% in outpatients compared with the previous audit. Additionally, a small group of patients commenced valproate with the Home Treatment Team, or in an external setting prior to transfer to our hospital. In these patients there was a very slight decrease in levels of valproate prescribing of 1.3% compared with the previous audit (Table 3).

7. Clinical Discussions in respect of Valproate Prescribing

The current study found a decline in the rate of clinical discussion carried out during commencement from 70% to 35% and at annual review from 50% to 22% compared with the 2005 audit. The 2012 audit found that, during initiation of valproate for inpatients, clinical discussions were carried out and documented 60% of the time. In the outpatient setting, clinical discussion was carried out only 10% of the time. There was a trend observed for clinical discussions to be carried out with less frequency in older patient groups (Table 4).

8. Documentation

The previous (2005) audit recommended that "yellow monitoring forms" were completed and filed in the case-notes for all women of child-bearing age commencing valproate. However, during clinic reviews in the 2012 audit, the yellow form was available in only 4.3% of cases. In patients without "Yellow Forms" there was nevertheless, evidence at review, of explaining teratogenic risks, giving of the contraceptive and collaborative pregnancy planning advice in 22% of cases and evidence of recording of last menstrual periods and communication of the clinical discussion to general practitioners in 13% (Table 4).

"Near Misses". Two women were identified during the 2012 audit who were classed as "near misses." These were women in the study sample who became pregnant during the study period. The first patient was commenced on valproate treatment without a clinical discussion. She however did have a clinical discussion at outpatient review, was appropriately counselled, and chose to discontinue valproate prior to becoming pregnant. A second patient had a clinical discussion at commencement of valproate treatment but defaulted from follow-up and hence did not have an outpatient review. She became pregnant and delivered a preterm baby with mild intracranial haemorrhage.

9. Survey

Following the reaudit, we carried out a survey among doctors locally, to uncover the reasons for the poor performance in respect of valproate prescribing advice. 17 doctors participated out of whom 23.5% were consultants, 29% were speciality trainee/speciality doctors, 23.5% were core trainees, 12% were foundation trainees, and 12% did not specify their grade.

94% of doctors in the sample stated that they would not consider valproate as first choice while treating women of child bearing age. 6% of doctors did not know what information ought to be given to women, and 41% admitted that they only gave partial information. 12% reported using yellow forms and only 35% said that they communicated their clinical discussion by letter to general practitioners in addition to documentation in case notes.

In carrying out clinical discussions, doctors identified a few barriers. These included time pressure (12%); patient factors like patient capacity and communication difficulties (12%), lack of knowledge (6%) and nonspecific factors (6%). More than 40% of doctors felt that they had low (12%) or moderate (30%) levels of confidence about their knowledge in respect of giving valproate prescribing advice.

10. Discussion

There is limited information in the literature regarding prescribing patterns of antiepileptic drugs in the United Kingdom. Specifically in patients with bipolar disorder, however, the trend has been for a steady increase in valproate prescribing since 1995, with increased psychotropic drug co-prescribing [17, 18]. In the United States, valproate prescription has remained the same amongst women of childbearing age, despite the teratogenic risks [19]. Our study results were similar to those of other studies in our finding of an overall rate of usage of valproate increased by 64% compared with the previous (2005) audit. An increased rate of usage from 24% to 62% was reported in a study in Newcastle, United Kingdom [20].

In the current study there was an increase in the prescription of sodium valproate by 8.5% when commenced in inpatients and a 6.5% decrease in outpatients—perhaps reflecting the requirement for effective medicines to manage severely ill patients in the inpatient setting. The trend appears to be shifting from the use of valproate predominantly for bipolar disorder to the use in several other psychiatric disorders like schizoaffective disorder, paranoid schizophrenia, and personality disorder showing flexible use for different conditions within psychiatry. This trend for off-license prescribing has been shown in other studies [21].

Valproate use was found to be reduced in our study, from 50% to 4.3% in women in younger age groups (≤25 years), compared with an increased use from 21.4% to 69.6% in women in the 36–45 years age group who might have completed their families. This trend is similar to that reported in other studies. An Australian study found that neurologists involved in the care of women with epilepsy had changed their pattern of prescribing based on knowledge of the teratogenic risks with valproate [22], prescribing less frequently and in lower dosage. A Primary Care study looking into trends of prescribing of valproate in adolescent females found increased prescribing of lamotrigine but decreased use of carbamazepine and a 3.1% reduction in the use of valproate [23].

It is not clear whether or not the results of our study in respect of younger women are a true reflection of improved prescribing practice or have arisen because our younger population is served by an Early Intervention team. It may be that this question would be addressed by doing similar valproate prescribing audits of Early Intervention teams which are more involved in the care of transition populations.

50% or more of pregnancies occur unplanned; hence it is generally recommended that contraception issues should be discussed regardless of whether or not women are planning a pregnancy [12]. The literature shows that women with bipolar disorder encounter problems engaging with health care professionals regarding their pregnancy planning. A survey among women with bipolar disorder showed that a preconceptual consultation, involving an explanation of the risks and benefits of maintenance or discontinuation of treatment in pregnancy, had an influence on patient's decisions. 37% of women chose not to pursue pregnancy while 63% decided to conceive following preconceptual consultation [24].

A 20-month Quality Improvement Programme in the South London and Maudsley NHS Foundation Trust demonstrated a significant improvement in information provision following the use of a multidisciplinary approach with both doctors and pharmacists involved in counselling women on the risks of medication in pregnancy. The study also found that ongoing identification of women prescribed valproate by the pharmacist and subsequent reminders to prescribers to counsel and advise women were effective [25]. We found a higher rate of discussion carried out during inpatient commencement (60%), compared to 10% in the outpatient setting. This could be attributed to the availability of a pharmacist on our wards and may highlight the need for employing a multidisciplinary approach in the outpatient setting as well.

The current reaudit showed an overall decline in rate of clinical discussions carried out during commencement from 70% to 35% and at review from 50% to 22%. Similar low rates of clinical discussion have been found in other published audits of mood stabiliser prescribing. An audit carried out in Bradford District Care Trust showed that in women of child bearing age using various mood stabilisers contraception advice was given, and risk of pregnancy was verbally communicated in 35% of cases and contraception advice was documented in only 24% of cases [26]. There were similarly low rates obtained in a survey of three Greater Manchester Teaching Hospitals [27] and a case-note review carried out in Kent [28].

The Bradford group found one of the main reasons for this low rate of clinical discussion was poor documentation [26]. Our survey of doctors found that a proportion of doctors claimed that they tended to hold discussions but did not usually indicate this by clear documentation in case notes. Our survey results also showed that more than 40% of doctors felt low to moderate levels of confidence about their knowledge in this area, indicating a training need. Other survey results suggest that, in addition to a lack of knowledge and confidence, factors specific to the doctor-patient interaction and a particular difficulty imparting the requisite information to women may be involved in the low rate of clinical discussion obtained in our audit.

The yellow monitoring forms introduced at the time of the initial audit in 2005 would have facilitated clinical discussion by serving as a template offering prompts for the various areas needing to be discussed. The reasons for the low rate of usage in our study population of the yellow monitoring forms are unclear. It may be that there is a role for local pharmacists in respect of increasing awareness and accessibility of the yellow monitoring forms and identifying women falling within the at-risk group [25].

In the current study there were two cases which were identified as being "near misses" in whom adverse outcomes due to valproate use during pregnancy were narrowly averted. One woman did not have a clinical discussion at commencement of valproate treatment but was identified at outpatient clinic review, discontinued valproate, and became pregnant. The consequences for the foetus may have been severe had there not been a clinical discussion at review. A second patient who received adequate information provided at commencement of valproate treatment, became pregnant having dropped out of services, and delivered a preterm baby with mild intracranial haemorrhage. This outcome may have been prevented had it been possible to have an outpatient review but in any case highlights the need for effective liaison and communication with general practitioners in respect of women prescribed valproate preparations. A similar study, reviewing mood stabiliser prescribing practice in Kent [28], found that 14 women (10%) became pregnant while taking lithium, carbamazepine, or valproate and 8 women had a complication of pregnancy.

One limitation of the current reaudit is that it only involved patients under the care of Adult Community Mental Health Teams. The current study did however involve all women prescribed valproate during the study period which extended from the time of the conclusion of the previous audit in 2005, to the current time (2012). There would no doubt be benefits from future studies involving a wider range of community services such as Early Intervention teams, Adult Intellectual Disability teams, and Child and Adolescent services. In addition, although the current reaudit involved patients prescribed valproate since 2005, the reaudit was done in 2012—7 years later. It is likely that an earlier reaudit would have helped to maintain awareness of the need for appropriate clinical discussion.

11. Conclusion

In the current audit, the level of clinical discussion with women prescribed valproate was found to be less than adequate. There is a need for strategic planning by Healthcare Trusts in accordance with national guidance in respect of valproate prescribing. We recommend a multidisciplinary approach involving pharmacists, increasing awareness by means of induction programmes for doctors, and the use of specific aids for the provision of information such as alert labels, patient leaflets, and the monitoring forms developed after the previous valproate audit.

Conflict of Interests

The authors declare that there is no conflict of interests regarding the publication of this paper.

References

[1] T. Tomson, D. Battino, E. Bonizzoni et al., "Dose-dependent risk of malformations with antiepileptic drugs: an analysis of data from the EURAP epilepsy and pregnancy registry," *The Lancet Neurology*, vol. 10, no. 7, pp. 609–617, 2011.

[2] European Medicines Agency, "PRAC recommends strengthening the restrictions on the use of valproate in women and girls. Review 612389," London, UK, European Medicines Agency, 2014.

[3] National Institute for Health and Care Excellence (NICE), "Antenatal and postnatal mental health: clinical management and service guidance," in *Clinical Guideline 192*, National Institute for Health and Care Excellence, 2014.

[4] S. J. Moore, P. Turnpenny, A. Quinn et al., "A clinical study of 57 children with fetal anticonvulsant syndromes," *Journal of Medical Genetics*, vol. 37, no. 7, pp. 489–497, 2000.

[5] N. Adab, U. Kini, J. Vinten et al., "The longer term outcome of children born to mothers with epilepsy," *Journal of Neurology, Neurosurgery and Psychiatry*, vol. 75, no. 11, pp. 1575–1583, 2004.

[6] K. J. Meador, G. A. Baker, N. Browning et al., "Cognitive function at 3 years of age after fetal exposure to antiepileptic drugs," *The New England Journal of Medicine*, vol. 360, no. 16, pp. 1597–1605, 2009.

[7] E. Gaily, E. Kantola-Sorsa, V. Hiilesmaa et al., "Normal intelligence in children with prenatal exposure to carbamazepine," *Neurology*, vol. 62, no. 1, pp. 28–32, 2004.

[8] J. Vinten, N. Adab, U. Kini, J. Gorry, J. Gregg, and G. A. Baker, "Neuropsychological effects of exposure to anticonvulsant medication in utero," *Neurology*, vol. 64, no. 6, pp. 949–954, 2005.

[9] E. Kantola-Sorsa, E. Gaily, M. Isoaho, and M. Korkman, "Neuropsychological outcomes in children of mothers with epilepsy," *Journal of the International Neuropsychological Society*, vol. 13, no. 4, pp. 642–652, 2007.

[10] R. L. Bromley, G. Mawer, J. Clayton-Smith, and G. A. Baker, "Autism spectrum disorders following in utero exposure to antiepileptic drugs," *Neurology*, vol. 71, no. 23, pp. 1923–1924, 2008.

[11] A. Ornoy, "Neuroteratogens in man: an overview with special emphasis on the teratogenicity of antiepileptic drugs in pregnancy," *Reproductive Toxicology*, vol. 22, no. 2, pp. 214–226, 2006.

[12] G. M. Goodwin, "Evidence-based guidelines for treating bipolar disorder: revised second edition-recommendations from the British association for psychopharmacology," *Journal of Psychopharmacology*, vol. 23, no. 4, pp. 346–388, 2009.

[13] O. Diav-Citrin, S. Shechtman, B. Bar-Oz, D. Cantrell, J. Arnon, and A. Ornoy, "Pregnancy outcome after *In Utero* exposure to valproate: evidence of dose relationship in teratogenic effect," *CNS Drugs*, vol. 22, no. 4, pp. 325–334, 2008.

[14] R. F. McKnight, M. Adida, K. Budge, S. Stockton, G. M. Goodwin, and J. R. Geddes, "Lithium toxicity profile: a systematic review and meta-analysis," *The Lancet*, vol. 379, no. 9817, pp. 721–728, 2012.

[15] Epilepsy Guidance Group, *Primary Care Guidance for the Management of Women taking Antiepileptic Drugs*, Epilepsy Guidance Group, 2011.

[16] National Institute for Health and Clinical Excellence (NICE), *Bipolar Disorder: The Management of Bipolar Disorder in Adults, Children and Adolescents, in Primary and Secondary Care*, NICE Clinical Guidelines, no. 38, NICE, 2006.

[17] J. Hayes, P. Prah, I. Nazareth et al., "Prescribing trends in bipolar disorder: cohort study in the United Kingdom THIN primary care database 1995–2009," *PLoS ONE*, vol. 6, no. 12, Article ID e28725, 2011.

[18] National Institute for Health and Clinical Excellence (NICE), *NICE Implementation Uptake Report: Bipolar Disorder Clinical Guideline 38*, NICE, 2009.

[19] D. A. Adedinsewo, D. J. Thurman, Y. H. Luo, R. S. Williamson, O. A. Odewole, and G. P. Oakley Jr., "Valproate prescriptions for nonepilepsy disorders in reproductive-age women," *Birth*

Defects Research, Part A—Clinical and Molecular Teratology, vol. 97, no. 6, pp. 403–408, 2013.

[20] A. J. Lloyd, C. L. Harrison, I. N. Ferrier, and A. H. Young, "The pharmacological treatment of bipolar affective disorder: practice is improving but could still be better," *Journal of Psychopharmacology*, vol. 17, no. 2, pp. 230–233, 2003.

[21] J. Langan, A. Perry, and M. Oto, "Teratogenic risk and contraceptive counselling in psychiatric practice: analysis of anticonvulsant therapy," *BMC Psychiatry*, vol. 13, article 234, 2013.

[22] F. J. E. Vajda, S. Hollingworth, J. Graham et al., "Changing patterns of antiepileptic drug use in pregnant Australian women," *Acta Neurologica Scandinavica*, vol. 121, no. 2, pp. 89–93, 2010.

[23] R. Ackers, F. M. C. Besag, A. Wade, M. L. Murray, and I. C. K. Wong, "Changing trends in antiepileptic drug prescribing in girls of child-bearing potential," *Archives of Disease in Childhood*, vol. 94, no. 6, pp. 443–447, 2009.

[24] A. C. Viguera, L. S. Cohen, S. Bouffard, T. H. Whitfield, and R. J. Baldessarini, "Reproductive decisions by women with bipolar disorder after prepregnancy psychiatric consultation," *The American Journal of Psychiatry*, vol. 159, no. 12, pp. 2102–2104, 2002.

[25] S. Mace and D. Taylor, "Improving adherence to NICE guidance for bipolar illness: valproate use in women of childbearing potential," *The Psychiatric Bulletin*, vol. 35, no. 2, pp. 63–67, 2011.

[26] M. Mothi, C. Chambers, S. Shora, and A. Jabeen, "2305—Audit on effects of mood stabilisers on women's health—informed decision making," *European Psychiatry*, vol. 28, supplement 1, p. 1, 2013.

[27] A. Wieck, S. Rao, K. Sein, and P. M. Haddad, "A survey of antiepileptic prescribing to women of childbearing potential in psychiatry," *Archives of Women's Mental Health*, vol. 10, no. 2, pp. 83–85, 2007.

[28] L. James, T. R. E. Barnes, P. Lelliott, D. Taylor, and C. Paton, "Informing patients of the teratogenic potential of mood stabilizing drugs: a case note review of the practice of psychiatrists," *Journal of Psychopharmacology*, vol. 21, no. 8, pp. 815–819, 2007.

14

Neuropsychological Profiles and Behavioral Ratings in ADHD Overlap Only in the Dimension of Syndrome Severity

Ádám Takács,[1] **Andrea Kóbor,**[1,2] **Zsanett Tárnok,**[3] **and András Vargha**[1,4]

[1] *Institute of Psychology, Eötvös Loránd University, Izabella u. 46., Budapest 1064, Hungary*
[2] *Brain Imaging Centre, Research Centre for Natural Sciences, Hungarian Academy of Sciences, Magyar Tudósok Körútja 2., Budapest 1117, Hungary*
[3] *Vadaskert Child Psychiatry Hospital, Hűvösvölgyi út 116., Budapest 1021, Hungary*
[4] *Institute of Psychology, Károli Gáspár University, Bécsi út 324., Budapest 1037, Hungary*

Correspondence should be addressed to Ádám Takács; takacs.adam@ppk.elte.hu

Academic Editor: Xingguang Luo

Objectives. The aim of this study was to compare the cognitive neuropsychological and the behavioral rating profiles of attention deficit/hyperactivity disorder (ADHD). *Methods.* Forty-two children diagnosed with ADHD (M = 11.5 years, SD = 1.1) and 43 typically developing children (M = 11.2 years, SD = 1.7) participated. We measured symptom severity with behavioral rating scales, and we administered neuropsychological tasks to measure inhibitory performance, updating/working memory, and shifting ability. *Results.* On the basis of the three neuropsychological variables, the hierarchical cluster analytic method yielded a six-cluster structure. The clusters, according to the severity of the impairment, were labeled as follows: none or few symptoms, Moderate inhibition and mild shifting, moderate to severe shifting with moderate updating, moderate updating, severe updating with mild shifting, and severe updating with severe shifting. There were no systematic differences in inattention and hyperactive-impulsive behavior across the clusters. The comorbid learning disorder appeared more likely only in severe neuropsychological forms of ADHD. *Conclusion.* In sum, our results suggest that behavioral ratings and neuropsychological profiles converge only in the dimension of symptom severity and that atypicalities in executive functions may manifest in nonspecific everyday problems.

1. Introduction

Attention deficit/hyperactivity disorder (ADHD) is one of the most frequent psychiatric disorders affecting approximately 5% of children [1, 2]. Despite its wide effects on social and academic achievements, the diagnosis has remained controversial [3]. The diagnosis of ADHD (DSM-5; [4]) is mostly based on clinical observations, parental (and rarely teacher) interviews, or rating scales, but the neuropsychological information is often missing from the protocol [5]. However, given the temporal and methodological instability (i.e., combining information from different sources) of the diagnosis [3], assessment cannot focus only on the behavioral ratings. Moreover, in order to develop a sufficient treatment plan, it is necessary to evaluate various impairments—including cognitive deficits in attention, executive functions (EF), and memory—affecting day-to-day functioning, and to

determine the presence of any deficiency in adaptive skills and key competences. To point at this shortcoming of the diagnostic protocol, the aim of this study was to compare the cognitive neuropsychological and the behavioral rating profiles of ADHD.

With respect to the neuropsychological impairments, children with ADHD show deviations in executive functions, including inhibitory control, delay aversion, and time estimation [6, 7]. Several studies proved the dysfunction of working memory (WM); however, this impairment is not specific to ADHD, and it can be observed in many other developmental psychiatric syndromes, such as autism spectrum disorder, conduct disorder, or oppositional defiant disorder [6, 8, 9]. EF assessments vary in a broad range; therefore, a selection of EF measures that is not theory-driven could increase the heterogeneity of neuropsychological findings in ADHD [9, 10]. Miyake et al. [11] used confirmatory factor analysis

(CFA) to understand the relationships among three types of executive functions: mental set shifting, inhibiting prepotent responses, and updating the contents of WM. The three functions were not only moderately correlated but also clearly separable. Further studies used this model in community based developmental and child clinical settings as well [12–14]. These studies used the three-factor model [11] with different EF tasks and corroborated the robustness of this model.

Though there is substantial research on this topic spanning a large period of time (with varying study designs), the relationship between symptoms of ADHD (inattentive, hyperactive-impulsive behavior) and EF is still unclear [9, 15]. Nigg et al. proposed an "executive deficit type" within the category of ADHD [16]. This suggestion was based on an estimation that only 35–50% of children with ADHD have inhibitory deficit. In line with the notion that ADHD can develop in multiple pathways [13, 17–19], a subtype with EF impairment as a potential endophenotype could lead to targeted etiological research and personalized treatment, as well. The study of Lambek et al. [20] investigated the cognitive and academic performance of children with ADHD with and without an executive function deficit (EFD). While the ADHD-EFD group was characterized by lower IQ and higher intraindividual response variability, children with ADHD without EFD showed more delay aversion but otherwise intact EF and IQ. The authors suggested [20] that an EFD subtype could represent different risk factors and different needs for educational and clinical care.

Another study used two-step cluster analysis to detect profiles of children with ADHD with distinguishable neuropsychological profiles [21]. They found a three-cluster structure, where the profiles represented children with poor inhibitory control, poor set shifting/speed, and intact task performance, respectively. Despite the importance of working memory in cognitive development [6, 8], they did not investigate WM. Participants from the poor set-shifting/speed cluster had more hyperactive-impulsive ADHD and ODD symptoms and lower IQ than children from the other clusters. Despite the fact that atypical inhibition is often described as a major cognitive characteristic of ADHD [6, 16, 22], the poor inhibitory control cluster did not show more risk for ADHD than the other two clusters [21]. At the same time, children with ADHD from the intact task performance cluster had more severe depression symptoms. The study targeted children with ADHD only; therefore, the cluster structure of EF in nonclinical children remained unfolded. However, other studies found mild or moderate EF impairments in nonreferred samples as well [13, 16].

Another cluster analytic study used a multimeasure, multi-informant approach based on ADHD rating scales with a preschooler community sample (hierarchical cluster analysis with Ward's method, [7]). They found four clusters, where the "high comorbidity risk" cluster showed the lowest inhibitory control performance and the "ADHD risk only" cluster showed the highest level of delay aversion. The two further clusters were characterized by few/none symptom and by sensorimotor deficits without EF impairments, respectively. Other studies could not present such clear

difference between ADHD and typically developing (TD) groups (e.g., [9, 13, 16]). Sjöwall et al. [13] found that children with ADHD had weaker performance than nonclinical children in working memory, inhibition, shifting, and emotion recognition in general, accompanied with greater reaction time variability. There were no group differences in delay aversion and in recognition of disgust. However, only one-third of the clinical participants had impairments in executive functions according to the 90th percentile of the nonclinical group's neuropsychological performance which was used as a cutoff criterion for what was regarded as impaired. More importantly, 26% of the nonclinical group had at least one neuropsychological deficit.

Our aim was to investigate whether subgroups characterized by various EF impairments are identifiable in a mixed sample of TD children and children with ADHD. Moreover, we tested how these expected clusters (see the following) differ in ADHD symptoms and comorbid conduct disorder (CD) and learning disorder (LD) problems. Given the diversity of EF [11] and the multifactorial heterogeneity of ADHD [21], we assumed that there would be at least five different cognitive clusters in our sample, and each one would be characterized by different symptom dimensions according to the rating scale scores. Our expectations were based on the conceptually relevant combinations of the three EF factors [11] and the two dimensions of ADHD symptoms. We expected a group of children with atypical inhibition, shifting, and updating associated with inattentive and hyperactive-impulsive symptoms, one cluster with solely updating problems and characterized by inattentive behavior, one with impairment in inhibition and high hyperactive-impulsive ratings, a group characterized by shifting problems related to both dimensions of ADHD symptoms, and a last group with normal neuropsychological profile and few or no behavioral problems.

2. Methods

2.1. Participants and Procedure. Eighty-five children were invited to participate in the present study. Clinical participants (38 boys, 4 girls, M = 11.5 years, SD = 1.1) were recruited from the Vadaskert Child Psychiatric Clinic where they were diagnosed with ADHD by a group consisting of a psychiatrist, a psychologist, a neuropsychologist, and an expert on special education. The diagnoses were based on the DSM-IV-TR [23]. All of the clinical participants met the criteria of ADHD-C in regard to their symptoms. The members of the typically developing group (36 boys, 7 girls, M = 11.2 years, SD = 1.7) were recruited from a primary and a high school in Budapest. The age range was from eight to fifteen years in both groups. Parents of all participants provided informed consent and the children made an oral agreement. The research was granted by the Medical Research Ethics Committee of Semmelweis University. Those children with ADHD, who strongly manifested comorbid disorders (autism spectrum disorder, obsessive-compulsive disorder, Tourette syndrome, or major depression) and/or low socioeconomic status, were excluded from the study. Children with learning disorder scored below appropriate age level of Hungarian Logopaedic Test Protocol [24], including tests of numerical cognition, communicative development, spontaneous speech, phonological awareness, and grammar and vocabulary. The children did not meet the criteria of specific language impairment, dyscalculia, or dyslexia. Participants of the TD group who possessed any psychiatric or neurological records were also excluded. An additional exclusion criterion was an estimated IQ below 80 (based on Raven Progressive Matrices [25]) in both groups. The two groups did not differ in gender $\chi^2(1) = .34, P = .56$. Members of the ADHD group were significantly older than those in the TD group, $t(195) = -7.64, P < .001$; by this reason we also tested the effect of age on cluster structure.

2.2. Measures

2.2.1. Questionnaires. The following questionnaires were administered: ADHD Rating Scale (ADHD-RS, [26]), the Children's Depression Inventory [27], the Yale Global Tic Severity Scale [28], and the Child Yale Brown Obsessive Compulsive Scale [29]. The children were examined in accordance with the MINI International Neuropsychiatric Interview for Children and Adolescents (MINI-KID, [30]) semistructured interview. The results of the questionnaires and interviews listed above are not presented in this paper, except for the ADHD Rating Scale.

2.2.2. Neuropsychological Measures

Golden Stroop Test. The Golden Stroop test [31] was administered in which participants were required to name as many items as they could in 45 seconds for each of the three cards (word, color, and color-word). The outcome variable used in the analyses was the interference score as an indicator of prepotent response inhibition or cognitive conflict.

Digit Span. To measure the updating factor, the digit span backward task of the Wechsler Intelligence Scale of Children (WISC-III, [32]) was administered, which is the most widely used test for working memory [33].

Wisconsin Card Sorting Test (WCST). The original 128-card version of the WCST was administered [34]. In this test participants saw four stimuli cards and two packs (2×64) of response cards. The stimuli cards differed in color, number, and form. Participants were asked to match the response cards to the stimuli cards with consideration of the feedback (correct/incorrect) given by the experimenter. The matching rules changed after every ten correct answers to which participants were blind. For analyses, we used the number of perseverative errors which is an indicator of problems in mental set shifting [11].

2.3. Statistical Methods. For identifying subgroups with distinct patterns of the three main executive factors, an agglomerative hierarchical cluster analysis was conducted, for which the interference score of the Golden Stroop test and the digit span backward score and the number of perseverative errors from the Wisconsin Card Sorting Test were used as clustering variables. We applied squared Euclidean distance

as the similarity measure and Ward's method as the type of cluster fusion, which was found to be more accurate and effective than solutions yielded by other techniques [35]. We did not use usual standardization methods on the three clustering variables but quasi-absolute scaling. This method can handle the extreme values, and, therefore, clinically meaningful ranges can be identified based on the distribution of the clustering variables (ranges of the quasi-absolute scaling were as follows: for digit span backward 0–2—severe (problems/impairment), 3—moderate, 4—mild, and 5–8—few or none; for WCST $T < 34$ moderately severe, $T = 35$–44 mild, $45 < T$ few or none; for the Stroop task $T = 32$–44 mild to moderate, $T = 45$–54 few or none, $55 < T$ above average) [36]. After conducting the hierarchical cluster analysis, we performed a K-means cluster analysis, which improves the obtained cluster solution by the relocation of cases. It starts from the initial classification and moves cases from one cluster to another if this leads to a reduction in the total error sum of squares of the cluster solution. In this method the "bad-fitting" cases are moved to other "better-fitting" clusters; thus, more homogeneous groups can be obtained. By reason of having clusters of different sample sizes, the differences across the final clusters in age and in hyperactive-impulsive and inattentive symptoms were analyzed with the robust Welch test of equality of means. Most of the analyses were performed in SPSS 17.0, but ROPStat ([37] for details see http://www.ropstat.com) was also applied for obtaining special pattern-oriented algorithms and features.

3. Results

3.1. The Executive Functions Clusters. The attributes for clustering participants were the three factors of executive functions: inhibition (interference score on the Golden Stroop), shifting (perseverative errors on the WCST), and WM/updating (digit span backward). We obtained six clusters explaining 78.03% of the variance (considering error sum of squares). The Silhouette coefficient (the Silhouette coefficient is an indicator of good cluster cohesion and separation, and it ranges between −1 and 1. Values greater than .5 indicate reasonable partitioning of data) of the cluster structure was .793. (For the detailed demographic and behavioral properties of the clusters see Table 1.)

The first cluster consists of well-performing participants ($n = 26$, 30.6% of the whole sample), so we called that none or few symptoms group. In the second cluster ($n = 8$, 9.4%) the performance of the children is moderately low on inhibition and mildly low on shifting. The third cluster ($n = 11$, 12.9%) is characterized by moderate to severe shifting impairment and moderately low working memory achievement. The fourth ($n = 15$, 17.6%) and sixth ($n = 13$, 15.3%) clusters consist of participants with severe WM problems which is associated with severe shifting impairments in cluster 6. On the other hand cluster 5 ($n = 12$, 14.2%) contains 12 children with moderately low WM capacity (for the detailed profiles see Figure 1).

Considering the properties of the six clusters (see Table 1) we can identify two groups with mostly TD children (none or few symptoms, moderate WM), two groups with mostly or

TABLE 1: Demographic and behavioral properties of the six clusters.

				Clusters			
		None or few	Mod Inh-Mild Shift	Mod/Sev Shift-Mod WM	Sev WM-Mild Shift	Mod WM	Sev WM-Sev Shift
Diagnosis	TD	20 (76.9%)	5 (62.5%)	7 (63.6%)	1 (6.7%)	10 (83.4%)	0 (0%)
	ADHD	6 (23%)	3 (37.5%)	4 (36.4%)	14 (93.3%)	2 (16.7%)	13 (100%)
Gender	Girls	4 (15.4%)	3 (38%)	2 (18.2%)	0 (0%)	1 (9%)	1 (7.7%)
	Boys	22 (84.6%)	5 (62%)	9 (81.8%)	15 (100%)	11 (91%)	12 (92.3%)
Age	Mean (SD)	11.5 (1.1)	11.2 (1.3)	12.6 (.9)	10.8 (2.1)	11.2 (.9)	10.8 (1.5)
Inattentive	Mean (SD)	6.04 (5.4)	9.63 (5.34)	10.91 (8.92)	13.93 (7.85)	5.55 (5.11)	15.55 (2.38)
Hyperactive-impulsive	Mean (SD)	4.46 (5.94)	8.75 (8.61)	7.09 (6.53)	13.86 (8.43)	2.91 (4.41)	13.36 (4.46)

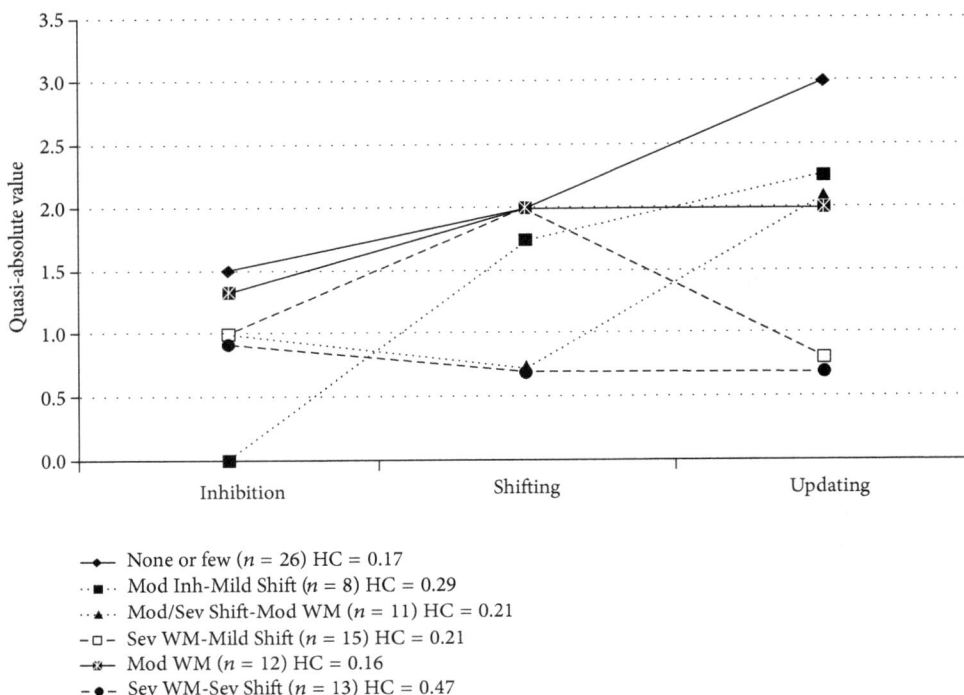

FIGURE 1: Neuropsychological profiles of the six clusters. Homogeneity coefficient (HC) is the average of the pairwise distances within a cluster. Larger values indicate more heterogeneous clusters. Inh: inhibition, Mod: moderate, Sev: severe, Shift: shifting.

solely children with ADHD (severe WM with mild shifting, severe WM with severe shifting), and two clusters with mixed samples (moderate inhibition with mild shifting, moderate to severe shifting with moderate WM). These last two groups could be named as subthreshold or subclinical clusters. In every group there are more boys than girls (this is an attribute of the whole sample), and this ratio is not different between the clusters, $\chi^2(5) = 7.46$, $P > .05$. The clusters differ in age, $W(5, 29.98) = 4.18$, MSE = .92, $P < .05$, but regarding the Games-Howell post hoc test, only the third group members (moderate to severe shifting and moderately low WM) are older than the others ($P < .05$), except for the second cluster (moderately low inhibition and mildly low shifting).

3.2. Cognitive and Behavioral Profiles. The cluster analysis revealed different cognitive neuropsychological profiles of the

sample. Then we investigated whether these profiles match the behavioral dimensions, and we analyzed the effect of frequent comorbid syndromes as conduct disorder (CD) and learning disorder (LD).

The cognitive clusters differ both in ADHD-RS inattention, $W(5, 28.26) = 13.82$, MSE = 41.78, $P < .01$, and in hyperactive-impulsive, $W(5, 28.27) = 8.39$, MSE = 50.2, $P < .01$, scales. Considering the Games-Howell post hoc tests, the two TD-like groups (none or few symptoms, moderate WM) have lower rating scale score than the two ADHD-like groups (severe WM with severe shifting, severe WM; in each case $P < .05$; see Table 1) but do not differ from one another or from the two subclinical clusters. The same pattern can be observed in the hyperactive-impulsive scale: the two TD-like clusters differ significantly ($P < .05$) only from the two ADHD-like groups.

TABLE 2: Comorbid diagnoses in the cognitive clusters.

| Clusters | Comorbid diagnosis | | | | | |
| | CD | | | LD | | |
	n	%	Adj. residual	n	%	Adj. residual
None or few	1	3.85	**−2.72**	2	7.69	**−2.29**
Mod Inh-Mild Shift	2	25	.19	0	0	−1.65
Mod/Sev Shift-Mod WM	3	27.27	.42	0	0	**−1.97**
Sev WM-Mild Shift	6	40	1.81	6	40	1.66
Mod WM	2	16.67	−.51	1	8.33	−1.34
Sev WM-Sev Shift	5	38.46	1.56	11	84.62	**5.64**

Note. LD = learning disorder, CD = conduct disorder. Adjusted residuals: the residual for a cell (observed minus expected value) divided by an estimate of its standard error. The resulting standardized residual is expressed in standard deviation units above or below the mean. When the absolute value of the residual is greater than 2, it can be concluded that the given cell had contribution to the chi-square result.

The clusters are different in the ratio of comorbid CD, $\chi^2(11.18)$, $P < .05$, and LD, $\chi^2(34.23)$, $P < .01$ indicated by Fisher's exact test (see Table 2). The proportions of additional CD and LD are lower in the none or few symptoms cluster than in the others. The ratio of comorbid LD is lower in the cluster with moderate to severe shifting achievement with moderate WM, but it is higher in the cluster with severe WM and shifting problems compared to the other four.

4. Discussion

In this study, we used a person-oriented statistical approach to understand the heterogeneity of EF in school-age children with or without ADHD. As we predicted, the three-factor model [11] was useful to segment children both in referred and nonreferred samples. Six different clusters were identified, where two were TD-like, two were ADHD-like groups, and two represented subthreshold categories. The executive factors were not totally independent in our sample: although shifting and updating composed separate clusters, the cognitive impairments were not severe. Interestingly, the updating factor was the most relevant in our obtained structure. While shifting could modulate the separation, inhibition had only a limited contribution to our model.

A previous research [21] presented a simpler cluster structure with three groups: children with poor inhibitory control, poor set-shifting/speed, and intact task performance. Our model was more elaborated with six clusters, which could reflect two differences between the studies. First, we measured WM, which is one of the most often found EF impairments in the developmental psychiatric literature [6]. Second, the previous study reported data from clinical sample only [21]. Another cluster analytic study [7] presented four clusters in a preschooler sample, where two represented clinical or at risk groups, while the two others showed neither ADHD risk nor EF deficits. Our cluster structure had two other groups with subclinical characteristics, in line with other studies which demonstrated mild EF deficits in nonclinical samples [13, 16].

Our clusters also varied in the severity of cognitive impairment. This result was also reflected by the latent class analysis (LCA) studies which reported different symptom severity classes in ADHD and in TD samples as well

[38–45]. Our results are in line with the study of Hudziak et al. [41], where severe behavioral symptoms existed only in the clinical setting; however, mild and moderate ones were in the TD sample as well. In accordance with the LCA studies, our cluster analytic approach supports more the continuum models rather than the categorical ones in regard to symptom severity. No rigorous borders are hypothesized in a continuum model, and only the number of symptom dimensions (hyperactivity, inattentive behavior, and impulsivity) affects the ADHD taxonomy to a large extent. LCA studies often suggest subtypes like impulsive behavior without hyperactivity, daydreaming, or excessive-talkative communication style. Importantly, these studies could also identify subthreshold groups with milder symptoms in epidemiological samples. LCA is part of the person-oriented statistical methods, whose approach is paraphrased by Bergman et al. [46]. Person-oriented methods (like hierarchical clustering, configural frequency analysis, latent structure models, and dense point analysis) can handle the phenomenon of symptom instability. The dynamic changes between ADHD and EF and their infinite variety may manifest in different profiles or clusters as types [47]. By using various forms of cluster analysis there is a beneficial way to test the similarity in a person-oriented way [46]. Nevertheless, in a therapeutic approach the personal focus could be relevant; however, group comparisons cannot serve this purpose.

We have hypothesized that the atypical neuropsychological clusters are differently characterized by ADHD symptoms. However, there was no difference between our clusters in the type of the symptoms ratings; that is, inattention and hyperactivity-impulsivity scales did not differ. The cognitive clusters and the behavioral dimensions only partially match in our sample. Nevertheless, both the cognitive neuropsychological and the behavioral rating scales were sensitive to symptom severity. Our clusters describe a cognitive dimension of the ADHD-TD continuum, where different types emerge from multiple EF components. This is in accordance with the transition from models of a single core deficit to multiple-deficit models that represents a paradigm shift in the way that the neuropsychology of ADHD is conceptualized. According to these changes, theoretical models emerged that attempted to account for the neuropsychological heterogeneity of ADHD [9, 18].

Comorbidity alone cannot explain the differences between the clusters. At the same time, we could see that comorbidity can transform the clusters' structure as it was previously demonstrated [7, 21, 43]. Considering that associations between ADHD-related comorbid symptoms and EF factors are not completely known [7], we should mention that in our study CD did not occur more frequently in any of the atypical cognitive clusters, and LD was obviously present only in the most severely impaired group (severe WM with severe updating). The difference in comorbid LD between our ADHD clusters could be a measurement bias due to a theoretical and cognitive overlap between the two diagnostic terms (i.e., LD and ADHD) [48]. It is still unclear whether the often reported learning problems in ADHD are parts of the core deficits or are caused by independent although cooccurring impairments in learning. Moreover, it is also possible that some children's symptoms of ADHD are secondary, caused by primary learning problems [48]. Therefore, conducting a similar cluster analytic study without comorbid LD would be important to understand this problem described above.

The three tasks used in this study are widely known and accessible for practitioners [9], which may ease implementing these findings in clinical practice (e.g., diagnostics and treatment). The Stroop task was repeatedly used to indicate the inhibition factor [10, 14]. The Wisconsin Card Sorting Test was originally proposed as a Shifting Paradigm [11]. Meanwhile, the digit span is analogous to many previously used verbal WM tasks in this line of literature [11, 13]. While our task selection was based on the three-factor model of EF [11], we would like to note that our results cannot be considered as an attempt to validate this model in ADHD. Due to the robustness of the model, we may assume that the present cluster structure would generally hold up; however, we do not expect exactly the same structure with different type of inhibition (Go/No-go, stop-signal), shifting (trail making, verbal fluency), or updating (operation span, spatial span) tasks. As another limitation, we should mention the relatively high male ratio in our sample. While the prevalence of ADHD is higher in boys than in girls, many authors suggest that epidemiological designs could balance this skewed pattern [49]. The relatively small number of participants in our clusters necessarily raises the question of reliability and generalizability of our findings. Despite the good clustering scores (ESS, HC, Silhouette) conducting a similar analysis on a larger sample is an important future task.

5. Conclusions

The behavioral ratings and the cognitive neuropsychological profiles of ADHD converged only in the dimension of symptom severity. In regard to the qualitative meaning of the clusters, the two types of information were mismatching, and there were no systematic relations among inattention, hyperactive-impulsive behavior, and the three components of executive functions. It is possible that atypicalities in EF may be manifested in nonspecific everyday problems (e.g., difficulties with turn taking in conversations, forgetfulness, losing things, etc.), similar to the comorbid learning disorder (e.g., listening or paying attention, doing math, etc.), which

appeared more likely in more severe neuropsychological forms of ADHD. However, neuropsychological profiles are unique and not replaceable with rating scales. We suggest that diagnostic description of behavior needs to be quantifiable and testable, taking into consideration both the cognitive neuropsychological and the behavioral profiles of symptomatology. We also propose adopting person-oriented statistical methods in neuropsychological studies, because those are more informative in developmental research than in the variable-oriented statistics.

Conflict of Interests

The authors declare that there is no conflict of interests regarding the publication of this paper.

References

[1] U. P. Ramtekkar, A. M. Reiersen, A. A. Todorov, and R. D. Todd, "Sex and age differences in attention-deficit/hyperactivity disorder symptoms and diagnoses: implications for DSM-V and ICD-11," *Journal of the American Academy of Child and Adolescent Psychiatry*, vol. 49, no. 3, pp. 217–228, 2010.

[2] L. Scahill, M. Schwab-Stone, K. R. Merikangas, J. F. Leckman, H. Zhang, and S. Kasl, "Psychosocial and clinical correlates of ADHD in a community sample of school-age children," *Journal of the American Academy of Child and Adolescent Psychiatry*, vol. 38, no. 8, pp. 976–984, 1999.

[3] S. Valo and R. Tannock, "Diagnostic instability of DSM-IV adhd subtypes: effects of informant source, instrumentation, and methods for combining symptom reports," *Journal of Clinical Child and Adolescent Psychology*, vol. 39, no. 6, pp. 749–760, 2010.

[4] American Psychiatric Association, *Diagnostic and Statistical Manual of Mental Disorders*, American Psychiatric Association, Arlington, Va, USA, 5th edition, 2013.

[5] I. S. Baron, "Attention-deficit/hyperactivity disorder: new challenges for definition, diagnosis, and treatment," *Neuropsychology Review*, vol. 17, no. 1, pp. 1–3, 2007.

[6] A. F. T. Arnsten and K. Rubia, "Neurobiological circuits regulating attention, cognitive control, motivation, and emotion: disruptions in neurodevelopmental psychiatric disorders," *Journal of the American Academy of Child and Adolescent Psychiatry*, vol. 51, no. 4, pp. 356–367, 2012.

[7] U. Pauli-Pott, S. Dalir, T. Mingebach, A. Roller, and K. Becker, "Attention deficit/hyperactivity and comorbid symptoms in preschoolers: differences between subgroups in neuropsychological basic deficits," *Child Neuropsychology*, vol. 20, no. 2, pp. 230–244, 2014.

[8] R. Martinussen and R. Tannock, "Working memory impairments in children with attention-deficit hyperactivity disorder with and without comorbid language learning disorders," *Journal of Clinical and Experimental Neuropsychology*, vol. 28, no. 7, pp. 1073–1094, 2006.

[9] E. G. Willcutt, A. E. Doyle, J. T. Nigg, S. V. Faraone, and B. F. Pennington, "Validity of the executive function theory of attention-deficit/ hyperactivity disorder: a meta-analytic review," *Biological Psychiatry*, vol. 57, no. 11, pp. 1336–1346, 2005.

[10] A. Miyake and N. P. Friedman, "The nature and organization of individual differences in executive functions: four general conclusions," *Current Directions in Psychological Science*, vol. 21, no. 1, pp. 8–14, 2012.

[11] A. Miyake, N. P. Friedman, M. J. Emerson, A. H. Witzki, A. Howerter, and T. D. Wager, "The unity and diversity of executive functions and their contributions to complex "Frontal Lobe" tasks: a latent variable analysis," *Cognitive Psychology*, vol. 41, no. 1, pp. 49–100, 2000.

[12] J. E. Lehto, P. Juujärvi, L. Kooistra, and L. Pulkkinen, "Dimensions of executive functioning: evidence from children," *British Journal of Developmental Psychology*, vol. 21, no. 1, pp. 59–80, 2003.

[13] D. Sjöwall, L. Roth, S. Lindqvist, and L. B. Thorell, "Multiple deficits in ADHD: executive dysfunction, delay aversion, reaction time variability, and emotional deficits," *The Journal of Child Psychology and Psychiatry*, vol. 54, no. 6, pp. 619–627, 2013.

[14] K. K. Wu, S. K. Chan, P. W. L. Leung, W.-S. Liu, F. L. T. Leung, and R. Ng, "Components and developmental differences of executive functioning for school-aged children," *Developmental Neuropsychology*, vol. 36, no. 3, pp. 319–337, 2011.

[15] L. Carr, J. Henderson, and J. T. Nigg, "Cognitive control and attentional selection in adolescents with ADHD versus ADD," *Journal of Clinical Child & Adolescent Psychology*, vol. 39, no. 6, pp. 726–740, 2010.

[16] J. T. Nigg, E. G. Willcutt, A. E. Doyle, and E. J. S. Sonuga-Barke, "Causal heterogeneity in attention-deficit/hyperactivity disorder: do we need neuropsychologically impaired subtypes?" *Biological Psychiatry*, vol. 57, no. 11, pp. 1224–1230, 2005.

[17] L. M. McGrath, B. F. Pennington, M. A. Shanahan et al., "A multiple deficit model of reading disability and attention-deficit/ hyperactivity disorder: searching for shared cognitive deficits," *Journal of Child Psychology and Psychiatry and Allied Disciplines*, vol. 52, no. 5, pp. 547–557, 2011.

[18] E. J. S. Sonuga-Barke, "Psychological heterogeneity in AD/HD—a dual pathway model of behaviour and cognition," *Behavioural Brain Research*, vol. 130, no. 1-2, pp. 29–36, 2002.

[19] E. G. Willcutt, R. S. Betjemann, L. M. McGrath et al., "Etiology and neuropsychology of comorbidity between RD and ADHD: the case for multiple-deficit models," *Cortex*, vol. 46, no. 10, pp. 1345–1361, 2010.

[20] R. Lambek, R. Tannock, S. Dalsgaard, A. Trillingsgaard, D. Damm, and P. H. Thomsen, "Validating neuropsychological subtypes of ADHD: how do children with and without an executive function deficit differ?" *The Journal of Child Psychology and Psychiatry*, vol. 51, no. 8, pp. 895–904, 2010.

[21] B. A. Roberts, M. M. Martel, and J. T. Nigg, "Are there executive dysfunction subtypes within ADHD?" *Journal of Attention Disorders*, 2013.

[22] R. A. Barkley, "Behavioral inhibition, sustained attention, and executive functions: constructing a unifying theory of ADHD," *Psychological Bulletin*, vol. 121, no. 1, pp. 65–94, 1997.

[23] American Psychiatric Association, *Diagnostic and Statistical Manual of Mental Disorders, Fourth Edition, Text Revision (DSM-IV-TR)*, American Psychiatric Association, Arlington, Va, USA, 2000.

[24] Á. Juhász, *Logopédiai vizsgálatok kézikönyve [The Manual of Examinations in Speech Therapy]*, Logopédiai Kiadó, Budapest, Hungary, 2007.

[25] J. C. Raven, *Guide to Using the Coloured Progressive Matrices*, H.K. Lewis, New York, NY, USA, 1965.

[26] G. J. DuPaul, T. J. Power, A. D. Anastopoulos, and R. Reid, *ADHD Rating Scale-IV: Checklists, Norms, and Clinical Interpretation*, Guilford Press, New York, NY, USA, 1998.

[27] A. T. Beck, R. A. Steer, and M. G. Carbin, "Psychometric properties of the Beck depression inventory: twenty-five years of evaluation," *Clinical Psychology Review*, vol. 8, no. 1, pp. 77–100, 1988.

[28] J. F. Leckman, M. A. Riddle, M. T. Hardin et al., "The yale global tic severity scale: initial testing of a clinician-rated scale of tic severity," *Journal of the American Academy of Child and Adolescent Psychiatry*, vol. 28, no. 4, pp. 566–573, 1989.

[29] L. Scahill, M. A. Riddle, M. McSwiggin-Hardin et al., "Children's yale-brown obsessive compulsive scale: reliability and validity," *Journal of the American Academy of Child and Adolescent Psychiatry*, vol. 36, no. 6, pp. 844–852, 1997.

[30] D. V. Sheehan, Y. Lecrubier, K. H. Sheehan et al., "The Mini-International Neuropsychiatric Interview (M.I.N.I.): the development and validation of a structured diagnostic psychiatric interview for DSM-IV and ICD-10," *Journal of Clinical Psychiatry*, vol. 59, supplement 20, pp. 22–33, 1998.

[31] C. J. Golden, *Stroop Color and Word Test: A Manual for Clinical and Experimental Uses*, Stoelting Co., Chicago, Ill, USA, 1978.

[32] D. Wechsler, *Wechsler Intelligence Scale for Children*, The Psychological Corporation, San Antonio, Tex, USA, 1991.

[33] S. Whitaker, "WISC–IV and low IQ: review and comparison with the WAIS–III," *Educational Psychology in Practice*, vol. 24, no. 2, pp. 129–137, 2008.

[34] R. K. Heaton, G. J. Chelune, J. L. Talley, G. G. Kay, and G. Curtiss, *Wisconsin Card Sorting Test Manual: Revised and Expanded*, Psychological Assessment Resources, Odessa, Fla, USA, 1993.

[35] L. C. Morey, R. K. Blashfield, and H. A. Skinner, "A comparison of cluster analysis techniques withing a sequential validation framework," *Multivariate Behavioral Research*, vol. 18, no. 3, p. 309, 1983.

[36] A. von Eye and L. R. Bergman, "Research strategies in developmental psychopathology: dimensional identity and the person-oriented approach," *Development and Psychopathology*, vol. 15, no. 3, pp. 553–580, 2003.

[37] A. Vargha, *Matematikai Statisztika Pszichológiai, Nyelvészetiés Biológiai Alkalmazásokkal. 2. Kiadás [Mathematical Statistics with Applications in Psychology, Linguistics, and Biology*, Pólya Kiadó, Budapest, Hungary, 2nd edition, 2007.

[38] P. F. A. de Nijs, R. F. Ferdinand, and F. C. Verhulst, "No hyper-active-impulsive subtype in teacher-rated attention-deficit/ hyperactivity problems," *European Child and Adolescent Psychiatry*, vol. 16, no. 1, pp. 25–32, 2007.

[39] J. Elia, M. Arcos-Burgos, K. L. Bolton, P. J. Ambrosini, W. Berrettini, and M. Muenke, "ADHD latent class clusters: DSM-IV subtypes and comorbidity," *Psychiatry Research*, vol. 170, no. 2-3, pp. 192–198, 2009.

[40] J. J. Hudziak, A. C. Heath, P. F. Madden et al., "Latent class and factor analysis of DSM-IV ADHD: a twin study of female adolescents," *Journal of the American Academy of Child and Adolescent Psychiatry*, vol. 37, no. 8, pp. 848–857, 1998.

[41] J. J. Hudziak, M. E. Wadsworth, A. C. Heath, and T. M. Achenbach, "Latent class analysis of child behavior checklist attention problems," *Journal of the American Academy of Child and Adolescent Psychiatry*, vol. 38, no. 8, pp. 985–991, 1999.

[42] A. Kóbor, Á. Takács, R. Urbán, and V. Csépe, "The latent classes of subclinical ADHD symptoms: convergences of multiple informant reports," *Research in Developmental Disabilities*, vol. 33, no. 5, pp. 1677–1689, 2012.

[43] R. J. Neuman, A. Heath, W. Reich et al., "Latent class analysis of ADHD and comorbid symptoms in a population sample

of adolescent female twins," *Journal of Child Psychology and Psychiatry*, vol. 42, no. 7, pp. 933–942, 2001.

[44] R. J. Neuman, R. D. Todd, A. C. Heath et al., "Evaluation of ADHD typology in three contrasting samples: a latent class approach," *Journal of the American Academy of Child and Adolescent Psychiatry*, vol. 38, no. 1, pp. 25–33, 1999.

[45] E. R. Rasmussen, R. J. Neuman, A. C. Heath, F. Levy, D. A. Hay, and R. D. Todd, "Replication of the latent class structure of attention-deficit/hyperactivity disorder (ADHD) subtypes in a sample of Australian twins," *Journal of Child Psychology and Psychiatry and Allied Disciplines*, vol. 43, no. 8, pp. 1018–1028, 2002.

[46] L. R. Bergman, D. Magnusson, and B. M. El-Khouri, *Studying Individual Development in an Interindividual Context: A Person-Oriented Approach*, Lawrence Erlbaum Associates, Mahwah, NJ, USA, 2003.

[47] L. R. Bergman and B. M. El-Khouri, "Developmental processes and the modern typological perspective," *European Psychologist*, vol. 6, no. 3, pp. 177–186, 2001.

[48] J. B. Hale, L. A. Reddy, M. Semrud-Clikeman et al., "Executive impairment determines ADHD medication response: implications for academic achievement," *Journal of Learning Disabilities*, vol. 44, no. 2, pp. 196–212, 2011.

[49] S. Jonsdottir, *ADHD and Its Relationship to Comorbidity and Gender*, Rijksuniversiteit Groningen, Groningen, The Netherlands, 2006.

15

Pharmacological Prevention of Posttraumatic Stress Disorder: A Systematic Review

Ravi Philip Rajkumar[1] and Balaji Bharadwaj[2]

[1] Department of Psychiatry, Disaster Management Committee, Jawaharlal Institute of
  Postgraduate Medical Education and Research (JIPMER), Puducherry 605 006, India
[2] Department of Psychiatry, Jawaharlal Institute of Postgraduate Medical Education and Research (JIPMER),
  Puducherry 605 006, India

Correspondence should be addressed to Ravi Philip Rajkumar; ravi.psych@gmail.com

Academic Editor: Takahiro Nemoto

Introduction. Various interventions, both psychological and pharmacological, have been studied for their efficacy in preventing posttraumatic stress disorder (PTSD) following trauma exposure. However, the preventive effect of pharmacotherapy has not been systematically assessed. *Methodology.* A systematic review of all clinical trials of drug therapy to prevent PTSD, available through the PubMed and EMBASE databases, was conducted. This included an assessment of each study's quality. *Results.* A total of 13 studies were reviewed. The drugs examined in these papers included propranolol, hydrocortisone, serotonin reuptake inhibitors, gabapentin, omega-3 fatty acids, and benzodiazepines. There was marked heterogeneity across studies in terms of quality, study populations, and methodology. Analysis of the outcomes revealed preliminary evidence for the efficacy of hydrocortisone, particularly in critical care settings. There was no consistent evidence to support the use of other drugs to prevent PTSD. *Discussion.* There may be a limited role for hydrocortisone in preventing the development of PTSD in specific settings. Results with other drugs are inconsistent. Further large-scale studies should assess the efficacy of these approaches in other contexts, such as natural disasters, and the time frame within which they should be used.

1. Introduction

Posttraumatic stress disorder (PTSD) is a common psychological consequence of exposure to trauma, particularly situations that threaten the safety or integrity of the self or loved ones. A wide range of traumatic situations has been associated with PTSD: combat situations, natural and man-made disasters, accidental injury, physical or sexual assault, and serious medical illnesses and their treatment [1–3]. PTSD consists of three distinctive groups of symptoms: *reexperiencing* the traumatic event, *avoidance* of reminders of the event, and *hyperarousal*. These symptoms should be present for at least one month and should cause significant impairment in social and occupational functioning [1, 4, 5]. Estimates of prevalence of PTSD in the general population have varied depending on study methodology, but rates as high as 12.3% have been reported, with prevalence in women generally higher than in men [1, 6]. Following exposure to

a natural or man-made disaster, prevalences as high as 40% have been reported [2].

The course of PTSD is variable, with some studies finding a favourable outcome and low rates of chronicity [7]; however, long-term studies have found that at least half the patients initially diagnosed with PTSD continue to experience symptoms after several years [6, 8, 9]. Chronic PTSD is associated with marked impairments in social and occupational functioning and is often associated with other mental disorders such as depression, anxiety disorders, and substance use disorders [10]. A variety of factors have been associated with the development or persistence of PTSD following a traumatic exposure: these include female gender, preexisting psychopathology, and the nature and severity of the exposure [10, 11].

One potential predictor of future PTSD is the appearance of initial PTSD-like symptoms following exposure to trauma.

These symptoms, sometimes referred to as *acute stress disorder* (ASD) [12], do not qualify for a diagnosis of PTSD unless they persist for over a month. Not all individuals who experience ASD are diagnosed with PTSD in the long term [13, 14], but severe ASD, particularly associated with high levels of hyperarousal, is associated with the subsequent emergence of PTSD [15, 16].

With this in mind, a variety of psychological interventions have been designed both to address these acute symptoms and to prevent the future development of PTSD [17, 18]; however, the efficacy of these interventions has been questioned [19, 20] and they may not be easily available in certain settings [21]. Recognition of these facts, as well as advances in understanding the biology of PTSD, has led to trials of various pharmacological agents immediately following a traumatic exposure to reduce the occurrence or severity of subsequent PTSD [22]. In this article, these approaches and the evidence for their efficacy are reviewed.

2. Methodology

2.1. Search Strategy. A search of the PubMed and EMBASE databases was carried out using the key words "posttraumatic stress disorder," "PTSD," "acute stress disorder," "pharmacotherapy," "drug therapy," and "prevention," including the PudMed medical subheadings "Stress Disorder, Posttraumatic/Drug Therapy" and "Stress Disorder, Posttraumatic/Prevention and Control." The references of these articles were checked for further papers of interest. Studies were included if they prospectively examined the effect of a pharmacological intervention on reducing the diagnosis or symptoms of PTSD at follow-up.

2.2. Outcomes. The primary outcome of interest was the diagnosis of PTSD as per standard criteria in patients receiving the intervention, as compared to those in the control group. Where this was not examined, secondary outcome measures, such as PTSD symptoms measured using a standardized rating scale, were assessed.

2.3. Data Extraction and Quality Assessment. All study data was extracted by the author and entered in the following format: study design, study duration, sample size, drug used with dose and duration, length of follow-up, outcome measures used, and results. The Jadad scoring system [23] was used to assess the methodological quality of these studies. This system assigns a score from 0 to 5 to a study, with higher scores indicating higher study quality, based on three items: randomization (0–2 points), blinding (0–2 points), and the handling of drop-outs (0-1 point). Each study was scored independently by the authors, who were blind to each other's assessments. The interrater reliability of these scores was good (Cohen's κ = 0.67). Where a discrepancy existed, this was resolved by a joint evaluation, and the consensus value was entered in Table 2.

3. Results

A total of 280 papers were examined, of which 13 fulfilled the criteria for inclusion in this review. A further seven papers were retrospective studies examining the possible protective effect of a given drug against PTSD; these papers were not included in the main review. These papers and their findings are summarized in Table 1. Only one of these papers, examining the effect of hydrocortisone on septic shock survivors, found an unequivocal effect of the study drug on PTSD prevention [24]; others reported negative results [25] or used indirect measures of drug efficacy [26–30], limiting the conclusions that could be drawn from them, though four studies did find a significant retrospective association between morphine treatment and reductions in PTSD symptoms [27–30].

The details of the thirteen papers included in this review, and their methodological quality, are summarized in Table 2. There was a wide variation in study quality (range 0–5, mean 2.3). Ten papers were randomized, double-blind, placebo-controlled drug trials, one was a randomized, placebo-controlled study without description of blinding, and two were open-label studies. Individual drugs examined included propranolol (4 studies), hydrocortisone (4 studies), selective serotonin reuptake inhibitors (SSRIs) (2 studies), benzodiazepines (2 studies), polyunsaturated fatty acids (1 study), and gabapentin (1 study). Only one study compared pharmacotherapy with psychological interventions [40].

Two studies included only children and adolescents [33, 39], while the remainder were conducted in adults. Studies were conducted across a wide range of settings. The commonest were emergency medical centres or services handling patients with physical trauma (n = 10); other settings included critical care settings (2) and paediatric burns units (1). None of the studies examined victims of disasters or mass casualties.

Treatment was initiated within 48 hours of a traumatic exposure in five studies; in a further two, preventive treatment was initiated immediately in an ICU setting. In the remaining studies, treatment was started several days or weeks after exposure to the traumatic event (range 6.7–29.35 days). Follow-up periods ranged from a minimum of 6 weeks to a maximum of 49 months after treatment.

Details of trials pertaining to specific drugs are summarized as shown in Table 2.

3.1. Propranolol. Four studies [31–34] examined the effect of propranolol (dose range 40–160 mg) in preventing PTSD; three of these were randomized controlled trials, and one was an open study. All these studies involved patients presenting to trauma centres for physical injuries, most commonly motor vehicle accidents. Jadad scores for these trials ranged from 0 to 3. Three studies were conducted in adults and one was conducted in children. The three adult studies [31, 32, 34] failed to find a significant effect of propranolol over placebo in reducing short- to medium-term rates of PTSD diagnoses (follow-up duration range, 2–8 months), though one study did find a significant effect of propranolol in reducing symptoms of PTSD [32]. The single study examining

TABLE 1: Papers excluded from the current review.

Study authors	Study population	Study design	Drug used	Outcome measure	Result
(1) Sharp et al., 2010 [25]	Children with severe burns, $n = 363$	Chart review	Propranolol	Diagnosis of ASD	No effect of propranolol in preventing ASD after 1 month
(2) Schelling et al., 1999 [24]	Adults surviving septic shock, $n = 54$ (27 receiving the drug, 27 controls)	Retrospective case-control	Hydrocortisone 100 mg, followed by 0.18 mg/kg/hr	Diagnosis of PTSD as per Posttraumatic Stress Syndrome-10 Inventory	Significantly lower rates of PTSD in patients receiving hydrocortisone (5/27 versus 16/27 controls, $P = .01$)
(3) Kobayashi et al., 2011 [26]	Adult victims of traffic accidents ($n = 255$; 23 receiving the drug, 232 controls)	Retrospective case-control	Salbutamol	PTSD symptoms as per CAPS	Lower CAPS scores in the salbutamol group at 6 weeks; only the re-experiencing sub-score was lower in this group after 1 year
(4) Saxe et al., 2001 [27]	Hospitalized children with burns, aged 6–16 ($n = 24$)	Prospective observational study	Morphine	PTSD symptoms as per Child PTSD Reaction Index	Significant correlation between morphine dose received and 6-month decrease in PTSD symptoms
(5) Bryant et al., 2009 [28]	Hospitalized patients with traumatic injuries ($n = 155$; 17 with PTSD, 138 without)	Chart review	Morphine	Amount of morphine used in patients with and without PTSD	Patients diagnosed with PTSD at 3 months received significantly less morphine
(6) Stoddard et al., 2009 [29]	Hospitalized children with burns, aged 1–4 ($n = 70$; complete data available only for 11 children)	Prospective observational study	Morphine	PTSD symptoms as per CDSC-B Child Stress Disorders Checklist-Burns Version	Significant correlation between morphine dose received and 6-month decrease in PTSD symptoms
(7) Holbrook et al., 2010 [30]	Military personnel with combat trauma ($n = 696$; 243 with PTSD, 453 without)	Chart review	Morphine	Rates of morphine use in patients with and without PTSD	Lower morphine use in those with PTSD (61%) than those without (76%; $P < .001$)

CAPS, clinician-assessed PTSD scale; CDSC-B, child stress disorders checklist-burns version.

the efficacy of propranolol in children [33] found no evidence of efficacy overall, but a significantly *higher* rate of PTSD in girls receiving the drug, suggesting an interaction between gender and drug effects in younger patients.

3.2. *Hydrocortisone.* Four studies [35–38] assessed the use of hydrocortisone in preventing PTSD. The Jadad scores for these studies ranged from 2 to 3. Two of these studies were conducted in critically ill patients admitted to intensive care facilities for septic shock [35] and cardiac surgery [36], respectively. These studies used an intravenous loading dose of hydrocortisone followed by a maintenance infusion during the course of hospitalization. One of these studies reported outcomes in terms of PTSD diagnosis and found a positive effect of the drug at long-term follow-up [35]; the other

found a significant decrease in PTSD symptoms in those who had received hydrocortisone, compared with a placebo group, after 6 months [36]. The remaining two studies both examined adult patients exposed to a traumatic event; both found significantly lower PTSD scores in the treatment group after 3 months. There was a trend towards lower rates of diagnosed PTSD in the hydrocortisone group in both these studies, but it failed to reach statistical significance.

3.3. *Selective Serotonin Reuptake Inhibitors (SSRIs).* Two studies examined the preventive effect of SSRIs against PTSD. The Jadad scores of these trials were 2 and 1 [39, 40]. The first, conducted in children and adolescents (mean age 12.35 ± 3.7 years) being treated in a burns unit, examined the effect of 24 weeks of treatment with sertraline (dosed flexibly

TABLE 2: Prospective clinical trials of pharmacotherapy to prevent PTSD.

Study authors	Study population	Study design	Drug used	Outcome measure	Interval between trauma and initiation of drug therapy	Follow-up period	Results	Jadad score
(1) Pitman et al., 2002 [31]	Emergency department attenders (n = 41; 20 male) exposed to a traumatic event	Randomized, double-blind, placebo-controlled trial	Propranolol, 160 mg/day for 10 days (n = 18 on propranolol, 23 on placebo)	PTSD diagnosis as per DSM-IV; PTSD symptoms as measured by CAPS	<6 hours	3 months	Nonsignificantly lower CAPS score in the propranolol group at 1 month; no difference in PTSD diagnosis across groups at 1 and 3 months	1
(2) Vaiva et al., 2003 [32]	Emergency department attenders (n = 19, 11 male) exposed to a traffic accident or physical assault	Nonrandomized open trial	Propranolol, 120 mg/day for 7 days (n = 11 on propranolol, 8 receiving treatment as usual)	PTSD diagnosis as per DSM-IV; PTSD symptoms as measured by Treatment Outcome PTSD Scale	9.5 ± 6 hours (range 2–20 hours)	2 months	Nonsignificantly lower PTSD diagnoses across groups (3/8 in controls, 1/11 in the propranolol group); significantly lower PTSD Scale symptoms in the propranolol group.	0
(3) Nugent et al., 2010 [33]	Pediatric trauma emergency department attenders (n = 29; 15 boys); the majority had traffic accidents	Randomized, double-blind, placebo-controlled trial	Propranolol, 40–80 mg/day (n = 14 on propranolol, 15 on placebo)	PTSD symptoms as measured by CAPS-CA	<12 hours	6 weeks	No significant difference in PTSD symptoms overall across groups; significantly increased PTSD symptoms in girls receiving propranolol	3
(4) Stein et al., 2007 [34]	Patients admitted to a surgical trauma centre (n = 48, 26 male); the majority had traffic accidents	Randomized, double-blind, placebo-controlled trial	Propranolol, 120 mg/day or gabapentin, 1200 mg/day for 14 days (n = 17 on propranolol, 14 on gabapentin, 17 on placebo)	PTSD diagnosis as per DSM-IV; PTSD symptoms as measured by PCL-C	<48 hours	8 months	No significant differences in PTSD diagnoses or PTSD symptoms across the three groups	4
(5) Schelling et al., 2001* [35]	Patients with septic shock admitted in a medical ICU (n = 40; only 20 available at follow-up; 8/20 male)	Randomized, double-blind, placebo-controlled trial	Hydrocortisone, 100 mg IV stat followed by 0.18 mg/kg/hr and then tapered (n = 9 on hydrocortisone, 11 on placebo)	PTSD diagnosis as per DSM-IV	Immediate$	31 months (median; range 21–49 months)	Significantly lower frequency of PTSD in the hydrocortisone group (1/9 versus 7/11 placebo; P = .02)	2

Table 2: Continued.

Study authors	Study population	Study design	Drug used	Outcome measure	Interval between trauma and initiation of drug therapy	Follow-up period	Results	Jadad score
(6) Schelling et al., 2004 [36]	Patients undergoing cardiac surgery (n = 48; 35 male)	Randomized, double-blind, placebo-controlled trial	Hydrocortisone, 100 mg IV stat followed by 10 mg/hr and then tapered (n = 26 on hydrocortisone, 22 on placebo)	PTSD symptoms as per PTSS-10	Immediate%	6 months	Significantly lower PTSD symptom scores in the hydrocortisone group ($P < .05$)	3
(7) Zohar et al., 2011 [37]	25 adults experiencing a traumatic stressor (20 had traffic accidents; only 17 completed the study; 9/17 male)	Randomized, double-blind, placebo-controlled trial	Hydrocortisone, 100–140 mg as a single dose (n = 9 on hydrocortisone, 8 on placebo)	PTSD symptoms as per CAPS	<6 hours	3 months	Significantly lower PTSD symptom scores in the hydrocortisone group at 2 weeks and 3 months, but not at 1 month; trend to less frequent PTSD diagnosis at 3 months in the hydrocortisone group (0/9 versus 3/8 on placebo)	3
(8) Delahanty et al., 2013 [38]	Inpatients at a trauma unit (n = 64, 42 male); only 42 completed the study	Randomized, double-blind, placebo-controlled trial	Hydrocortisone, 40 mg/d orally for 10 days (n = 31 on hydrocortisone, 33 on placebo)	PTSD diagnosis and PTSD symptoms as per CAPS	<12 hours	3 months	Significantly lower PTSD symptom scores in the hydrocortisone group at 1 and 3 months ($P < .05$); less frequent PTSD diagnosis in the hydrocortisone group at 3 months, but not significant	3
(9) Stoddard et al., 2011 [39]	Children and adolescents with burns (age 6–20 years; n = 26)	Randomized, placebo-controlled, double-blind study	Sertraline, 25–150 mg/day for 24 weeks (n = 17 on sertraline, 9 on placebo)	PTSD symptoms as per parental report and self-report	Variable&	24 weeks	Significantly greater decrease in parent-rated PTSD symptoms at 8, 12, and 24 weeks in the sertraline group; no difference in self-rated PTSD symptoms	2

TABLE 2: Continued.

Study authors	Study population	Study design	Drug used	Outcome measure	Interval between trauma and initiation of drug therapy	Follow-up period	Results	Jadad score
(10) Shalev et al., 2012# [40]	Adult survivors of trauma admitted to emergency services ($n = 242$; 107 male)	Randomized, double-blind, placebo-controlled study	Escitalopram, 20 mg/day for 12 weeks ($n = 23$ on escitalopram, 23 on placebo; 93 wait-list controls; 63 on prolonged exposure; 40 on cognitive therapy)	PTSD diagnosis and PTSD symptoms as per CAPS	29.35 ± 4.91 days	9 months	Similar rates of PTSD in the escitalopram and placebo groups at 5 months (61.9% versus 55.6% placebo) and 9 months (42.1% versus 47.1% placebo); no difference in PTSD symptoms	1
(11) Gelpin et al., 1996 [41]	Adult trauma survivors ($n = 26$)	Nonrandomized, controlled study	Benzodiazepines, either clonazepam ($n = 10$, mean dose 2.7 mg/day) or alprazolam ($n = 3$, mean dose 2.5 mg/day). 13 gender-matched trauma survivors formed the control group	PTSD diagnosis and PTSD symptoms as per CAPS	6.7 ± 5.8 days (range 2–18 days)	6 months	Higher rates of PTSD in the benzodiazepine group at 6 months (9/13 versus 3/13 in controls; $P = .047$)	0
(12) Mellman et al., 2002 [42]	Adult trauma centre admissions ($n = 22$; 14 male; 15 had traffic accidents)	Randomized, placebo-controlled study	Temazepam, 30 mg for 7 days ($n = 11$ on temazepam, 11 on placebo)	PTSD diagnosis and PTSD symptoms as per CAPS	14.3 ± 10 days	6 weeks	Nonsignificantly higher rates of PTSD in the benzodiazepine group at 6 weeks (6/11 versus 3/11 in controls; no significant effect of treatment on PTSD symptoms)	1
(13) Matsuoka et al., 2011 [43]	Patients presenting to an ICU with accidental injuries ($n = 15$; 11 completed the study)	Open-label study	PUFA capsules, 7/day for 12 weeks; no control group	PTSD diagnosis as per DSM-IV; PTSD symptoms as per CAPS	<240 hours (10 days)	12 weeks	Only 1/11 subjects developed PTSD at 4 weeks, and retained the diagnosis at 12 weeks.	1

PTSD: posttraumatic stress disorder, CAPS: clinician-assessed PTSD scale; CAPS-CA: clinician-assessed PTSD scale for children and adolescents, PCL-C: posttraumatic stress disorder checklist-civilian version, ICU: intensive care unit, and PTSS-10: posttraumatic 10 stress symptom inventory.
*Study initially conducted to study the haemodynamic effects of hydrocortisone in septic shock; PTSD assessed at long-term follow-up.
#Study compared prolonged exposure (PE), cognitive therapy (CT), escitalopram and placebo.
$Hydrocortisone given as a loading dose at ICU admission.
%Hydrocortisone given as a loading dose during induction of anaesthesia.
&This study included 12 children with acute burns and 14 admitted for reconstructive surgery, so time between trauma and sertraline initiation could not be computed.

between 25–150 mg/day) on self- and parent-reported PTSD symptoms. This study found a significant effect in favour of sertraline at 8, 12, and 24 weeks for parent-reported symptoms, but not for child-reported symptoms. Of note, this study included 12 children with acute burns and 14 seeking reconstructive surgery; this heterogeneity may have accounted for the equivocal results obtained [39]. A second study was part of a larger, multiarm trial of interventions to prevent PTSD in adult trauma patients. This study found no effect of treatment with escitalopram (dose 20 mg/day) on preventing PTSD when compared with placebo; on the other hand, psychological interventions (prolonged exposure and cognitive therapy) showed significant efficacy in the other arms of this study [40].

3.4. Benzodiazepines. Two small studies, one open-label [41] and one randomized [42], assessed the efficacy of benzodiazepines in adult trauma patients; the Jadad scores of these trials were 0 and 1, respectively. In both these studies, drug treatment was started several days after trauma exposure in most patients. Both studies found an unfavourable outcome for the study drug, with higher rates of PTSD at follow-up in the treatment groups (pooled rates 15/24 in the benzodiazepine groups, 6/24 in the placebo groups; $P = .01$). Of all the treatments examined in this review, benzodiazepines appear to be the only ones which paradoxically increase PTSD rates.

3.5. Gabapentin. A single study of high quality (Jadad score 4) compared the effects of gabapentin, propranolol, and placebo, initiated within 48 hours of exposure, in preventing PTSD in adult patients following a physical injury. At 8 months, there was no significant difference between the three groups in terms of PTSD diagnosis or PTSD symptoms [34].

3.6. Polyunsaturated Fatty Acids (PUFA). A small open-label study examined the effects of 12 weeks of treatment with fixed dose PUFA capsules, each containing 1470 mg docosahexaenoic acid and 147 mg eicosapentaenoic acid (7 capsules/day) on PTSD outcomes in 15 adult patients exposed to an accidental injury [43]. This study had a Jadad score of 1. 11 patients who completed the study, and only 1 patient developed PTSD; however, due to the lack of a control group, a true preventive effect could not be demonstrated.

4. Discussion

Factors affecting study results are as follows.

4.1. Outcome Measures. Of thirteen trials reviewed, twelve provided information that could be used to make inferences regarding efficacy. Nine studies reported outcomes in terms of PTSD diagnoses using the DSM-IV criteria. Of these studies, only one—a trial of hydrocortisone in patients hospitalized for septic shock—reported an unequivocally lower frequency of PTSD in the treatment group [35]. On the other hand, seven papers reported outcomes in terms of PTSD symptoms measured on a standardized, clinical-rated

scale; of these, three found consistently lower PTSD symptom scores in the drug group [32, 36, 38], and a fourth found lower PTSD scores at two out of three assessments [37]. The drugs used in these studies were propranolol [32] or hydrocortisone [36–38]. Three of these four papers also reported outcomes for PTSD diagnoses, and all found lower rates of PTSD in their respective treatment groups, though these differences were not statistically significant. This suggests that even when pharmacotherapy with hydrocortisone or propranolol does not prevent PTSD, it may reduce its severity in some cases; alternately, these studies may have been underpowered to detect differences in the frequency of categorical diagnoses.

4.2. Study Quality. There was significant variation in quality across studies. The mean Jadad score was 1.85, indicating a generally poor study quality. Using a cut-off Jadad score of 3, five papers could be categorized as being of good quality [33, 34, 36–38]. Two of these studies reported outcomes in terms of PTSD diagnosis, with a negative result in one case [34] and a nonsignificantly lower rate of PTSD in the other [38]. All five studies reported outcomes in terms of PTSD symptoms on standard rating scales; of these, three studies, all involving hydrocortisone, had a positive outcome [36–38].

In comparison, of eight studies scoring below 3 on the Jadad scale, one of seven measuring this outcome demonstrated a positive effect in terms of PTSD diagnoses [35], and two of four measuring PTSD symptoms had findings in favour of the study drug [32, 39]. This suggests that study design had little effect on the results obtained; furthermore, the best-designed study, with a Jadad score of 4, was negative in terms of drug effects on either PTSD diagnosis or symptom severity [34].

4.3. Time Interval between Trauma Exposure and Treatment Initiation. There is evidence from animal research that there may be a "window of opportunity" immediately after a traumatic event [37, 44] during which the use of medications may prevent PTSD and that administering treatment after this period may be ineffective. This period may last only for a few hours [37]. Four studies began drug administration within 6 hours of trauma exposure; of these, a trial of propranolol was negative [31], two trials of hydrocortisone in medical settings were positive [35, 36], and a trial of hydrocortisone in adult trauma patients found some evidence of efficacy [37]. In seven other studies in which treatments were administered over 6 hours after trauma exposure, only two reported an effect of the drug in attenuating PTSD symptoms [32, 38]; in both these studies, the drug was administered within 12 hours of trauma exposure. Studies in which treatment was begun 48 hours or more after trauma exposure were uniformly negative [34, 40–42]. Though the small numbers preclude a meaningful comparison, these findings suggest that even if effective, pharmacotherapy to prevent PTSD may work best when given no more than 12 hours after a traumatic exposure. On the other hand, psychological interventions may be effective even when administered several days after an exposure [40].

4.4. Nature of the Study Population. Of the thirteen studies reviewed above, the majority recruited patients who had experienced physical trauma, most commonly in the form of motor vehicle accidents. Two studies were conducted in patients in ICU settings who were at risk for PTSD owing to the grave nature of their illness and/or invasive medical procedures [35, 36], and two studies were conducted in children with either physical trauma [33] or burns [39]. It is not possible, with the existing data, to comment on whether the type of trauma or the age of the study population had a significant effect on outcomes; however, there was some evidence of a gender effect in the trial of propranolol in children exposed to physical trauma, with girls in the treatment group showing a paradoxically worse outcome [33].

4.5. Nature of the Drug Used. The two trials of benzodiazepines [41, 42] showed uniformly poor results, with trends towards worse outcomes in the form of higher rates of PTSD in the treatment groups. This unexpected negative effect may arise from the fact that benzodiazepines block the normal cortisol response to trauma, and this response may be important in fear responses [45]; alternately, benzodiazepines may need to be given before rather than after a traumatic event if they are to have a preventive effect [22].

Results with propranolol were largely negative, with only one small study (out of four reviewed) finding a significant difference in PTSD scores [32]. Though this may result from the individual studies being underpowered, research in animals suggests that the ineffectiveness of propranolol may be due to the fact that traumatic stress-related processes are not correlated with the effects of propranolol on either autonomic activity or learning [46].

All four studies of hydrocortisone reported positive results, though only one demonstrated a clear reduction in PTSD diagnosis [35]. Though promising and neurobiologically plausible [22, 45], the interpretation of these results is confounded by the fact that two of these studies were conducted in ICU settings, in which hydrocortisone may have corrected an underlying physiological imbalance [35, 36], and effects on PTSD may have been indirect. However, one of the non-ICU studies was probably underpowered [37] and the other suffered from high dropout rates [38]; when the 3-month outcomes of these two studies were combined, a significant difference in favour of hydrocortisone for the diagnosis of PTSD was found (pooled frequencies: 0/33 for 3-month PTSD diagnosis in the hydrocortisone group; 6/30 for placebo; $P = .009$, Fisher's exact test), suggesting that this drug may be effective even outside critical care settings.

Though SSRIs are effective treatments for established PTSD [4], their preventive efficacy cannot be established from the above studies. This may reflect the relatively long period between trauma exposure and initiation of treatment in both studies, as discussed above. Given the apparent efficacy of SSRIs in an animal model of PTSD [47], trials of more immediate treatment with these drugs in the aftermath of trauma may be indicated.

5. Ethical Issues

Following initial reports of the use of propranolol to prevent PTSD, concerns were raised about the possible undesirable effects of such a form of treatment to "erase" unpleasant memories, as well as the medicalization of negative life events by the medical profession or drug manufacturers. More fancifully, it has been argued that such treatments may even disrupt a person's sense of self, or lead to a dystopic society [48]. Given the evidence reviewed above about the actual efficacy of propranolol and other drugs in preventing PTSD, such concerns seem premature; moreover, in high-risk groups, such as military veterans experiencing combat trauma, withholding an effective preventive treatment—if one existed—could itself be unethical [49]. If and when such treatments are approved and available on a large scale, they will need to be handled carefully, and informed consent should be obtained in all cases [48].

6. Applicability of the Existing Research to Clinical Practice

As of now, it is premature to recommend any of the treatment approaches reviewed above—including hydrocortisone—in routine clinical practice. Further research, involving larger numbers of patients exposed to different sorts of trauma in various settings, needs to be conducted before this can be done. There is little evidence for the use of other drugs, and benzodiazepines in particular should be avoided as they may actually worsen patient outcomes. In patients presenting days or weeks after a traumatic exposure, psychological interventions may be more beneficial [40]. Similar caveats apply to the use of these drugs in disaster or mass casualty settings, where they have never been tested.

7. Future Directions

A variety of other pharmacological agents have shown promise in animal models of PTSD; these include corticotropin-releasing factor (CRF) antagonists [50], cannabinoids [51], inhibitors of protein synthesis [52], and inhibitors of steroid synthesis, such as ketoconazole [53]. The safety, efficacy, and feasibility of these approaches in humans have yet to be established. In the meantime, large-scale clinical trials of hydrocortisone and of SSRIs during the "window period" may clarify the role of these drugs in clinical practice, as well as their efficacy compared to psychological interventions. Systematic trials of morphine, which has shown promise in observational studies [27–30], are also required.

8. Conclusion

The field of pharmacotherapy for the prevention of PTSD is still in its infancy. The early enthusiasm for propranolol therapy has not been justified by the results of controlled trials. The existing literature suggests that hydrocortisone therapy is promising, both in and outside intensive care settings, and this approach should be tested on a larger scale. However, no specific drug therapy can be routinely recommended yet for the prevention of PTSD in clinical or disaster settings.

Conflict of Interests

The authors declare that there is no conflict of interests regarding the publication of this paper.

References

[1] R. Yehuda, "Post-traumatic stress disorder," *The New England Journal of Medicine*, vol. 346, no. 2, pp. 108–114, 2002.

[2] Y. Neria, A. Nandi, and S. Galea, "Post-traumatic stress disorder following disasters: a systematic review," *Psychological Medicine*, vol. 38, no. 4, pp. 467–480, 2008.

[3] J. C. Jackson, R. P. Hart, S. M. Gordon, R. O. Hopkins, T. D. Girard, and E. W. Ely, "Post-traumatic stress disorder and posttraumatic stress symptoms following critical illness in medical intensive care unit patients: assessing the magnitude of the problem," *Critical Care*, vol. 11, no. 1, p. R27, 2007.

[4] B. D. Grinage, "Diagnosis and management of post-traumatic stress disorder," *American Family Physician*, vol. 68, no. 12, pp. 2401–2409, 2003.

[5] F. Lamprecht and M. Sack, "Posttraumatic stress disorder revisited," *Psychosomatic Medicine*, vol. 64, no. 2, pp. 222–237, 2002.

[6] A. Perkonigg, H. Pfister, M. B. Stein et al., "Longitudinal course of posttraumatic stress disorder and posttraumatic stress disorder symptoms in a community sample of adolescents and young adults," *The American Journal of Psychiatry*, vol. 162, no. 7, pp. 1320–1327, 2005.

[7] I. R. Galatzer-Levy, Y. Ankri, S. Freedman et al., "Early PTSD symptom trajectories: persistence, recovery, and response to treatment: results from the Jerusalem trauma outreach and prevention study (J-TOPS)," *PLoS ONE*, vol. 8, Article ID e70084, 2013.

[8] D. Koren, I. Arnon, and E. Klein, "Long term course of chronic posttraumatic stress disorder in traffic accident victims: a three-year prospective follow-up study," *Behaviour Research and Therapy*, vol. 39, no. 12, pp. 1449–1458, 2001.

[9] Z. Solomon and M. Mikulincer, "Trajectories of PTSD: a 20-year longitudinal study," *American Journal of Psychiatry*, vol. 163, no. 4, pp. 659–666, 2006.

[10] N. Breslau, "Outcomes of posttraumatic stress disorder," *Journal of Clinical Psychiatry*, vol. 62, supplement 17, pp. 55–59, 2001.

[11] C. S. North, J. Oliver, and A. Pandya, "Examining a comprehensive model of disaster-related posttraumatic stress disorder in systematically studied survivors of 10 disasters," *The American Journal of Public Health*, vol. 102, no. 10, pp. e40–e48, 2012.

[12] S. P. Cahill and K. Pontoski, "Post-traumatic stress disorder and acute stress disorder I: their nature and assessment considerations," *Psychiatry*, vol. 2, no. 4, pp. 14–25, 2005.

[13] R. A. Bryant, "Acute stress disorder as a predictor of posttraumatic stress disorder: a systematic review," *Journal of Clinical Psychiatry*, vol. 72, no. 2, pp. 233–239, 2011.

[14] R. A. Bryant, M. Creamer, M. O'Donnell, D. Silove, and A. C. McFarlane, "The capacity of acute stress disorder to predict posttraumatic psychiatric disorders," *Journal of Psychiatric Research*, vol. 46, no. 2, pp. 168–173, 2012.

[15] M. Hansen and A. Elklit, "Does acute stress disorder predict posttraumatic stress disorder following bank robbery?" *Journal of Interpersonal Violence*, vol. 28, no. 1, pp. 25–44, 2013.

[16] M. Shevlin, P. Hyland, and A. Elklit, "Different profiles of acute stress disorder differentially predict posttraumatic stress disorder in a large sample of female victims of sexual trauma," *Psychological Assessment*. In press.

[17] K. Ponniah and S. D. Hollon, "Empirically supported psychological treatments for adult acute stress disorder and posttraumatic stress disorder: a review," *Depression and Anxiety*, vol. 26, no. 12, pp. 1086–1109, 2009.

[18] S. E. Hobfoll, P. Watson, C. C. Bell et al., "Five essential elements of immediate and mid-term mass trauma intervention: empirical evidence," *Psychiatry*, vol. 70, no. 4, pp. 283–315, 2007.

[19] S. C. Rose, J. Bisson, R. Churchill, and S. Wessely, "Psychological debriefing for preventing post traumatic stress disorder," *Cochrane Database of Systematic Reviews*, no. 2, Article ID CD000650, 2002.

[20] C. A. Forneris, G. Gartlehner, K. A. Brownley et al., "Interventions to prevent post-traumatic stress disorder: a systematic review," *American Journal of Preventive Medicine*, vol. 44, no. 6, pp. 635–650, 2013.

[21] M. van Ommeren, S. Saxena, and B. Saraceno, "Aid after disasters," *British Medical Journal*, vol. 330, no. 7501, pp. 1160–1161, 2005.

[22] R. K. Pitman and D. L. Delahanty, "Conceptually driven pharmacologic approaches to acute trauma," *CNS Spectrums*, vol. 10, no. 2, pp. 99–106, 2005.

[23] A. R. Jadad, R. A. Moore, D. Carroll et al., "Assessing the quality of reports of randomized clinical trials: is blinding necessary?" *Controlled Clinical Trials*, vol. 17, no. 1, pp. 1–12, 1996.

[24] G. Schelling, C. Stoll, H.-P. Kapfhammer et al., "The effect of stress doses of hydrocortisone during septic shock on posttraumatic stress disorder and health-related quality of life in survivors," *Critical Care Medicine*, vol. 27, no. 12, pp. 2678–2683, 1999.

[25] S. Sharp, C. Thomas, L. Rosenberg, M. Rosenberg, and W. Meyer III, "Propranolol does not reduce risk for acute stress disorder in pediatric burn trauma," *The Journal of trauma*, vol. 68, no. 1, pp. 193–197, 2010.

[26] I. Kobayashi, E. Sledjeski, W. Fallon, E. Spoonster, D. Riccio, and D. Delahanty, "Effects of early albuterol (salbutamol) administration on the development of posttraumatic stress symptoms," *Psychiatry Research*, vol. 185, no. 1-2, pp. 296–298, 2011.

[27] G. Saxe, F. Stoddard, D. Courtney et al., "Relationship between acute morphine and the course of PTSD in children with burns," *Journal of the American Academy of Child and Adolescent Psychiatry*, vol. 40, no. 8, pp. 915–921, 2001.

[28] R. A. Bryant, M. Creamer, M. O'Donnell, D. Silove, and A. C. McFarlane, "A study of the protective function of acute morphine administration on subsequent posttraumatic stress disorder," *Biological Psychiatry*, vol. 65, no. 5, pp. 438–440, 2009.

[29] F. J. Stoddard, E. A. Sorrentino, T. A. Ceranoglu et al., "Preliminary evidence for the effects of morphine on posttraumatic stress disorder symptoms in one- to four-year-olds with burns," *Journal of Burn Care and Research*, vol. 30, no. 5, pp. 836–843, 2009.

[30] T. L. Holbrook, M. R. Galarneau, J. L. Dye, K. Quinn, and A. L. Dougherty, "Morphine use after combat injury in Iraq and posttraumatic stress disorder," *The New England Journal of Medicine*, vol. 362, no. 2, pp. 110–117, 2010.

[31] R. K. Pitman, K. M. Sanders, R. M. Zusman et al., "Pilot study of secondary prevention of posttraumatic stress disorder with propranolol," *Biological Psychiatry*, vol. 51, no. 2, pp. 189–192, 2002.

[32] G. Vaiva, F. Ducrocq, K. Jezequel et al., "Immediate treatment with propranolol decreases posttraumatic stress disorder two months after trauma," *Biological Psychiatry*, vol. 54, no. 9, pp. 947–949, 2003.

[33] N. R. Nugent, N. C. Christopher, J. P. Crow, L. Browne, S. Ostrowski, and D. L. Delahanty, "The efficacy of early propranolol administration at reducing PTSD symptoms in pediatric injury patients: a pilot study," *Journal of Traumatic Stress*, vol. 23, no. 2, pp. 282–287, 2010.

[34] M. B. Stein, C. Kerridge, J. E. Dimsdale, and D. B. Hoyt, "Pharmacotherapy to prevent PTSD: Results from a randomized controlled proof-of-concept trial in physically injured patients," *Journal of Traumatic Stress*, vol. 20, no. 6, pp. 923–932, 2007.

[35] G. Schelling, J. Briegel, B. Roozendaal, C. Stoll, H.-B. Rothenhäusler, and H.-P. Kapfhammer, "The effect of stress doses of hydrocortisone during septic shock on posttraumatic stress disorder in survivors," *Biological Psychiatry*, vol. 50, no. 12, pp. 978–985, 2001.

[36] G. Schelling, E. Kilger, B. Roozendaal et al., "Stress doses of hydrocortisone, traumatic memories, and symptoms of posttraumatic stress disorder in patients after cardiac surgery: a randomized study," *Biological Psychiatry*, vol. 55, no. 6, pp. 627–633, 2004.

[37] J. Zohar, H. Yahalom, N. Kozlovsky et al., "High dose hydrocortisone immediately after trauma may alter the trajectory of PTSD: interplay between clinical and animal studies," *European Neuropsychopharmacology*, vol. 21, no. 11, pp. 796–809, 2011.

[38] D. L. Delahanty, C. Gabert-Quillen, S. A. Ostrowski et al., "The efficacy of initial hydrocortisone administration at preventing posttraumatic distress in adult trauma patients: a randomized trial," *CNS Spectrums*, vol. 18, no. 2, pp. 103–111, 2013.

[39] F. J. Stoddard Jr., R. Luthra, E. A. Sorrentino et al., "A randomized controlled trial of sertraline to prevent posttraumatic stress disorder in burned children," *Journal of Child and Adolescent Psychopharmacology*, vol. 21, no. 5, pp. 469–477, 2011.

[40] A. Y. Shalev, Y. Ankri, Y. Israeli-Shalev, T. Peleg, R. Adessky, and S. Freedman, "Prevention of posttraumatic stress disorder by early treatment: results from the Jerusalem trauma outreach and prevention study," *Archives of General Psychiatry*, vol. 69, no. 2, pp. 166–176, 2012.

[41] E. Gelpin, O. Bonne, T. Peri, D. Brandes, and A. Y. Shalev, "Treatment of recent trauma survivors with benzodiazepines: a prospective study," *Journal of Clinical Psychiatry*, vol. 57, no. 9, pp. 390–394, 1996.

[42] T. A. Mellman, V. Bustamante, D. David, and A. I. Fins, "Hypnotic medication in the aftermath of trauma," *Journal of Clinical Psychiatry*, vol. 63, no. 12, pp. 1183–1184, 2002.

[43] Y. Matsuoka, D. Nishi, N. Yonemoto, K. Hamazaki, T. Hamazaki, and K. Hashimoto, "Potential role of brain-derived neurotrophic factor in omega-3 fatty acid supplementation to prevent posttraumatic distress after accidental injury: an open-label pilot study," *Psychotherapy and Psychosomatics*, vol. 80, no. 5, pp. 310–312, 2011.

[44] H. Cohen, M. A. Matar, D. Buskila, Z. Kaplan, and J. Zohar, "Early post-stressor intervention with high-dose corticosterone attenuates posttraumatic stress response in an animal model of posttraumatic stress disorder," *Biological Psychiatry*, vol. 64, no. 8, pp. 708–717, 2008.

[45] J. Zohar, R. Sonnino, A. Juven-Wetzler, and H. Cohen, "Can posttraumatic stress disorder be prevented?" *CNS spectrums*, vol. 14, supplement 1, pp. 44–51, 2009.

[46] H. Cohen, Z. Kaplan, O. Koresh, M. A. Matar, A. B. Geva, and J. Zohar, "Early post-stressor intervention with propranolol is ineffective in preventing posttraumatic stress responses in an animal model for PTSD," *European Neuropsychopharmacology*, vol. 21, no. 3, pp. 230–240, 2011.

[47] M. A. Matar, H. Cohen, Z. Kaplan, and J. Zohar, "The effect of early poststressor intervention with sertraline on behavioral responses in an animal model of post-traumatic stress disorder," *Neuropsychopharmacology*, vol. 31, no. 12, pp. 2610–2618, 2006.

[48] M. Henry, J. R. Fishman, and S. J. Youngner, "Propranolol and the prevention of post-traumatic stress disorder: is it wrong to erase the "sting" of bad memories?" *The American Journal of Bioethics*, vol. 7, no. 9, pp. 12–20, 2007.

[49] E. Donovan, "Propranolol use in the prevention and treatment of posttraumatic stress disorder in military veterans: forgetting therapy revisited," *Perspectives in Biology and Medicine*, vol. 53, no. 1, pp. 61–74, 2010.

[50] R. Adamec, D. Fougere, and V. Risbrough, "CRF receptor blockade prevents initiation and consolidation of stress effects on affect in the predator stress model of PTSD," *International Journal of Neuropsychopharmacology*, vol. 13, no. 6, pp. 747–757, 2010.

[51] E. Ganon-Elazar and I. Akirav, "Cannabinoids prevent the development of behavioral and endocrine alterations in a rat model of intense stress," *Neuropsychopharmacology*, vol. 37, no. 2, pp. 456–466, 2012.

[52] H. Cohen, Z. Kaplan, M. A. Matar, U. Loewenthal, N. Kozlovsky, and J. Zohar, "Anisomycin , a protein synthesis inhibitor, disrupts traumatic memory consolidation and attenuates posttraumatic stress response in rats," *Biological Psychiatry*, vol. 60, no. 7, pp. 767–776, 2006.

[53] H. Cohen, J. Benjamin, Z. Kaplan, and M. Kotler, "Administration of high-dose ketoconazole, an inhibitor of steroid synthesis, prevents posttraumatic anxiety in an animal model," *European Neuropsychopharmacology*, vol. 10, no. 6, pp. 429–435, 2000.

16

Aggression in Psychoses

Jan Volavka

New York University School of Medicine, P.O. Box 160663, Big Sky, MT 59716, USA

Correspondence should be addressed to Jan Volavka; janvolavka@gmail.com

Academic Editor: Jane E. Boydell

Most individuals diagnosed with a mental illness are not violent, but some mentally ill patients commit violent acts. PubMed database was searched for articles published between 1980 and November 2013 using the combination of key words "schizophrenia" or "bipolar disorder" with "aggression" or "violence." In comparison with the general population, there is approximately a twofold increase of risk of violence in schizophrenia without substance abuse comorbidity and ninefold with such comorbidity. The risk in bipolar disorder is at least as high as in schizophrenia. Most of the violence in bipolar disorder occurs during the manic phase. Violence among adults with schizophrenia may follow two distinct pathways: one associated with antisocial conduct and another associated with the acute psychopathology, particularly anger and delusions. Clozapine is the most effective treatment of aggressive behavior in schizophrenia. Emerging evidence suggests that olanzapine may be the second most effective treatment. Treatment nonadherence greatly increases the risk of violent behavior, and poor insight as well as hostility is associated with nonadherence. Nonpharmacological methods of treatment of aggression in schizophrenia and bipolar disorder are increasingly important. Cognitive behavioral approaches appear to be effective in cases where pharmacotherapy alone is not sufficient.

1. Introduction

Many people believe that psychiatric patients are dangerous, and fear of violence is the most important part of the stigma of mental illness. This belief persists despite the fact that most psychiatric patients are in fact not violent and that they are much more likely to be victims rather than perpetrators of aggressive behavior.

Although the public fear of patients is overblown, there is a general consensus among experts that severe mental illness does increase the risk of violence. Indeed, violent behavior of the mentally ill presents a multitude of problems. There is the risk of injuries or death of victims and perpetrators. Caring for violent psychiatric patients challenges the clinician. It elicits fear, countertransference problems, and eventual burnout. It complicates the efforts of all caregivers. Caring for a violent relative is emotionally exhausting; it is obviously very difficult to live with an assaultive patient.

Importantly, violence affects the cost of treatment. Today, violent behavior is a leading cause of hospitalization, which may be prolonged if that behavior persists. Staff time is costly, and violent patients require a lot of it. Finally, there are societal costs such as the time spent by the police that have to

deal with assaultive patients in the community, and the enormous stress imposed on the jails and prisons where many assaultive psychiatric patients are incarcerated.

This review will examine the epidemiology, underlying mechanisms and pathways to violence, and the management of aggression in schizophrenia and bipolar disorder.

2. Methods

PubMed database was searched for articles published between 1980 and November 2012. For the general searches on aggression in psychoses, the combinations of key words "schizophrenia" or "bipolar disorder" with "aggression" or "violence" were used. For the treatment searches, generic names of medications were used in combination with key words "schizophrenia" or "bipolar disorder" and "aggression." No language constraint was applied. Only articles dealing with adults were included. The lists of references were searched manually to find additional articles.

Additionally, the review draws on the author's own experimental and other studies in the area of violence in psychoses over the past 30 years. Published and unpublished materials were included.

3. Definitions and Assessment Methods

Many definitions of *aggression* have been offered [1]. The most useful and parsimonious (albeit imperfect) definition states that aggression is overt action intended to harm. This term may describe animal or human behavior. Human aggression can be assessed quantitatively with various rating scales designed for this purpose. The overt aggression scale (OAS) [2] and its modification (modified overt aggression scale (MOAS)) [3, 4] have been frequently used to separately assess verbal aggression and physical aggression against objects, against self, and against others. Aggression against self is outside the scope of this review and it will not be discussed here. The term *aggression* is typically used in biomedical and psychological literature.

Aggressive behavior has been classified into various subgroups. A useful classification defines two subtypes: impulsive or premeditated aggression. Impulsive aggression is a hair-trigger aggressive response to environmental provocation, characterized by a loss of behavioral control. This is in contrast with premeditated aggression which is defined as a planned aggressive act that lacks spontaneity and behavioral agitation.

This discussion leads us back to the definition of aggression stated above: "an overt action *intended* to harm." Without the intent, the definition would make no sense: any unintentional error resulting in an injury to another person would be misclassified as aggression. But some cases of impulsive aggression represent a response to provocation that comes so fast that we may have some doubts about the assailant's ability to fully form an intent in a fraction of a second. Even more seriously, that ability may be impaired or lost in cases of intoxication. The ability to form an intent is in doubt in psychotic or demented persons. To make things even more difficult, we do not fully understand the term "intent." Thus, the definition of aggression offered here is imperfect. But so are all the other definitions that have been published. We have to keep these imperfections in mind when using the definition of aggression. A more extensive discussion of these issues can be found elsewhere [1].

Violence is defined as physical aggression among humans. This term tends to be more commonly used in sociology and criminology (e.g., *violent crime*). Some authors use the terms *violence* and *aggression* interchangeably, depending on context and style.

Violence perpetrated by psychiatric patients in the community can be assessed (and defined) by the MacArthur community violence interview that distinguishes two levels of severity: minor violence, corresponding to simple assault without injury or weapon use, and serious violence, corresponding to any assault using a lethal weapon or resulting in injury, any threat with a lethal weapon in hand, or any sexual assault [5–8].

The US Bureau of Justice Statistics's definition of violent crime includes murder, rape and sexual assault, robbery, and assault (http://www.bjs.gov/index.cfm?ty=tp&tid=31 accessed 11 20 2013).

Agitation is excessive motor and/or verbal activity. It may include verbal aggression manifested by threats, abuse,

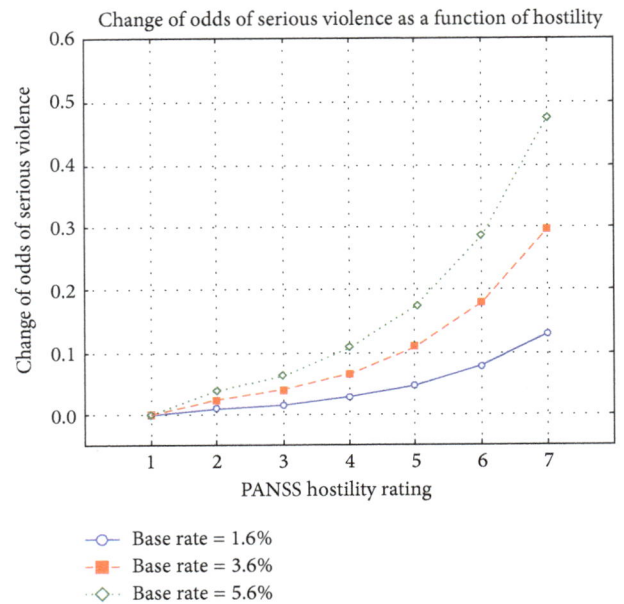

FIGURE 1: Change of odds of serious violence as a function of hostility. The computation and display were provided by Pal Czobor, PhD, using the data published by Swanson et al. [8].

or incoherent screams. Agitation may be assessed using the excited component of the positive and negative syndrome scale (PANSS) [9]. The excited component consists of five PANSS items: tension, excitement, hostility, uncooperativeness, and poor impulse control; each item is rated from 1 (absent) to 7 (extreme).

Hostility signifies unfriendly attitudes. Manifestations of hostility include overt irritability, anger, resentment, or verbal aggression. Hostility is assessed and operationally defined by rating scales. The most frequently used method to assess hostility is the "hostility" item in the PANSS [9] or in the brief psychiatric rating scale (BPRS) [10]. The principal clinical importance of hostility is in its close association with violence. Hostility item in the PANSS is rated from 1 (absent) to 7 (extreme). For each unit increase on this 7-point rating of hostility, the odds of serious aggression (assessed with MacArthur community violence interview) were reported to increase by a factor of 1.65 ($P < 0.001$) [8] (see Figure 1).

The association of hostility rating with overt physical aggression has led to its widespread use as a proxy measure of violence. Hostility is also associated with nonadherence to medication [11] and difficulties in psychological treatments. Hostility interferes with therapeutic alliance.

Psychopathy is currently defined by assessment instruments developed by Hare and his group. The psychopathy checklist-revised (PCL-R) [12] is a 20-item instrument. Each item is scored on a three-point scale (0 = does not apply, 1 = applies to an extent, and 2 = applies). Items are summed, the total score range is 0–40. PCL-R can be used as a dimensional instrument (employing the total score) or as a categorical classifier using a cut-off score. The recommended cut-off score is 30 [12], but sometimes lower cut-off scores are used [13].

Psychopathy Checklist. Screening version (PCL:SV) was developed as a shorter variant of PCL-R, suitable for administration to individuals with major psychiatric disorders [14]. It has 12 items that are scored in the same way as the PCL-R. The total score range is 0–24. The cut-off score for the diagnosis of psychopathy is 18. Analyses of the PCL:SV (and PCL-R) yielded two factors: factor 1 reflects personal and affective characteristics. Some of these items, such as lack of remorse and empathy, cannot be reliably distinguished from blunted affect in persons with schizophrenia. Factor 2 comprises behaviors manifesting continued socially deviant, unstable lifestyle and thus may be indexing the same syndrome as diagnoses of conduct disorder and antisocial personality disorder. Much of the research work on comorbidity of psychopathy with schizophrenia used the PCL:SV.

It should be noted that the antisocial personality disorder in the DSM-IV-TR and the DSM-5 [15] is partly defined by acts of violence, but the diagnosis can be given in the absence of aggressive behavior.

The American Psychiatric Association Board of Trustees recognized the numerous shortcomings of the current DSM-5 system for the classification of personality disorders. Nevertheless, the decision was to preserve the current system to maintain continuity with clinical practice. At the same time, an alternative DSM-5 model for personality disorders was developed and presented [15, page 761]. For the Antisocial Personality Disorder, the alternative system introduces "psychopathic features" as a diagnostic specifier, and "psychopathy" is introduced as a "distinct variant." The main new alternative criteria for antisocial personality disorder are somewhat closer to Hare's concept of psychopathy in that they pay more attention to personality functioning than the current system.

These modifications introduced in the alternative model represent partial improvements in comparison with the current system. Hopefully, work on these modifications will continue, and DSM-6 will switch from the current model to a new system for the diagnosis of personality disorders.

4. Schizophrenia

4.1. Prevalence of Violent Behavior in Schizophrenia. The National Institute of Mental Health (NIMH) supported the epidemiological catchment area surveys (ECA), an epidemiological study that provided prevalence estimates for mental disorders in the United States [16, 17]. The data were based on structured diagnostic household interviews conducted at five sites in the United States. It should be noted that this classical study had different sampling and time frames than most other studies. It included prisoners and it was conducted in the early 1980s before deinstitutionalization was fully completed and when antipsychotic medications differed from those used today.

The surveys included questions pertaining to any history of violent behavior. Analyses of these data yielded a one-year prevalence of violent behavior of 8.4% in persons diagnosed with schizophrenia and 2.1% in those without any mental disorder [18, 19]. Males were more violent than females. Comorbid substance abuse substantially increased the prevalence of violent behavior in schizophrenia.

A longitudinal study assessed the population rates of violence in schizophrenia linking nationwide Swedish registry data of hospital admissions for schizophrenia and data on criminal convictions between 1973 and 2006 [20]. The study comprised a total of 80,025 individuals, 8,003 of whom were diagnosed with schizophrenia. In this schizophrenia subset, 13.2% of individuals had a record of at least one violent criminal offense, compared with 5.3% of individuals in general population (odds ratio (OR) = 2.0, 95% confidence interval (CI) = 1.8–2.2). The risk of violence was particularly elevated in individuals with schizophrenia and comorbid substance abuse: in individuals without substance abuse, OR = 1.2 (95% CI = 1.1–1.4), whereas with substance abuse OR = 4.4 (95% CI = 3.9–5.0) [20].

To study familial confounding, Fazel et al. also investigated risk of violence among unaffected siblings ($n = 8123$) of patients with schizophrenia. The risk increase among the patients with substance abuse comorbidity was significantly less pronounced when unaffected siblings were used as controls (28.3% of those with schizophrenia had a violent offense compared with 17.9% of their unaffected siblings; adjusted OR = 1.8; 95% CI = 1.4–2.4; $P < .001$ for interaction), suggesting significant familial confounding of the association between schizophrenia and violence [20]. These results are further discussed in a subsequent section on genetic influences.

A meta-analysis of 20 studies comparing risk of violence in schizophrenia and other psychosis with general population controls [21] confirmed and expanded the results reviewed above [20]. The meta-analysis comprised data from 18,423 individuals diagnosed with schizophrenia that were compared with 1,714,904 individuals in general population. There was a modest but statistically significant increase of risk of violence in schizophrenia (OR = 2.1, 95% CI = 1.7–2.7) without comorbidity and OR = 8.9 (95% CI = 5.4–14.7) with substance abuse comorbidity. Risk estimate of violence in individuals with substance abuse (but without psychosis) showed an OR of 7.4 (95% CI = 4.3–1) [21].

The national epidemiologic survey on alcohol and related conditions (NESARC) was a two-wave project conducted in the United States ($N = 34,653$: Wave 1: 2001–2003; Wave 2: 2004-2005). Indicators of mental illness in the year prior to Wave 1 were used to predict violence between Waves 1 and 2 [22]. Violence was assessed by self-report in a structured interview. Contrary to prior published evidence, severe mental illness did not independently predict violent behavior. Comorbid substance use disorder was one of the independent predictors.

We reanalyzed the same NESARC data using different methods [23]. Contrary to the results reported by Elbogen and Johnson [22], we found that individuals with severe mental illness with or without comorbid substance abuse were significantly more likely to be violent than those with no mental or substance use disorders. As expected, those with comorbid mental and substance use disorders had the highest risk of violence. Male gender, history of childhood abuse and neglect, household antisocial behavior, binge drinking, and stressful life events were also associated with violence [23].

The epidemiological studies reviewed above used samples that aimed to represent populations. Other studies, however, used samples that were selected clinically; that is, they selected individuals who were ascertained to be diagnosed with schizophrenia.

The MacArthur violence risk assessment study enrolled 1136 patients with mental disorders at three acute inpatient facilities in the United States and followed them up during their first year after discharge from the hospital to monitor their violent behavior [5]. The comparison group consisted of 519 people residing in the same neighborhoods. A special assessment tool, the MacArthur community violence interview, was developed for this project (see above). The interview was conducted with the subjects and collateral informants. The one-year prevalence of violence was 17.9% for patients with a major mental disorder and without a substance abuse diagnosis and 31.1% for patients with a major mental disorder and a substance abuse diagnosis. The results showed no significant difference between the prevalence of violence by patients without substance abuse and the prevalence of violence by comparison group members who were also without substance abuse. Substance abuse raised the rate of violence in both groups. The methods and interpretation of this influential study raised certain concerns [24].

The NIMH supported clinical antipsychotic trials of intervention effectiveness (CATIE) [25] enrolled a national sample of 1,445 schizophrenia patients from 57 United States sites. Information on violent behavior during the 6 months prior to enrollment was collected using a version of the MacArthur Community Violence Interview (see above). The results showed that 4% had committed serious acts of violence involving weapons or causing injury to another individual, and 16% had engaged in less serious acts that would be described as simple battery, such as slapping, pushing, and shoving [8]. Minor violence was associated with co-occurring substance abuse. Females were significantly more likely to be violent than males; this effect appeared to be attributable to a group of young women with a history of substance abuse and arrest.

Homicide is the violent crime that is almost always reported to the police, and its investigation results more frequently in the identification of the perpetrator in comparison with other crimes. The Finnish police have been able to solve about 95% of all homicides committed during several decades. The prevalence of various mental disorders among 693 Finnish homicide offenders was determined [26]. The prevalence of schizophrenia and schizophreniform psychoses was 6.4% in male and 6.0% in female offenders. Primary or secondary diagnosis of alcoholism was detected in 32.9% of male and 32.1% of female offenders. Comparing the prevalence of schizophrenia and schizophreniform psychoses in offenders with the general population, the age-adjusted OR = 9.7, 95% CI = 7.4–12.6 for males and 9.0, 95% CI = 3.6–22.2 for females.

Other data suggested that females diagnosed with schizophrenia may be more at risk for committing homicide than their male counterparts. A study of 1087 homicide offenders

(convicted or exculpated) in Austria [27] detected that 4.3% male and 13.5% female offenders had schizophrenia. Comorbid substance abuse/dependence was diagnosed in 46.3% of the male (39% alcohol and 24.4% nonalcohol) and 11.8% of the female schizophrenics (5.9% alcohol and 11.8% nonalcohol). A comparison of risk for schizophrenia or schizophreniform disorder in offenders with the general population in Austria showed age-adjusted ORs in men 5.85, 95% CI = 4.3–8.0; in women OR = 18.4, 95% CI = 11.2–31.6 [27]. For males and females combined, the proportion of offenders with schizophrenia or schizophreniform disorder (with or without alcohol use or abuse comorbidity) was 5.3%, OR = 8.8, 95% CI = 6.6–11.5. For those *without* that comorbidity, the respective numbers were 3.8%, OR = 7.1, 95% CI = 5.1–9.8. The numbers for subjects with alcohol comorbidity were substantially higher.

Psychiatric diagnoses of 2005 individuals convicted of homicide or attempted homicide in Sweden were analyzed [28]. It was found that 8.9% of homicide offenders had schizophrenia, 2.5% had bipolar disorder, and 6.5% had other psychoses. It should be noted that 47.5% of offenders with complete information had a primary or secondary diagnosis of substance use disorder. A meta-analysis of 10 studies indicated that the risk of homicide in psychosis is maximal during the first episode before the start of treatment [29].

Thus, schizophrenia may be associated with a somewhat higher risk for homicide than for less serious violent behavior. However, caution is required when comparing the homicide studies with the other studies of violence risk in mental illness. It should be noted that, except for Schanda et al. [27], the homicide studies do not present separate estimates of the risk for homicide in schizophrenia without substance abuse comorbidity. That comorbidity is high in homicide offenders and may be responsible for a substantial proportion of risk variance. There may be a gender difference in the risk for homicide in schizophrenia patients, but the evidence is unreliable (note the large CI for the OR in females in the Schanda et al. study [27]). The risk elevation in the first episode of psychosis is well supported and it underscores the need for early treatment and monitoring.

When interpreting the prevalence and risk data reviewed above, it is important to remember that they largely apply to schizophrenia patients dwelling in the community. Except for the ECA study [18, 19], hospitalized and incarcerated patients did not contribute to these estimates. Violent behavior is a frequent reason for hospitalization and arrest of schizophrenia patients. Thus, the estimates of prevalence and risk of violent behavior in the community are lowered by a constant removal of the most violent schizophrenia patients to hospitals and jails. In many cases, violent behavior continues inside these institutions [30, 31]. Furthermore, it is important to point out that only some incidents of aggressive behavior lead to prosecution. Therefore, studies based on self-reports must be distinguished from those based on convictions.

In summary, prevalence estimates of violent behavior in patients diagnosed with schizophrenia vary depending on the severity of violence. The six-month prevalence of serious violence perpetrated by community-dwelling schizophrenia patients in the United States is approximately 4%.

Schizophrenia patients without substance abuse comorbidity are about twice as likely to perpetrate violent acts as their counterparts in the general population and about nine times as likely if that comorbidity is present. Thus, substance abuse is a major risk factor for violence in schizophrenia. Future efforts at tertiary prevention and management of schizophrenia should be targeted at the diagnosis and systematic treatment of comorbid substance use disorder.

4.2. Comorbidity of Schizophrenia and Psychopathy/Antisocial Personality Disorder.

Studies in prisoners have established that psychopathy alone (without any comorbidity) is associated with violent behavior [32]. A meta-analysis involving 15,826 individuals indicated that the PCL-R had a moderate effect size in predicting interpersonal violence [33]. Another meta-analysis showed a similar result [34].

The PCL:SV was administered to 26 persistently violent patients and 25 matched nonviolent patients, all diagnosed with schizophrenia or schizoaffective disorder [35]. Mean psychopathy scores were higher for violent patients than nonviolent patients. Higher psychopathy scores were associated with earlier age of onset of illness and more arrests for both violent and nonviolent offenses.

The relationship between schizophrenia/psychopathy comorbidity and violence was addressed with ratings on the PCL-R that were used to test the hypothesis that psychopathy predicts violent recidivism in a Swedish forensic cohort of 202 male violent offenders with schizophrenia. Psychopathy was strongly associated with violent recidivism [13].

Interestingly, Finnish homicide offenders with schizophrenia ($N = 72$) had significantly *lower* mean score on PCL-R than a comparison sample of homicide offenders without schizophrenia [36].

The relationship between psychopathy and violence was confirmed in a sample of 94 Australian men diagnosed with schizophrenia-spectrum disorders [37]. The predictive validity of PCL-R scores remained significant after controlling for substance abuse.

Several studies examined relative contributions of psychopathy, psychotic symptoms, and other factors to the development of aggressive behavior. One of them assessed the contributions of psychosis, disordered impulse control, and psychopathy to assaults perpetrated by inpatients with schizophrenia or schizoaffective disorder [38]. A semistructured interview aimed to elicit reasons for assaults from assailants and victims. Consensus ratings indicated that approximately 20 percent of the assaults were directly related to positive psychotic symptoms. Factor analysis revealed two psychosis-related factors, one related to positive psychotic symptoms and the other to psychotic confusion and disorganization, as well as a third factor that differentiated impulsive from psychopathic assaults [38].

In an English study, 33 violent and 49 nonviolent forensic patients were assessed using neuropsychological tasks and measures of psychotic symptoms and psychopathy (PCL:SV) [39]. The "violent" group had significantly higher psychopathy scores. Personality factors (factor 1 of PCK:SV) rather than symptoms and neuropsychological function predicted violence [39].

A multisite study examined the correlates of antisocial personality disorder among 232 men with schizophrenic disorders and comorbid antisocial personality disorder [40]. Comparisons of the men with and without antisocial personality disorder revealed no differences in the course or symptomatology of schizophrenia. By contrast, individuals with antisocial comorbidity committed significantly more crimes and significantly more nonviolent crimes than those without that comorbidity. The mean total number of *violent* crimes was 5.1 (SD = 8.6) for patients with antisocial comorbidity and 1.9 (SD = 3.0) without antisocial comorbidity; $t = 2.6$, $P = 0.01$. This P value was uncorrected for multiple comparisons; the significance was lost after Bonferroni correction [40].

Thus, comorbid psychopathy or antisocial personality disorder in patients with schizophrenia or schizoaffective disorder is associated with violent behavior. This risk increase is statistically independent of comorbid substance use disorders and the severity of psychotic symptoms that also elevate the risk.

As stated above in the section on definitions and assessment methods, Factor 2 of the PCL:SV may be indexing a pattern of aggressive behavior since childhood that is captured by a diagnosis of conduct disorder in childhood. Recent imaging findings suggest that schizophrenia preceded by conduct disorder represents a distinct subtype of schizophrenia [41].

4.3. Risk Factors and Pathways to Violence in Schizophrenia.

Risk factors for violence can be classified in several ways. One of them is a classification depending on the temporal proximity to a violent event: proximal factors act to some extent as triggers, whereas the role of distal factors is less direct. Another classification is based on the factor's modifiability: static factors such as genotype and demographics are not modifiable, whereas dynamic factors such as symptoms are amenable to change. The latter classification is somewhat more clinically oriented.

4.3.1. Static Factors.

These factors include age, gender, genetic influences, childhood maltreatment, development of childhood conduct disorder, history of arrest and conviction, and history of adult victimization.

There is robust evidence indicating that young age is a risk factor for violence in general population as well as in psychotic patients [1, 42]. As mentioned in the preceding section on prevalence, the effect of gender is somewhat equivocal. A large recent review reported that male gender was modestly associated with violence in psychotic patients (OR = 1.6, 95% CI = 1.2–2.1) [43]. This systematic review and metaregression analyzed 110 studies involving 45,533 psychotic individuals, 87.8% of whom were diagnosed with schizophrenia. A total of 8,439 of these individuals (18.5%) were violent [43].

Genetic Influences. In a nonpatient sample, heritability of assaultiveness was shown to be approximately 50% [44]. A large epidemiological project focusing primarily on the risk of violent crime among schizophrenia patients had a genetic component to study familial confounding [20]. This project was reviewed in the section on prevalence. The main genetic finding was that the variation in violence risk depended on the degree of relatedness between the patient and the control group. Compared with unrelated general population controls, the risk of violent crime in individuals with schizophrenia and violent crime was increased approximately 4-fold. However, unaffected siblings had higher rates of substance abuse compared with unrelated general population. Therefore, the risk increase for schizophrenia with substance abuse comorbidity compared with these siblings was substantially reduced from 4-fold to approximately 2-fold. This reduction suggested familial confounding of this association. It is not clear if this familial confounding occurred through genetic susceptibility or early environmental effects [20].

Efforts to explore a molecular basis of genetic influences in this area have focused on neurotransmitters and their genes. Enhancement of central dopaminergic or noradrenergic function facilitates aggressive behavior in most animal studies [45]. Drugs that increase central dopaminergic transmission, such as amphetamines and cocaine, may elicit psychosis with violent behavior [1]. Furthermore, drugs that diminish noradrenergic activity (such as propranolol) have antiaggressive effects in humans [46, 47]. Thus, the preponderance of the evidence suggests that catecholamines generally enhance violence.

However, the information on genetic influences on violence in schizophrenia is limited. Much of the molecular genetic work in schizophrenia and violence has focused on catechol-O-methyltransferase (COMT), one of the enzymes involved in the catabolism of catecholamines; amines in the brain. A functional single nucleotide polymorphism involves a Val (valine) to Met (methionine) substitution at codon 158 of the COMT gene. The Val allele at this locus is associated with high enzymatic activity, whereas the Met allele is associated with low enzymatic activity. Homozygosity for the Met allele confers a 3- to 4-fold reduction in COMT activity relative to Val homozygotes; heterozygotes have intermediate activity.

Male heterozygous COMT knockout mice exhibit increased aggressive behavior [48]. When mouse strains were ranked according to their aggressivity, the ranking correlated with the expression of the COMT gene in the hippocampus: the lower the level of expression, the more aggressive the strain [49]. Thus, consistent with the enhancing effects of catecholamines on aggression, low expression of the COMT is associated with increased aggression in animal models. Based on the findings discussed above, it would seem appropriate to hypothesize that, in general, the COMT polymorphism would exert an effect in humans such that the Met allele would be associated with increased violent behavior.

COMT had originally been explored as a candidate gene for schizophrenia, and the association of COMT polymorphism with violence in schizophrenia patients was first tested in this context. Initial association studies yielded encouraging results [50, 51], and numerous attempts at replication followed. Two meta-analyses of such association studies have been published to date. One of them included 15 studies comprising 2,370 individuals with schizophrenia [52]. Evidence of a significant association between the presence of

a Met allele and violence was found such that men's violence risk increased by approximately 50% for those with at least one Met allele compared with homozygous Val individuals (diagnostic OR = 1.45; 95% CI = 1.05–2.00; z = 2.37, P = 0.02). No significant association between the presence of a Met allele and violence was found for women [52].

A meta-analysis testing the same association in 14 studies was independently conducted by another group [53]. Similarly, it was found that the Met158 allele of the COMT gene confers a significantly increased risk for violent behavior in schizophrenia. Taken together, these findings have potential implications for pharmacogenetics of schizophrenia. Future research could test the usefulness of this genetic information for personalized treatment.

Childhood Maltreatment. In a classical cohort study of 908 child abuse and neglect court cases, Widom established that being maltreated as a child increases risk for delinquency, adult criminal behavior, and violent criminal behavior [54]. However, she observed that the majority of abused and neglected do not become delinquent, criminal, or violent. The interaction between childhood maltreatment and MAOA polymorphism described above [55] partially explained the differences in the effects of maltreatment on violent behavior [56]. More recent reports confirm the association between childhood maltreatment and adult criminal violence in individuals without schizophrenia [57, 58].

The evidence for that association in schizophrenia is more tentative, although individuals with schizophrenia report more childhood adversities than controls [59]. History of childhood physical abuse was one of the factors associated with the occurrence of incidents of assaultive behavior among 183 male patients of a forensic psychiatric hospital, 106 of whom were diagnosed with schizophrenia [30]. A group of 60 male psychotic patients legally detained at a forensic unit was assessed for history of violence; the participants were also asked about any history of childhood abuse, substance use, medication adherence, and current insight in terms of awareness of mental illness [60]. Multiple regression analysis indicated that the history of childhood abuse was associated with the severity of violence independently of substance use, medication adherence, and insight (beta = 0.18, P < 0.01) [60]. In a group of 28 schizophrenia patients with a history of violence, 46% had experienced child abuse and/or neglect [61]. Childhood physical (OR = 2.2, 95% CI = 1.5–3.1) or sexual abuse (OR = 1.9, 95% CI = 1.5–2.4) was moderately associated with violence [43].

Thus, similar to robust evidence in general population indicating a relationship between childhood maltreatment and violent behavior in adulthood, there are data indicating that this relationship also exists in psychotic patients. Interactions between genes and environment that affect risk for violent behavior have been studied in general population.

Childhood Conduct Problems. Males diagnosed with schizophrenia are at increased risk to have exhibited conduct disorder before age 15. A study examined the consequences of conduct disorder among 248 adult men with schizophrenia or schizoaffective disorder [62]. Participants were assessed at hospital discharge and repeatedly during the subsequent two years. In adulthood, the diagnosis and symptoms of conduct disorder were associated with increased nonviolent and violent criminal offending, after adjusting for diagnoses of substance use disorders. During the 2-year follow-up period, conduct disorder diagnosis and the number of conduct disorder symptoms were associated with aggressive behavior, controlling for lifetime diagnoses of substance use disorders, substance misuse measured objectively and subjectively, and medication compliance. During the two-year follow-up period, neither the diagnosis of conduct disorder nor the number of conduct disorder symptoms was associated with levels of positive and negative symptoms, compliance with medication, substance use, or readmission. Thus, it appears that conduct disorder is a distinct comorbid disorder proceeding alongside the course of schizophrenia and elevating the risk of violent behavior independently of psychotic symptoms [62].

These results have implications for understanding etiology and for treatment. If the relationship between the history of conduct disorder and aggression in schizophrenia is independent of comorbid substance use disorder and of medication, then "reduction of substance use disorder would reduce violent behavior only among patients with no history of aggressive behavior prior to the onset of schizophrenia. Among adults with schizophrenia and a history of conduct disorder, treatments designed to reduce aggressive and antisocial behaviors, in addition to treatment of substance use disorder, may be necessary to reduce violence" [63]. These implications for treatment remain to be tested experimentally.

The findings reported by the Hodgins group are consistent with evidence suggesting that violence among adults with schizophrenia may follow at least two distinct pathways: one associated with premorbid conditions, including antisocial conduct, and another associated with the acute psychopathology of schizophrenia. That evidence came from a reanalysis of data from the CATIE [64]. The prevalence of violence was higher among patients with a history of childhood conduct problems than among those without this history (28.2% versus 14.6%; $P < 0.001$). In the conduct-problems group, violence was associated with current substance use at levels below diagnostic criteria. Positive psychotic symptoms were linked to violence only in the group without conduct problems. Adherence with antipsychotic medications was associated with significantly reduced violence only in the group without a history of conduct problems. In the conduct problems group, violence remained higher and did not significantly differ between patients who were adherent with medications and those who were not [64].

History of Violent and Criminal Behavior. Past violence is one of the strongest predictors of future violence [1]. Detailed confirmation of this rule has been provided in a recent analysis demonstrating that history of assault, imprisonment, arrest, and conviction for any offense were all showing strong associations with violent behavior, with ORs ≥ 4.2 [43].

Most offenders diagnosed with schizophrenia get their first conviction before their first psychotic episode [65].

A study examined offending among 301 individuals experiencing their first episode of psychosis [66]. The results showed that 33.9% of the men and 10.0% of the women had a record of criminal convictions, and 19.9% of the men and 4.6% of the women had been convicted of at least one violent crime. This increased their risk for future violent behavior. These findings have important implications for the understanding, prevention, and treatment of violent behavior in psychotic patients.

Adult Victimization. Relationships between victimization and offending were addressed by several studies. In individuals diagnosed with serious mental illness, history of a criminal conviction was associated with having been robbed ($r = 0.09$, $P < 0.05$), threatened with a weapon ($r = 0.12$, $P < 0.001$), and beaten ($r = 0.10$, $P < 0.01$) [67].

Relationships between victimization and crime were examined in a sample of 331 involuntarily admitted patients with serious mental illness [68]. Being a victim of a crime predicted patients' violence significantly and independently of age and substance use (OR = 1.76 [95% CI = 1.11–2.79], $P < 0.05$).

Logistic regression was used to estimate the bivariate association between being violent towards others and violent victimization. The OR = 7.12 ($P \leq 0.001$) [69]. Patients with serious mental illness charged with a criminal offense were more likely (OR = 4.80 [95% CI = 3.71–6.20], $P \leq 0.001$) than patients who were nonoffenders ($n = 2,413$) to have a record of violent victimization and more likely (OR = 3.07 [95% CI = 2.55–3.69], $P \leq 0.001$) to have a record of nonviolent victimization, controlling for the effects of age, gender, and substance use disorders [70]. Thus, relationship between victimization and violent behavior by patients with serious mental illness has been established.

4.3.2. Dynamic Factors. These factors include psychotic symptoms, comorbid substance use disorders and psychopathy, lack of insight, and nonadherence to treatment. Some of these factors that are in close temporal proximity to a violent assault act as triggers. Immediate environmental provocation, intoxication, and current clinical symptoms play a role.

The environmental provocation can be real. A study using video recordings of interactions between psychiatric inpatients has revealed that threatening and intrusive behaviors in assailants and victims preceded 60% of assaults [71]. When psychiatric inpatients are asked by staff to do (or to stop doing) something, they may respond by assaulting the staff member. Such situation was in fact listed by staff members as the most frequent reason for assaults on a maximum security psychiatric unit [72]. However, the assaulters in the same study listed being teased or "bugged" as the most frequent reason. Some of this "bugging" may have been delusional.

Intoxication. As discussed repeatedly in previous sections, comorbid substance use disorders substantially elevate the risk of violence in individuals diagnosed with schizophrenia. Acute intoxication is one of the mechanisms for this effect. Binge drinking, the pattern of alcohol consumption that is most likely to lead to intoxication, was significantly related to violence in an analysis of the NESARC data mentioned earlier [23]. Recent alcohol misuse was moderately associated with violence in psychotic patients (OR = 2.2, 95% CI = 1.6–2.9) in a recent meta-analysis of risk factors for violence in psychosis [43].

Schizophrenic individuals who also abuse drugs may be particularly likely to become assaultive under the influence of alcohol [73]. Furthermore, the lifetime prevalence of comorbidity between schizophrenia and any substance use or dependence was estimated at 47.0% (OR = 4.6), and the analogous numbers for alcohol abuse or dependence were 33.7% (OR = 3.3) [74]. These data were determined from 20,291 interviews in the ECA study mentioned earlier in the section on prevalence. Thus, schizophrenia patients may be more vulnerable to acute alcohol effects and are more likely to abuse alcohol than members of the general population.

Current Clinical Symptoms. Current clinical psychotic symptoms play a role in the development of violent behavior in schizophrenia. As described in the preceding section, approximately 20% of assaults perpetrated by psychotic inpatients are attributable to positive psychotic symptoms [38]. Positive symptoms of schizophrenia were associated with an increased risk of violence, whereas negative symptoms showed the opposite relationship [8]. In a large metaregression study, the relation between positive symptoms and violence was very modest (OR = 1.2, 95% CI = 1.0–1.5), whereas negative symptoms had no effect on violence [43]. Command hallucinations to harm others may increase risk of violence, although the level of compliance with such commands varies [75, 76].

Mentally ill patients sometimes make threats to kill, and such threats need to be evaluated by clinicians. An Australian study addressed this problem [77]. A total of 613 individuals convicted of threats to kill had their prior contact with public mental health services established at the time of this offense. The group's subsequent criminal convictions were established 10 years later using the police database. Within 10 years, 44% of threateners were convicted of further violent offending, including 19 (3%) homicides. Those with histories of psychiatric contact (40%) had a higher rate (58%) of subsequent violence. Homicidal violence was most frequent among threateners with a schizophrenic illness. Sixteen threateners (2.6%) killed themselves, and three were murdered. Thus, this study revealed high rates of assault and even homicide following threats to kill [77].

A group of delusional psychotic symptoms—so-called threat/control-override (TCO) symptoms—was reported to lead to violence [78, 79]. These symptoms are elicited by questions like "dominated by forces beyond you," "thoughts put into your head," and "people who wished you harm".

An analysis of the data from the MacArthur violence risk assessment study [5] suggested that although delusions can precipitate violence in individual cases, they do not increase the overall risk of violence. An early analysis suggested that the threat/control-override symptoms were not associated with violent behavior in that study [80].

However, when the same MacArthur data set was reanalyzed using methods that considered the temporal proximity of the symptoms to violent events, the results indicated relationships between specific delusions and violence [81]. The delusions included being spied upon (OR = 1.62, 95% CI = 1.06–2.47, P = 0.027), being followed (OR = 1.90, 95% CI = 1.29–2.80, P = 0.001), being plotted against (OR = 1.70, 95% CI = 1.14–2.52, P = 0.009), being under control of person/force (OR = 1.92, 95% CI = 1.24–2.97, P = 0.003), thought insertion (OR = 1.63, 95% CI = 1.00–2.66, P = 0.048), and having special gifts/powers (OR = 1.95, 95% CI = 1.31–2.92, P = 0.001). All these delusions were associated with angry affect (P < 0.05). Inclusion of anger in the model significantly attenuated the main effects (except grandiose delusions), indicating an indirect pathway. Thus, temporal proximity is important when investigating relationships between delusions and violence. Anger due to delusions is the key factor in this pathway [81]. The importance of temporal proximity for research on causes of violence is now being increasingly accepted [23].

Similar findings were reported by the same group of investigators using data from the East London first episode psychosis study [42]. The participants were 458 patients with first episode psychosis who were 18 to 64 years of age. Patients were clinically assessed and interviewed about their overt violent behavior while experiencing psychotic symptoms during the 12-month period prior to interview. The prevalence of violence was 38% during the 12-month period, and 12% of the sample engaged in serious violence. Anger was the only affect due to delusions that was positively associated with violence. Three highly prevalent delusions demonstrated pathways to serious violence mediated by anger due to delusional beliefs: persecution, being spied on, and conspiracy. Thus, anger due to delusions is a key factor that explains the relationship between violence and acute psychosis [42].

Patients with first episode of psychosis who had a record of criminal convictions prior to contact with mental health services showed impaired performance on neuropsychological studies in comparison with their nonoffending patient counterparts. Offenders had significantly lower IQ scores than nonoffenders, both current and premorbid. The offenders were further distinguished by significantly poorer performance on the verbal learning and short-term verbal recall, visual recall memory, a measure of visual-spatial perception and organization, and three subtests of the WAIS, digit symbol, which assesses processing speed and vocabulary and comprehension, which index verbal intelligence [66].

Lack of Insight. A prospective study of 63 inpatients diagnosed with schizophrenia or schizoaffective disorder provided what was probably the first rigorous demonstration of the relationship between insight and violence [82]. Similar observations regarding the lack of insight into illness and into legal consequences of their illness were described in a sample of 115 violent patients with schizophrenia in a jail or court psychiatric clinic [83].

The German national crime register was searched for records of criminal offenses committed by 1662 patients with schizophrenia treated between 1990 and 1995 at a German hospital. Analyses were performed to determine predictors of later criminal behavior, and psychopathology was assessed. Sixty-two (3.7%) patients were convicted for physical injury offenses in the 7–12 years after discharge. Significantly higher rates of criminal conviction and recidivism were found for patients with lack of insight at discharge. Analyses also showed a significantly higher risk of nonviolent and violent crimes in patients with a hostility syndrome at admission and discharge. There was a significantly lower incidence of criminal behavior in subjects with a depressive syndrome [84].

In a study of pretrial detainees that was described in the segment on childhood maltreatment [60], impaired insight (lack of awareness of having a mental illness) was significantly related to the severity of reported violence, and that relationship was statistically independent of the effects of substance use, medication adherence, and childhood abuse. Schizophrenia patients without concomitant substance abuse or Axis II disorders ($N = 133$) were recruited for a Turkish study of violence [85]. History of violence, lower self-reflectiveness, worse insight, and delusion severity were significant predictors of violence in a comparison of 47 violent with 86 nonviolent patients.

In a study of 168 psychotic patients (86 with schizophrenia and 43 with bipolar disorder) in Spain, it was found that patients showing poor insight showed higher hostility and impaired impulse control; these variables were assessed as PANSS items [86]. The authors hypothesized that lack of insight was the primary problem, leading to increased hostility and impairment of impulse control. Lack of insight was moderately associated with violence in a large metaregression analysis (OR = 2.7, 95% CI = 1.4–5.2) [43].

However, a study of 209 schizophrenia patients has shown that while insight was associated with aggression in univariate analysis, the association was no longer significant after controlling for psychopathy scores and positive symptoms [87].

In summary, preponderance of evidence links violence in psychotic individuals to their impaired insight into mental illness. This effect may be indirect, mediated through the reduced adherence to treatment that is associated with poor insight.

Nonadherence to Treatment. Nonadherence to antipsychotic medication treatment is a major problem in treating schizophrenia. Less than 50% of schizophrenia patients are adherent to their medication [88, 89]. Nonadherence has been associated with symptom worsening, including aggressive behavior [90]. Non-adherence with medication was modestly associated with violence in a large metaregression study (OR = 2.0, 95% CI = 1.0–3.7) [43]. Somewhat surprisingly, the effect of non-adherence with psychological therapies on violence appeared considerably stronger (OR = 6.7, 95% CI = 2.4–19.2) [43]. It should be noted that only three studies of non-adherence to psychological therapies were used for the computation of the OR, whereas nine studies were used for medication non-adherence.

Comorbidity of alcohol or other drug abuse with poor adherence to medication further elevates the risk of violent behavior among persons with severe mental illness [91]. As discussed in the preceding section, impaired insight may lead to reduced adherence. Canadian researchers noted that

poor insight was one of the predictors of poor adherence to medication in a sample of 200 patients with first episode psychosis [92]. Furthermore, medication adverse effects such as parkinsonism, weight gain, and loss of libido may additionally reduce the patients' willingness to take medication [88].

While non-adherence to medication certainly elevates the risk for violence, hostility also appears to contribute to the development of non-adherence in patients with schizophrenia or schizoaffective disorder [11]. However, rising hostility may be the result of inadequate treatment or inadequate antipsychotic response, leading to patient's unwillingness to continue treatment.

Antisocial personality disorder/psychopathy is perhaps also affecting adherence to medication treatment. This is suggested by the fact that history of aggressive behavior, arrest, or incarceration was strongly related to non-adherence to treatment in a large prospective naturalistic study of schizophrenia patients [93].

In the CATIE study [25], higher levels of insight at baseline were significantly associated with lower levels of schizophrenia symptoms at followup, and more positive medication attitudes, which were in turn associated with better adherence with medication treatment [94].

Relationships between insight, hostility, and adherence were examined in a post hoc analysis of the data obtained in the European First Episode Schizophrenia Trial (EUFEST) [95]. EUFEST was a randomized, one-year open trial comparing the effectiveness of haloperidol, amisulpride, olanzapine, quetiapine, and ziprasidone in first episode schizophrenia, schizoaffective disorder, or schizophreniform disorder. The primary outcome measure was all-cause treatment discontinuation. Secondary measures included the PANSS and the Hayward scale [96], a measure of adherence.

The reanalysis investigated concurrent and predictive associations to determine whether medication adherence varies as a function of hostility and lack of insight [97]. Predictive association of hostility and lack of insight (assessed as PANSS items) with non-adherence to medication (Hayward scale) was statistically significant at one month of treatment (Figure 2).

Thus, non-adherence to treatment is of central importance among pathways to violence in schizophrenia. It is closely related to substance use disorder. Furthermore, impaired insight and probably increased hostility are among the symptoms that are impairing adherence. Also, comorbid antisocial features are linked with non-adherence.

4.4. Treatment of Violent Behavior in Schizophrenia

4.4.1. Atypical Antipsychotics. Atypical antipsychotics are currently the principal treatment of aggressive behavior in schizophrenia.

Aripiprazole was compared with placebo in five randomized, double-blind studies of patients with schizophrenia or schizoaffective disorder, and haloperidol was used as a comparator in three of these studies. A meta-analysis of these five studies showed that aripiprazole was significantly superior to placebo, but not to haloperidol, in reducing hostility [98].

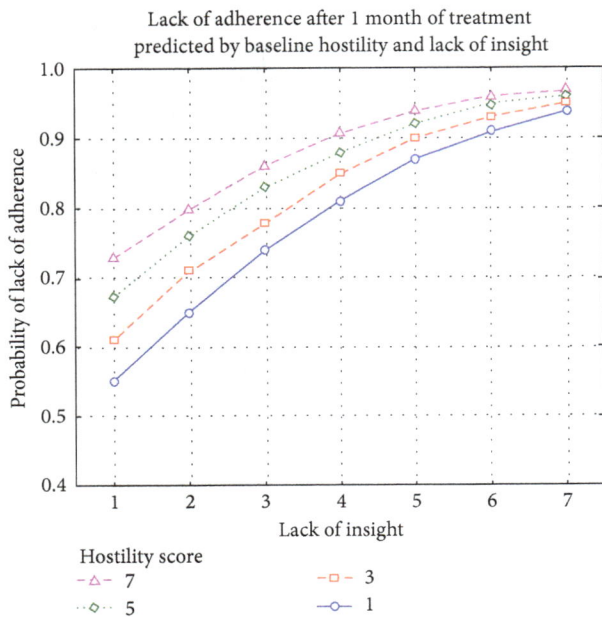

FIGURE 2: Lack of adherence after one month of treatment predicted by baseline hostility and lack of insight. Predictive relationship of hostility and lack of insight at baseline with medication adherence at 1 month of treatment in the study. Logistic regression analysis indicated that both predictor variables reached significance (hostility $P = 0.027$, lack of insight $P < 0.0001$). The figure illustrates the combined effect of the two predictors, that is, the probability of lack of full adherence at 1 month (any score of <7 on the Hayward scale) both as a function of lack of insight at baseline (*x*-axis) and hostility (*y*-axis strata depicting additive effects with increasing severity of hostility). Display and computations were provided by Pal Czobor, PhD, who used data collected in the EUFEST study [95, 97].

Clozapine is the most effective, evidence-based treatment for schizophrenia patients exhibiting violent behavior. The evidence for clozapine superiority in antiaggressive effects is based, in part, on randomized, double-blind, controlled trials. One trial compared clozapine, haloperidol, olanzapine, and risperidone in 157 treatment-resistant patients diagnosed with schizophrenia or schizoaffective disorder [99]. The scores on hostility item of the PANSS were used as the dependent variable in analyses that have demonstrated superior efficacy of clozapine in comparison with risperidone and haloperidol [100]. However, neither risperidone nor olanzapine was superior to haloperidol.

Further analyses of the same trial [99] examined incidents of overt physical aggression [101]. The results demonstrated superiority of clozapine over haloperidol, but this effect only became significant after 24 days of treatment when an effective dose of clozapine—around 500 mg/day—was reached. A principal limitation of this trial [99] was that the patients were not selected for being violent.

A more recent double-blind randomized controlled trial compared clozapine, olanzapine, and risperidone in 110 patients diagnosed with schizophrenia or schizoaffective disorder who *were* selected for being violent [102]. Efficacy of clozapine to reduce the number and severity of aggressive

incidents was superior to olanzapine, which was in turn superior to haloperidol.

Numerous observational studies and uncontrolled trials have indicated superior antiaggressive affectiveness of clozapine in psychotic patients [103–107]. These studies and similar literature are discussed elsewhere [108, 109].

Although its antiaggressive efficacy is firmly established [110, 111], clozapine is not appropriate or effective in all patients [112]. Perhaps as many as 50% of patients fail to respond to clozapine [113]. Patients whose aggressive behavior continues despite clozapine treatment are sometimes those with a history of conduct disorder and comorbid personality disorder [64, 114].

Furthermore, as mentioned above, clozapine is not fully effective during the dose escalation period [101]. The principal risk of clozapine is agranulocytosis which develops in approximately 1% of patients during the first three months of treatment [115]. This requires regular monitoring of white cell counts, which is one of the reasons why patients sometimes refuse or discontinue clozapine. Finally, some patients cannot receive or continue clozapine treatment for medical contraindications or adverse effects.

Olanzapine is effective against hostility [99] and overt physical aggression [102] in long-term schizophrenia patients. Olanzapine was less effective against aggression than clozapine [102]. In the CATIE study [25], its effects in reducing violence during the first 6 months of the study were not distinguishable from other atypical antipsychotics [116].

However, when the treatment effects on PANSS hostility item scores acquired during the 18-month Phase 1 of the CATIE study were analyzed, significant differences between treatments were discovered ($F_{4,1487} = 7.78$, $P < 0.0001$). Olanzapine was significantly superior to perphenazine and quetiapine at months 1, 3, 6, and 9. It was also significantly superior to ziprasidone at months 1, 3, and 6 and to risperidone at months 3 and 6 [117]. These results were similar to those obtained in the EUFEST study [95], where olanzapine was superior to haloperidol, quetiapine, and amisulpride in its effect against hostility [118].

Quetiapine reduced hostility and aggression in open studies [119, 120]. These observations were confirmed by post-hoc analyses of randomized double-blind trials demonstrating superior antiaggressive effect of quetiapine in comparison with placebo in schizophrenia patients [121]. In CATIE patients, quetiapine's antiaggressive effects were similar to other atypical antipsychotics, but they were weaker than those of perphenazine [116].

Risperidone showed superiority over placebo in reducing hostility in a post-hoc analysis of a randomized double-blind study [122]. Reduction of hostility and violent behavior was seen as an effect of risperidone in open studies of schizophrenia [123, 124]. Other comparisons of risperidone with various antipsychotics in randomized trials showed mostly no significant differences in antiaggressive effects [116].

Ziprasidone effects on hostility were studied using data from a randomized, open-label study comparing ziprasidone with haloperidol in schizophrenia and schizoaffective disorder [125]. Post-hoc analyses showed that both drugs reduced hostility; ziprasidone was superior to haloperidol only during the first week of the study [126]. Ziprasidone's antiaggressive effect was not significantly different from other antipsychotics in CATIE patients [116].

In summary, clozapine is the most effective antipsychotic in reducing hostility and aggression in patients diagnosed with schizophrenia or schizoaffective disorder. However, its use in clinical practice is limited by its adverse effects, particularly the risk of agranulocytosis. Olanzapine's effectiveness against hostility is inferior to clozapine, but superior to other antipsychotics. Other atypical antipsychotics are also effective, and there are apparently no major differences among them in terms of antiaggressive activity.

4.4.2. Other Medications. *Adrenergic beta-blockers* were demonstrated to possess antiaggressive properties [127–131], but cardiovascular adverse effects such as reduced blood pressure and pulse rate occurring at doses required for anti-aggressive effect have limited their clinical use for this indication. Beta-blockers have been supplanted by antipsychotics. Nevertheless, antipsychotics are not always effective and have adverse effects of their own. Therefore, efficacy of adjunctive beta-blockers in the treatment of persistently aggressive schizophrenia patients should be studied further.

Recently published meta-analyses indicating an association between the polymorphism of the catechol-o-methyl transferase (COMT) gene and violence in schizophrenia [52, 53] have pointed to a role of catecholamines in the pathogenesis of violence in schizophrenia. These meta-analyses may therefore rekindle future interest in influencing noradrenergic system as a potential treatment for violent behavior in schizophrenia.

Anticonvulsants are widely used for the adjunctive treatment of aggressive behavior in schizophrenia patients. However, empirical evidence supporting efficacy of this treatment is missing. Although it may perhaps be effective in individual patients, such treatment must be monitored, and it must be discontinued if it fails to show benefits or if adverse effects develop [132].

4.4.3. Nonpharmacological Treatment. Pharmacological treatment of aggressive behavior in schizophrenia has variable effectiveness. Etiological heterogeneity of this behavior (and probably of schizophrenia itself) plays a role in this variability of treatment response [133, 134]. As discussed above, history of conduct disorder and current comorbidity with antisocial personality disorder or psychopathy constitute alternative pathways to violence in schizophrenia [64]. Aggressive behavior in schizophrenia patients with these problems may not be directly caused by psychosis, and therefore it is less likely to respond to antipsychotics.

Non-adherence to treatment constitutes a crucially important limit to the effectiveness of pharmacological treatment. Non-adherence to pharmacological treatment and substance abuse elevate the risk of relapse and violence in schizophrenia [60, 134, 135].

Standard psychiatric treatment programs relying only on pharmacological approaches have therefore limited success in reducing recidivistic violent and criminal behaviors. Some

studies show that outpatient civil commitment may reduce violence in such cases [136].

Various cognitive behavioral treatment programs were developed for recidivistically violent and criminal patients. One such program has been operating at a state hospital providing treatment to the severely mentally ill in New York City. The cognitive skills training course is the principal component of the program. Substance abuse programs are included. The program has effects after discharge from the hospital: its graduates exhibit reduced rates of arrest and rehospitalization, as well as improved adherence to treatment [137]. Reports of similar programs operating elsewhere have been published [138, 139]. Programs of this type have a potential to break the revolving-door cycle of hospitalization-discharge-nonadherence to medication and drug abuse-relapse with violent behavior-arrest-jail-hospitalization, and so on. Developing more of these programs in the future could improve the lives of patients and their families and reduce the cost of management of the chronically ill and violent individuals.

Promising practices for psychosocial treatment of schizophrenia include cognitive adaptive therapy, cognitive behavioral therapy for posttraumatic stress disorder, first-episode psychosis intervention, healthy lifestyle interventions, integrated treatment for co-occurring disorders, peer support services, physical disease management, prodromal stage intervention, social cognition training, supported education, and supported housing [140].

5. Bipolar Disorder

5.1. Prevalence of Violent Behavior in Bipolar Disorder. Clinical observations indicated that the risk of violence is particularly high during acute manic episodes during hospitalization and immediately prior to it [141, 142].

Between 1990 and 1992, diagnoses and history of aggressive behavior during the preceding year were determined by interviews in a representative US sample for the national comorbidity survey [143]. Aggressive behavior or "trouble with the police or the law" was endorsed by 12.2% of individuals with the lifetime diagnosis of bipolar disorder, 8.2% with alcohol abuse, 10.9% with drug abuse, and 1.9% with no disorder. The analogous numbers for "last year" diagnoses were 16.0%, 9.1%, 19.8%, and 2.0% [143].

The NESARC study (described in the previous segment on schizophrenia) determined that the lifetime prevalence of aggressive behavior after age 15 was 0.66% in persons without lifetime psychiatric disorder, but 25.3% and 13.6% in bipolar disorders I and II, respectively. The odds ratios were 3.72 (2.94–4.70) and 1.77 (1.26–2.49). These numbers represent a mixture of bipolar disorders with or without comorbid diagnoses. The prevalence of aggressive behavior in pure bipolars I and II (without comorbidity) was, respectively, 2.52% and 5.12%. Comparable prevalence of aggressive behavior for pure alcohol dependence and drug dependence was, respectively, 7.22% and 11.32% [144]. High rates of comorbidity of bipolar disorder with alcohol dependence, drug dependence, paranoid personality disorder, and antisocial personality disorder were reported [145]. These comorbidities substantially increase the risk of violence.

A total of 3,743 individuals diagnosed with bipolar disorder were compared with 37,429 general population controls in a study using official Swedish records [146]. After the diagnosis, 9.5% of individuals with bipolar disorder committed violent crime compared with 629 general population controls (1.7%) (adjusted OR = 6.6, 95% CI = 5.8–7.6) [147]. Substance abuse comorbidity further increased the risk (adjusted OR = 19.9, 95% CI = 14.7–26.9). In patients without substance abuse comorbidity, there was still a significant risk increase (adjusted OR = 3.1, 95% CI = 2.6–3.8) [147].

Prevalence of criminal justice involvement during episodes of mania and contribution of manic symptoms to such involvement were the subject of additional analyses of NESARC data. Among the 1,044 respondents with bipolar I who experienced a manic episode, 13.0% reported legal involvement (being arrested or jailed) during the most severe manic episode [148]. Legal involvement was associated with symptoms of increased self-esteem and libido, high-risk pleasurable activities, more manic symptoms, and social and occupational impairment [148].

Prevalence of aggressive behavior was compared in a sample of 255 individuals with bipolar I and bipolar II disorder, 85 individuals with other psychopathology, and 84 healthy controls [149]. Lifetime aggression was assessed using a questionnaire that was administered by interviewers in the subjects' homes. Bipolar patients showed significantly higher scores on an aggression questionnaire than the other groups. Subjects who were currently psychotic showed significantly higher total aggression scores, hostility, and anger than those who were not. Patients experiencing a current mood episode showed significantly higher aggression scores than those not in a mood episode. This effect was independent of the severity of bipolar disorder and polarity of the episode [149].

In summary, the prevalence of violent behavior in bipolar disorder is comparable to the prevalence in schizophrenia; it may be even higher. The risk is increased during manic episodes. Similar to schizophrenia, comorbidity of bipolar disorder with substance use disorders further increases the risk. Although the problems caused by violent behavior of bipolar patients are not less important than those caused by similar behavior in schizophrenia, violence in bipolars has received considerably less research attention [150–152].

5.2. Risk Factors for Violence in Bipolar Disorder

5.2.1. Static Factors. Risk factors for aggression were examined in a sample of 100 consecutively evaluated patients with bipolar disorder [153]. The 32-item Brown-Goodwin Aggression scale (BGA) [154] was used to assess lifetime history of aggression. Age was significantly related to BGA scores ($r = -0.236$ and $P = 0.020$), indicating that younger patients were more aggressive. Gender had no significant relation to aggression.

History of *childhood trauma* was retrieved using the childhood trauma questionnaire which examines 5 types of maltreatment (physical abuse, physical neglect, emotional abuse, emotional neglect, and sexual abuse) [155]. The bivariate correlation coefficient between the BGA and the total score on the childhood trauma questionnaire was 0.325 ($P = 0.001$). When specific subtypes of childhood trauma were explored, physical abuse and emotional abuse were found to be significantly correlated with BGA.

Biological and psychological links between suicide and outward aggression have been intensively studied. Patients with bipolar disorder who had a *history of suicide attempt* scored higher on scales assessing hostility and lifetime history of aggression than those without such a history [156]. In a similar study of bipolar patients, suicide attempters scored significantly higher than nonattempters on a hostility scale [157], particularly on the subscale measuring overt physical aggression [158]. The attempters also showed higher level of impulsiveness. Furthermore, impulsiveness and hostility were correlated in the attempter subset.

5.2.2. Dynamic Factors. Comorbidities of bipolar disorder with other disorders are frequent, and some of them substantially elevate the risk of violence. A study of 983 bipolar patients showed that the prevalence of comorbidity between bipolar disorder and alcohol abuse/dependence ranged between 31.9% and 47.3%; drug abuse/dependence abuse range was 15.1%–34.2%, depending on age of onset [159]. Early onset was associated with higher risk of comorbidity. Other studies yield a range of 17%–64% for substance abuse comorbidity with bipolar disorder [160].

The impact of alcohol abuse on symptoms was assessed in patients with bipolar mania with and without current alcohol abuse [161]. The comorbid group showed higher levels of impulsivity and aggressive behavior. In general, the evidence for the role of substance use disorders in the pathophysiology of aggression in the mentally ill is robust [91, 147], even though much of the aggression in this population is attributable to other factors as well [162].

As mentioned in the preceding section on prevalence, comorbidity of bipolar disorder with antisocial personality disorder was demonstrated in the NESARC sample [145]. It was also observed in forensic facilities and prisons [163] and described in case reports [164]. This comorbidity would be expected to elevate the risk of aggression since the diagnosis of antisocial personality disorder is partly defined by it.

Bipolar disorder and borderline personality disorder share several clinical features, such as affective lability, impulsiveness, and aggressiveness. These and other shared features have led to discussions debating whether borderline personality disorder should belong to the bipolar spectrum. These disorders co-occur, and there are overlaps as well as important differences in phenomenology and in medication response. A detailed discussion of the relationship between these two disorders and its impact on the risk of violence in psychotic patients can be found elsewhere [114].

Comorbidity with borderline personality disorder elevates risk of aggression while it is also associated with higher impulsiveness in patients with bipolar disorder [165]. This is consistent with the fact that impulsive aggression is a core component of borderline personality disorder [166].

In the study of 100 bipolar patients reviewed above [153], comorbid substance use disorder, posttraumatic stress disorder, borderline personality disorder, and antisocial personality disorder were all found to be associated with elevated BGA scores in bivariate analyses.

In a stepwise multiple regression, after iterative entries it was found that the combination of three variables provided the best-fit model for the data: diagnosis of borderline personality disorder, total score on the Hamilton depression rating scale [167], and total score on the Young mania rating scale [168]. The model significantly predicted the BGA scores [$F(3, 91) 1/4 21.763, P < 0.001$]. The sample multiple correlation coefficient (r) was 0.646, indicating that approximately 41.8% of the variance of the aggression score in the sample could be accounted for by the linear combination of these three predictors.

Similar to schizophrenia, bipolar disorder is associated with *poor insight* [169]. The predictive effect of insight on clinical outcomes was investigated in a 2-year prospective study of 65 remitted bipolar I disorder patients [170] who were administered the schedule of assessment of insight [171] to assess baseline insight and then received follow-up assessments during subsequent 2 years. Impaired insight into treatment significantly increased the risk of adverse clinical outcomes with bipolar disorder in the 2-year period. The most frequent adverse outcome observed was occurrence of violent behavior. This observation is consistent with the literature on aggression in bipolar disorder. This finding is consistent with the literature on aggression in bipolar disorder [150]. Thus, impaired insight may be one of the mechanisms that raise the risk of violence in bipolar disorder.

Finally, *executive dysfunction* predicted aggressive behavior among psychiatric inpatients with various diagnoses, including bipolar disorder [172]. Stable and euthymic bipolar patients performed significantly worse than controls on neuropsychological tests of executive function and showed an impairment of inhibition [173]. Thus, stable and remitted euthymic bipolar patients have distinct impairments of executive function, verbal memory, psychomotor speed, and sustained attention [174]. It is possible that some of these dysfunctions, perhaps present as traits, predispose bipolar patients to aggressive behavior. These neuropsychological impairments, plus the elevated trait hostility and impulsivity mentioned before, may form a diathesis that predisposes some bipolar patients to respond by aggression to the experience of stress. A manic episode would be a typical stressful experience of these patients, but other stresses that may occur during remissions can have a similar effect.

5.3. Treatment of Violent Behavior in Bipolar Disorder

5.3.1. Treatment of Agitation in Acute Manic Episode.
Acute agitation is common in manic episodes. Staff training in the management of agitated patients is important, since their intervention may prevent an escalation of agitation into violence. The first interventions include removing the nonagitated patients from the room, having several staff members available to assist, and encouraging the patient to talk about his\her needs and concerns. Prompt use of sedating or calming agents is important [108].

Benzodiazepines are frequently administered. They are particularly useful in patients who are in withdrawal from alcohol or sedatives. *Lorazepam* is a benzodiazepine that is typically used as injections for nonspecific treatment of agitation since it is reliably absorbed intramuscularly. Its half-life ranges between 10 and 20 hours; usual dose is 0.5–2.0 mg every 1–6 hours. It has no active metabolites. Respiratory depression is a potential adverse effect. Similar to other benzodiazepines, lorazepam has a potential for developing tolerance and dependence. It is therefore not recommended for long-term use.

Antipsychotics. First-generation antipsychotics, mostly haloperidol, have been used to treat agitated behavior in acute mania. These agents are associated with extrapyramidal adverse effects, including acute dystonia and akathisia. These extrapyramidal symptoms are difficult to tolerate. Akathisia can be confused by the staff with underlying agitation; if that happens, it may be erroneously concluded that the dose of haloperidol is too low to be effective. Raising the dose under these conditions is a major error; it will make akathisia worse. Adverse effects of haloperidol can be mitigated by the administration of promethazine [175].

Short-acting intramuscular formulations of atypical antipsychotics aripiprazole, olanzapine, and ziprasidone are available to treat acute agitation. The effects for the reduction of agitation are similar to that observed for haloperidol or lorazepam [176]. These atypical antipsychotics have lower propensity for extrapyramidal adverse effects, which is an advantage in comparison with haloperidol. A recent unpublished randomized double-blind placebo-controlled trial suggests that sublingual tablets of another atypical antipsychotic, asenapine, can be used for treatment of acutely agitated patients [177].

Loxapine, a typical antipsychotic, has recently become available in an inhalation form. The drug is delivered using a device that produces an aerosol, resulting in rapid delivery into the lung and then into the systemic circulation [178, 179]. Inhaled loxapine was demonstrated to be a rapid, well-tolerated treatment for agitation in patients with bipolar I disorder [180].

5.3.2. Long-Term Treatment of Violent Behavior in Bipolar Disorder.
Typical symptoms of mania include aggression and irritability. Thus, the treatment of the underlying manic episode should reduce or eliminate the concurrent aggressive behavior. Long-term antiaggressive pharmacological treatment of manic patients is therefore implied in the general management of bipolar disorder. Such general information is not in the scope of this review. General guidelines for the pharmacological treatment of bipolar disorder are available [181–183].

Nonpharmacological management of bipolar disorder frequently uses cognitive behavioral therapy (CBT) that can address many aspects of bipolar disorder elevating the risk of aggression, including comorbid personality disorders and substance use disorders as well as treatment nonadherence. A randomized controlled study of CBT in bipolar patients addressed treatment adherence [184]. The patients who received six CBT sessions showed better adherence to medication, better insight, and fewer hospitalizations than a control group. The use of CBT in bipolar disorder has been manualized [185]. Parts of the manuals are directed at treatment adherence and substance use.

Family members are the most likely victims of assaults by psychotic patients. Psychoeducational programs for the patients' families focus on information about the illness, lack of skills in conflict resolution, and communication problems in the family [186].

6. Conclusions

Most patients with schizophrenia and bipolar disorder are not violent. Nevertheless, the risk of violence in patients with these disorders is greater than in general population. This represents a major public health problem and contributes to the stigma of mental illness. The risk of violence is further increased if schizophrenia or bipolar disorder patients concurrently suffer with substance use disorders and personality disorders, but it exists even without such comorbidities. Pharmacological treatments, particularly clozapine, are the principal tools for the long-term management of violence in schizophrenia. However, the effectiveness of pharmacotherapy is limited due to treatment resistance, treatment nonadherence, adverse effects, and the fact that some violent behavior in patients diagnosed with schizophrenia or bipolar disorder is not directly caused by psychosis. Comorbidities are frequently implicated in violent behavior of psychotic patients, and the detection and treatment of comorbidities, particularly substance abuse, are therefore of primary importance. Psychosocial treatments are necessary components of the management of violence in psychosis.

Conflict of Interests

The author declares that there is no conflict of interests regarding the publication of this paper.

References

[1] J. Volavka, *Neurobiology of Violence*, American Psychiatric Publishing, Washington, DC, USA, 2nd edition, 2002.

[2] S. C. Yudofsky, J. M. Silver, W. Jackson, J. Endicott, and D. Williams, "The overt aggression scale for the objective rating of verbal and physical aggression," *The American Journal of Psychiatry*, vol. 143, no. 1, pp. 35–39, 1986.

[3] S. R. Kay, F. Wolkenfeld, and L. M. Murrill, "Profiles of aggression among psychiatric patients—I. Nature and prevalence," *The Journal of Nervous and Mental Disease*, vol. 176, no. 9, pp. 539–546, 1988.

[4] D. W. Knoedler, "The modified overt aggression scale," *The American Journal of Psychiatry*, vol. 146, no. 8, pp. 1081–1082, 1989.

[5] H. J. Steadman, E. P. Mulvey, J. Monahan et al., "Violence by people discharged from acute psychiatric inpatient facilities and by others in the same neighborhoods," *Archives of General Psychiatry*, vol. 55, no. 5, pp. 393–401, 1998.

[6] J. W. Swanson, M. S. Swartz, and E. B. Elbogen, "Effectiveness of atypical antipsychotic medications in reducing violent behavior among persons with schizophrenia in community-based treatment," *Schizophrenia Bulletin*, vol. 30, no. 1, pp. 3–20, 2004.

[7] J. W. Swanson, M. S. Swartz, E. B. Elbogen, and R. A. van Dorn, "Reducing violence risk in persons with schizophrenia: olanzapine versus risperidone," *The Journal of Clinical Psychiatry*, vol. 65, no. 12, pp. 1666–1673, 2004.

[8] J. W. Swanson, M. S. Swartz, R. A. van Dorn et al., "A national study of violent behavior in persons with schizophrenia," *Archives of General Psychiatry*, vol. 63, no. 5, pp. 490–499, 2006.

[9] S. R. Kay, L. A. Opler, and J.-P. Lindenmayer, "The positive and negative syndrome scale (PANSS): rationale and standardisation," *The British Journal of Psychiatry*, vol. 155, no. 7, pp. 59–65, 1989.

[10] W. Guy, *ECDEU Assessment Manual for Psychopharmacology*, National Institute of Mental Health, Rockville, Md, USA, 1986.

[11] J.-P. Lindenmayer, H. Liu-Seifert, P. M. Kulkarni et al., "Medication nonadherence and treatment outcome in patients with schizophrenia or schizoaffective disorder with suboptimal prior response," *The Journal of Clinical Psychiatry*, vol. 70, no. 7, pp. 990–996, 2009.

[12] R. D. Hare, *The Hare Psychopathy Checklist-Revised (PCL-R)*, Multi-Health Systems, Toronto, Canada, 2003.

[13] A. Tengström, M. Grann, N. Långström, and G. Kullgren, "Psychopathy (PCL-R) as a predictor of violent recidivism among criminal offenders with schizophrenia," *Law and Human Behavior*, vol. 24, no. 1, pp. 45–58, 2000.

[14] S. D. Hart, R. D. Hare, and A. E. Forth, "Psychopathy as a risk marker for violence: development and validation of a screening version of the revised psychopathy checklist," in *Violence and Mental Disorder: Developments in Risk Assessment*, J. Monahan and H. J. Steadman, Eds., pp. 81–98, The University of Chicago Press, Chicago, Ill, USA, 1994.

[15] American Psychiatric Association, *Diagnostic and Statistical Manual of Mental Disorders*, American Psychiatric Association, Arlington, Va, USA, 5th edition, 2013.

[16] D. A. Regier, J. H. Boyd, J. D. Burke Jr. et al., "One-month prevalence of mental disorders in the United States, based on five epidemiologic catchment area sites," *Archives of General Psychiatry*, vol. 45, no. 11, pp. 977–986, 1988.

[17] D. A. Regier, J. K. Myers, M. Kramer et al., "The NIMH epidemiologic catchment area program. Historical context, major objectives, and study population characteristics," *Archives of General Psychiatry*, vol. 41, pp. 934–941, 1984.

[18] J. W. Swanson, C. E. Holzer III, V. K. Ganju, and R. T. Jono, "Violence and psychiatric disorder in the community: evidence from the epidemiologic catchment area surveys," *Hospital and Community Psychiatry*, vol. 41, no. 7, pp. 761–770, 1990.

[19] J. W. Swanson, "Mental disorder, substance abuse, and community violence: an epidemiological approach," in *Violence and Mental Disorder: Developments in Risk Assessment*, J. Monahan and H. J. Steadman, Eds., pp. 101–136, The University of Chicago Press, Chicago, Ill, USA, 1994.

[20] S. Fazel, N. Langstrom, A. Hjern, M. Grann, and P. Lichtenstein, "Schizophrenia, substance abuse, and violent crime," *The Journal of the American Medical Association*, vol. 301, no. 19, pp. 2016–2023, 2009.

[21] S. Fazel, G. Gulati, L. Linsell, J. R. Geddes, and M. Grann, "Schizophrenia and violence: systematic review and meta-analysis," *PLoS Medicine*, vol. 6, no. 8, Article ID e1000120, 2009.

[22] E. B. Elbogen and S. C. Johnson, "The intricate link between violence and mental disorder: results from the national epidemiologic survey on alcohol and related conditions," *Archives of General Psychiatry*, vol. 66, no. 2, pp. 152–161, 2009.

[23] R. van Dorn, J. Volavka, and N. Johnson, "Mental disorder and violence: is there a relationship beyond substance use?" *Social Psychiatry and Psychiatric Epidemiology*, vol. 47, no. 3, pp. 487–503, 2011.

[24] P. Czobor, J. Volavka, H. J. Steadman et al., "Violence in the mentally ill: questions remain," *Archives of General Psychiatry*, vol. 56, no. 2, pp. 193–194, 1999.

[25] J. A. Lieberman, S. T. Stroup, J. P. McEvoy et al., "Effectiveness of antipsychotic drugs in patients with chronic schizophrenia," *The New England Journal of Medicine*, vol. 353, no. 12, pp. 1209–1223, 2005.

[26] M. Eronen, P. Hakola, and J. Tiihonen, "Mental disorders and homicidal behavior in Finland," *Archives of General Psychiatry*, vol. 53, no. 6, pp. 497–501, 1996.

[27] H. Schanda, G. Knecht, D. Schreinze, T. Stompe, G. Ortwein-Swoboda, and T. Waldhoer, "Homicide and major mental disorders: a 25-year study," *Acta Psychiatrica Scandinavica*, vol. 110, no. 2, pp. 98–107, 2004.

[28] S. Fazel and M. Grann, "Psychiatric morbidity among homicide offenders: a Swedish population study," *The American Journal of Psychiatry*, vol. 161, no. 11, pp. 2129–2131, 2004.

[29] O. Nielssen and M. Large, "Rates of homicide during the first episode of psychosis and after treatment: a systematic review and meta-analysis," *Schizophrenia Bulletin*, vol. 36, no. 4, pp. 702–712, 2010.

[30] M. J. Hoptman, K. F. Yates, M. B. Patalinjug, R. C. Wack, and A. Convit, "Clinical prediction of assaultive behavior among male psychiatric patients at a maximum-security forensic facility," *Psychiatric Services*, vol. 50, no. 11, pp. 1461–1466, 1999.

[31] R. B. Flannery, A. Staffieri, S. Hildum, and A. P. Walker, "The violence triad and common single precipitants to psychiatric patient assaults on staff: 16-Year analysis of the assaulted staff action program," *Psychiatric Quarterly*, vol. 82, no. 2, pp. 85–93, 2011.

[32] R. D. Hare and L. M. McPherson, "Violent and aggressive behavior by criminal psychopaths," *International Journal of Law and Psychiatry*, vol. 7, no. 1, pp. 35–50, 1984.

[33] A.-M. R. Leistico, R. T. Salekin, J. DeCoster, and R. Rogers, "A large-scale meta-analysis relating the hare measures of psychopathy to antisocial conduct," *Law and Human Behavior*, vol. 32, no. 1, pp. 28–45, 2008.

[34] G. D. Walters, R. A. Knight, M. Grann, and K.-P. Dahle, "Incremental validity of the psychopathy checklist facet scores: predicting release outcome in six samples," *Journal of Abnormal Psychology*, vol. 117, no. 2, pp. 396–405, 2008.

[35] K. A. Nolan, J. Volavka, P. Mohr, and P. Czobor, "Psychopathy and violent behavior among patients with schizophrenia or schizoaffective disorder," *Psychiatric Services*, vol. 50, no. 6, pp. 787–792, 1999.

[36] T. Laajasalo, S. Salenius, N. Lindberg, E. Repo-Tiihonen, and H. Häkkänen-Nyholm, "Psychopathic traits in Finnish homicide offenders with schizophrenia," *International Journal of Law and Psychiatry*, vol. 34, no. 5, pp. 324–330, 2011.

[37] K. McGregor, D. Castle, and M. Dolan, "Schizophrenia spectrum disorders, substance misuse, and the four-facet model of psychopathy: the relationship to violence," *Schizophrenia Research*, vol. 136, no. 1–3, pp. 116–121, 2012.

[38] K. A. Nolan, P. Czobor, B. B. Roy et al., "Characteristics of assaultive behavior among psychiatric inpatients," *Psychiatric Services*, vol. 54, no. 7, pp. 1012–1016, 2003.

[39] R. S. Fullam and M. C. Dolan, "Executive function and inpatient violence in forensic patients with schizophrenia," *The British Journal of Psychiatry*, vol. 193, no. 3, pp. 247–253, 2008.

[40] P. Moran and S. Hodgins, "The correlates of comorbid antisocial personality disorder in schizophrenia," *Schizophrenia Bulletin*, vol. 30, no. 4, pp. 791–802, 2004.

[41] B. Schiffer, N. Leygraf, B. W. Muller et al., "Structural brain alterations associated with schizophrenia preceded by conduct disorder: a common and distinct subtype of schizophrenia?" *Schizophrenia Bulletin*, vol. 39, no. 5, pp. 1115–1128, 2012.

[42] J. W. Coid, S. Ullrich, C. Kallis et al., "The relationship between delusions and violence: findings from the east London first episode psychosis study," *Journal of the American Medical Association Psychiatry*, vol. 70, no. 5, pp. 465–471, 2013.

[43] K. Witt, R. van Dorn, and S. Fazel, "Risk factors for violence in psychosis: systematic review and meta-regression analysis of 110 studies," *PLoS ONE*, vol. 8, no. 2, Article ID e55942, 2013.

[44] E. F. Coccaro, C. S. Bergeman, R. J. Kavoussi, and A. D. Seroczynski, "Heritability of aggression and irritability: a twin study of the Buss-Durkee aggression scales in adult male subjects," *Biological Psychiatry*, vol. 41, no. 3, pp. 273–284, 1997.

[45] S. Comai, M. Tau, and G. Gobbi, "The psychopharmacology of aggressive behavior: a translational approach—part 1: neurobiology," *Journal of Clinical Psychopharmacology*, vol. 32, no. 1, pp. 83–94, 2012.

[46] E. R. Allan, M. Alpert, C. E. Sison, L. Citrome, G. Laury, and I. Berman, "Adjunctive nadolol in the treatment of acutely aggressive schizophrenic patients," *The Journal of Clinical Psychiatry*, vol. 57, no. 10, pp. 455–459, 1996.

[47] J. M. Silver, S. C. Yudofsky, J. A. Slater et al., "Propranolol treatment of chronically hospitalized aggressive patients," *The Journal of Neuropsychiatry & Clinical Neurosciences*, vol. 11, no. 3, pp. 328–335, 1999.

[48] J. A. Gogos, M. Morgan, V. Luine et al., "Catechol-O-methyltransferase-deficient mice exhibit sexually dimorphic changes in catecholamine levels and behavior," *Proceedings of the National Academy of Sciences of the United States of America*, vol. 95, no. 17, pp. 9991–9996, 1998.

[49] C. Fernandes, J. L. Paya-Cano, F. Sluyter, U. D'Souza, R. Plomin, and L. C. Schalkwyk, "Hippocampal gene expression profiling across eight mouse inbred strains: towards understanding the molecular basis for behaviour," *European Journal of Neuroscience*, vol. 19, no. 9, pp. 2576–2582, 2004.

[50] H. M. Lachman, K. A. Nolan, P. Mohr, T. Saito, and J. Volavka, "Association between catechol O-methyltransferase genotype and violence in schizophrenia and schizoaffective disorder," *The American Journal of Psychiatry*, vol. 155, no. 6, pp. 835–837, 1998.

[51] R. D. Strous, N. Bark, S. S. Parsia, J. Volavka, and H. M. Lachman, "Analysis of a functional catechol-O-methyltransferase gene polymorphism in schizophrenia: evidence for association with aggressive and antisocial behavior," *Psychiatry Research*, vol. 69, no. 2-3, pp. 71–77, 1997.

[52] J. P. Singh, J. Volavka, P. Czobor, and R. A. van Dorn, "A meta-analysis of the Val158Met COMT polymorphism and violent behavior in schizophrenia," *PLoS ONE*, vol. 7, no. 8, Article ID e43423, 2012.

[53] S. G. Bhakta, J. P. Zhang, and A. K. Malhotra, "The COMT Met158 allele and violence in schizophrenia: a meta-analysis," *Schizophrenia Research*, vol. 140, no. 1–3, pp. 192–197, 2012.

[54] C. S. Widom, "The cycle of violence," *Science*, vol. 244, no. 4901, pp. 160–166, 1989.

[55] A. Caspi, J. McCray, T. E. Moffitt et al., "Role of genotype in the cycle of violence in maltreated children," *Science*, vol. 297, no. 5582, pp. 851–854, 2002.

[56] C. S. Widom and L. M. Brzustowicz, "MAOA and the "cycle of violence:" childhood abuse and neglect, MAOA genotype, and risk for violent and antisocial behavior," *Biological Psychiatry*, vol. 60, no. 7, pp. 684–689, 2006.

[57] T. C. Silva, P. Larm, F. Vitaro, R. E. Tremblay, and S. Hodgins, "The association between maltreatment in childhood and criminal convictions to age 24: a prospective study of a community sample of males from disadvantaged neighbourhoods," *European Child & Adolescent Psychiatry*, vol. 21, no. 7, pp. 403–413, 2012.

[58] N. J. Kolla, C. Malcolm, S. Attard, T. Arenovich, N. Blackwood, and S. Hodgins, "Childhood maltreatment and aggressive behaviour in violent offenders with psychopathy," *Canadian Journal of Psychiatry*, vol. 58, no. 8, pp. 487–494, 2013.

[59] K. L. McCabe, E. A. Maloney, H. J. Stain, C. M. Loughland, and V. J. Carr, "Relationship between childhood adversity and clinical and cognitive features in schizophrenia," *Journal of Psychiatric Research*, vol. 46, no. 5, pp. 600–607, 2012.

[60] N. Alia-Klein, T. M. O'Rourke, R. Z. Goldstein, and D. Malaspina, "Insight into illness and adherence to psychotropic medications are separately associated with violence severity in a forensic sample," *Aggressive Behavior*, vol. 33, no. 1, pp. 86–96, 2007.

[61] M. Bennouna-Greene, V. Bennouna-Greene, F. Berna, and L. Defranoux, "History of abuse and neglect in patients with schizophrenia who have a history of violence," *Child Abuse & Neglect*, vol. 35, no. 5, pp. 329–332, 2011.

[62] S. Hodgins, J. Tiihonen, and D. Ross, "The consequences of conduct disorder for males who develop schizophrenia: associations with criminality, aggressive behavior, substance use, and psychiatric services," *Schizophrenia Research*, vol. 78, no. 2-3, pp. 323–335, 2005.

[63] S. Hodgins, "Parental violent crime, previous violence and substance abuse predict future violence in people with schizophrenia," *Evidence-Based Mental Health*, vol. 12, no. 4, article 127, 2009.

[64] J. W. Swanson, R. A. van Dorn, M. S. Swartz, A. Smith, E. B. Elbogen, and J. Monahan, "Alternative pathways to violence in persons with schizophrenia: the role of childhood antisocial behavior problems," *Law and Human Behavior*, vol. 32, no. 3, pp. 228–240, 2008.

[65] C. Wallace, P. E. Mullen, and P. Burgess, "Criminal offending in schizophrenia over a 25-year period marked by deinstitutionalization and increasing prevalence of comorbid substance use disorders," *The American Journal of Psychiatry*, vol. 161, no. 4, pp. 716–727, 2004.

[66] S. Hodgins, M. Calem, R. Shimel et al., "Criminal offending and distinguishing features of offenders among persons experiencing a first episode of psychosis," *Early Intervention in Psychiatry*, vol. 5, no. 1, pp. 15–23, 2011.

[67] J. A. Lam and R. Rosenheck, "The effect of victimization on clinical outcomes of homeless persons with serious mental illness," *Psychiatric Services*, vol. 49, no. 5, pp. 678–683, 1998.

[68] V. A. Hiday, J. W. Swanson, M. S. Swartz, R. Borum, and H. R. Wagner, "Victimization: a link between mental illness and violence?" *International Journal of Law and Psychiatry*, vol. 24, no. 6, pp. 559–572, 2001.

[69] E. Silver, "Mental disorder and violent victimization: the mediating role of involvement in conflicted social relationships," *Criminology*, vol. 40, no. 1, pp. 191–212, 2002.

[70] T. B. Short, S. Thomas, S. Luebbers, P. Mullen, and J. R. Ogloff, "A case-linkage study of crime victimisation in schizophrenia-spectrum disorders over a period of deinstitutionalisation," *BMC Psychiatry*, vol. 13, article 66, 2013.

[71] M. L. Crowner, G. Peric, F. Stepcic, and S. Lee, "Assailant and victim behaviors immediately preceding inpatient assault," *Psychiatric Quarterly*, vol. 76, no. 3, pp. 243–256, 2005.

[72] G. T. Harris and G. W. Varney, "A ten-year study of assaults and assaulters on a maximum security psychiatric unit," *Journal of Interpersonal Violence*, vol. 1, no. 2, pp. 173–191, 1986.

[73] J. A. Yesavage and V. Zarcone, "History of drug abuse and dangerous behavior in inpatient schizophrenics," *The Journal of Clinical Psychiatry*, vol. 44, no. 7, pp. 259–261, 1983.

[74] D. A. Regier, M. E. Farmer, D. S. Rae et al., "Comorbidity of mental disorders with alcohol and other drug abuse. Results from the epidemiologic catchment area (ECA) study," *The Journal of the American Medical Association*, vol. 264, no. 19, pp. 2511–2518, 1990.

[75] J. Junginger, "Command hallucinations and the prediction of dangerousness," *Psychiatric Services*, vol. 46, no. 9, pp. 911–914, 1995.

[76] J. Junginger, L. McGuire, D. E. McNiel, J. P. Eisner, and R. L. Binder, "The paradox of command hallucinations," *Psychiatric Services*, vol. 52, no. 3, article 385, 2001.

[77] L. J. Warren, P. E. Mullen, S. D. M. Thomas, J. R. P. Ogloff, and P. M. Burgess, "Threats to kill: a follow-up study," *Psychological Medicine*, vol. 38, no. 4, pp. 599–605, 2008.

[78] B. G. Link and A. Stueve, "Psychotic symptoms and the violent/illegal behavior of mental patients compared to community controls," in *Violence and Mental Disorder: Developments in Risk Assessment*, J. Monahan and H. J. Steadman, Eds., pp. 137–159, The University of Chicago Press, Chicago, Ill, USA, 1994.

[79] B. G. Link, A. Stueve, and J. Phelan, "Psychotic symptoms and violent behaviors: probing the components of "threat/control-override" symptoms," *Social Psychiatry and Psychiatric Epidemiology*, vol. 33, no. 1, supplement, pp. S55–S60, 1998.

[80] P. S. Appelbaum, P. C. Robbins, and J. Monahan, "Violence and delusions: data from the MacArthur violence risk assessment study," *The American Journal of Psychiatry*, vol. 157, no. 4, pp. 566–572, 2000.

[81] S. Ullrich, R. Keers, and J. W. Coid, "Delusions, anger, and serious violence: new findings from the MacArthur violence risk assessment study," *Schizophrenia Bulletin*, 2013.

[82] C. Arango, A. C. Barba, T. González-Salvador, and A. C. Ordóñez, "Violence in inpatients with schizophrenia: a prospective study," *Schizophrenia Bulletin*, vol. 25, no. 3, pp. 493–503, 1999.

[83] P. F. Buckley, D. R. Hrouda, L. Friedman, S. G. Noffsinger, P. J. Resnick, and K. Camlin-Shingler, "Insight and its relationship to violent behavior in patients with schizophrenia," *The American Journal of Psychiatry*, vol. 161, no. 9, pp. 1712–1714, 2004.

[84] M. Soyka, C. Graz, R. Bottlender, P. Dirschedl, and H. Schoech, "Clinical correlates of later violence and criminal offences in schizophrenia," *Schizophrenia Research*, vol. 94, no. 1-3, pp. 89–98, 2007.

[85] O. Ekinci and A. Ekinci, "Association between insight, cognitive insight, positive symptoms and violence in patients with schizophrenia," *Nordic Journal of Psychiatry*, vol. 67, no. 2, pp. 116–123, 2013.

[86] G. L. Calatayud, N. H. Sebastián, E. A. García-Iturrospe, J. C. G. Piqueras, J. S. Arias, and C. L. Cercós, "Relationship between insight, violence and diagnoses in psychotic patients," *Revista de Psiquiatria y Salud Mental*, vol. 5, no. 1, pp. 43–47, 2012.

[87] T. M. Lincoln and S. Hodgins, "Is lack of insight associated with physically aggressive behavior among people with schizophrenia living in the community?" *The Journal of Nervous and Mental Disease*, vol. 196, no. 1, pp. 62–66, 2008.

[88] D. I. Velligan, P. J. Weiden, M. Sajatovic et al., "The expert consensus guideline series: adherence problems in patients with serious and persistent mental illness," *The Journal of Clinical Psychiatry*, vol. 70, supplement 4, pp. 1–46, 2009.

[89] A. Berger, J. Edelsberg, K. N. Sanders, J. M. Alvir, M. A. Mychaskiw, and G. Oster, "Medication adherence and utilization in patients with schizophrenia or bipolar disorder receiving aripiprazole, quetiapine, or ziprasidone at hospital discharge: a retrospective cohort study," *BMC Psychiatry*, vol. 12, no. 1, article 99, 2012.

[90] H. Ascher-Svanum, D. E. Faries, B. Zhu, F. R. Ernst, M. S. Swartz, and J. W. Swanson, "Medication adherence and long-term functional outcomes in the treatment of schizophrenia in usual care," *The Journal of Clinical Psychiatry*, vol. 67, no. 3, pp. 453–460, 2006.

[91] M. S. Swartz, J. W. Swanson, V. A. Hiday, R. Borum, H. Ryan Wagner, and B. J. Burns, "Violence and severe mental illness: the effects of substance abuse and nonadherence to medication," *The American Journal of Psychiatry*, vol. 155, no. 2, pp. 226–231, 1998.

[92] E. L. Coldham, J. Addington, and D. Addington, "Medication adherence of individuals with a first episode of psychosis," *Acta Psychiatrica Scandinavica*, vol. 106, no. 4, pp. 286–290, 2002.

[93] H. Ascher-Svanum, B. Zhu, D. Faries, J. P. Lacro, and C. R. Dolder, "A prospective study of risk factors for nonadherence with antipsychotic medication in the treatment of schizophrenia," *The Journal of Clinical Psychiatry*, vol. 67, no. 7, pp. 1114–1123, 2006.

[94] S. Mohamed, R. Rosenheck, J. McEvoy, M. Swartz, S. Stroup, and J. A. Lieberman, "Cross-sectional and longitudinal relationships between insight and attitudes toward medication and clinical outcomes in chronic schizophrenia," *Schizophrenia Bulletin*, vol. 35, no. 2, pp. 336–346, 2009.

[95] R. S. Kahn, W. W. Fleischhacker, H. Boter et al., "Effectiveness of antipsychotic drugs in first-episode schizophrenia and schizophreniform disorder: an open randomised clinical trial," *The Lancet*, vol. 371, no. 9618, pp. 1085–1097, 2008.

[96] R. Kemp, P. Hayward, G. Applewhaite, B. Everitt, and A. David, "Compliance therapy in psychotic patients: randomised controlled trial," *British Medical Journal*, vol. 312, no. 7027, pp. 345–349, 1996.

[97] P. Czobor, J. Volavka, E. M. Derks et al., "Insight and hostility as predictors and correlates of nonadherence in the European first episode schizophrenia trial," *Journal of Clinical Psychopharmacology*, vol. 33, no. 2, pp. 258–261, 2013.

[98] J. Volavka, P. Czobor, L. Citrome et al., "Efficacy of aripiprazole against hostility in schizophrenia and schizoaffective disorder: data from 5 double-blind studies," *The Journal of Clinical Psychiatry*, vol. 66, no. 11, pp. 1362–1366, 2005.

[99] J. Volavka, P. Czobor, B. Sheitman et al., "Clozapine, olanzapine, risperidone, and haloperidol in the treatment of patients with chronic schizophrenia and schizoaffective disorder," *The American Journal of Psychiatry*, vol. 159, no. 2, pp. 255–262, 2002.

[100] L. Citrome, J. Volavka, P. Czobor et al., "Effects of clozapine, olanzapine, risperidone, and haloperidol on hostility among patients with schizophrenia," *Psychiatric Services*, vol. 52, no. 11, pp. 1510–1514, 2001.

[101] J. Volavka, P. Czobor, K. Nolan et al., "Overt aggression and psychotic symptoms in patients with schizophrenia treated with clozapine, olanzapine, risperidone, or haloperidol," *Journal of Clinical Psychopharmacology*, vol. 24, no. 2, pp. 225–228, 2004.

[102] M. I. Krakowski, P. Czobor, L. Citrome, N. Bark, and T. B. Cooper, "Atypical antipsychotic agents in the treatment of violent patients with schizophrenia and schizoaffective disorder," *Archives of General Psychiatry*, vol. 63, no. 6, pp. 622–629, 2006.

[103] W. H. Wilson, "Clinical review of clozapine treatment in a state hospital," *Hospital and Community Psychiatry*, vol. 43, no. 7, pp. 700–703, 1992.

[104] J. Volavka, J. M. Zito, J. Vitrai, and P. Czobor, "Clozapine effects on hostility and aggression in schizophrenia," *Journal of Clinical Psychopharmacology*, vol. 13, no. 4, pp. 287–289, 1993.

[105] T.-P. Su, J. Tuskan, L. Tsao, and D. Pickar, "Aggression during drug-free and antipsychotic treatment in inpatients with chronic schizophrenia, using the overt aggression scale," in *Proceedings of the 33rd Annual Meeting of the American College of Neuropsychopharmacology*, vol. 229, San Juan, Puerto Rico, December 1994.

[106] P. Buckley, J. Bartell, K. Donenwirth, S. Lee, F. Torigoe, and S. C. Schulz, "Violence and schizophrenia: clozapine as a specific antiaggressive agent," *Bulletin of the American Academy of Psychiatry and the Law*, vol. 23, no. 4, pp. 607–611, 1995.

[107] W. H. Wilson and A. M. Claussen, "18-month outcome of clozapine treatment for 100 patients in a state psychiatric hospital," *Psychiatric Services*, vol. 46, no. 4, pp. 386–389, 1995.

[108] J. Volavka, J. W. Swanson, and L. L. Citrome, "Understanding and managing violence in schizophrenia," in *Comprehensive Care of Schizophrenia: A Textbook of Clinical Management*, J. A. Lieberman and R. M. Murray, Eds., pp. 262–290, Oxford University Press, New York, NY, USA, 2012.

[109] S. Comai, M. Tau, Z. Pavlovic, and G. Gobbi, "The psychopharmacology of aggressive behavior: a translational approach—part 2: clinical studies using atypical antipsychotics, anticonvulsants, and lithium," *Journal of Clinical Psychopharmacology*, vol. 32, no. 2, pp. 237–260, 2012.

[110] A. Topiwala and S. Fazel, "The pharmacological management of violence in schizophrenia: a structured review," *Expert Review of Neurotherapeutics*, vol. 11, no. 1, pp. 53–63, 2011.

[111] C. Frogley, D. Taylor, G. Dickens, and M. Picchioni, "A systematic review of the evidence of clozapine's antiaggressive effects," *The International Journal of Neuropsychopharmacology*, vol. 15, no. 9, pp. 1351–1371, 2012.

[112] J. Volavka, "Clozapine is gold standard, but questions remain," *The International Journal of Neuropsychopharmacology*, vol. 15, no. 9, pp. 1201–1204, 2012.

[113] J. A. Lieberman, A. Z. Safferman, S. Pollack et al., "Clinical effects of clozapine in chronic schizophrenia: response to treatment and predictors of outcome," *The American Journal of Psychiatry*, vol. 151, no. 12, pp. 1744–1752, 1994.

[114] J. Volavka, "Comorbid personality disorders and violent behavior in psychotic patients," *Psychiatric Quarterly*, 2013.

[115] J. M. J. Alvir, J. A. Lieberman, A. Z. Safferman, J. L. Schwimmer, and J. A. Schaaf, "Clozapine-induced agranulocytosis: incidence and risk factors in the United States," *The New England Journal of Medicine*, vol. 329, no. 3, pp. 162–167, 1993.

[116] J. W. Swanson, M. S. Swartz, R. A. van Dorn et al., "Comparison of antipsychotic medication effects on reducing violence in people with schizophrenia," *The British Journal of Psychiatry*, vol. 193, no. 1, pp. 37–43, 2008.

[117] J. Volavka, P. Czobor, L. Citrome, and R. A. van Dorn, "Effectiveness of antipsychotic drugs against hostility in patients with schizophrenia in the clinical antipsychotic trials of intervention effectiveness (CATIE) study," *CNS Spectrums*, 2013.

[118] J. Volavka, P. Czobor, E. M. Derks et al., "Efficacy of antipsychotic drugs against hostility in the European first-episode schizophrenia trial (EUFEST)," *The Journal of Clinical Psychiatry*, vol. 72, no. 7, pp. 955–961, 2011.

[119] L. Citrome, M. Krakowski, W. M. Greenberg, E. Andrade, and J. Volavka, "Antiaggressive effect of quetiapine in a patient with schizoaffective disorder," *The Journal of Clinical Psychiatry*, vol. 62, no. 11, p. 901, 2001.

[120] V. Villari, P. Rocca, V. Fonzo, C. Montemagni, P. Pandullo, and F. Bogetto, "Oral risperidone, olanzapine and quetiapine versus haloperidol in psychotic agitation," *Progress in Neuro-Psychopharmacology and Biological Psychiatry*, vol. 32, no. 2, pp. 405–413, 2008.

[121] C. Arango and M. Bernardo, "The effect of quetiapine on aggression and hostility in patients with schizophrenia," *Human Psychopharmacology*, vol. 20, no. 4, pp. 237–241, 2005.

[122] P. Czobor, J. Volavka, and R. C. Meibach, "Effect of risperidone on hostility in schizophrenia," *Journal of Clinical Psychopharmacology*, vol. 15, no. 4, pp. 243–249, 1995.

[123] K. N. R. Chengappa, J. Levine, R. Ulrich et al., "Impact of risperidone on seclusion and restraint at a state psychiatric hospital," *Canadian Journal of Psychiatry*, vol. 45, no. 9, pp. 827–832, 2000.

[124] I. Bitter, P. Czobor, M. Dossenbach, and J. Volavka, "Effectiveness of clozapine, olanzapine, quetiapine, risperidone, and haloperidol monotherapy in reducing hostile and aggressive behavior in outpatients treated for schizophrenia: a prospective naturalistic study (IC-SOHO)," *European Psychiatry*, vol. 20, no. 5-6, pp. 403–408, 2005.

[125] S. Brook, J. Walden, I. Benattia, C. O. Siu, and S. J. Romano, "Ziprasidone and haloperidol in the treatment of acute exacerbation of schizophrenia and schizoaffective disorder: comparison of intramuscular and oral formulations in a 6-week, randomized, blinded-assessment study," *Psychopharmacology*, vol. 178, no. 4, pp. 514–523, 2005.

[126] L. Citrome, J. Volavka, P. Czobor, S. Brook, A. Loebel, and F. S. Mandel, "Efficacy of ziprasidone against hostility in schizophrenia: post hoc analysis of randomized, open-label study data," *The Journal of Clinical Psychiatry*, vol. 67, no. 4, pp. 638–642, 2006.

[127] N. J. Yorkston, J. H. Gruzelier, and S. A. Zaki, "Propranolol as an adjunct to the treatment of schizophrenia," *The Lancet*, vol. 2, no. 8038, pp. 575–578, 1977.

[128] G. P. Sheppard, "High-dose propranolol in schizophrenia," *The British Journal of Psychiatry*, vol. 134, no. 5, pp. 470–476, 1979.

[129] J. R. Whitman, G. J. Maier, and B. Eichelman, "Beta-adrenergic blockers for aggressive behavior in schizophrenia," *The American Journal of Psychiatry*, vol. 144, no. 4, pp. 538–539, 1987.

[130] N. Caspi, I. Modai, P. Barak et al., "Pindolol augmentation in aggressive schizophrenic patients: a double-blind crossover randomized study," *International Clinical Psychopharmacology*, vol. 16, no. 2, pp. 111–115, 2001.

[131] W. J. Newman and B. E. McDermott, "Beta blockers for violence prophylaxis: case reports," *Journal of Clinical Psychopharmacology*, vol. 31, no. 6, pp. 785–787, 2011.

[132] L. Citrome, "Adjunctive lithium and anticonvulsants for the treatment of schizophrenia: what is the evidence?" *Expert Review of Neurotherapeutics*, vol. 9, no. 1, pp. 55–71, 2009.

[133] J. Volavka and L. Citrome, "Heterogeneity of violence in schizophrenia and implications for long-term treatment," *The International Journal of Clinical Practice*, vol. 62, no. 8, pp. 1237–1245, 2008.

[134] J. Volavka and L. Citrome, "Pathways to aggression in schizophrenia affect results of treatment," *Schizophrenia Bulletin*, vol. 37, no. 5, pp. 921–929, 2011.

[135] M. S. Swartz, J. W. Swanson, V. A. Hiday, R. Borum, R. Wagner, and B. J. Burns, "Taking the wrong drugs: the role of substance abuse and medication noncompliance in violence among severely mentally ill individuals," *Social Psychiatry and Psychiatric Epidemiology*, vol. 33, no. 1, pp. S75–S80, 1998.

[136] J. W. Swanson, M. S. Swartz, R. Borum, V. A. Hiday, H. R. Wagner, and B. J. Burns, "Involuntary out-patient commitment and reduction of violent behaviour in persons with severe mental illness," *The British Journal of Psychiatry*, vol. 176, pp. 324–331, 2000.

[137] K. F. Yates, M. Kunz, A. Khan, J. Volavka, and S. Rabinowitz, "Psychiatric patients with histories of aggression and crime five years after discharge from a cognitive-behavioral program," *Journal of Forensic Psychiatry & Psychology*, vol. 21, no. 2, pp. 167–188, 2010.

[138] G. Haddock, C. Barrowclough, J. J. Shaw, G. Dunn, R. W. Novaco, and N. Tarrier, "Cognitive-behavioural therapy *v.* social activity therapy for people with psychosis and a history of violence: randomised controlled trial," *The British Journal of Psychiatry*, vol. 194, no. 2, pp. 152–157, 2009.

[139] A. E. Cullen, A. Y. Clarke, E. Kuipers, S. Hodgins, K. Dean, and T. Fahy, "A multi-site randomized controlled trial of a cognitive skills programme for male mentally disordered offenders: violence and antisocial behavior outcomes," *Journal of Consulting and Clinical Psychology*, vol. 80, no. 6, pp. 1114–1120, 2012.

[140] K. T. Mueser, F. Deavers, D. L. Penn, and J. E. Cassisi, "Psychosocial treatments for schizophrenia," *Annual Review of Clinical Psychology*, vol. 9, pp. 465–497, 2013.

[141] R. L. Binder and D. E. McNiel, "Effects of diagnosis and context on dangerousness," *The American Journal of Psychiatry*, vol. 145, no. 6, pp. 728–732, 1988.

[142] K. Barlow, B. Grenyer, and O. Ilkiw-Lavalle, "Prevalence and precipitants of aggression in psychiatric inpatient units," *Australian & New Zealand Journal of Psychiatry*, vol. 34, no. 6, pp. 967–974, 2000.

[143] P. W. Corrigan and A. C. Watson, "Findings from the national comorbidity survey on the frequency of violent behavior in individuals with psychiatric disorders," *Psychiatry Research*, vol. 136, no. 2-3, pp. 153–162, 2005.

[144] A. J. Pulay, D. A. Dawson, D. S. Hasin et al., "Violent behavior and DSM-IV psychiatric disorders: results from the national epidemiologic survey on alcohol and related conditions," *The Journal of Clinical Psychiatry*, vol. 69, no. 1, pp. 12–22, 2008.

[145] B. F. Grant, F. S. Stinson, D. S. Hasin et al., "Prevalence, correlates, and comorbidity of bipolar I disorder and axis I and II disorders: results from the national epidemiologic survey on alcohol and related conditions," *The Journal of Clinical Psychiatry*, vol. 66, no. 10, pp. 1205–1215, 2005.

[146] S. Fazel, P. Lichtenstein, M. Grann, G. M. Goodwin, and N. Långström, "Bipolar disorder and violent crime: new evidence from population-based longitudinal studies and systematic review," *Archives of General Psychiatry*, vol. 67, no. 9, pp. 931–938, 2010.

[147] S. Fazel, P. Lichtenstein, T. Frisell, M. Grann, G. Goodwin, and N. Långström, "Bipolar disorder and violent crime: time at risk reanalysis," *Archives of General Psychiatry*, vol. 67, no. 12, pp. 1325–1326, 2010.

[148] P. P. Christopher, P. J. McCabe, and W. H. Fisher, "Prevalence of involvement in the criminal justice system during severe mania and associated symptomatology," *Psychiatric Services*, vol. 63, no. 1, pp. 33–39, 2012.

[149] J. Ballester, T. Goldstein, B. Goldstein et al., "Is bipolar disorder specifically associated with aggression?" *Bipolar Disorders*, vol. 14, no. 3, pp. 283–290, 2012.

[150] K. Latalova, "Bipolar disorder and aggression," *The International Journal of Clinical Practice*, vol. 63, no. 6, pp. 889–899, 2009.

[151] K. Latalova, *Aggression in Psychiatry*, Grada, Prague, Czech Republic, 2013, (Czech).

[152] K. Latalova, *Bipolar Affective Disorder*, Grada, Prague, Czech Republic, 2011, (Czech).

[153] J. L. Garno, N. Gunawardane, and J. F. Goldberg, "Predictors of trait aggression in bipolar disorder," *Bipolar Disorders*, vol. 10, no. 2, pp. 285–292, 2008.

[154] G. L. Brown, F. K. Goodwin, J. C. Ballenger, P. F. Goyer, and L. F. Major, "Aggression in humans correlates with cerebrospinal fluid amine metabolites," *Psychiatry Research*, vol. 1, no. 2, pp. 131–139, 1979.

[155] D. P. Bernstein, L. Fink, L. Handelsman et al., "Initial reliability and validity of a new retrospective measure of child abuse and neglect," *The American Journal of Psychiatry*, vol. 151, no. 8, pp. 1132–1136, 1994.

[156] M. A. Oquendo, C. Waternaux, B. Brodsky et al., "Suicidal behavior in bipolar mood disorder: clinical characteristics of attempters and nonattempters," *Journal of Affective Disorders*, vol. 59, no. 2, pp. 107–117, 2000.

[157] A. H. Buss and A. Durkee, "An inventory for assessing different kinds of hostility," *Journal of Consulting Psychology*, vol. 21, no. 4, pp. 343–349, 1957.

[158] B. H. Michaelis, J. F. Goldberg, G. P. Davis, T. M. Singer, J. L. Garno, and S. J. Wenze, "Dimensions of impulsivity and aggression associated with suicide attempts among bipolar patients: a preliminary study," *Suicide and Life-Threatening Behavior*, vol. 34, no. 2, pp. 172–176, 2004.

[159] R. H. Perlis, S. Miyahara, L. B. Marangell et al., "Long-term implications of early onset in bipolar disorder: data from the first 1000 participants in the systematic treatment enhancement program for bipolar disorder (STEP-BD)," *Biological Psychiatry*, vol. 55, no. 9, pp. 875–881, 2004.

[160] C. F. Baldassano, "Illness course, comorbidity, gender, and suicidality in patients with bipolar disorder," *The Journal of Clinical Psychiatry*, vol. 67, supplement 11, pp. 8–11, 2006.

[161] I. M. Salloum, J. R. Cornelius, J. E. Mezzich, and L. Kirisci, "Impact of concurrent alcohol misuse on symptom presentation of acute mania at initial evaluation," *Bipolar Disorders*, vol. 4, no. 6, pp. 418–421, 2002.

[162] J. Volavka and J. Swanson, "Violent behavior in mental illness: the role of substance abuse," *The Journal of the American Medical Association*, vol. 304, no. 5, pp. 563–564, 2010.

[163] M. I. Good, "Primary affective disorder, aggression, and criminality. A review and clinical study," *Archives of General Psychiatry*, vol. 35, no. 8, pp. 954–960, 1978.

[164] W. F. Thorneloe and E. L. Crews, "Manic depressive illness concomitant with antisocial personality disorder: six case reports and review of the literature," *The Journal of Clinical Psychiatry*, vol. 42, no. 1, pp. 5–9, 1981.

[165] B. Carpiniello, L. Lai, S. Pirarba, C. Sardu, and F. Pinna, "Impulsivity and aggressiveness in bipolar disorder with comorbid borderline personality disorder," *Psychiatry Research*, vol. 188, no. 1, pp. 40–44, 2011.

[166] K. Látalová and J. Praško, "Aggression in borderline personality disorder," *Psychiatric Quarterly*, vol. 81, no. 3, pp. 239–251, 2010.

[167] M. Hamilton, "Development of a rating scale for primary depressive illness," *British Journal of Social and Clinical Psychology*, vol. 6, no. 4, pp. 278–296, 1967.

[168] R. C. Young, J. T. Biggs, V. E. Ziegler, and D. A. Meyer, "A rating scale for mania: reliability, validity and sensitivity," *The British Journal of Psychiatry*, vol. 133, no. 11, pp. 429–435, 1978.

[169] K. Latalova, "Insight in bipolar disorder," *Psychiatric Quarterly*, vol. 83, no. 3, pp. 293–310, 2012.

[170] C.-F. Yen, C.-S. Chen, J.-Y. Yen, and C.-H. Ko, "The predictive effect of insight on adverse clinical outcomes in bipolar I disorder: a two-year prospective study," *Journal of Affective Disorders*, vol. 108, no. 1-2, pp. 121–127, 2008.

[171] A. S. David, "Insight and psychosis," *The British Journal of Psychiatry*, vol. 156, pp. 798–808, 1990.

[172] M. Serper, D. R. Beech, P. D. Harvey, and C. Dill, "Neuropsychological and symptom predictors of aggression on the psychiatric inpatient service," *Journal of Clinical and Experimental Neuropsychology*, vol. 30, no. 6, pp. 700–709, 2008.

[173] M. Mur, M. J. Portella, A. Martínez-Arán, J. Pifarré, and E. Vieta, "Persistent neuropsychological deficit in euthymic bipolar patients: executive function as a core deficit," *The Journal of Clinical Psychiatry*, vol. 68, no. 7, pp. 1078–1086, 2007.

[174] K. Latalova, J. Prasko, T. Diveky, and H. Velartova, "Cognitive impairment in bipolar disorder," *Biomedical Papers*, vol. 155, no. 1, pp. 19–26, 2011.

[175] G. Huf, J. Alexander, M. H. Allen, and N. S. Raveendran, "Haloperidol plus promethazine for psychosis-induced aggression," *Cochrane Database of Systematic Reviews*, no. 3, Article ID CD005146, 2009.

[176] L. Citrome, "Comparison of intramuscular ziprasidone, olanzapine, or aripiprazole for agitation: a quantitative review of efficacy and safety," *The Journal of Clinical Psychiatry*, vol. 68, no. 12, pp. 1876–1885, 2007.

[177] M. Pratts, W. Grant, L. A. Opler et al., "Treating acutely agitated patients with asenapine sublingual tablets: a single-dose, randomized, double-blind placebo controlled trial," in *Proceedings of the 53rd Annual NCDEU Meeting*, pp. 28–31, Hollywood, Calif, USA, May 2013.

[178] L. Citrome, "Inhaled loxapine for agitation revisited: focus on effect sizes from 2 phase III randomised controlled trials in persons with schizophrenia or bipolar disorder," *The International Journal of Clinical Practice*, vol. 66, no. 3, pp. 318–325, 2012.

[179] L. Citrome, "Addressing the need for rapid treatment of agitation in schizophrenia and bipolar disorder: focus on inhaled loxapine as an alternative to injectable agents," *Therapeutics and Clinical Risk Management*, vol. 2013, article 9, pp. 235–245, 2013.

[180] J. Kwentus, R. A. Riesenberg, M. Marandi et al., "Rapid acute treatment of agitation in patients with bipolar I disorder: a

multicenter, randomized, placebo-controlled clinical trial with inhaled loxapine," *Bipolar Disorders*, vol. 14, no. 1, pp. 31–40, 2012.

[181] N. Collins, T. R. E. Barnes, A. Shingleton-Smith, D. Gerrett, and C. Paton, "Standards of lithium monitoring in mental health trusts in the UK," *BMC Psychiatry*, vol. 10, article 80, 2010.

[182] A. Podawiltz, "A review of current bipolar disorder treatment guidelines," *The Journal of Clinical Psychiatry*, vol. 73, no. 3, article e12, 2012.

[183] K. N. Fountoulakis, S. Kasper, O. Andreassen et al., "Efficacy of pharmacotherapy in bipolar disorder: a report by the WPA section on pharmacopsychiatry," *European Archives of Psychiatry and Clinical Neuroscience*, vol. 262, no. 1, supplement, pp. 1–48, 2012.

[184] S. D. Cochran, "Preventing medical noncompliance in the outpatient treatment of bipolar affective disorders," *Journal of Consulting and Clinical Psychology*, vol. 52, no. 5, pp. 873–878, 1984.

[185] M. R. Basco and A. J. Rush, *Cognitive-Behavioral Therapy for Bipolar Disorder*, Guilford Press, New York, NY, USA, 2nd edition, 2007.

[186] E. Herman, P. Grof, J. Hovorka, J. Prasko, and P. Doubek, "Bipolar disorder," in *Postupy v Lecbe Psychickych Poruch*, D. Seifertova, J. Prasko, and C. Hoschl, Eds., pp. 93–120, Academia Medica Pragensis, Prague, Czech Republic, 2004, (Czech).

17

Demographic and Clinical Characteristics of Patients with Dementia in Greece

Eleni Jelastopulu,[1] Evangelia Giourou,[1] Konstantinos Argyropoulos,[1,2] Eleftheria Kariori,[3] Eleftherios Moratis,[4] Angeliki Mestousi,[4] and John Kyriopoulos[5]

[1] Department of Public Health, School of Medicine, University of Patras, 26500 Rio Patras, Greece
[2] Psychiatric Hospital of Tripoli, 5th Km Tripolis-Kalamatas, 22100 Tripoli, Greece
[3] Health Center of Erymanthia, 25015 Erymanthia, Greece
[4] Department of Medical Affairs, Janssen-Cilag, 56 Eirinis Avenue, Pefki, 15121 Athens, Greece
[5] Department of Health Economics, National School of Public Health, 196 Alexandras Avenue, 11521 Athens, Greece

Correspondence should be addressed to Evangelia Giourou; egiourou@upatras.gr

Academic Editor: Takahiro Nemoto

Introduction. Dementia's prevalence increases due to population aging. The purpose of this study was to determine the demographic profile of Greek patients with dementia and the differences in management between the urban and rural population. *Methods.* A cross sectional study was carried out including 161 randomly selected specialists from different regions in Greece who filled in a structured questionnaire relating to patients with dementia, regarding various sociodemographic and clinical characteristics. *Results.* A total of 4580 patients (52% males) with dementia were recorded. Mean age was 73.6 years and 31% lived in rural areas. The Mini Mental Status Examination (MMSE) was used in 87% of cases. In the urban areas the diagnosis of dementia was made in an earlier stage of the disease in comparison to the rural areas ($P = 0.013$). Higher comorbidity and a higher percentage of low education were evident in rural residents ($P < 0.001$), while higher medication usage was observed in urban patients ($P = 0.04$). *Conclusions.* The results implicate the need for improvement in health care delivery in Greek rural areas and health care professionals' training to achieve a proper treatment of dementias and increase the quality of life among the elderly habitants of remote areas.

1. Introduction

Old age seems to be the main risk factor for dementia [1, 2]. Higher prevalence rates are observed in people over 65 years old showing steadily increasing rates in each following five-year age group. About 14% of people aged 71 and older are affected by dementia, with women demonstrating higher rates in prevalence, but not in incidence [3].

Socioeconomic features [1], low educational level [3–6], cardiovascular comorbidity, and coexistence of other medical conditions increase the prevalence [2, 7] and the mortality of dementia [7] while the quality of life of patients decreases. Moreover, mental disorders often affect patients with dementia [8] and their caregivers [9, 10] influencing even more their

diminished quality of life and need for institutionalization. Therefore, neuropsychiatric symptoms and mental disorders of patients with dementia need to be assessed and treated independently [11].

Given the persistent prolongation of life expectancy, the impact of dementia on healthcare systems [1], on families and caregivers [12, 13], and the mortality directly linked to Alzheimer's disease (AD) and other dementias [1], it is imperative for current epidemiological data to be available to primary and secondary health care systems. A report of Turner et al. showed that general practitioners' lack of knowledge of the epidemiology of dementia had the consequence of overdiagnosing cases during their practice [14]. In a survey conducted in Greece considering the attitudes of physicians, caregivers, and patients regarding AD, specialists admit lacking the expertise in distinguishing normal symptoms of aging from AD [15].

Epidemiological data are rare and have shown an inability to assess some basic parameters in Greece. In an epidemiological study of the municipality of Pilea, Greece, conducted on people over 70 years ($N = 277$), the estimated prevalence of Alzheimer's disease and vascular dementia was 5.3% and 2.5%, respectively [16]. In another study conducted at a primary health center in Northern Greece on people over 65 years ($N = 536$), 37.6% males and 41.6% females were found with cognitive impairment [17]. However, data concerning the sociodemographic and clinical profile, the therapeutic approach followed by physicians, and other important information regarding patients with dementia in Greece are scarce in the literature [18, 19].

In the United States one in four people older than 65 years who is living in rural environments is at greater risk of developing dementia [20]. Other studies have reported that the prevalence of cognitive impairment is higher in rural compared to urban populations [2] and there is a higher rate of hospitalization. This is probably related to distance and to limited access to health care providers compared to metropolitan citizens [21].

Moreover, most studies that include rural and remote needs within a broader national focus highlight the limited access to specialist health services and community services, compared to those living in metropolitan regions [22].

Noteworthy inefficiencies exist in the healthcare services delivery in rural areas of Greece as well. Certain disadvantages of quality and quantity of available health care providers to the residents of remote areas as well as the distinctiveness of rural-urban diversity in Greece [23] and the large proportion of elderly in rural areas, leads to the need of an update of the available epidemiological data of dementia.

The purpose of this study was to gather information to determine the demographic profile of Greek patients with dementia, to identify risk factors, and to record the screening tools used by specialists. Moreover, there was an emphasis to assess the differences in diagnostic and treatment management of dementia between urban and rural population in Greece.

2. Methods

2.1. Population and Setting. Medical and demographic data of 4580 patients in outpatient setting (2276 males, 2112 females, and 192 missing) who had a diagnosis of dementia by their treating physicians were included. The relevant data of participants were retrospective and they were obtained by 161 randomly selected specialists (i.e., neurologists $n = 82$; psychiatrists $n = 45$; neuropsychiatrists $n = 32$; missing $N = 2$; response rate 89.4%) using the medical records they kept in public and private healthcare facilities all over the country. The physicians were randomly selected by the Panhellenic Medical Association's database. The treating physicians were qualified specialists (neurologists and psychiatrists) by board examinations and appropriate clinical practice. They were

professionally trained in diagnosing and treating dementia according to the requirements concerning the formal residency training and the license to practice the certified specialty. The mandatory residency program requires the use of certain criteria and guidelines in diagnosing disorders. Primary care physicians were excluded because they are usually not formally trained in diagnosing and treating dementia. No other excluding criteria were used. All forms of dementia were included: Alzheimer's disease, vascular dementia, mixed, and other forms. The physicians used the information collected to fill a structured questionnaire provided by the research team.

2.2. Procedures. The study was conducted within a period of one year (1.7.2007 to 31.7.2008). During the 12-month study period, the specialist physicians enrolled a total of 4580 diagnosed patients. The patients agreed to participate in the study and provided written informed consent (mostly by their caregiver). Diagnosis of dementia was made by the treating physicians on the basis of objective cognitive tests and additional general informal tests for cognitive assessment (i.e., clinical evaluation and assessment of cognitive features such as working memory, e.g., digit span tasks, serial sevens and serial threes tasks; complex attention, e.g., months in reverse order, and orientation, e.g., time, location, and autobiographical data). For the patients' assessment, the included measure was a structured questionnaire supplied by the research team and filled by the treating doctors. The aim was to investigate the usual procedures followed by specialists in assessing and treating dementia in urban and rural areas of Greece. The questionnaire was designed by the researchers to assess differences in demographic characteristics, diagnostic procedures, and comorbid factors of dementia between urban and rural population in Greece. The questionnaire also contained items that assessed information regarding (a) sociodemographic data (age, sex, educational level, type of caregiver, and place of residence). Rural was defined as the population of those municipalities and communes in which the inhabitants of the largest population center were less than 10,000; urban was defined, respectively, as not less than 10,000 inhabitants; (b) type of dementia (Alzheimer's disease, vascular dementia, mixed form, or other); (c) comorbid factors to dementia (hypertension and other cardiological disorders, diabetes mellitus, psychiatric disorders, Parkinson disease, and other neurological disorders); (d) usage of diagnostic tools (MMSE, Clock Drawing test, Neuropsychiatry Inventory, Clinical Dementia Rating, Disability Assessment for Dementia, Global Deterioration Scale, Cambridge Cognitive Examination, or other); (e) disease's severity and symptomatology; (f) clinical and diagnostic features (i.e., clinical impression evaluation according to the physician judgment and cognitive decline evaluation according to the Mini Mental State Examination, MMSE, if the treating physician used it); and (g) drugs the treating physicians prescribed for the pharmaceutical palliative treatment of dementia, for each patient. The treating physicians were qualified specialists (i.e., neurologists and psychiatrists) professionally trained in diagnosing and treating dementia and they were randomly selected. The information collected was obtained by the medical records kept by the randomly selected treating physicians.

2.3. Data Analysis. All data were analyzed using descriptive statistics. Differences among subgroups (urban and rural population) were evaluated using chi-square and t-tests. All significance tests were two-sided using $P < 0.05$ as the level of significance. Data analyses were performed using SPSS software, version 15.1.0 (SPSS, Inc., Chicago, IL, USA).

3. Results

3.1. Demographic and Clinical Characteristics. The majority of the studied patients (N = 4580) were diagnosed with Alzheimer's disease (N = 1664) or mixed form (N = 1378). No statistical difference was observed among genders regarding dementia's forms. Patients' mean age was 74 years, while the majority of patients were over 70 years (N = 3248), living in urban areas (N = 2696), being illiterate or of lower education (n = 2020). Mean duration of disease was 27.6 months (median = 12 months, maximum = 192 months). Mean duration of treatment was 24 months. (For further details see Table 1.)

Cardiovascular risk factors, that is, hypertension (N = 2209), other cardiovascular diseases (N = 1779), and diabetes (N = 1286) were the most frequent comorbidities. A positive family history of dementia was present in 34.6% of patients (N = 1587).

Memory decline (87.4%) and orientation disability (61%) were present in the vast majority of patients, while critical judgment disability (53.8%), difficulty in planning and in complex task completion (49.8%), and cognitive ability decline (47.4%) followed (for further details see Table 2). Fifty-eight percent of patients were found with mood, behavior, and personality disorders while a personal history of mental disease was present in 19.5%.

To assess the functional, cognitive, and behavioral status of the patients the Mini Mental Status Examination (MMSE) was the tool mostly used by physicians in their everyday practice among the screening tools (Table 3).

Nearly 50% of patients (N = 2172) received medication in the past, including nootropics (N = 963, 44.3%) and acetylcholinesterase inhibitors (AchEIs) (donepezil N = 742, 34.2%; rivastigmine N = 651, 30%). 71.5% were on monotherapy.

Table 4 presents the clinical impression evaluation according to the physicians' judgment and the cognitive decline evaluation according to the Mini Mental State Examination (MMSE) scale.

3.2. Rural-Urban Differences. The recruiting specialists distribution by specialty was similar between urban (51.7% neurologists; 31.1% psychiatrists; 17.2% neuropsychiatrists) and rural areas (49.7% neurologists; 25.3% psychiatrists; 25% neuropsychiatrists). The diagnosis of dementia in the urban areas was made in an earlier stage of the disease in comparison to the rural areas (40.8% versus 36.2%, P = 0.013). Increased medication usage (three or more drugs) was

TABLE 1: Demographic and disease characteristics of study population (n = 4580).

Sex (n = 4388)[*]	n (%)
Male (%)	2276 (49.7)
Female (%)	2112 (46.1)
Age	Years
Mean age	73.6
Nationality (n = 3758)[*]	n (%)
Greek	3630 (96.6)
Other	128 (3.4)
Education[†] (n = 4128)[*]	n (%)
Illiterate or low	2020 (48.9)
Middle	1761 (42.7)
Higher	347 (8.4)
Residence (n = 3911)[*]	n (%)
Urban	2696 (68.9)
Rural	1215 (31.1)
Caregiver (n = 3805)[*]	n (%)
Relative	3199 (84.1)
Other	606 (15.9)
Type of dementia (n = 4156)[*]	n (%)
Alzheimer's disease	1664 (40.0)
Vascular dementia	1018 (24.5)
Mixed form	1378 (33.2)
Other	96 (2.3)

[*] Valid answers.
[†] Low education (first 6 years of formal education), middle education (secondary education consisting of 7–12 years of formal education), and higher education (tertiary education towards a degree-level qualification).

monitored in urban patients, although higher comorbidity (cardiological disorders, $P < 0.001$; diabetes mellitus, P = 0.001; neurological disorders, P = 0.001) was evident in rural residents. Regarding the educational level, a very high percentage of low education was observed in rural population in comparison to the urban ($P < 0.001$). For further details see Table 5.

4. Discussion

Given the lack of epidemiological data in Greece, this study provides new insights into the epidemiological pattern of dementia in Greece. It also examines the health care inequalities as they are demonstrated through the treatment present during the time patients turned to specialists. Finally it examines the urban/rural differences in healthcare delivery in regard to patients with dementia.

In previous studies, age [1, 2], educational level [3, 6], cardiovascular comorbidity [2, 24], and familiar predisposition are identifiable risk factors to dementia. The present study supports these data, since the majority of patients were over 70 years, they were diagnosed with Alzheimer's disease or mixed form, they lived in urban areas and they had achieved the lower education or were illiterate.

TABLE 2: Estimation of severity and symptomatology of dementia (%).

Symptomatology	Severity[‡]					
	0 (%)	0.5 (%)	1 (%)	2 (%)	3 (%)	Total (in %)
Memory decline	0	1.4	22.1	59.0	17.4	87.4
Orientation disability	1.6	3.8	30.0	49.0	15.5	61.0
Judgment disability	1.2	4.0	30.3	48.3	16.1	53.8
Difficulty in planning and in complex task completion	2.1	4.4	30.4	47.0	16.2	49.8
Cognitive ability decline	2.6	4.7	30.9	46.3	15.5	47.4
Mood, behavioral, and personality disorders	1.0	4.0	31.0	47.9	16.1	58.1

[‡]0 (no decline), 0.5 (undefined decline), 1 (minor decline), 2 (modest decline), and 3 (severe decline).

TABLE 3: Dementia screening tools used by setting (%).

Screening tools	Urban	Rural	Total
Mini Mental State Examination (MMSE)	89.9	92.9	90.9
Clock Drawing test (CDT)	41.2	46.3	42.8
Neuropsychiatry Inventory (NPI)	14.6	11.9	13.7
Clinical Dementia Rating (CDR)	2.7	3.0	2.8
Disability Assessment for Dementia (DAD)	3.6	1.6	3.0
Global Deterioration Scale, Reisberg (GDS)	2.0	3.3	2.4
Cambridge Cognitive Examination (CAMCOG)	1.1	1.2	1.2

TABLE 4: Cognitive decline according to clinical impression evaluation (CIE)[§] and the Mini Mental State Examination (MMSE) (in %).

CIE	$n = 2217$	MMSE[‖]	$n = 2107$
Very good/good	7.8	**30–27**	2.3
Satisfactory	21.4	**26–18**	66.5
Moderate	47.0	**17–11**	26.5
Bad	23.7	**<10**	4.6

[§]CIE stands for the diagnostic procedures the treating physicians followed based on clinical features and by performing additional general additional informal tests for cognitive assessment (cognitive features were assessed such as working memory, e.g., digit span tasks, serial sevens and serial threes tasks; complex attention, e.g., months in reverse order, and orientation, e.g., time, location, and autobiographical data).

[‖]Cut-off score under the Consensus Statements "Dementia" of the Austrian Alzheimer Society. 30–27 = no cognitive decline; 26–18 = mild cognitive decline; 17–11 = moderate cognitive decline; <10 = severe cognitive decline.

TABLE 5: Differences of dementia patients in rural and urban areas (in %).

	Urban	Rural	P value
Early stage diagnosis	40.8	36.2	*0.040*
Lower educational level[**]	35.8	76.3	*<0.001*
Polypharmacy (3 or more medications)	39.3	31.2	*0.004*
Comorbidity			
Hypertension	49.6	54.4	*0.005*
Other cardiological disorders	38.4	44.9	*<0.001*
Diabetes mellitus	27.4	32.8	*0.001*
Psychiatric disorders	20.4	23.2	*0.044*
Morbus Parkinson	11.5	13.1	0.147
Neurological disorders	5.9	8.8	*0.001*

[**]First 6 years of formal education.

In the literature female gender has been associated with increased risk of development of Alzheimer's disease [25, 26]. Of the total 4580 patients with all dementia forms recorded, 52% were males but no statistical difference was observed among genders regarding dementia's forms.

To assess the functional, cognitive, and behavioral status of the patients the physicians used in 90.9% the MMSE, only in 42.8% the Clock Drawing test (CDT), and in even lower proportion other scales. MMSE and CDT are sensitive and easy to use; however, cognitive decline remains underestimated even among hospitalized elderly patients by treating physicians as a recent study of Douzenis et al.

displayed [27]. Even if the MMSE reflects the main cognitive domains affected in AD, additional scales are important, such as the CDT, for screening domains that are less assessed by the MMSE. Neuropsychiatric symptoms are common in dementias [28]. As this study displayed, 58.1% of patients were found with mood, behavior, and personality disorders while a personal history of mental disease was present in only 19.5%. Despite that the Neuropsychiatric Inventory (NPI) provides a clinical screening examination of frequent neuropsychiatric signs which appear in dementia, it was only used in 13.5% of cases.

A large proportion (61.2%) of the enrolled patients was newly diagnosed. According to the MMSE screening 66.5% of patients displayed Mild Cognitive Impairment (MCI; score = 26–18), which is composed of an evident cognitive decline in screening tests and others without interfering with patients' daily life. Overall prevalence of MCI among elderly is high [29]; of those a notable percentage will convert to AD at an accelerated rate [1, 29, 30]. Today there is a trend towards early diagnosis and treatment, towards altering progression of MCI. Patients and caregivers though abstain from confirming the existence of dementia [31] and many physicians (i.e., general practitioners and specialists) overlook symptoms of MCI attributing them to normal aging manifestations [14, 31]. While the Global Deterioration Scale (GDS) and the Clinical Dementia Rating (CDS) are important instruments in scaling patients among normal aging and severe dementia, they were only used in 2.4% and 2.8%, respectively.

Nootropics were present in medication patients received in the past, in a relatively large proportion. Furthermore, the vast majority were on monotherapy. As far as the urban/rural diversity in health care delivery is concerned, some statistically important differences were noted. Firstly, in the rural areas dementia was diagnosed in a later stage of the disease in comparison to the urban areas, which may lead to negative effects in altering the progression of the disease itself as well as to the general well-being of patients. High mortality has been directly linked to AD and other dementias. Indeed, higher comorbidity was evident, in rural residents, which was expected due to certain inefficiencies of the health care system in rural areas of Greece [23, 32]. Rural population is characterized as being less healthy overall in comparison to urban residents [33] with a higher rate of hospitalization, for a range of causes, probably related to the often limited and delayed access to health care services [21]. In a recent study of Tountas et al., rural patients' contacts with health care professionals were less than urban residents' especially among the less educated [32]. Indeed, 76.3% of patients in our study recorded in rural areas were low educated or illiterate. An increasing number of immigrants living in remote areas, carrying a low socioeconomic profile as well as the large proportion of elderly habitants of the rural areas, often illiterate [34], add to the result. Patients' and caregivers' training to recognize the early symptoms of dementia needs to be addressed in order to ensure adequate health care.

Increased medication usage (three and more drugs), as to counterbalance, was monitored in urban patients, something that enhances the need for more rational and targeted drug usage in Greece. In a recent study of Pappa et al., 2011, advanced age (>65 years) visits to physician and comorbidity were associated with high rate of drug use or polypharmacy [35].

There are some limitations that merit particular consideration. The study was not a population-based cross-sectional study with a representative sample size of dementia patients. Furthermore, the physicians did not provide drop out percentages of the patients they recruited in the study. That limits the generalizability of the results. However, the specialists participating in this study were selected from various urban and rural regions from the whole country. A further weakness may arise from the fact that the questionnaire was not formally validated. On the other hand the questions were specific, well-defined, and completed by experienced and professionally qualified physicians in diagnosing and treating dementia patients. The exclusion of general practitioners may pose an extra limitation since general practitioners are more likely to encounter patients with dementia in rural areas. However, the scope of this study was to assess the demographic and clinical characteristics of patients with dementia and the diagnostic and treatment procedures used by specialists (i.e., neurologists and psychiatrists) and to describe the differences in the special care management of dementia between urban and rural population. The weak primary care sector in Greece would pose further issues concerning the validity of the diagnostic procedures followed. Furthermore comorbidities other than vascular disorders, metabolic disorders, and neuropsychiatric conditions have been correlated with dementia, such as periodontal pathogenesis or thyroid disease, which might have aggravated patients' condition. However, since there is a lack of multidisciplinary teams in the healthcare system, especially in rural areas, and also a lack of a systematic data collection, the validity of medical records could be questionable. Therefore there was an aim to describe comorbidities within broad categories of conditions which could be easily identified by the vast majority of physicians or they could be retrieved from patients' prescriptions on medications used and from medical certificates of other speciality attending physicians.

There is a growing need for interventions regarding the provision of services to patients with dementia and a growing need for the implementation of strategies to raise the awareness of the disease and to develop structures and capacities to manage the growing burden of dementia. Several issues must be addressed, such as the development of formal diagnostic and treating guidelines, the reinforcement of community support services and housing options accessible to patients and caregivers, and the creation of a national plan for dementia focused on the particular needs of the patients with dementia in Greece. This can facilitate the development of a more efficient and personalized healthcare plan for patients with dementia and high risk population living across the country.

5. Conclusions

In conclusion, there are considerable differences concerning dementia health care delivery among specialists practicing in urban and rural areas in Greece. Insufficiencies are observed in specialists' care to make an early diagnosis of dementia in order to prevent or slow the transition in more severe forms of the disease. There is an increasing need for improvement in health care delivery in rural areas and health care professionals' training as well as caregivers' education, in focused and proper treatment of dementias, so that substantial quality of life and general wellbeing are to be achieved even among the elderly habitants of remote areas.

Ethical Approval

Ethics approval was given from the Board of the Medical School of Patras, the Research Committee of the University of Patras, and the National Organization for Medicines, Greece. All participants and their caregivers were informed about the study and provided written informed consent for participation.

Conflict of Interests

Authors Eleftherios Moratis and Angeliki Mestousi are employed by Janssen-Cilag. All other authors declare that they have no competing interests.

Authors' Contribution

Eleni Jelastopulu participated in the design of the study, collected, analyzed, and interpreted the data, and wrote the first draft of the paper. Evangelia Giourou contributed to interpreting the data and to developing and writing subsequent drafts. Konstantinos Argyropoulos and Eleftheria Kariori contributed to drafting the paper and revising it critically. Eleftherios Morati and Angeliki Mestousi developed the idea for the study and were involved in the conception and design of the study and in the critical review of the paper. John Kyriopoulos participated in the design, coordinated the study, and was involved in revising the paper critically for important intellectual content. All authors read and approved the final paper. Eleni Jelastopulu is the guarantor.

Acknowledgments

This study was supported by a research grant received from the Janssen-Cilag Greece. The authors sincerely thank the physicians for all their work and contribution and all patients who kindly participated in this study.

References

[1] Alzheimer's Association, "2010 Alzheimer's disease facts and figures," *Alzheimer's and Dementia*, vol. 6, no. 2, pp. 158–194, 2010.

[2] B. Nunes, R. D. Silva, V. T. Cruz, J. M. Roriz, J. Pais, and M. C. Silva, "Prevalence and pattern of cognitive impairment in rural and urban populations from Northern Portugal," *BMC Neurology*, vol. 10, article 42, 2010.

[3] B. L. Plassman, K. M. Langa, G. G. Fisher et al., "Prevalence of dementia in the United States: the aging, demographics, and memory study," *Neuroepidemiology*, vol. 29, no. 1-2, pp. 125–132, 2007.

[4] Y. Stern, B. Gurland, T. K. Tatemichi, M. X. Tang, D. Wilder, and R. Mayeux, "Influence of education and occupation on the incidence of Alzheimer's disease," *The Journal of the American Medical Association*, vol. 271, no. 13, pp. 1004–1010, 1994.

[5] D. A. Evans, L. E. Hebert, L. A. Beckett et al., "Education and other measures of socioeconomic status and risk of incident Alzheimer disease in a defined population of older persons," *Archives of Neurology*, vol. 54, no. 11, pp. 1399–1405, 1997.

[6] W. A. Kukull, R. Higdon, J. D. Bowen et al., "Dementia and Alzheimer disease incidence: a prospective cohort study," *Archives of Neurology*, vol. 59, no. 11, pp. 1737–1746, 2002.

[7] C. Helmer, P. Joly, L. Letenneur, D. Commenges, and J.-F. Dartigues, "Mortality with dementia: results from a French prospective community-based cohort," *American Journal of Epidemiology*, vol. 154, no. 7, pp. 642–648, 2001.

[8] J. Calleo and M. Stanley, "Anxiety disorders in later life: differentiated diagnosis and treatment strategies," *Psychiatric Times*, vol. 25, no. 8, pp. 24–27, 2008.

[9] K. Yaffe, P. Fox, R. Newcomer et al., "Patient and caregiver characteristics and nursing home placement in patients with dementia," *The Journal of the American Medical Association*, vol. 287, no. 16, pp. 2090–2097, 2002.

[10] D. H. Taylor Jr., M. Ezell, M. Kuchibhatla, T. Østbye, and E. C. Clipp, "Identifying trajectories of depressive symptoms for women caring for their husbands with dementia," *Journal of the American Geriatrics Society*, vol. 56, no. 2, pp. 322–327, 2008.

[11] D. Shub and M. E. Kunik, "Psychiatric comorbidity in persons with dementia: assessment and treatment strategies," *Psychiatric Times*, vol. 26, no. 4, pp. 32–36, 2009.

[12] M. Raivio, U. Eloniemi-Sulkava, M.-L. Laakkonen et al., "How do officially organized services meet the needs of elderly caregivers and their spouses with Alzheimer's disease?" *American Journal of Alzheimer's Disease and other Dementias*, vol. 22, no. 5, pp. 360–368, 2007.

[13] L. Froelich, N. Andreasen, M. Tsolaki et al., "Long-term treatment of patients with Alzheimer's disease in primary and secondary care: results from an international survey," *Current Medical Research and Opinion*, vol. 25, no. 12, pp. 3058–3068, 2009.

[14] S. Turner, S. Iliffe, M. Downs et al., "General practitioners' knowledge, confidence and attitudes in the diagnosis and management of dementia," *Age and Ageing*, vol. 33, no. 5, pp. 461–467, 2004.

[15] M. Tsolaki, S. Paraskevi, N. Degleris, and S. Karamavrou, "Attitudes and perceptions regarding alzheimer's disease in Greece," *The American Journal of Alzheimer's Disease and other Dementias*, vol. 24, no. 1, pp. 21–26, 2009.

[16] K. N. Fountoulakis, M. Tsolaki, R. C. Mohs, and A. Kazis, "Epidemiological Dementia Index: A screening instrument for Alzheimer's disease and other types of dementia suitable for use in populations with low education level," *Dementia and Geriatric Cognitive Disorders*, vol. 9, no. 6, pp. 329–338, 1998.

[17] S. Argyriadou, H. Melissopoulou, E. Krania, A. Karagiannidou, I. Vlachonicolis, and C. Lionis, "Dementia and depression: two frequent disorders of the aged in primary health care in Greece," *Family Practice*, vol. 18, no. 1, pp. 87–91, 2001.

[18] M. Tsolaki, K. Fountoulakis, E. Chantzi, and A. Kazis, "Risk factors for clinically diagnosed Alzheimer's disease: a case-control study of a Greek population," *International Psychogeriatrics*, vol. 9, no. 3, pp. 327–341, 1997.

[19] M. Tsolaki, C. Fountoulakis, I. Pavlopoulos, E. Chatzi, and A. Kazis, "Prevalence and incidence of Alzheimer's disease and other dementing disorders in Pylea, Greece," *American Journal of Alzheimer's Disease*, vol. 14, no. 3, pp. 138–148, 1999.

[20] R. W. Keefover, E. D. Rankin, P. M. Keyl, J. C. Wells, J. Martin, and J. Shaw, "Dementing illnesses in rural populations: the need for research and challenges confronting investigators," *Journal of Rural Health*, vol. 12, no. 3, pp. 178–187, 1996.

[21] J. Byles, J. Powers, C. Chojenta, and P. Warner-Smith, "Older women in Australia: ageing in urban, rural and remote environments," *Australasian Journal on Ageing*, vol. 25, no. 3, pp. 151–157, 2006.

[22] H. Brodaty, C. Thomson, C. Thompson, and M. Fine, "Why caregivers of people with dementia and memory loss don't use services," *International Journal of Geriatric Psychiatry*, vol. 20, no. 6, pp. 537–546, 2005.

[23] N. Kontodimopoulos, P. Nanos, and D. Niakas, "Balancing efficiency of health services and equity of access in remote areas in Greece," *Health Policy*, vol. 76, no. 1, pp. 49–57, 2006.

[24] Alzheimer's Association, "Alzheimer's disease facts and figures," *Alzheimer's and Dementia*, vol. 5, no. 3, pp. 234–270, 2009.

[25] N. A. Azad, M. Al Bugami, and I. Loy-English, "Gender differences in dementia risk factors," *Gender Medicine*, vol. 4, no. 2, pp. 120–129, 2007.

[26] P. S. Mathuranath, P. J. Cherian, R. Mathew et al., "Dementia in Kerala, South India: prevalence and influence of age, education and gender," *International Journal of Geriatric Psychiatry*, vol. 25, no. 3, pp. 290–297, 2010.

[27] A. Douzenis, I. Michopoulos, R. Gournellis et al., "Cognitive decline and dementia in elderly medical inpatients remain

underestimated and underdiagnosed in a recently established university general hospital in Greece," *Archives of Gerontology and Geriatrics*, vol. 50, no. 2, pp. 147–150, 2010.

[28] C. G. Lyketsos, O. Lopez, B. Jones, A. L. Fitzpatrick, J. Breitner, and S. Dekosky, "Prevalence of neuropsychiatric symptoms in dementia and mild cognitive impairment: results from the cardiovascular health study," *The Journal of the American Medical Association*, vol. 288, no. 12, pp. 1475–1483, 2002.

[29] G. Ravaglia, P. Forti, F. Montesi et al., "Mild cognitive impairment: epidemiology and dementia risk in an elderly Italian population," *Journal of the American Geriatrics Society*, vol. 56, no. 1, pp. 51–58, 2008.

[30] P. Fischer, S. Jungwirth, S. Zehetmayer et al., "Conversion from subtypes of mild cognitive impairment to Alzheimer dementia," *Neurology*, vol. 68, no. 4, pp. 288–291, 2007.

[31] G. Waldemar, K. T. T. Phung, A. Burns et al., "Access to diagnostic evaluation and treatment for dementia in Europe," *International Journal of Geriatric Psychiatry*, vol. 22, no. 1, pp. 47–54, 2007.

[32] Y. Tountas, N. Oikonomou, G. Pallikarona et al., "Sociodemographic and socioeconomic determinants of health services utilization in Greece: the Hellas Health I study," *Health Services Management Research*, vol. 24, no. 1, pp. 8–18, 2011.

[33] M. P. R. DesMeules, C. Lagace, D. Heng, D. Manuel, and R. Pitblado, "How healthy are rural Canadians? An assessment of their health status and health determinants," in *Book How Healthy Are Rural Canadians? An Assessment of Their Health Status and Health Determinants*, Canadian Institute for Health Information, Ottawa, Canada, 2006.

[34] N. Bouzas, "Poverty and social exclusion in rural areas," in *Book Poverty and Social Exclusion in Rural Areas*, European Communities, 2008.

[35] E. Pappa, N. Kontodimopoulos, A. A. Papadopoulos, Y. Tountas, and D. Niakas, "Prescribed-drug utilization and polypharmacy in a general population in Greece: association with sociodemographic, health needs, health-services utilization, and lifestyle factors," *European Journal of Clinical Pharmacology*, vol. 67, no. 2, pp. 185–192, 2011.

18

The Knowledge Concealed in Users' Narratives, Valuing Clients' Experiences as Coherent Knowledge in Their Own Right

Ragnfrid Kogstad,[1] Tor-Johan Ekeland,[2] and Jan Kaare Hummelvoll[1]

[1] *Hedmark University College, 2418 Elverum, Norway*
[2] *Volda University College, 6101 Volda, Norway*

Correspondence should be addressed to Ragnfrid Kogstad; ragnfrid.kogstad@hihm.no

Academic Editor: Christine M. Blasey

Objective. As the history of psychiatry has been written, users have told their stories and often presented pictures incompatible with the professional or official versions. We ask if such a gap still exists and what the ethical as well as epistemological implications may be. *Study Design*. The design is based on a hermeneutic-phenomenological approach, with a qualitative content analysis of the narratives. *Data Sources*. The paper draws on user narratives written after the year 2000, describing positive and negative experiences with the mental health services. *Extraction Methods*. Among 972 users answering a questionnaire, 492 also answered the open questions and wrote one or two stories. We received 715 stories. 610 contained enough information to be included in this narrative analysis. *Principal Findings*. The stories are coherent, containing traditional narrative plots, but reports about miscommunication, rejection, lack of responsiveness, and humiliation are numerous. *Conclusions*. The picture drawn from this material has ethical as well as epistemological implications and motivates reflections upon theoretical and practical consequences when users' experiences do not influence professional knowledge to a larger degree.

1. Introduction

The stories from a subjective or patient perspective have followed the official story of psychiatry like a side stream [1–3]. Listening to the nonexperts, "ordinary people" or "victims of history" [4], has a long tradition in social science. Women, workers, the colonialized, religious minorities, prisoners, the ill, and also the "mad" have in turn had their voices heard. But listening to valuing and appreciating the stories of the mentally disabled has been a more complicated case and has needed more time for reasons we will return to. As expressed by Molinari [5] there has been a kind of an unequal relationship between the client who writes to express his/her truth and the professional reader who reads the story to confirm his/her diagnosis.

Even if users' perspective gradually has been set on the agenda and user involvement is established as a method for improving the health services [6–8], user involvement in the field of mental health care still does not avoid the asymmetrical relations between users and professionals, not the least because of the possibility of diagnosing users' opinions [9]

rather than receiving their feedback and narratives as helpful corrections necessary in the process of improving the delivery of health services. As a consequence user involvement may be regarded only as an empowerment strategy for users and not a method by which professionals may also achieve new insights [10]. Then, necessary changes in the health services aiming at mutual collaboration may be neglected. Barker [11] holds that it is not the professionals who empower the patient; it is the person with mental illness who is in position to empower the professional. The only way to be of real service is to learn from the person. Having learned what to do for the patient, from him/her, the professionals can gain some understanding or insights, which changes them, however imperceptibly. This change in professional attitude influences the next interactions and so on (page 321).

2. The Aim of the Study

The study aims to analyse clients' stories written after the year 2000 and reflect upon the message in the stories as well as how clients experience that their stories are received and used in the process of improving the health services. Further, clients' variegated experiences and the need to communicate those experiences to leaders and professional experts are discussed from ethical and epistemological perspectives.

3. Methodology

The paper refers to a data material consisting of 492 users' narratives about meetings with the mental health service system [12]. The narratives were written in response to two open questions at the end of a comprehensive questionnaire: (1) Would you like to tell a story from a special meeting with a helper or a health service system that represented a turning point in your life? and (2) If you have had strong negative experiences, would you like to describe such an event?

Our methodology is anchored in a hermeneutic-phenomenological tradition, focusing on individuals' subjective experiences and interpretations, where credibility depends on the coherence in the argument [13, 14]. Further, we use elements from narrative methods in order to shed light on common narrative plots, power relations, and the implications of speaking from a nonhegemonic position [15].

Narratives can be defined in different ways, but in this paper we use the much employed definitions of Hydén [16], Edwards [17], and Mishler [18] who define narratives as stories written in a coherent way, aiming at explaining and making sense of events, legitimating actions and reactions, confirming identity, and adding meaning to experiences. Mishler [18] also maintains that the presentation and confirmation of identity is a constant factor in all personal narratives and is related to the creation of meaning. The construction of plots, understood as phrases describing a cause, an effect, and a link between them, informs the kind of meaning that is added to the experience and how cause, effect, and meaning are perceived [19].

4. Respondents

The data we refer to was selected from a larger study carried out in cooperation with the national user organization, Mental Health Norway (MHN). MHN was chosen because it is the largest user organization. The organization has a reasonable well-functioning relationship with the government; for example, MHN regularly serves as a consultative body and an administrative system which could assist in the collection of data. During the period of data collection, there were about 5000 members spread over the whole country. About 4000 of them, chosen randomly, were invited to take part in the study. Nearly 1/4 responded. The user organization Mental Health Norway could not provide any information about the profile of their member group (like age, gender, occupation, social security support, or experiences with the help service system), but the spread we found regarding the mentioned indicators tells that the experiences are applicable for several groups of people. 492 of the respondents (151 men and 341 women, aged 19–90 years) also answered one or both of the two open questions at the end of the questionnaire. 223 of

the respondents reported both a positive and a negative story, while 112 wrote only a negative story and 157 wrote only a positive story. In total we got 715 stories, some with a lot of information and others with not enough information to have them categorised in any way. The latter stories were excluded from the analysis and consequently 610 stories remained for the categorisation process. The respondents who were included in the categorisation process have experiences from all parts of the mental health care system, traditional psychiatric institutions, outpatient clinics, day centres, and individual therapy. 67% received disability pension, 13% had a job, and 20% combined disability pension with a job or studies.

The narratives were analysed by qualitative content analysis [20]. The stories were read through several times in order to discover themes embedded in the texts and to obtain a sense of the whole. Manifest content in the texts is presented as categories that may also be seen as expressions of the latent content. The presentation of meaning units in categories is based on the researcher's judgment and validated in a process where the researchers proposed categorization independently of each other.

5. The Narratives

In the following we present an overview of themes emerging from the stories and thereafter some example stories, chosen from all the four main categories as shown in Table 1 and which also illustrate two overriding narrative plots: the search for meaning and the confirmation of identity. Recognizing clients' stories as coherent and valuable knowledge is then discussed from ethical and epistemological perspectives.

When studying the therapeutic framework described in the stories we found—as shown in the table—two main themes: a mainly psychiatric medical approach and a humanistic-existential psychosocial approach [21]. Under each theme there were two main categories: (1) the help service experienced as being beneficial and (2) negative experiences related to rejection, humiliation, or threats. The majority of positive experiences were found where a humanistic-existential psychosocial approach was dominating and the majority of negative experiences were found in a medical context where diagnoses and medicines were the dominating means by which the clients were met.

5.1. The Creation of Meaning as a Narrative Feature. From a humanistic perspective the meaning dimension is essential to human beings [19, 22, 23]. By telling our stories we can create meaning by establishing a culture-specific sense of order, which makes life worth living [24–26]. The following stories illustrate how the mental health clients' stories display deeply human traits and deserve status as coherent knowledge in their own right and how the experience of meaning is related to (a) regaining a feeling of worth and dignity, (b) realizing that hardships can give insights and increased ability to understand and help other people, (c) discovering connections between earlier assaults and depression or anxiety, and (d) putting life experiences together in a story which can be imparted and contribute to the richness of life stories.

TABLE 1: A summary of all the narrative themes under four main categories.

Psychiatric medical approach	Humanistic-existential psychosocial approach
Medical-instrumental help experienced as beneficial ($n = 18$)	Positive experiences with psychosocial and social help and support ($n = 297$)
Beneficial medication practice	Traumas worked through
Medicines and following up	Working through traumas
Medicines that functioned ok	Obtained selfinsight
Helped to reduce medicines	A new start and quality of life
Diagnosis experienced as a relief	Experienced community
Enough time for diagnosis	Trust, confidence, and feeling of worth
Diagnosis and following up	Spiritual experiences
The experience that service is available	Peer support and network
Access to hospital	Welfare/socio-economic help
Hospital as a place of refuge in crisis	Practical help
	Housing and activities
Psychiatric-medical help experienced as threatening and humiliating ($n = 225$)	Rejection and encroachment in therapeutic relations with a humanistic-existential psychosocial approach ($n = 70$)
Experienced rejection and isolation in treatment context	
Not taken seriously	Bad communication
Rejection, lack of treatment	Miscommunication
Just stored away, no following up	No understanding
Strain caused by treatment	Client's dilemma rejected
Medicines abruptly removed	Childhood/trauma rejected
Negative side effects of medicines	Persuasion to divorce
Wrong diagnosis	Children not cared about when parents were sent to hospital/received help
Disrespect and threat to integrity	Unethical behavior from the therapist
Compulsion, punishment	Inappropriate behavior from the therapist
Treated violently	Appointments not respected
Accusations, infringements	

I had taken an overdose of medicines and was an in-patient at a local hospital. I made very good contact with a nurse there. She sat down at my bedside and talked to me. Gave me a good lotion after I had cut my arms with a broken piece of mirror and gave me the whole tube and a hug when I was sent to the psychiatric ward. I will never forget her! Woman, age 31.

To me the organisation MHN (Mental Health Norway) meant more than "the good helpers" I met in hospital 1.5 years ago. To experience fellowship and the feeling that you are doing something useful for others means quite a lot. Woman, age 45.

In the hospital I took part in body-oriented therapy. Then I got into contact with forgotten experiences from my childhood, experiences that my body remembered. It was a very painful experience and I needed years to heal the wounds. But this experience was a breakthrough in the effort to recover, and many questions were answered. Woman, age 54.

The narratives contain several plots describing relations between being labelled as a psychiatric patient and various kinds of rejections. The meaning dimension appeared when the clients were given the opportunity to present their own coherent stories about what had happened:

The chief physician wanted to give me 16 mg Trilafon. My experience told me that I then would be totally unable to think. 8 mg was enough to get me on my feet again. Then I was medicated by force, held by 4-5 persons while I got an injection in my buttocks. Gradually they discovered that I did not resist. Because I was also sexually abused as a child this was a horrible experience that still causes me to shiver as I write it down. It was good to have the opportunity to write about it. Man, aged 50.

5.2. The Confirmation of Identity. Narrative properties like efforts to confirm or protect identity and also to give rational reasons for the way of acting are clearly projecting in this material, but in addition some extra dimensions related to the confirmation of identity were discovered; the expressions of disempowerment and the unusual strong efforts to confirm identity and justify oneself as a rational being are as follows.

I was afraid and thought someone would kill me. I was prevented from talking to the doctor and locked myself into the bathroom. The water warmed and comforted me. They came in. I said: Do not touch me; I will go to my room. They did touch me. I got angry. I am sad I did not write this when I was angry and felt I was not listened to. I bit the woman who touch me and tore up her blouse. She got angry and wouldn't let me talk. I was awake the whole night because of anxiety. She reported how hopeless I was. I think she should have listened to me; maybe we could have avoided the episode in the bathroom if she had called the doctor. I did not trust her, that's the reason I could not tell her anything. When I locked the door to the bathroom I can understand that they maybe were worried about me, but it was not necessary to touch me, because I would have gone myself and, furthermore, I was in a humiliating situation there in the bathtub. I did pay for the blouse. Woman, age 62.

Most of the negative stories are reports about the lack of responsiveness, which invoke feelings of rejection as well as humiliation. Besides they illustrate that feedback from clients is neither necessarily welcomed nor used to improve the quality of the services.

To be taken care of, listened to, respected, and supported means that pain and suffering is made bearable and several informants reported that relations marked by these qualities helped them back to a normal life and even to a richer life than before.

For 13 years I had the help line number for the anxiety self-help organisation on my bulletin board. I did not dare to call. But then I decided that I had to. I called. After the talk I dared to visit them. When meeting the leader I for the first time experienced not to be alone with my bottomless shame. Other people had the same experiences. This happened one year ago and today I feel that life is opening up. Woman, age 44.

The need to confirm or reestablish identity seems to be of special importance when a client's dignity has been threatened or lost due to a humiliating process in the course of treatment. The disempowered client language and the efforts several informants spend on confirming identity emerge as the most interesting discoveries when looking for narrative plots in the clients' stories. An underlying message is about the need to reclaim dignity, which in turn means integration of the experience of lost honour [27, 28]. Reshaping identity may involve a new kind of honesty meaning that there is no reason to pretend, thus being willing to reveal what has threatened the self-image and sense of dignity. A main question concerns the health service system's ability to understand the processes that represent a threat to the person's integrity and the implications of lost dignity.

It is a paradox that the experience of lost honour is often related to being a client in the health service system. Important information about the social order is embedded in this paradox. Stories about compassionate encounters marked by responsiveness, genuine care, and empathetic understanding do not have the same need of strong legitimating explanations.

After having fought with all kinds of bureaucracy and systems I at last considered committing suicide as a final escape. In desperation and by accident I passed a house where Catholic monks lived. I am not a Catholic, but was met with incredible

warmth and not least, respect. The brother invited me inside and we talked until I felt able to walk home. Later we had several talks about thoughts I was struggling with. The brother's genuine wish to help showed through and he offered to engage himself also beyond the conversations. Until this day I have never met a person with an equivalent capacity to look into the soul and meet another person on this person's premise. I could also contact him whenever I wanted. This caused me to restrain myself, but I still experienced the feeling of security. Man, age 43.

The stories have illustrated the search for meaning as well as efforts to confirm identity. The composition of plots is an overall demonstration about rationally described connections between the users' earlier or recent experiences and their present situation and exemplifies the strong need of experiencing meaning and confirming identity. At the same time they inform on personal experiences and knowledge which can benefit the health service system if listened to and taken seriously.

The efforts to demonstrate rationality appeared as extra strong when the users described situations where their identity and honour were threatened. Very detailed descriptions about what happened and why tell about feelings of powerlessness or that understanding cannot be taken for granted. Situations of powerlessness and threatened identity also informed about a distance gap experienced between the way services were delivered and what the users themselves regarded as beneficial.

6. Ethical Reasons for Recognising Clients' Stories as Coherent Knowledge

Ethics concerns protecting dignity and respecting integrity and represents fundamental values in human relations. In research, these ethical principles should always be considered. Schaanning [29] has suggested that in a situation where we can no longer relate to a final truth as being the "last instance" ethics should take on the role of being this "last instance." Research will then be evaluated by its ability to facilitate the implementation of actions to the good, improve human conditions and preserve dignity, and empower patients to exercise increased control over their lives [30–32]. But in the field of mental health care ethical guidelines can also contribute to the silencing of clients' voices, as protection barriers are set up against discussing personal subjects with "vulnerable" persons [33]. This emerges as a paradox as there are no indications that mental health clients themselves want this special protection. In fact, being able to relate their tales of suffering could be a way for the person to find an opening to their inner worlds and interpretations of what has been experienced and thus serve an essential path towards its alleviation (cf. [34]). The mentioned ethical guidelines stem from a paternalistic attitude saying that vulnerability in this field may be related to lack of self-insight or ability to handle one's own emotions. So, ethical guidelines by themselves do not necessarily protect clients' interests, which further points to the importance of upholding clients' right to tell their stories and making dialogic communication a main ethical concern [35–37]. As underlined by Bachtin [38] dialogic communication is the essential realm of humans and "to deny the dialogue is to deny the human being" ([38]: 282).

Users' perspectives and users' choices have been on the agenda for some decades, but there have been unsaid reservations, as highlighted by Morrison et al. [39], asking, antipsychotics, is it time to introduce patient choice? As mental health services have for decades been dominated by the psychopharmacological "revolution," stigmatisation, and lack of response to clients' expressed needs can hardly be understood without observing the tradition which allows professionals to medicate clients without their free and informed consent [40]. To Barker and Buchanan-Barker [41] this concerns the major ethical dilemma, that is, autonomy versus paternalism in the field of mental health. They criticise the ethical literature for avoiding dilemmas raised by the use of coercion, for contributing to the confusion over the nature of "mental disorder," and for embracing the misplaced paternalism they see as part of the medical tradition. If there is a single psychiatric "truth" they say, "it is that people had a better chance of recovery from a psychiatric 'breakdown' *before* the advent of psychiatric drugs 60 years ago, than they do today" ([41]: 455, see also [42]). Given this knowledge the use of coercion as well as a nonresponsive attitude in general raises serious ethical questions concerning autonomy and lack of reciprocity in therapeutic settings. A disputable scientific fundament is not, according to human rights' legislation [43], able to justify the serious encroachments into peoples' lives we talk about here. The convention on the rights of people with disabilities [44] then takes further steps to transform mental health users' status according to ethical standards, by among others underlining legal capacity as a universal property (art 12) and the universal right to healthcare including being on the basis of free and informed consent (art 25). Ethical reasons then also have become legal reasons, which will support the process of implementing ethical standards related to the recognition of clients' voices.

7. Epistemological Tensions in the Field of Mental Health Care

Users' own stories have challenged the history of psychiatry and also become assimilated into it so that tensions between users' and professionals' understandings are partly transformed into tensions between two different professional and epistemological approaches where roughly spoken the first one sees the evolution of psychiatry as associated with progress made in biomedicine while the other contributes by reflecting about context and how society influences the development of mental illness and how we perceive it [3]. The division may be traced back to different sources. By the writings of Foucault [45], Scheff [46], and Goffman [47] the ideological aspects behind all historical analyses became visible and also the relations between broader social trends like social disciplining, regulations, division of labour, definitions of deviation, and stigma processes on one hand and how we define and handle mental disabilities on the other hand. In philosophy and psychology a new concept of

Self originated as studies into rationality and consciousness revealed human beings as less rational and with a less stable Self than presumed earlier [29, 48]. This new concept of Self also contributed to changed attitudes about madness and influenced treatment institutions. Both critical approaches advocating contextual understanding and new insights into human beings' limited rationality seem to have strengthened the arguments for listening to the "voices from below" and confirmed patients' right to possess their own clinical experience [3].

Along with controversies over the rationality of human beings in general, the dispute between professional approaches concerning mental patients' lack of self-insight still goes on. Even if attempts at defining the insight phenomenon are scarce [49, 50], information about the opinions and experiences of mental health clients is lost to a greater degree compared to information obtained from other groups of clients, which may be explained by the fact that the voice of the client is often seen as less valid because he/she is receiving mental health care [51].

In the postpsychiatry movement, it seems like clients' perspectives emerge as a critical element without denying traditional psychiatry as a science [52]. Maybe this movement can bridge the gap between the two approaches. But looking at the different ways psychoses are understood: as from outside, as biological defects which can be objectified, independent of the individual, or as a phenomenon anchored in fundamental human conditions and something that should be understood from inside, in the light of the subject's own experiences [53, 54], the bridge is not easily discovered.

Psychoses seen as pure irrationality sustain the impression that mental health clients lack self-insight to a larger degree than other groups of clients. In order to have clients' experiences accepted as coherent knowledge in their own right, it seems important to accept the need of reciprocity and trust that the dialogue can be reestablished also in situations of confusion and seemingly irrationality.

8. Conclusion

The clients' narratives emerge as coherent and with obvious plots and are also often marked by less typical characteristics like the very strong efforts to confirm identity and demonstrate rationality and sometimes a kind of honesty or self-exposure which can best be understood in relation to a need of integrating the experience of lost honour. The common factor is the need to, and the importance of, being recognized as a subject. Several narratives—by illustrating the lack of responsiveness—repeatedly demonstrate the existence of a gap between users' and professionals' discourses. A main reason seems to be a hegemonic, professional discourse creating distance to users' own experiences and counteracting equal dialogues. Users' voices are still to a large degree silenced by an objectifying epistemology. Thereby the health services are also deprived of information that would be essential for planning, management, and further improvements in the field of mental health care.

Ethical Approval

The project was registered at the Norwegian Social Science Database (NSD) which has delegated authority from the Data Inspectorate of Norway to accept investigations in which sensitive, personal information is involved. The collecting of data organised in such a way that the researchers were unable to identify the informants. In practice the user organisation had ownership of the investigation and asked its own members to participate.

Conflict of Interests

The authors declare that there is no conflict of interests regarding the publication of this paper.

References

[1] R. Porter, *A Social History of Madness. Stories of the Insane*, Weidenfeld and Nicholson, London, UK, 1987.

[2] A. J. W. Andersen and I. B. Larsen, "Hell on earth: textual reflections on the experience of mental illness," *Journal of Mental Health*, vol. 21, no. 2, pp. 174–181, 2012.

[3] R. Huertas, "Another history for another psychiatry. The patient's view," *Culture & History*, vol. 2, no. 1, 2013.

[4] G. Lefevbre, *Les Payans Du Nord Pendant La Revolution Francaise*, C. Robbe, Lille, France, 1924.

[5] A. Molinari, "Autobiografias de mujeres en un manicomio italiano a principios del siglo XX," in *Letras Bajo Sospecha. Escritura y Lectura en Centros de Internamiento*, A. Castillo, V. Sierra, and G. Trea, Eds., pp. 79–96, 2005.

[6] B. Williams and G. Grant, "Defining people-centredness: making the implicit explicit," *Health and Social Care in the Community*, vol. 6, no. 2, pp. 84–94, 1998.

[7] T. A. Andreassen, *User Involvement, Policy and the Welfare State. Dr. Polit Dissertation [Ph.D. thesis]*, Institute of Sociology and Social Geography, University of Oslo, 2004.

[8] Health Directorate of Norway, *User Involvement in Mental Health Care. Objectives, Recommendations and Actions*, The Norwegian Directorate of Health, 2006.

[9] P. Beresford and A. Wilson, "Genes spell danger: mental health service users/survivors, bioethics and control," *Disability & Society*, vol. 17, no. 5, pp. 541–553, 2002.

[10] T. A. Andreassen, "When users are not taken seriously," *Journal of Welfare Research*, vol. 10, no. 1, pp. 3–14, 2007.

[11] P. Barker, *Assessment in Psychiatric and Mental Health Nursing. In Search of the Whole Person*, Stanley Thornes, Cheltenham, UK, 1997.

[12] R. Kogstad, *Stories from other positions [Ph.D. thesis]*, Faculty of Medicine, University of Oslo, 2011.

[13] J. K. Hummelvoll and A. B. da Silva, "The use of the qualitative research interview to uncover the essence of community psychiatric nursing: methodological reflections," *Journal of Holistic Nursing*, vol. 16, no. 4, pp. 453–478, 1998.

[14] H. Starks and S. B. Trinidad, "Choose your method: a comparison of phenomenology, discourse analysis, and grounded theory," *Qualitative Health Research*, vol. 17, no. 10, pp. 1372–1380, 2007.

[15] A. Jaworski and N. Coupland, "Introduction: perspectives on discourse analysis," in *The Discourse Reader*, A. Jaworski and N. Coupland, Eds., Taylor & Francis Group, Routledge, New York, NY, USA, 2nd edition, 2006.

[16] L. C. Hydén, "The numerous stories," in *To Study Narratives*, L. C. Hydén and M. Hydén, Eds., Liber AB, Stockholm, Sweden, 1997.

[17] D. Edwards, "Narrative analysis," in *The Discourse Reader*, A. Jaworski and N. Coupland, Eds., Taylor & Francis, Routledge, New York, NY, USA, 2nd edition, 2006.

[18] E. G. Mishler, *Research Interviewing: Context and Narrative*, Harvard University Press, Cambridge, Mass, USA, 1986.

[19] D. E. Polkinghorne, *Narrative Knowing and the Human Sciences*, State University of New York, New York, NY, USA, 1988.

[20] U. H. Graneheim and B. Lundman, "Qualitative content analysis in nursing research: concepts, procedures and measures to achieve trustworthiness," *Nurse Education Today*, vol. 24, no. 2, pp. 105–112, 2004.

[21] R. E. Kogstad, J. K. Hummelvoll, and B. G. Eriksson, "User experiences of different treatment cultures in mental health care," *Ethical Human Psychology and Psychiatry*, vol. 11, no. 2, pp. 97–111, 2009.

[22] A. Giddens, *New Rules of Sociological Method: A Positive Critique of Interpretative Sociologies*, Stanford University Press, 1993.

[23] C. Mattingly and L. C. Garro, *Narrative and the Cultural Construction of Illness and Healing*, Berkeley University of California Press, 2000.

[24] J. Lacan, *The Symbolic*, Selected Drafts, By Svein Haugsgjerd, Gyldendal, Oslo, Norway, 1985.

[25] L. J. Kirmayer, "Healing and the invention of metaphor: the effectiveness of symbols revisited," *Culture, Medicine and Psychiatry*, vol. 17, no. 2, pp. 161–195, 1993.

[26] U. Wikan, "With life on one's lap," in *Narrative and the Cultural Construction of Health and Illness*, C. Mattingly and L. Garro, Eds., Berkeley University of California Press, 2000.

[27] P. Deegan, "Recovery as a journey of the heart," in *Recovery from Severe Mental Illnesses: Research Evidence and Implications for Practice*, L. Davidson, C. Harding, and L. Spaniol, Eds., Center for Psychiatric Rehabilitation, Boston University, 2005.

[28] S. J. Onken, C. M. Craig, P. Ridgway, R. O. Ralph, and J. A. Cook, "An analysis of the definitions and elements of recovery: a review of the literature," *Psychiatric Rehabilitation Journal*, vol. 31, no. 1, pp. 9–22, 2007.

[29] E. Schaanning, *Dissolving Modernity*, Spartacus, Oslo, Norway, 1992.

[30] Y. S. Lincoln and E. Guba, *Naturalistic Inquiry*, Sage, Beverly Hills, Calif, USA, 1985.

[31] S. Kvale, *InterViews. An Introduction To Qualitative Research Inquiry*, Sage, Thousand Oaks, Calif, USA, 1996.

[32] M. W. Jørgensen and L. Philips, *Discourse Analysis as Theory and Method*, Roskilde Universitetsforlag, 1999.

[33] J. K. Hummelvoll, "Forskningsetikk i handlingsorientert forskningssamarbeid med mennesker med psykiske problemer," in *Etiske Utfordringer i Praksisnær Forskning*, J. K. Hummelvoll, E. Andvig, and A. Lyberg, Eds., Gyldendal Akademisk, Oslo, Norway, 2010.

[34] M. Arman and A. Rehnsfeldt, "How can we research human suffering?" *Scandinavian Journal of Caring Sciences*, vol. 20, no. 3, pp. 239–240, 2006.

[35] E. Levinas, *The Other's Humanism*, Thorleif Dahl's Cultural Library, Aschehoug, Oslo, Norway, 1993.

[36] I. B. Neumann, "Meaning, materiality and power," in *An Introduction To Discourse Analysis*, Fagbokforlaget, Bergen, Norway, 2001.

[37] A. Johnsen, R. Sundet, and V. W. Torsteinsson, *Interaction and Self Experience. New Ways in Relation Oriented Therapies*, Tano Aschehoug, Oslo, Norway, 2000.

[38] M. Bachtin, *The Dialogic Word*, Bokfirlaget Anthropos AB, Graabo, Sweden, 1997.

[39] A. P. Morrison, P. Hutton, D. Shiers, and D. Turkington, "Antipsychotics: is it time to introduce patient choice?" *The British Journal of Psychiatry*, vol. 201, pp. 83–84, 2012.

[40] P. Tyrer, "From the editor's desk, The end of the psychopharmacological revolution," *British Journal of Psychiatry*, vol. 201, article 168, 2012.

[41] P. Barker and P. Buchnan-Barker, "First, do no harm: confronting the myths of psychiatric drugs," *Nursing Ethics*, vol. 19, no. 4, pp. 451–463, 2012.

[42] D. Healy, M. Harris, P. Michael et al., "Service utilization in 1896 and 1996: morbidity and mortality data from North Wales," *History of Psychiatry*, vol. 16, no. 1, pp. 27–41, 2005.

[43] ECHR (European Convention on Human Rights), Council of Europe, 1950.

[44] "CRPD (Convention on the Rights of Persons with Disabilities)," Adopted by the United Nation's General Assembly on December 2006.

[45] M. Foucault, *History of Madness in the Classical Age*, Translated by: J. Khalfa & J. Murphy, First Published 1961, Routledge, 2006.

[46] T. J. Scheff, *Being Mentally Ill: A Sociology Theory*, Aldine, Chicago, Ill, USA, 1966.

[47] E. Goffman, *Asylums*, Doubleday, New York, NY, USA, 1961.

[48] D. Kaufmann, *Aufklärung, Selbsterfahrung und Die Erfindung der Psychiatrie in Deutschland, 1770-1850*, Vandenhoeck & Ruprecht, Göttingen, Germany, 1995.

[49] G. Høyer, "On the justification for civil commitment," *Acta Psychiatrica Scandinavica, Supplement*, vol. 101, no. 399, pp. 65–71, 2000.

[50] T. Grisso and P. S. Appelbaum, "Structuring the debate about ethical predictions of future violence," *Law and Human Behavior*, vol. 17, no. 4, pp. 482–485, 1993.

[51] B. Williams, "Users' views of community mental health care," in *Community Care: Evaluation of the Provision of Mental Health Services*, C. Crosby and M. M. Barry, Eds., Brookfield, Avebury, UK, 1995.

[52] P. Bracken and P. Thomas, "Postpsychiatry: a new direction for mental health," *British Medical Journal*, vol. 322, no. 7288, pp. 724–727, 2001.

[53] T.-J. Ekeland, "Ny kunnskap—ny praksis. Et nytt psykisk helsevern," Erfaringskompetanse, nr. 1, 2011.

[54] T.-J. Ekeland, "Kampen om kunnskapen," Morgenbladet, 2013.

19

D-Serine in Neuropsychiatric Disorders: New Advances

Andrea R. Durrant[1] and Uriel Heresco-Levy[1,2]

[1] *Research and Psychiatry Departments, Ezrath Nashim-Herzog Memorial Hospital, P.O. Box 3900, 91035 Jerusalem, Israel*
[2] *Hadassah Medical School, Hebrew University, Jerusalem, Israel*

Correspondence should be addressed to Uriel Heresco-Levy; urielh@ekmd.huji.ac.il

Academic Editor: Raphael J. Braga

D-Serine (DSR) is an endogenous amino acid involved in glia-synapse interactions that has unique neurotransmitter characteristics. DSR acts as obligatory coagonist at the glycine site associated with the N-methyl-D-aspartate subtype of glutamate receptors (NMDAR) and has a cardinal modulatory role in major NMDAR-dependent processes including NMDAR-mediated neurotransmission, neurotoxicity, synaptic plasticity, and cell migration. Since either over- or underfunction of NMDARs may be involved in the pathophysiology of neuropsychiatric disorders; the pharmacological manipulation of DSR signaling represents a major drug development target. A first generation of proof-of-concept animal and clinical studies suggest beneficial DSR effects in treatment-refractory schizophrenia, movement, depression, and anxiety disorders and for the improvement of cognitive performance. A related developing pharmacological strategy is the indirect modification of DSR synaptic levels by use of compounds that alter the function of main enzymes responsible for DSR production and degradation. Accumulating data indicate that, during the next decade, we will witness important advances in the understanding of DSR role that will further contribute to elucidating the causes of neuropsychiatric disorders and will be instrumental in the development of innovative treatments.

1. Introduction

Although the enzyme D-amino-acid oxidase (DAAO) has been identified in higher organisms in 1935 [1], historically, D-amino acids were thought to be absent in mammalian tissue. This dogma was revolutionized at the beginning of 1990's when it was found that abundant quantities of free D-serine (DSR) occur in the mammalian brain, at concentrations comparable with those of classical neurotransmitters and higher than those of most essential amino acids [2, 3]. Presently, DSR is considered the most biologically active D-amino acid described in mammalian systems [4]. Phylogenetically, its concentrations appear to be extremely low in the brains of fish, amphibians, and birds, suggesting that endogenous DSR is specifically maintained at high levels in the mammalian brain among vertebrates [5].

In the late 1990s, it was demonstrated that DSR is an obligatory endogenous coagonist of the N-methyl-D-aspartate receptor (NMDAR), functioning *in vivo* as a specific and potent full agonist at the NMDAR-associated glycine (GLY)

modulatory site (GMS). The NMDAR subtype of glutamate (GLU) receptors is widely expressed in the central nervous system (CNS) and has a cardinal role in activity-dependent changes in synaptic strength and connectivity underlying higher brain functions such as memory and learning [6, 7]. Unlike other neurotransmitter receptors, which are activated by individual neurotransmitters, NMDARs activation requires, in addition to the agonist GLU, the binding of a coagonist which was originally thought to be GLY [8, 9]. However, research over the last decade indicates that significant amounts of DSR are produced in the CNS [10–12], where DSR is converted from L-serine by serine racemase (SR) and is degraded by DAAO [11–13]. Furthermore, functional studies demonstrate that DSR represents the physiological ligand for the GMS in different brain areas including cortex and hippocampus [14–18], hypothalamus [19], and the retina [20, 21].

DSR has a cardinal modulatory role in major NMDAR-dependent processes, including NMDAR neurotransmission [22], neurotoxicity [23, 24], synaptic plasticity, [21] and cell migration [25]. Either over- or underfunction of NMDAR neurotransmission may elicit neurotoxicity, leading to behavioral and cognitive dysfunction. NMDAR hyperactivity can cause cell death mediated by excitotoxic calcium overload [26, 27] in stroke and neurodegenerative disorders such as Alzheimer's disease (AD) [28, 29]. By contrast, synaptic NMDAR hypoactivity leads to apoptosis [30, 31] and may contribute to the generation of psychotic symptoms and cognitive deficits. The long standing paradox that NMDARs can both promote neuronal health and kill neurons [32] highlights the importance of a strictly regulated optimal NMDAR function. Within this context, DSR modulation appears to play a critical role in the achievement of balanced NMDAR activity. Furthermore, compelling evidence suggests that dysfunctional DSR signaling may be involved in the pathophysiology of neuropsychiatry disorders.

2. D-Serine Neurobiology: An Overview

Despite notable progress in the 20 years since DSR was first identified, many aspects of DSR neurobiology remain enigmatic and are presently the focus of intense research. In contrast to classic neurotransmitters, DSR was originally shown to be exclusively produced and released from astrocytes *via* a vesicular release mechanism [33–35]. However, although glial DSR is prominent, DSR presence was subsequently identified in neurons as well [23]. Some studies have found DSR in most or in a subset of neurons in the cerebral cortex [36], whereas others observed DSR mainly in hindbrain neurons [37, 38]. Recent data indicate that DSR is predominantly expressed in glutamatergic neurons further challenging the notion that DSR is exclusively released from astrocytes [23, 39–41]. Furthermore, it was reported that neurons robustly release endogenous DSR [42] and that neuronal DSR release *via* the amino acid transporter Asc-1 enhances NMDAR potentials and long term potentiation (LTP), a cellular mechanism that underlies learning and memory [43]. The presence of DSR in neurons led to an updated DSR signaling model (rev. in [34, 44]) which incorporates the release and uptake of DSR from both neurons and astrocytes (see Figure 1). This model emphasizes DSR role in the neuron-glia cross-talk relevant to NMDAR function modulation and allows for conceivably distinct roles of glial and neuronal DSR in both physiological and disturbed NMDAR function.

NMDAR is a tetramer composed of two NR1 subunits and two NR2 subunits or less commonly two NR3 subunits. NMDAR activation requires the binding of either GLY or DSR at the GMS on the NR1 subunit [45, 46]. DSR is enriched in corticolimbic regions of the brain where its localization closely parallels that of NMDARs [46] and is thought to be the primary forebrain NMDAR coagonist. SR is considered the primary endogenous source of DSR (using L-serine as a substrate), while DAAO is generally regarded as its primary mechanism of degradation. This view is however confounded by the fact that SR also degrades both DSR and L-serine irreversibly to pyruvate and ammonia, appearing thus to provide a bidirectional regulation of free serine levels *in vivo* [4]. Synaptic DSR is taken up into glia

and neurons differentially *via* Asc-1 and ASCT-2 transporters and is broken down mainly by peroxisomal DAAO forming the alpha-keto acid (AKA), ammonia, and hydrogen peroxide (Figure 1).

As a physiological coagonist of NMDARs, DSR may play a role in NMDAR-dependent neurodegeneration and can mediate neurotoxicity in primary cultures and hippocampal slices [23, 24]. Selective DSR degradation by DAAO markedly reduces NMDAR neurotransmission in cortical and hippocampal preparations [22, 47]. Moreover, DSR depletion in the medial prefrontal cerebral cortex diminishes NMDAR synaptic potentials and prevents LTP inhibition [48]. Recent data suggests that DSR release from astrocytes controls NMDAR-dependent plasticity and LTP in many thousands of excitatory synapses nearby [49], while in adulthood, neuronally-derived DSR regulates neuronal dendritic architecture in the somatosensory cortex [39].

Although they are both endogenous NMDAR coagonists, GLY and DSR seem to act at distinct receptor populations, with DSR present at synaptic NMDARs and GLY at their extrasynaptic counterparts [47], which may constitute a functionally distinct pool of receptors (rev. in [32, 47]). Synaptic NMDARs are responsible for inducing the most common forms of synaptic plasticity found in the brain, namely, LTP and long-term depression (LTD). Whether specific subsets of synaptic NMDARs mediate LTP or LTD [50–54] and whether extrasynaptic receptors also play a role in these processes [55] are controversial. Extrasynaptic NMDARs contribute to neuronal synchronization [56, 57] but have mostly been implicated in neurodegenerative disorders, including stroke, AD, and Huntington's disease [58–60]. Recent evidence suggests that synaptic NMDARs are neuroprotective, whereas extrasynaptic receptors may promote cell death [32].

Overall, the complexities involved in the neurobiology of DSR-based signaling in the human brain are expected to further unravel during the coming decade and contribute to the understanding of a novel and complex neurotransmitter system and to the development of innovative pharmacotherapy for neuropsychiatric disorders.

3. D-Serine Therapeutic Potential

NMDARs crucial role in both physiological and pathophysiological processes has generated massive clinical interest in the development of novel pharmacological interventions aiming at NMDAR-related therapeutic targets. Since direct stimulation of NMDAR with GLU or aspartate, agonists of the primary GLU receptor site, is associated with neurotoxicity [68], most of the efforts to date have focused on the GMS. The main compounds directly acting at this site that have been so far assessed in clinical trials include GLY, DSR, and D-cycloserine (DCS), a tuberculostatic antibiotic having also complex agonist/antagonist action at the GMS [69]. In this context, a number of advantages are associated with DSR use, including better blood-brain-barrier penetration and stronger affinity at the GMS *versus* GLY [70] and, in contrast to DCS, specific and potent full agonist action at this site. Accordingly, during the last two decades, the first proof-of-concept animal and clinical studies have been performed with

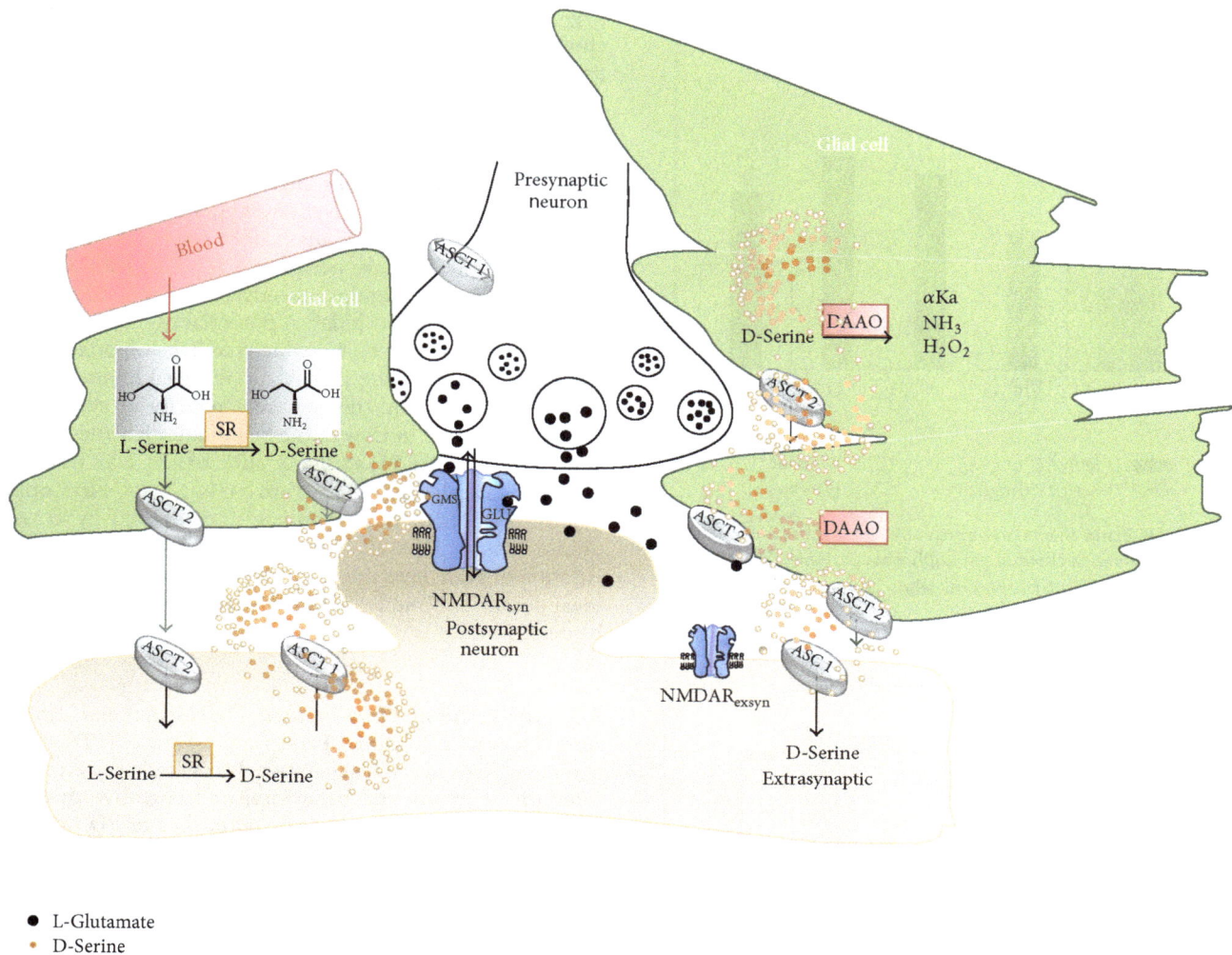

- ● L-Glutamate
- • D-Serine

FIGURE 1: Schematic diagram of D-serine signaling at a glutamatergic synapse. $NMDAR_{syn}$ and $NMDAR_{exsyn}$ = synaptic and extrasynaptic N-methyl-D-aspartate receptor; GMS = Glycine modulatory site; GLU = L-glutamate binding site; SR = serine racemase; ASC 1 and ASCT 2 = neutral amino acid transporters; DAAO = D-amino-acid oxidase; αKa = alpha-Keto acid; NH_3 = ammonia; H_2O_2 = hydrogen peroxide.

DSR in the context of neuropsychiatric disorders including schizophrenia, Parkinson's disease, depression, and anxiety disorders.

3.1. Schizophrenia. Over the last 20 years, glutamatergic models of schizophrenia have become increasingly accepted as etiopathological models of this disorder, mainly based on the observation that the cyclohexylamine "dissociative anesthetics" phencyclidine (PCP) and ketamine induce schizophrenia-like positive and negative symptoms and cognitive deficits by blocking NMDAR neurotransmission (rev. in [66, 71]). The PCP/NMDAR model implies that treatments which aimed at potentiating NMDAR function should be therapeutically beneficial. Furthermore, pharmacological manipulation of DSR signaling represents a particularly attractive candidate strategy since convergent lines of evidence suggest an involvement of dysfunctional DSR transmission in schizophrenia [72–75]. Single polymorphisms for SR and DAAO have been linked to schizophrenia

[76–78], in rodents genetic loss of DAAO activity reverses schizophrenia-like phenotypes [79, 80] and reduced DSR serum and cerebrospinal fluid (CSF) levels were documented in chronic schizophrenia patients [81–85]. Moreover, supporting the hypo-NMDAR hypothesis of schizophrenia, DSR selectively blocks PCP-induced hyperactivity and stereotypic behavior [86, 87].

A number of clinical studies [62, 65, 88–90] have demonstrated that adjuvant DSR (30–120 mg/kg/day) added to ongoing treatment with non-clozapine antipsychotics results in significant symptom improvements in chronic schizophrenia patients. The most significant changes were registered in the negative symptom cluster (Figure 2). Nevertheless, two recent meta-analytic reviews indicate that additional dysfunction domains may be affected by DSR. S. P. Singh and V. Singh [91] reported medium effect sizes of DSR for negative symptoms (standardized mean difference (SMD), −0.53) and total symptomatology (SMD, −0.40). Tsai and Lin [92] found DSR effective for negative symptoms (effect size (ES), 0.48),

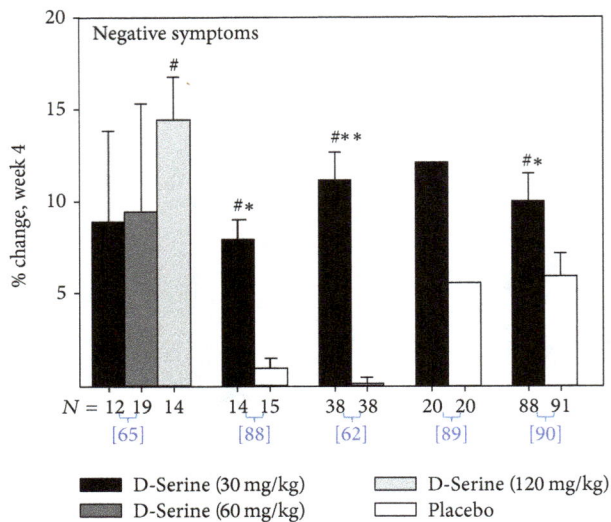

FIGURE 2: D-serine effects on negative symptoms in controlled add-on clinical trials with chronic schizophrenia patients. $^*P < 0.05$ versus placebo; $^{**}P < 0.001$ versus placebo; $^{#}P < 0.05$ versus baseline.

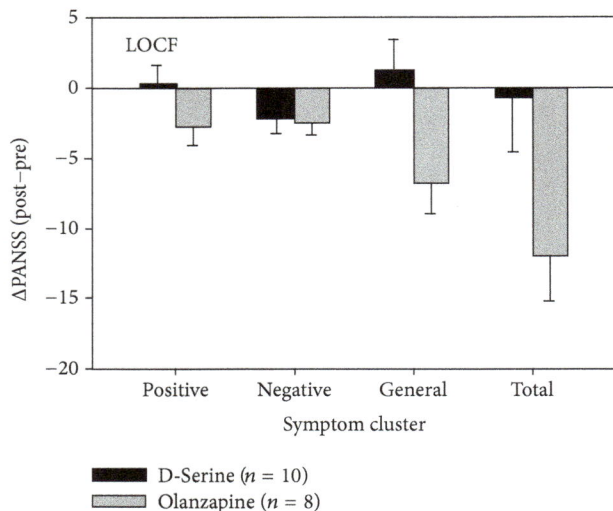

FIGURE 3: Positive and Negative Syndrome Scale (PANSS) symptom clusters score changes during monotherapy with high dose olanzapine and D-serine ($^*F = 6.60$, d.f. $= 1.16$, $P = 0.012$).

cognitive symptoms (ES, 0.42), and total psychopathology (ES, 0.40).

Two schizophrenia treatment issues stemming from these findings are the potential use of DSR for improving cognition and as stand-alone pharmacotherapy in this disorder. In a preliminary four week open-label study [65], it was shown that high dose DSR ($\geq$60 mg/kg/day) improves neurocognitive functions as measured by the Measurement and Treatment Research to Improve Cognition in Schizophrenia (MATRICS) battery. An additional controlled pilot investigation [93] compared the effectiveness of DSR

(3 g/day) versus high-dose olanzapine (30 mg/day) as antipsychotic monotherapy in 18 treatment-resistant schizophrenia patients. The primary LOCF analysis indicated a lack of efficacy of DSR as compared to high-dose olanzapine (Figure 3). However, DSR was not inferior to the prestudy antipsychotic drug treatment. Furthermore, among the patients who completed the nine study weeks, high dose olanzapine and DSR did not differ in their effectiveness, suggesting that a subgroup of patients may be successfully maintained on DSR.

In all clinical trials performed to date with DSR in schizophrenia, no significant adverse events have been observed at doses of $\leq$4 g/day. A potential concern with DSR use is nephrotoxicity [94, 95] which has been reported in one patient receiving 120 mg/kg/day and resolved following DSR discontinuation [65]. This apparent paucity of side effects seems remarkable in view of the fact that both acute [65, 96] and chronic [62, 88, 93] administration of 1-2 g DSR results in $\geq$100 times increases in DSR serum levels. Nevertheless, orally administered DSR is substantially metabolized by DAAO diminishing its bioavailability and necessitating the administration of gram level doses. In view of these limitations, the ideal dosage and mode of administration of DSR remain to be determined.

3.2. Parkinsonism, Drug-Induced Dyskinesia, and Parkinson's Disease. Idiopathic Parkinson's disease (PD) is an age-dependent neurodegenerative disorder characterized by intertwined motor and behavioral and cognitive dysfunctions. Current pharmacological approaches to PD predominantly target the dopamine system. Although dopaminergic medications are effective, a significant number of patients show continued motor symptoms, drug-induced dyskinesia, and "on/off" phenomena, even during treatment. Furthermore, the treatment of nonmotor symptoms represents an additional major therapeutic challenge in PD. Among these manifestations, apathy and cognitive impairment respond poorly to presently available medications, pose increased management difficulties, and contribute significantly to caregiver burden. An innovative pharmacological approach for PD presently under investigation is the modulation of NMDAR-mediated glutamatergic neurotransmission (rev. in [97]).

We have hypothesized that direct or indirect augmentation of synaptic GLY or DSR levels may represent a novel type of treatment for PD [63]. This line of thought stems mainly from the clinical data obtained in schizophrenia research, indicating GLY and DSR efficacy against negative symptoms (rev. in [91, 92]). To the extent that negative symptoms of schizophrenia overlap with components of the apathy syndrome characteristic of PD (e.g., reduced motivation/initiative/volition and anhedonia) and have similar underlying etiology, that is, prefrontal dopaminergic deficit [98], the beneficial effect of DSR on negative symptoms would predict potential beneficial effects against apathy in PD. Moreover, therapeutic effects of NMDAR agonists are not confined to behavioral symptoms of schizophrenia but extend to motor symptoms as well. Some GLY and DSR schizophrenia clinical trials have included subjects that had

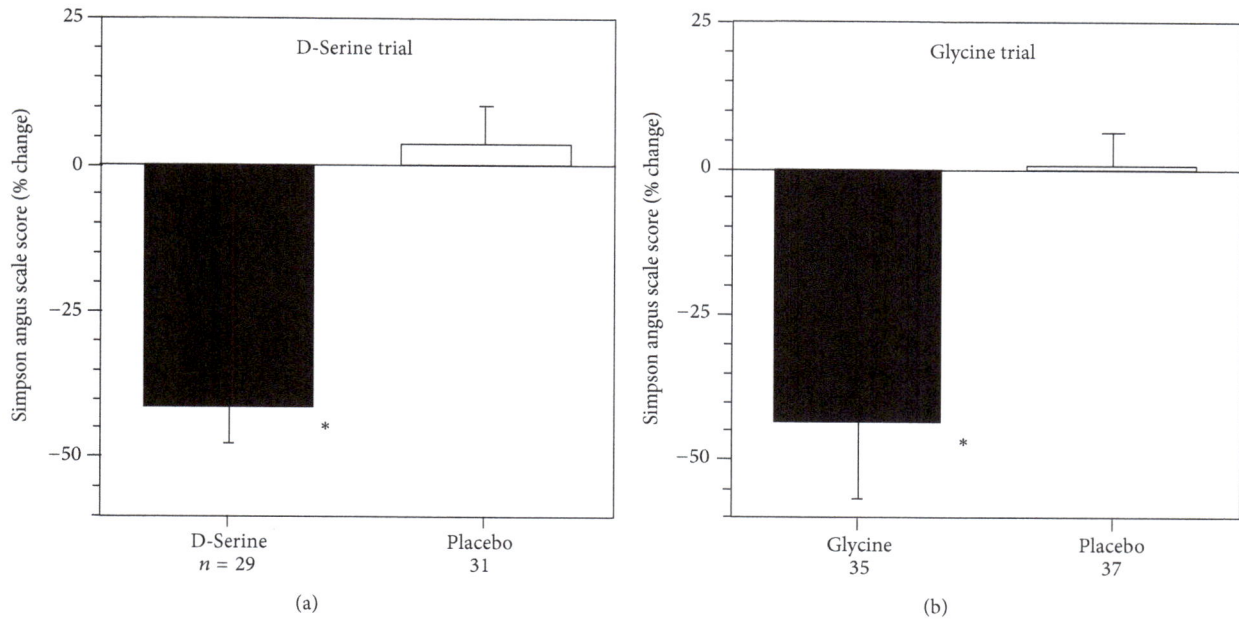

FIGURE 4: Effect of NMDAR-glycine site agonists on extrapyramidal symptoms as reflected in Simpson Angus Scale for Extrapyramidal Symptoms (SAS) change scores. Data are from glycine [61] and D-serine [62] studies. $^*P < 0.0001$ *versus* placebo. (Reproduced from [63]).

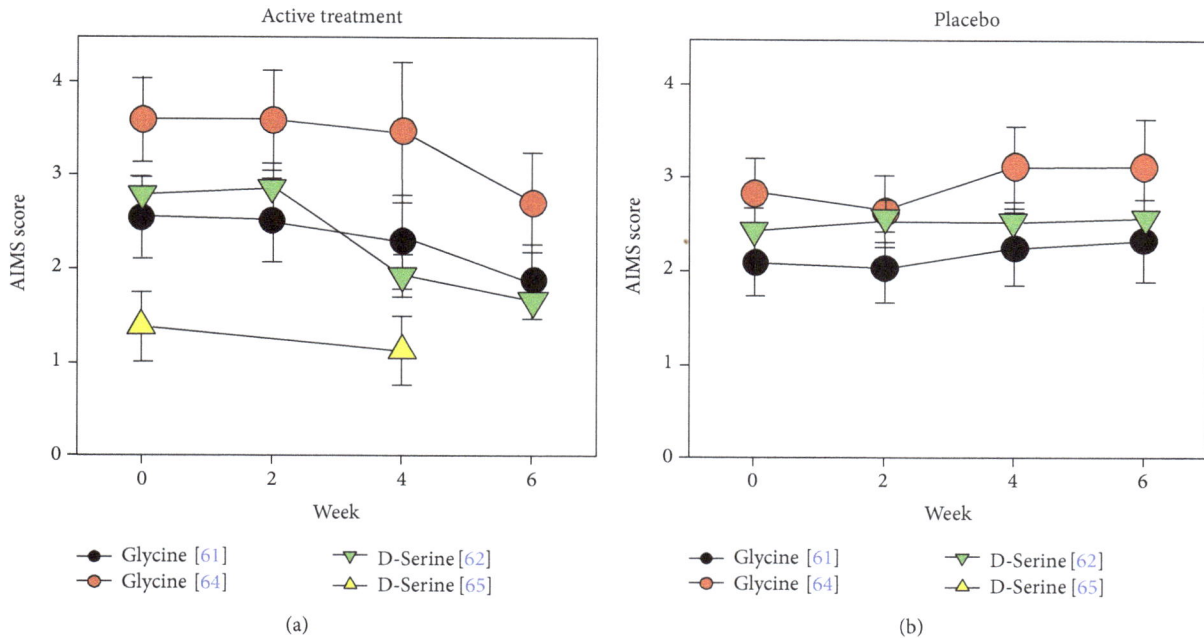

FIGURE 5: Effect of NMDAR-glycine-site agonists on dyskinesia symptoms as reflected in Abnormal Involuntary Movement Scale (AIMS) score. Data are from studies of glycine [61, 64] and D-serine [62, 65]. Across all studies, D-serine treatment led to a highly significant ($t = 4.86$, d.f. = 192, $P < 0.00001$, $d = 0.83$) improvement in AIMS scores. (Reproduced from [66]).

significant antipsychotic drugs-induced parkinsonian [62, 64] and tardive dyskinesia [61, 62, 64, 65] symptoms. In these studies, highly significant, large effect size improvements were registered in these symptom domains (Figures 4 and 5). Thus, since GMS agonists affect motor and nonmotor clinical domains that overlap significantly with PD phenomenology,

it is hypothesized that NMDAR neurotransmission modulation specifically *via* DSR administration may represent an innovative treatment approach in PD.

This hypothesis accords well with current theories on the role of NMDAR in modulation of brain dopaminergic systems relevant to PD [99]. NMDARs are divided into

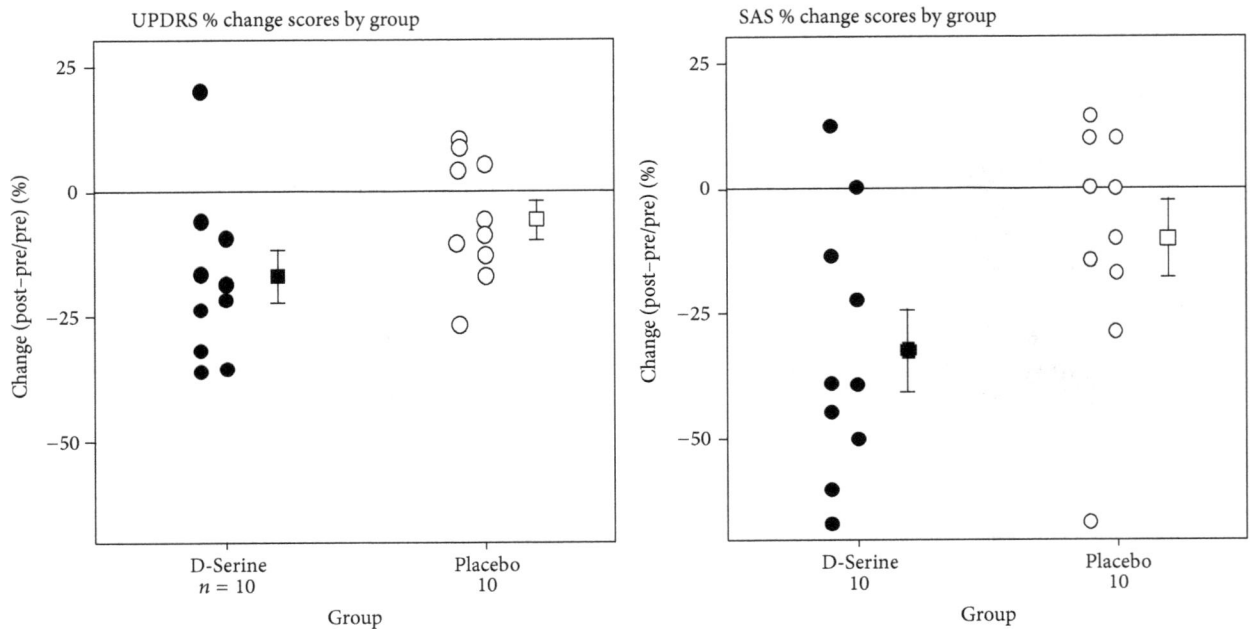

FIGURE 6: Subject-by-subject change scores in Simpson Angus Scale for Extrapyramidal Symptoms (SAS) and Unified Parkinson's Disease Rating Scale (UPDRS) by treatment group. Squares show group means. Data are from pilot trial with D-serine in Parkinson's disease [67]. (Reproduced from [63]).

subtypes based upon the presence of specific modulatory subunits. In adults, NMDARs are primarily of types NR2A and NR2B and research in PD has focused predominantly upon development of NR2B antagonists based upon the observation that dopaminergic denervation leads to specific upregulation of striatal NR2B *versus* NR2A receptors [100]. Significantly, in animal models, NR2B selective antagonists have proven more effective than nonselective drugs, such as MK-801, that target both NR2A and NR2B receptors [101], indicating that NR2A blockade, in fact, may be deleterious, but that NR2A stimulation might be beneficial. NMDAR subtypes show differing sensitivity to GMS agonists such that NR2B receptors are saturated under physiological conditions, whereas NR2A are not [102]. Thus, GMS agonists may function *in vivo* as selective NR2A agonists. Consequently, activation of NR2A *versus* NR2B receptors may restore the balance between NR2A- and NR2B-containing NMDARs similarly to the effects of NR2B antagonists.

We recently addressed the hypothesis that GMS agonists might be beneficial for motor and negative-like symptoms in PD in a 6-week controlled adjuvant treatment trial of DSR (30 mg/day) *versus* placebo in advanced PD patients (age, 64.3 ± 7.4 years; disease duration, 8.9 ± 5.4 years; Hoehn & Yahr staging II–IV) [67]. The ~2 g/day DSR regimen was well tolerated and resulted in significant reductions in Unified Parkinson's Disease Rating Scale (UPDRS) and Simpson-Angus Scale for Extrapyramidal Symptoms (SAS) total scores. Five of 10 completers had >20% improvement in total UPDRS scores during DSR treatment versus 1 of 10 subjects during placebo administration ($\chi^2 = 4.07$, $P = 0.04$). For SAS scores, 7 subjects had >20% improvement during DSR treatment versus 2 during placebo administration ($\chi^2 = 5.3$, $P = 0.02$)

(Figure 6). Significant benefits relative to placebo were also observed in the Positive and Negative Syndrome Scale (PANSS) and in both the motor (III) and mental (I) UPDRS subscales. In view of these novel concepts and findings, additional larger-scale studies are presently warranted to further determine whether motor and nonmotor PD components are significantly affected by GMS modulators.

3.3. Depression and Anxiety. The antidepressant potential of NMDAR antagonism has been unambiguously established during the last decade. Already in the early 1990s, preclinical studies indicated that several types of NMDAR antagonists exert antidepressant-like effects in animal models of depression [103–105]. Subsequently, a series of animal studies demonstrated that long-term antidepressant treatment produces adaptive changes in the binding profile of NMDARs [106]. The translational confirmation of these findings was achieved by the demonstration of a robust, rapid, and long-lasting antidepressant effect of ketamine in, usually treatment-resistant, unipolar or bipolar depression patients (rev. in [107, 108]). Furthermore, in addition to ketamine which acts as a noncompetitive antagonist at the intra-NMDAR channel PCP site, similar effects seem achievable with mechanistically diverse NMDAR antagonists. Recently, we reported that treatment with high-dose DCS, potentially having a net antagonistic effect at the GMS, also improves major depression symptomatology in treatment-resistant patients [109].

Nevertheless, an apparently contradictory body of data advocates in favor of NMDAR agonists efficacy as antidepressants. GLY and DSR adjuvant treatment results in alleviation of depressive symptoms in schizophrenia patients [91,

92], and SSR504734, a reversible GLY-transporter inhibitor, as well as DSR, has been shown to have antidepressant/anxiolytic effects in depression/anxiety models [110, 111]. Moreover, expression of NMDAR 1 and 2A subunit is decreased in postmortem brains of patients with major depression [112], and NMDAR binding is also reduced in suicide victims [113]. Taken together, these findings imply that NMDAR hypofunction may contribute to the pathophysiology of depression. Moreover, this hypothesis is supported by recent clinical data, although systematic investigation of antidepressant effects of NMDAR enhancement is still in an early phase. Acute administration of 2.1 g DSR to 35 healthy university students was reported to reduce, in a placebo-controlled challenge paradigm study, subjective feelings of depression and anxiety as measured by Visual Analog Scales [114]. The GLY-transporter-1 (GLYT1) inhibitor sarcosine [115] and the DAAO inhibitor sodium benzoate [116] were reported to be beneficial in depressed patients who were drug-naïve for at least 3 months and had no history of treatment-resistance.

Present explanations for the discordant observations of antidepressant effect of both NMDAR agonists and antagonists include, theoretically, common α-amino-3-hydroxy-5-methyl-4-isoxazolepropionic acid (AMPA) receptor-mediated mechanisms [117] and similar net effects achieved by differential action at synaptic versus extrasynaptic NMDARs [29, 32]. A stratified model of psychiatric phenomenology, as function of suboptimal/decreased versus overactive/increased NMDAR function, may also contribute to the conceptualization of available data by taking into account the vast heterogeneity underlying the overinclusive concept of depression. While schizophrenia is a typical NMDAR hypofunction disorder, responsive to treatment with NMDAR agonists, the opposite may be characteristic of treatment-resistant depression. Nevertheless, milder, nonrefractory forms of depression may represent predominately suboptimal NMDAR functioning and could be responsive to GMS agonism. Interestingly, depression feelings are improved in both schizophrenia [91, 92] and normal subjects [114] by DSR and in schizophrenia [92] and nonrefractory depression [115] by sarcosine. On the other hand, ketamine characteristically exacerbates schizophrenia manifestations [118], while it has antidepressant, mood stabilizing and procognitive effects in treatment-resistant depression [119].

Anxiety disorders represent an additional domain in which treatment aiming at augmentation of DSR synaptic levels may prove beneficial. Brain regions extensively implicated in the mediation of fear and anxiety (i.e., amygdala, hippocampus, and prefrontal cortex) are characterized by high NMDAR levels [120] and may show morphological changes as a result of stress-related disorders [121, 122]. NMDARs play a central role in stress response [123] and are critically involved in learning and memory formation which may be impaired in anxiety disorder (e.g., post-traumatic stress disorder, PTSD) [124].

Following a series of studies indicating that extinction learning is NMDAR- dependent, Davis and colleagues first demonstrated that DCS can enhance retention of fear extinction in rats and subsequently showed that DCS enhances

the outcome of extinction-based therapy (i.e., virtual reality exposure therapy) for height phobia [125, 126]. These findings were replicated and are cardinal for the concept that DCS may enhance the outcomes of exposure-based cognitive behavioral therapy (CBT). Furthermore, clinical trials accumulated across a range of anxiety-related disorders including specific phobia, social phobia, panic disorders, obsessive-compulsive disorder, and PTSD confirm that single dose (25–500 mg) DCS acutely administered prior to the psychotherapeutic sessions shows promise in augmenting the effects of exposure-based therapy (rev. in [127]). However, the efficacy of DCS has been variable across studies, with several evidencing strong augmentative effects and several showing either relatively weak or no effects [128].

The potential of acute DSR administration in conjunction with CBT interventions has not yet been explored, although it may hold several advantages. DCS is a partial agonist at the GMS of NMDARs bearing the GluN2A and GluN2B subunits (previously NR2A and NR2B subunits) and a full agonist of NMDARs containing the GluN2C and GluN2D subunits [69, 129]. Furthermore, its net effect is affected by the concentration of endogenous GMS modulators (e.g., GLY, DSR, and kynurenic acid), which may be differentially altered in pathophysiological states. In contrast, DSR acts as a specific and potent full agonist at GMS and DSR-induced improvements in cognition parameters have been reported in healthy subjects [114] and schizophrenia patients [65]. Furthermore, Horio et al. [130] recently proposed that DCS may act as a prodrug for DSR in the brain. In an in vivo microdialysis study using free-moving mice, these researchers reported significantly increased extracellular DSR levels in mouse hippocampus following oral or intracerebroventricular (ICV) administration of DCS. Therefore, it was proposed that the DSR produced in the brain after DCS treatment may play at least a partial role in the therapeutic effects of DCS seen in patients with anxiety disorders [130].

While chronic use of DCS for facilitation of exposure sessions is known to lead to negative effects [131, 132], the use of DSR as continuous pharmacology unrelated to CBT interventions may prove rewarding. In long-standing PTSD, in which learning deficits may impair normal extinction of aversive memories, NMDAR agonists may hold a therapeutic potential [133–135]. Accordingly, the demonstrated efficacy of DSR against negative and cognitive symptoms of chronic treatment-resistant schizophrenia patients [91, 92] may also be of relevance to PTSD therapeutics, since PTSD impairments include cognitive dysfunction and features such as affective numbing, anhedonia, and withdrawal from social/vocational activities. Consequently, we have conducted a 6-week controlled proof-of-concept trial that examined the effects of 30 mg/kg/day DSR used as mono- or add-on pharmacotherapy with twenty-two chronic PTSD patients [136]. Compared with placebo administration, DSR treatment resulted in significantly reduced Hamilton Rating Scale for Depression (HAM-D) ($P = 0.007$) and Mississippi Scale for Combat-Related PTSD-civilian version (MISS-PTSD-CV) ($P = 0.001$) scores and a trend towards improved Clinician-Administered PTSD Scale (CAPS) total scores. These preliminary findings suggest that GMS-based pharmacotherapy may be effective in PTSD and warrant larger-sized clinical trials with optimized DSR dosages.

Obsessive-compulsive disorder (OCD) represents an additional clinical entity for which enhancement of GMS-mediated neurotransmission *via* continuous pharmacological treatment is presently assessed [137]. A case report of a young adult male patient who was disabled with OCD and body dysmorphic disorder illustrates the use of high-dose GLY (0.8 mg/kg), with gradual improvement of clinical status [138]. In a placebo-controlled double-blind trial including 24 adult outpatients with OCD, who were treated with adjunctive GLY 60 g/day for 12 weeks, 14 patients completed the study and two patients in the GLY group were considered responders [139]. The Hoffmann-LaRoche GLYT1 inhibitor bitopertin is presently assessed as add-on treatment in conjunction with selective serotonin reuptake inhibitors in OCD in a Phase II multicenter study [140]. The use of DSR or indirect elevation of DSR levels in OCD has not yet been reported.

3.4. Cognitive Impairment and Dementia.

Cognitive impairment is a cardinal feature of dementia and NMDAR dysfunction is hypothesized to play a cardinal role in AD which is the most common type of dementia [141]. NMDAR overactivation by GLU leads to cell death mediated by calcium overload [31, 32]. This process, known as excitotoxicity, is one of the accepted neurochemical models of AD. Furthermore, there are mutual interactions between NMDAR and Amyloid-β peptide (Aβ) which is a hallmark of AD pathogenesis [142]. Aβ increases NMDAR activity [143, 144] and induces inwards Ca^{2+} current and neurotoxicity [145]. Reciprocally, NMDAR activation stimulates Aβ production [146–148] and Aβ associated synaptic loss may be NMDAR-dependent [149].

On the contrary, NMDAR signaling pathways in the cerebral cortex and hippocampus are impaired in the aging brain [150]. NMDAR neurotransmission is crucial to neuronal survival and NMDAR hypofunction is known to lead to apoptosis [29, 30]. Blockade of NMDAR function by gene deletion or using NMDAR antagonists increases apoptotic cell death [151, 152]. This type of NMDAR hypoactivity-induced neurodegeneration is postulated to contribute to AD pathogenesis [153, 154]. Furthermore, NMDAR hypofunction may also be involved in the progression of the aging brain from mild cognitive impairment (MCI) to AD (rev. in [155]). Individuals with AD or MCI have fewer NMDARs in the frontal cortex and hippocampus [156, 157]. In the genetic mouse model of AD, expression of surface NMDARs in neurons is decreased [158] and NMDAR-mediated response is impaired progressively with age [159, 160]. In addition to reduced number of NMDARs, disrupted glutamatergic neurotransmission [146], decreased CSF concentrations of excitatory amino acids [161], decreased serum levels of DSR [162], and reduced D-aspartate uptake [163] are also noted in AD.

Thus, balanced NMDAR activity is required for optimal cognitive performance and both over- or underfunction of NMDAR neurotransmission may contribute to cognitive dysfunction or neurotoxicity. This NMDAR function paradox may be related to different composition of NR subunits and receptor localization [164, 165]. Accordingly, normalizing NMDAR dysfunction by selectively enhancing NR1/NR2B NMDARs, while avoiding excitotoxicity mediated at NR1/NR2B receptors, could be a better therapeutic approach than nonselective NMDAR antagonism which may actually impair cognitive functioning (rev. in [155]).

During the 1990s, we have witnessed the development of NMDAR antagonists as neuroprotective agents for AD. However, with the exception of memantine, this type of compounds failed to show neuroprotective effects in large scale Phase II/III studies. Memantine is a weak uncompetitive NMDAR partial antagonist of low affinity, which hypothetically can block NMDAR overactivation by preventing excessive influx of calcium without affecting physiological NMDAR activity [166, 167]. Consistently, therapeutically relevant plasma concentrations of memantine produce only 30% NMDAR occupancy [168]. Pharmacological intervention at GMS may represent an additional therapeutic mechanism for AD. NMDAR function enhancement *via* GMS may avoid the excitotoxicity mediated through the GLU site. Furthermore, in mouse models, the learning deficits caused by NMDAR hypofunction in mice with point mutations in GMS can be rescued by administration of DSR [169, 170]. Supporting neurotrophic/cognitive effects, DCS can improve cognitive functions in animal studies [171, 172] and is used clinically in conjunction with CBT interventions [127]. However, cognition-enhancing effects of DCS in AD have not been conclusively demonstrated [173–175].

The potential efficacy of DSR for the treatment of cognitive impairments has not yet been assessed. Nevertheless, in preliminary investigations, DSR was shown to improve recognition and working memory parameters in mice [176] and cognitive tasks performance in healthy subjects [114]. Thus, DSR may improve cognitive parameters, while NMDAR antagonists (e.g., ketamine) may worsen them in the healthy human organism. Furthermore, it was recently reported that sodium benzoate administration, which hypothetically results in increased synaptic DSR levels is beneficial in patients with MCI or mild AD [177]. In contrast, memantine is approved for use in moderate to severe AD [178], but its efficacy in MCI or mild AD is questionable [179].

3.5. Amyotrophic Lateral Sclerosis.

Recent data suggest that DSR is involved in the neurodegenerative processes associated with amyotrophic lateral sclerosis (ALS). This neurodegenerative disease targets motor neurons in the spinal cord, brain stem, and cerebral cortex, leading to death within a few years of onset [180, 181]. In ALS, DSR may mediate motoneuron cell death caused by excessive NMDAR stimulation [182]. A missense mutation that inactivates DAAO results in increased DSR in the spinal cord of patients and causes a familial form of ALS. The affected patients with the DAAO mutation exhibit much lower DAAO activity in spinal cord and significantly increased DSR levels [183]. Furthermore, in sporadic ALS cases elevated DSR may also arise from induction of SR, the DSR synthetic enzyme, caused by cell stress and inflammation [181]. Thus, both anabolic and catabolic DSR-related abnormalities may lead to increased synaptic DSR levels and contribute to disease pathogenesis. Pharmacological interventions aiming at inhibiting DSR synthesis or release may represent an innovative treatment strategy in ALS and potentially other neurodegenerative disorders characterized by NMDAR overactivation.

4. Indirect Augmentation of DSR Function

Regulation of GMS function *via* pharmacological manipulation of GLYT1 and DAAO represents presently an important research and development target. Although DSR may be effective for treatment of various psychiatric symptom domains, DSR is substantially neutralized by DAAO, diminishing its oral bioavailability and necessitating the administration of high doses. Moreover, a concern with high doses may be potential nephrotoxicity, although no significant adverse events have yet been observed at DSR doses of ≤4 g/day [65, 91, 92].

High levels of DAAO expression and enzyme activity are found in the mammalian liver, kidney, and brain although the expression pattern can vary between species. Humans express DAAO in both liver and kidney, whereas mice, for example, express DAAO in the kidney but not the liver [184]. The physiological role of DAAO in the kidney and liver is detoxification of accumulated D-amino acids [185]. Collectively, the limited preclinical experience with a small number of structurally diverse DAAO inhibitors indicates that extensive inhibition of peripheral and central DAAO has a limited effect on brain or extracellular DSR concentration. Furthermore, in contrast to the fairly robust effects reported with DSR administration in animal models, the reported behavioral effects of DAAO inhibitors are fairly modest and inconsistent (rev. in [186]).

Given the moderate efficacy of DAAO inhibitors on brain DSR and behavior, several authors have investigated the effects of coadministering DAAO inhibitors in conjunction with DSR. Ferraris et al. [187] showed that the 6-chloro analog (CBIO) had quite pronounced effects on brain and plasma DSR when coadministered with 30 mg/kg DSR, relative to either CBIO or DSR administered alone. Hashimoto et al. [188] extended this finding by showing effects on cortical DSR and also demonstrated that coadministration of DSR (30 mg/kg) and CBIO reversed an MK-801-induced deficit in prepulse inhibition (PPI), whereas the 30 mg/kg dose of DSR had no effect on its own. Smith et al. [186] showed that coadministration of compound 4 in conjunction with DSR elevates CSF and cortical DSR levels to a greater extent than administration of DSR alone in male rats. Overall, these findings suggest that DAAO inhibitors could be useful clinically for reducing the dose of DSR necessary for symptom improvement. Moreover, the coadministration of DAAO inhibitors with DSR could ameliorate potential side effects associated with the administration of high DSR doses, for example, nephrotoxicity [189].

Recently, the first results of clinical research with sodium benzoate have been reported. Benzoic acid and its salts, including sodium benzoate, exist in many plants and are widely used as food preservatives [190]. Sodium benzoate also acts as a DAAO inhibitor and has favorable effects in

NMDAR-based models such as pain relief [191, 192] and glial cell death [193]. The potential molecular mechanisms of action of sodium benzoate remain to be determined. Since DAAO activity is high in the adult brain cerebellum, it is possible that DSR cerebellar levels may be increased following sodium benzoate administration. Furthermore, recent findings suggest that sodium benzoate may upregulate brain-derived neurotrophic factor (BDNF) *via* protein kinase A- (PKA-)mediated activation of cAMP response element binding (CREB) protein [194].

In two controlled trials, the administration of up to 1 g/day sodium benzoate proved beneficial for schizophrenia [195] and MCI or mild AD [177] patients. Furthermore, partial remission within 6 weeks was reported with a major depressive disorder patient treated with 500 g/day sodium benzoate [116]. These preliminary findings show promise for DAAO inhibition as a novel treatment approach. Nevertheless, at present, the therapeutic potential of DAAO inhibitors is still relatively unexplored and preclinical studies have primarily addressed the relevance of these compounds mainly for schizophrenia. Further research is warranted given that the few published studies characterizing novel DAAO inhibitors have yielded conflicting results.

5. Conclusions and Future Directions

The scientific view about DSR has changed drastically during the last decade. Converging data strongly suggest a complex and unique neurotransmitter function of DSR which is likely to include an important role in glia-synapse interactions. Furthermore, the demonstration of a DSR modulatory role in cardinal NMDAR-dependent processes has been a driving force for the conceptualization of novel treatment strategies involving the direct or indirect manipulation of DSR signaling. These concepts are likely to undergo further integration and development in the context of the need for strictly balanced NMDAR functioning, with either over- or under-NMDAR function potentially involved in the pathogenesis of neuropsychiatric dysfunctions. A first generation of proof-of-concept animal and clinical studies indicate beneficial DSR effects in refractory schizophrenia, movement, depression, and anxiety disorders and for the improvement of cognitive performance. An additional presently developing strategy is the indirect modulation of DSR synaptic levels by use of compounds that alter the function of main enzymes responsible for DSR production and degradation.

Future research on DSR is likely to further develop along three main axes: (1) characterization of the DSR neurotransmitter system and its role throughout lifespan; (2) the implication of DSR in pathological states characterized by either hypo- or hyper- NMDAR function; and (3) direct or indirect pharmacological manipulation of DSR signaling. The accumulated data suggest that, during the next decade, we will witness important advances in DSR research that will further contribute to elucidate the causes of neuropsychiatric disorders and will be instrumental in the development of innovative treatments.

Conflict of Interests

Dr. Heresco-Levy is inventor in patents for the use of NMDAR-glycine site modulators in movement disorders and in patent applications for the use of NMDAR-glycine site modulators in depression and autoimmune-induced NMDAR dysfunctions. Dr. Durrant reports no conflict of interests.

Acknowledgments

Part of the work reviewed in this paper has been supported by research Grants to Dr. Heresco-Levy from The Stanley Medical Research Institute (SMRI), USA, The Brain and Behavior Research Foundation (formerly National Alliance for Research on Schizophrenia and Depression (NARSAD)), USA, and The Israel Science Foundation (ISF), Israel.

References

[1] H. A. Krebs, "Metabolism of amino-acids: deamination of amino-acids," *Biochemical Journal*, vol. 29, no. 7, pp. 1620–1644, 1935.

[2] A. Hashimoto, T. Nishikawa, T. Hayashi et al., "The presence of free D-serine in rat brain," *FEBS Letters*, vol. 296, no. 1, pp. 33–36, 1992.

[3] A. Hashimoto, T. Nishikawa, T. Oka, and K. Takahashi, "Endogenous D-serine in rat brain: N-methyl-D-aspartate receptor-related distribution and aging," *Journal of Neurochemistry*, vol. 60, no. 2, pp. 783–786, 1993.

[4] J. P. Crow, J. C. Marecki, and M. Thompson, "D-Serine production, degradation, and transport in ALS: critical role of methodology," *Neurology Research International*, vol. 2012, Article ID 625245, 8 pages, 2012.

[5] Y. Nagata, K. Horiike, and T. Maeda, "Distribution of free D-serine in vertebrate brains," *Brain Research*, vol. 634, no. 2, pp. 291–295, 1994.

[6] N. Rebola, B. N. Srikumar, and C. Mulle, "Activity-dependent synaptic plasticity of NMDA receptors," *Journal of Physiology*, vol. 588, no. 1, pp. 93–99, 2010.

[7] R. C. Malenka and M. F. Bear, "LTP and LTD: an embarrassment of riches," *Neuron*, vol. 44, no. 1, pp. 5–21, 2004.

[8] P. Paoletti and J. Neyton, "NMDA receptor subunits: function and pharmacology," *Current Opinion in Pharmacology*, vol. 7, no. 1, pp. 39–47, 2007.

[9] J. W. Johnson and P. Ascher, "Glycine potentiates the NMDA response in cultured mouse brain neurons," *Nature*, vol. 325, no. 6104, pp. 529–531, 1987.

[10] A. Hashimoto and T. Oka, "Free D-aspartate and D-serine in the mammalian brain and periphery," *Progress in Neurobiology*, vol. 52, no. 4, pp. 325–353, 1997.

[11] L. Pollegioni and S. Sacchi, "Metabolism of the neuromodulator D-serine," *Cellular and Molecular Life Sciences*, vol. 67, no. 14, pp. 2387–2404, 2010.

[12] M. Martineau, G. Baux, and J.-P. Mothet, "D-Serine signalling in the brain: friend and foe," *Trends in Neurosciences*, vol. 29, no. 8, pp. 481–491, 2006.

[13] H. Wolosker, "NMDA receptor regulation by D-serine: new findings and perspectives," *Molecular Neurobiology*, vol. 36, no. 2, pp. 152–164, 2007.

[14] J.-P. Mothet and S. H. Snyder, "Brain D-amino acids: a novel class of neuromodulators," *Amino Acids*, vol. 43, no. 5, pp. 1809–1810, 2012.

[15] Y. Yang, W. Ge, Y. Chen et al., "Contribution of astrocytes to hippocampal long-term potentiation through release of D-serine," *Proceedings of the National Academy of Sciences of the United States of America*, vol. 100, no. 25, pp. 15194–15199, 2003.

[16] A. C. Basu, G. E. Tsai, C.-L. Ma et al., "Targeted disruption of serine racemase affects glutamatergic neurotransmission and behavior," *Molecular Psychiatry*, vol. 14, no. 7, pp. 719–727, 2009.

[17] Z. Zhang, N. Gong, W. Wang, L. Xu, and T.-L. Xu, "Bell-shaped d-serine actions on hippocampal long-term depression and spatial memory retrieval," *Cerebral Cortex*, vol. 18, no. 10, pp. 2391–2401, 2008.

[18] J. P. Mothet, E. Rouaud, P.-M. Sinet et al., "A critical role for the glial-derived neuromodulator D-serine in the age-related deficits of cellular mechanisms of learning and memory," *Aging Cell*, vol. 5, no. 3, pp. 267–274, 2006.

[19] A. Panatier, D. T. Theodosis, J.-P. Mothet et al., "Glia-derived D-serine controls NMDA receptor activity and synaptic memory," *Cell*, vol. 125, no. 4, pp. 775–784, 2006.

[20] E. R. Stevens, M. Esguerra, P. M. Kim et al., "D-serine and serine racemase are present in the vertebrate retina and contribute to the physiological activation of NMDA receptors," *Proceedings of the National Academy of Sciences of the United States of America*, vol. 100, no. 11, pp. 6789–6794, 2003.

[21] T. L. Kalbaugh, J. Zhang, and J. S. Diamond, "Coagonist release modulates NMDA receptor subtype contributions at synaptic inputs to retinal ganglion cells," *The Journal of Neuroscience*, vol. 29, no. 5, pp. 1469–1479, 2009.

[22] J.-P. Mothet, A. T. Parent, H. Wolosker et al., "D-serine is an endogenous ligand for the glycine site of the N-methyl-D-aspartate receptor," *Proceedings of the National Academy of Sciences of the United States of America*, vol. 97, no. 9, pp. 4926–4931, 2000.

[23] E. Kartvelishvily, M. Shleper, L. Balan, E. Dumin, and H. Wolosker, "Neuron-derived D-serine release provides a novel means to activate N-methyl-D-aspartate receptors," *The Journal of Biological Chemistry*, vol. 281, no. 20, pp. 14151–14162, 2006.

[24] M. Shleper, E. Kartvelishvily, and H. Wolosker, "D-serine is the dominant endogenous coagonist for NMDA receptor neurotoxicity in organotypic hippocampal slices," *The Journal of Neuroscience*, vol. 25, no. 41, pp. 9413–9417, 2005.

[25] P. M. Kim, H. Aizawa, P. S. Kim et al., "Serine racemase: activation by glutamate neurotransmission via glutamate receptor interacting protein and mediation of neuronal migration," *Proceedings of the National Academy of Sciences of the United States of America*, vol. 102, no. 6, pp. 2105–2110, 2005.

[26] S. A. Lipton and P. A. Rosenberg, "Mechanisms of disease: excitatory amino acids as a final common pathway for neurologic disorders," *The New England Journal of Medicine*, vol. 330, no. 9, pp. 613–622, 1994.

[27] D. W. Choi, "Excitotoxic cell death," *Journal of Neurobiology*, vol. 23, no. 9, pp. 1261–1276, 1992.

[28] J. A. Kemp and R. M. McKernan, "NMDA receptor pathways as drug targets," *Nature Neuroscience*, vol. 5, pp. 1039–1042, 2002.

[29] G. E. Hardingham and H. Bading, "The Yin and Yang of NMDA receptor signalling," *Trends in Neurosciences*, vol. 26, no. 2, pp. 81–89, 2003.

[30] C. Ikonomidou, F. Bosch, M. Miksa et al., "Blockade of NMDA receptors and apoptotic neurodegeneration in the developing brain," *Science*, vol. 283, no. 5398, pp. 70–74, 1999.

[31] B. K. Fiske and P. C. Brunjes, "NMDA receptor regulation of cell death in the rat olfactory bulb," *Journal of Neurobiology*, vol. 47, no. 3, pp. 223–232, 2001.

[32] G. E. Hardingham and H. Bading, "Synaptic versus extrasynaptic NMDA receptor signalling: implications for neurodegenerative disorders," *Nature Reviews Neuroscience*, vol. 11, no. 10, pp. 682–696, 2010.

[33] M. J. Schell, M. E. Molliver, and S. H. Snyder, "D-serine, an endogenous synaptic modulator: localization to astrocytes and glutamate-stimulated release," *Proceedings of the National Academy of Sciences of the United States of America*, vol. 92, no. 9, pp. 3948–3952, 1995.

[34] H. Wolosker, "Serine racemase and the serine shuttle between neurons and astrocytes," *Biochimica et Biophysica Acta—Proteins and Proteomics*, vol. 1814, no. 11, pp. 1558–1566, 2011.

[35] J.-P. Mothet, L. Pollegioni, G. Ouanounou, M. Martineau, P. Fossier, and G. Baux, "Glutamate receptor activation triggers a calcium-dependent and SNARE protein-dependent release of the gliotransmitter D-serine," *Proceedings of the National Academy of Sciences of the United States of America*, vol. 102, no. 15, pp. 5606–5611, 2005.

[36] E. Yasuda, N. Ma, and R. Semba, "Immunohistochemical evidences for localization and production of D-serine in some neurons in the rat brain," *Neuroscience Letters*, vol. 299, no. 1-2, pp. 162–164, 2001.

[37] S. M. Williams, C. M. Diaz, L. T. Macnab, R. K. P. Sullivan, and D. V. Pow, "Immunocytochemical analysis of D-serine distribution in the mammalian brain reveals novel anatomical compartmentalizations in glia and neurons," *GLIA*, vol. 53, no. 4, pp. 401–411, 2006.

[38] J. Puyal, M. Martineau, J.-P. Mothet, M.-T. Nicolas, and J. Raymond, "Changes in D-serine levels and localization during postnatal development of the rat vestibular nuclei," *Journal of Comparative Neurology*, vol. 497, no. 4, pp. 610–621, 2006.

[39] D. T. Balu and J. T. Coyle, "Neuronal d-serine regulates dendritic architecture in the somatosensory cortex," *Neuroscience Letters*, vol. 517, no. 2, pp. 77–81, 2012.

[40] M. A. Benneyworth, Y. Li, A. C. Basu, V. Y. Bolshakov, and J. T. Coyle, "Cell selective conditional null mutations of serine racemase demonstrate a predominate localization in cortical glutamatergic neurons," *Cellular and Molecular Neurobiology*, vol. 32, no. 4, pp. 613–624, 2012.

[41] K. Miya, R. Inoue, Y. Takata et al., "Serine racemase is predominantly localized in neurons in mouse brain," *Journal of Comparative Neurology*, vol. 510, no. 6, pp. 641–654, 2008.

[42] D. Rosenberg, E. Kartvelishvily, M. Shleper, C. M. C. Klinker, M. T. Bowser, and H. Wolosker, "Neuronal release of D-serine: a physiological pathway controlling extracellular D-serine concentration," *The FASEB Journal*, vol. 24, no. 8, pp. 2951–2961, 2010.

[43] D. Rosenberg, S. Artoul, A. C. Segal et al., "Neuronal D-serine and glycine release via the Asc-1 transporter regulates NMDA receptor-dependent synaptic activity," *The Journal of Neuroscience*, vol. 33, no. 8, pp. 3533–3544, 2013.

[44] H. Wolosker, "D-serine regulation of NMDA receptor activity," *Science's STKE: Signal Transduction Knowledge Environment*, vol. 2006, no. 356, p. pe41, 2006.

[45] N. Kishi and J. D. Macklis, "MECP2 is progressively expressed in post-migratory neurons and is involved in neuronal maturation rather than cell fate decisions," *Molecular and Cellular Neuroscience*, vol. 27, no. 3, pp. 306–321, 2004.

[46] M. J. Schell, R. O. Brady Jr., M. E. Molliver, and S. H. Snyder, "D-serine as a neuromodulator: regional and developmental localizations in rat brain glia resemble NMDA receptors," *The Journal of Neuroscience*, vol. 17, no. 5, pp. 1604–1615, 1997.

[47] T. Papouin, L. Ladépêche, J. Ruel et al., "Synaptic and extrasynaptic NMDA receptors are gated by different endogenous coagonists," *Cell*, vol. 150, no. 3, pp. 633–646, 2012.

[48] P. Fossat, F. R. Turpin, S. Sacchi et al., "Glial D-serine gates NMDA receptors at excitatory synapses in prefrontal cortex," *Cerebral Cortex*, vol. 22, no. 3, pp. 595–606, 2012.

[49] C. Henneberger, T. Papouin, S. H. R. Oliet, and D. A. Rusakov, "Long-term potentiation depends on release of d-serine from astrocytes," *Nature*, vol. 463, no. 7278, pp. 232–236, 2010.

[50] L. Liu, T. P. Wong, M. F. Pozza et al., "Role of NMDA receptor subtypes in governing the direction of hippocampal synaptic plasticity," *Science*, vol. 304, no. 5673, pp. 1021–1024, 2004.

[51] P. V. Massey, B. E. Johnson, P. R. Moult et al., "Differential roles of NR2A and NR2B-containing NMDA receptors in cortical long-term potentiation and long-term depression," *The Journal of Neuroscience*, vol. 24, no. 36, pp. 7821–7828, 2004.

[52] W. Morishita, W. Lu, G. B. Smith, R. A. Nicoll, M. F. Bear, and R. C. Malenka, "Activation of NR2B-containing NMDA receptors is not required for NMDA receptor-dependent long-term depression," *Neuropharmacology*, vol. 52, no. 1, pp. 71–76, 2007.

[53] S. Berberich, P. Punnakkal, V. Jensen et al., "Lack of NMDA receptor subtype selectivity for hippocampal long-term potentiation," *The Journal of Neuroscience*, vol. 25, no. 29, pp. 6907–6910, 2005.

[54] C. Weitlauf, Y. Honse, Y. P. Auberson, M. Mishina, D. M. Lovinger, and D. G. Winder, "Activation of NR2A-containing NMDA receptors is not obligatory for NMDA receptor-dependent long-term potentiation," *The Journal of Neuroscience*, vol. 25, no. 37, pp. 8386–8390, 2005.

[55] D. A. Rusakov, A. Scimemi, M. C. Walker, and D. M. Kullmann, "Comment on "Role of NMDA receptor subtypes in governing the direction of hippocampal synaptic plasticity"," *Science*, vol. 305, no. 5692, p. 1912, 2004.

[56] T. Fellin, O. Pascual, S. Gobbo, T. Pozzan, P. G. Haydon, and G. Carmignoto, "Neuronal synchrony mediated by astrocytic glutamate through activation of extrasynaptic NMDA receptors," *Neuron*, vol. 43, no. 5, pp. 729–743, 2004.

[57] M. C. Angulo, A. S. Kozlov, S. Charpak, and E. Audinat, "Glutamate released from glial cells synchronizes neuronal activity in the hippocampus," *The Journal of Neuroscience*, vol. 24, no. 31, pp. 6920–6927, 2004.

[58] M. Arundine and M. Tymianski, "Molecular mechanisms of calcium-dependent neurodegeneration in excitotoxicity," *Cell Calcium*, vol. 34, no. 4-5, pp. 325–337, 2003.

[59] A. J. Milnerwood, C. M. Gladding, M. A. Pouladi et al., "Early increase in extrasynaptic NMDA receptor signaling and expression contributes to phenotype onset in Huntington's disease mice," *Neuron*, vol. 65, no. 2, pp. 178–190, 2010.

[60] K. Bordji, J. Becerril-Ortega, O. Nicole, and A. Buisson, "Activation of extrasynaptic, but not synaptic, NMDA receptors modifies amyloid precursor protein expression pattern and increases amyloid-β production," *The Journal of Neuroscience*, vol. 30, no. 47, pp. 15927–15942, 2010.

[61] U. Heresco-Levy, D. C. Javitt, C. Ermilov, C. Mordel, G. Silipo, and M. Lichtenstein, "Efficacy of high-dose glycine in the treatment of enduring negative symptoms of schizophrenia," *Archives of General Psychiatry*, vol. 56, no. 1, pp. 29–36, 1999.

[62] U. Heresco-Levy, D. C. Javitt, R. Ebstein et al., "D-serine efficacy as add-on pharmacotherapy to risperidone and olanzapine for treatment-refractory schizophrenia," *Biological Psychiatry*, vol. 57, no. 6, pp. 577–585, 2005.

[63] U. Heresco-Levy, S. Shoham, and D. C. Javitt, "Glycine site agonists of the N-methyl-d-aspartate receptor and Parkinson's disease: a hypothesis," *Movement Disorders*, vol. 28, no. 4, pp. 419–424, 2013.

[64] U. Heresco-Levy, M. Ermilov, P. Lichtenberg, G. Bar, and D. C. Javitt, "High-dose glycine added to olanzapine and risperidone for the treatment of schizophrenia," *Biological Psychiatry*, vol. 55, no. 2, pp. 165–171, 2004.

[65] J. T. Kantrowitz, A. K. Malhotra, B. Cornblatt et al., "High dose D-serine in the treatment of schizophrenia," *Schizophrenia Research*, vol. 121, no. 1–3, pp. 125–130, 2010.

[66] D. C. Javitt, S. R. Zukin, U. Heresco-Levy, and D. Umbricht, "Has an angel shown the way? Etiological and therapeutic implications of the PCP/NMDA model of schizophrenia," *Schizophrenia Bulletin*, vol. 38, no. 5, pp. 958–966, 2012.

[67] E. Gelfin, Y. Kaufman, I. Korn-Lubetzki et al., "D-serine adjuvant treatment alleviates behavioural and motor symptoms in Parkinson's disease," *International Journal of Neuropsychopharmacology*, vol. 15, no. 4, pp. 543–549, 2012.

[68] J. T. Coyle and P. Puttfarcken, "Oxidative stress, glutamate, and neurodegenerative disorders," *Science*, vol. 262, no. 5134, pp. 689–695, 1993.

[69] S. M. Dravid, P. B. Burger, A. Prakash et al., "Structural determinants of D-cycloserine efficacy at the NR1/NR2C NMDA receptors," *The Journal of Neuroscience*, vol. 30, no. 7, pp. 2741–2754, 2010.

[70] T.-A. Matsui, M. Sekiguchi, A. Hashimoto, U. Tomita, T. Nishikawa, and K. Wada, "Functional comparison of D-serine and glycine in rodents: the effect on cloned NMDA receptors and the extracellular concentration," *Journal of Neurochemistry*, vol. 65, no. 1, pp. 454–458, 1995.

[71] U. Heresco-Levy, "Glutamatergic neurotransmission modulators as emerging new drugs for schizophrenia," *Expert Opinion on Emerging Drugs*, vol. 10, no. 4, pp. 827–844, 2005.

[72] C. A. Ross, R. L. Margolis, S. A. J. Reading, M. Pletnikov, and J. T. Coyle, "Neurobiology of Schizophrenia," *Neuron*, vol. 52, no. 1, pp. 139–153, 2006.

[73] L. Verrall, M. Walker, N. Rawlings et al., "D-Amino acid oxidase and serine racemase in human brain: normal distribution and altered expression in schizophrenia," *European Journal of Neuroscience*, vol. 26, no. 6, pp. 1657–1669, 2007.

[74] V. Labrie, R. Fukumura, A. Rastogi et al., "Serine racemase is associated with schizophrenia susceptibility in humans and in a mouse model," *Human Molecular Genetics*, vol. 18, no. 17, pp. 3227–3243, 2009.

[75] S. Sacchi, M. Bernasconi, M. Martineau et al., "pLG72 modulates intracellular D-serine levels through its interaction with D-amino acid oxidase: effect on schizophrenia susceptibility," *The Journal of Biological Chemistry*, vol. 283, no. 32, pp. 22244–22256, 2008.

[76] J. Schumacher, R. Abon Jamra, J. Freudenberg et al., "Examination of G72 and D-amino-acid oxidase as genetic risk factors for schizophrenia and bipolar affective disorder," *Molecular Psychiatry*, vol. 9, no. 2, pp. 203–207, 2004.

[77] S. D. Detera-Wadleigh and F. J. McMahon, "G72/G30 in Schizophrenia and bipolar disorder: review and meta-analysis," *Biological Psychiatry*, vol. 60, no. 2, pp. 106–114, 2006.

[78] A. M. Addington, M. Gornick, A. L. Sporn et al., "Polymorphisms in the 13q33.2 gene G72/G30 are associated with childhood-onset schizophrenia and psychosis not otherwise specified," *Biological Psychiatry*, vol. 55, no. 10, pp. 976–980, 2004.

[79] S. L. Almond, R. L. Fradley, E. J. Armstrong et al., "Behavioral and biochemical characterization of a mutant mouse strain lacking d-amino acid oxidase activity and its implications for schizophrenia," *Molecular and Cellular Neuroscience*, vol. 32, no. 4, pp. 324–334, 2006.

[80] V. Labrie, W. Wang, S. W. Barger, G. B. Baker, and J. C. Roder, "Genetic loss of D-amino acid oxidase activity reverses schizophrenia-like phenotypes in mice," *Genes, Brain and Behavior*, vol. 9, no. 1, pp. 11–25, 2010.

[81] K. Hashimoto, T. Fukushima, E. Shimizu et al., "Decreased serum levels of D-serine in patients with schizophrenia: evidence in support of the N-methyl-D-aspartate receptor hypofunction hypothesis of schizophrenia," *Archives of General Psychiatry*, vol. 60, no. 6, pp. 572–576, 2003.

[82] K. Hashimoto, G. Engberg, E. Shimizu, C. Nordin, L. H. Lindström, and M. Iyo, "Reduced D-serine to total serine ratio in the cerebrospinal fluid of drug naive schizophrenic patients," *Progress in Neuro-Psychopharmacology and Biological Psychiatry*, vol. 29, no. 5, pp. 767–769, 2005.

[83] M. A. Calcia, C. Madeira, F. V. Alheira et al., "Plasma levels of D-serine in Brazilian individuals with schizophrenia," *Schizophrenia Research*, vol. 142, no. 1–3, pp. 83–87, 2012.

[84] K. Yamada, T. Ohnishi, K. Hashimoto et al., "Identification of multiple serine racemase (SRR) mRNA isoforms and genetic analyses of SRR and DAO in schizophrenia and D-serine levels," *Biological Psychiatry*, vol. 57, no. 12, pp. 1493–1503, 2005.

[85] I. Bendikov, C. Nadri, S. Amar et al., "A CSF and postmortem brain study of d-serine metabolic parameters in schizophrenia," *Schizophrenia Research*, vol. 90, no. 1–3, pp. 41–51, 2007.

[86] Y. Tanii, T. Nishikawa, A. Hashimoto, and K. Takahashi, "Stereoselective antagonism by enantiomers of alanine and serine of phencyclidine-induced hyperactivity, stereotypy and ataxia in the rat," *Journal of Pharmacology and Experimental Therapeutics*, vol. 269, no. 3, pp. 1040–1048, 1994.

[87] P. C. Contreras, "D-serine antagonized phencyclidine- and MK-801-induced stereotyped behavior and ataxia," *Neuropharmacology*, vol. 29, no. 3, pp. 291–293, 1990.

[88] G. Tsai, P. Yang, L.-C. Chung, N. Lange, and J. T. Coyle, "D-serine added to antipsychotics for the treatment of schizophrenia," *Biological Psychiatry*, vol. 44, no. 11, pp. 1081–1089, 1998.

[89] H.-Y. Lane, Y.-C. Chang, Y.-C. Liu, C.-C. Chiu, and G. E. Tsai, "Sarcosine or D-serine add-on treatment for acute exacerbation of schizophrenia: a randomized, double-blind, placebo-controlled study," *Archives of General Psychiatry*, vol. 62, no. 11, pp. 1196–1204, 2005.

[90] M. Weiser, U. Heresco-Levy, M. Davidson et al., "A multicenter, add-on randomized controlled trial of low-dose D-serine for negative and cognitive symptoms of schizophrenia," *Journal of Clinical Psychiatry*, vol. 73, no. 6, pp. e728–e734, 2012.

[91] S. P. Singh and V. Singh, "Meta-analysis of the efficacy of adjunctive NMDA receptor modulators in chronic schizophrenia," *CNS Drugs*, vol. 25, no. 10, pp. 859–885, 2011.

[92] G. E. Tsai and P.-Y. Lin, "Strategies to enhance N-Methyl-D-Aspartate receptor-mediated neurotransmission in schizophrenia, a critical review and meta-analysis," *Current Pharmaceutical Design*, vol. 16, no. 5, pp. 522–537, 2010.

[93] M. Ermilov, E. Gelfin, R. Levin et al., "A pilot double-blind comparison of d-serine and high-dose olanzapine in treatment-resistant patients with schizophrenia," *Schizophrenia Research*, vol. 150, no. 2-3, pp. 604–605, 2013.

[94] J. P. Kaltenbach, C. E. Ganote, and F. A. Carone, "Renal tubular necrosis induced by compounds structurally related to D-serine," *Experimental and Molecular Pathology*, vol. 30, no. 2, pp. 209–214, 1979.

[95] F. A. Carone, S. Nakamura, and B. Goldman, "Urinary loss of glucose, phosphate, and protein by diffusion into proximal straight tubules injured by D-serine and maleic acid," *Laboratory Investigation*, vol. 52, no. 6, pp. 605–610, 1985.

[96] G. E. Tsai, H.-Y. Lane, C. M. Vandenberg, Y.-C. Liu, P. Tsai, and M. W. Jann, "Disposition of D-serine in healthy adults," *Journal of Clinical Pharmacology*, vol. 48, no. 4, pp. 524–527, 2008.

[97] K. A. Johnson, P. J. Conn, and C. M. Niswender, "Glutamate receptors as therapeutic targets for Parkinson's disease," *CNS and Neurological Disorders—Drug Targets*, vol. 8, no. 6, pp. 475–491, 2009.

[98] R. S. Marin, "Apathy: a neuropsychiatric syndrome," *Journal of Neuropsychiatry and Clinical Neurosciences*, vol. 3, no. 3, pp. 243–254, 1991.

[99] M. S. Starr, "Glutamate/dopamine D1/D2 balance in the basal ganglia and its relevance to Parkinson's disease," *Synapse*, vol. 19, no. 4, pp. 264–293, 1995.

[100] S. S. Nikam and L. T. Meltzer, "NR2B selective NMDA receptor antagonists," *Current Pharmaceutical Design*, vol. 8, no. 10, pp. 845–855, 2002.

[101] P. J. Blanchet, S. Konitsiotis, E. R. Whittemore, Z. L. Zhou, R. M. Woodward, and T. N. Chase, "Differing effects of N-methyl-D-aspartate receptor subtype selective antagonists on dyskinesias in levodopa-treated 1-methyl-4-phenyl-tetrahydropyridine monkeys," *Journal of Pharmacology and Experimental Therapeutics*, vol. 290, no. 3, pp. 1034–1040, 1999.

[102] J. N. C. Kew, J. G. Richards, V. Mutel, and J. A. Kemp, "Developmental changes in NMDA receptor glycine affinity and ifenprodil sensitivity reveal three distinct populations of NMDA receptors in individual rat cortical neurons," *The Journal of Neuroscience*, vol. 18, no. 6, pp. 1935–1943, 1998.

[103] R. Trullas and P. Skolnick, "Functional antagonists at the NMDA receptor complex exhibit antidepressant actions," *European Journal of Pharmacology*, vol. 185, no. 1, pp. 1–10, 1990.

[104] R. Trullas, T. Folio, A. Young, R. Miller, K. Boje, and P. Skolnick, "1-Aminocyclopropanecarboxylates exhibit antidepressant and anxiolytic actions in animal models," *European Journal of Pharmacology*, vol. 203, no. 3, pp. 379–385, 1991.

[105] R. T. Layer, P. Popik, T. Olds, and P. Skolnick, "Antidepressant-like actions of the polyamine site NMDA antagonist, eliprodil (SL-82.0715)," *Pharmacology Biochemistry and Behavior*, vol. 52, no. 3, pp. 621–627, 1995.

[106] P. Skolnick, P. Popik, and R. Trullas, "Glutamate-based antidepressants: 20 years on," *Trends in Pharmacological Sciences*, vol. 30, no. 11, pp. 563–569, 2009.

[107] J. H. Krystal, G. Sanacora, and R. S. Duman, "Rapid-acting glutamatergic antidepressants: the path to ketamine and beyond," *Biological Psychiatry*, vol. 73, no. 12, pp. 1133–1141, 2013.

[108] A. J. Rush, "Ketamine for treatment-resistant depression: ready or not for clinical use?" *The American Journal of Psychiatry*, vol. 170, no. 10, pp. 1079–1081, 2013.

[109] U. Heresco-Levy, G. Gelfin, B. Bloch et al., "A randomized add-on trial of high-dose d-cycloserine for treatment-resistant depression," *International Journal of Neuropsychopharmacology*, vol. 16, no. 3, pp. 501–506, 2013.

[110] R. Depoortère, G. Dargazanli, G. Estenne-Bouhtou et al., "Neurochemical, electrophysiological and pharmacological profiles of the selective inhibitor of the glycine transporter-1 SSR504734, a potential new type of antipsychotic," *Neuropsychopharmacology*, vol. 30, no. 11, pp. 1963–1985, 2005.

[111] O. Malkesman, D. R. Austin, T. Tragon et al., "Acute d-serine treatment produces antidepressant-like effects in rodents," *International Journal of Neuropsychopharmacology*, vol. 15, no. 8, pp. 1135–1148, 2012.

[112] M. Beneyto and J. H. Meador-Woodruff, "Lamina-specific abnormalities of NMDA receptor-associated postsynaptic protein transcripts in the prefrontal cortex in schizophrenia and bipolar disorder," *Neuropsychopharmacology*, vol. 33, no. 9, pp. 2175–2186, 2008.

[113] G. Nowak, G. A. Ordway, and I. A. Paul, "Alterations in the N-methyl-D-aspartate (NMDA) receptor complex in the frontal cortex of suicide victims," *Brain Research*, vol. 675, no. 1-2, pp. 157–164, 1995.

[114] U. Heresco-Levy, "D-serine effects in healthy volunteers and neuropsychiatric disorders," in *Proceedings of the CINP Thematic Meeting: Pharmacogenomics and Personalized Medicine*, Jerusalem, Israel, April 2013.

[115] C. C. Huang, I. H. Wei, C. L. Huang et al., "Inhibition of glycine transporter-I as a novel mechanism for the treatment of depression," *Biological Psychiatry*, vol. 74, no. 10, pp. 734–741, 2013.

[116] C.-H. Lai, H.-Y. Lane, and G. E. Tsai, "Clinical and cerebral volumetric effects of sodium benzoate, a d-amino acid oxidase inhibitor, in a drug-nave patient with major depression," *Biological Psychiatry*, vol. 71, no. 4, pp. e9–e10, 2012.

[117] S. Maeng, C. A. Zarate Jr., J. Du et al., "Cellular mechanisms underlying the antidepressant effects of ketamine: Role of α-amino-3-hydroxy-5-methylisoxazole-4-propionic acid receptors," *Biological Psychiatry*, vol. 63, no. 4, pp. 349–352, 2008.

[118] A. C. Lahti, B. Koffel, D. LaPorte, and C. A. Tamminga, "Subanesthetic doses of ketamine stimulate psychosis in schizophrenia," *Neuropsychopharmacology*, vol. 13, no. 1, pp. 9–19, 1995.

[119] D. R. Lara, L. W. Bisol, and L. R. Munari, "Antidepressant, mood stabilizing and procognitive effects of very low dose sublingual ketamine in refractory unipolar and bipolar depression," *International Journal of Neuropsychopharmacology*, vol. 16, no. 9, pp. 2111–2117, 2013.

[120] A. J. McDonald, "Glutamate and aspartate immunoreactive neurons of the rat basolateral amygdala: colocalization of excitatory amino acids and projections to the limbic circuit," *Journal of Comparative Neurology*, vol. 365, no. 3, pp. 367–379, 1996.

[121] B. S. McEwen, "Plasticity of the hippocampus: adaptation to chronic stress and allostatic load," *Annals of the New York Academy of Sciences*, vol. 933, pp. 265–277, 2001.

[122] B. H. Harvey, F. Oosthuizen, L. Brand, G. Wegener, and D. J. Stein, "Stress-restress evokes sustained iNOS activity and altered GABA levels and NMDA receptors in rat hippocampus," *Psychopharmacology*, vol. 175, no. 4, pp. 494–502, 2004.

[123] B. S. McEwen, "Gonadal and adrenal steroids regulate neurochemical and structural plasticity of the hippocampus via cellular mechanisms involving NMDA receptors," *Cellular and Molecular Neurobiology*, vol. 16, no. 2, pp. 103–116, 1996.

[124] M. D. Horner and M. B. Hamner, "Neurocognitive functioning in posttraumatic stress disorder," *Neuropsychology Review*, vol. 12, no. 1, pp. 15–30, 2002.

[125] M. Davis and K. M. Myers, "The role of glutamate and gamma-aminobutyric acid in fear extinction: clinical implications for exposure therapy," *Biological Psychiatry*, vol. 52, no. 10, pp. 998–1007, 2002.

[126] M. Davis, K. Ressler, B. O. Rothbaum, and R. Richardson, "Effects of D-cycloserine on extinction: translation from preclinical to clinical work," *Biological Psychiatry*, vol. 60, no. 4, pp. 369–375, 2006.

[127] M. M. Norberg, J. H. Krystal, and D. F. Tolin, "A meta-analysis of D-cycloserine and the facilitation of fear extinction and exposure therapy," *Biological Psychiatry*, vol. 63, no. 12, pp. 1118–1126, 2008.

[128] J. A. J. Smits, D. Rosenfield, M. W. Otto et al., "D-cycloserine enhancement of exposure therapy for social anxiety disorder depends on the success of exposure sessions," *Journal of Psychiatric Research*, vol. 47, no. 10, pp. 1455–1461, 2013.

[129] A. Sheinin, S. Shavit, and M. Benveniste, "Subunit specificity and mechanism of action of NMDA partial agonist D-cycloserine," *Neuropharmacology*, vol. 41, no. 2, pp. 151–158, 2001.

[130] M. Horio, H. Mori, and K. Hashimoto, "Is D-cycloserine a prodrug for D-serine in the brain?" *Biological Psychiatry*, vol. 73, no. 12, pp. e33–e34, 2013.

[131] R. Richardson, L. Ledgerwood, and J. Cranney, "Facilitation of fear extinction by D-cycloserine: theoretical and clinical implications," *Learning and Memory*, vol. 11, no. 5, pp. 510–516, 2004.

[132] K. J. Ressler, B. O. Rothbaum, L. Tannenbaum et al., "Cognitive enhancers as adjuncts to psychotherapy: use of D-cycloserine in phobic individuals to facilitate extinction of fear," *Archives of General Psychiatry*, vol. 61, no. 11, pp. 1136–1144, 2004.

[133] M. J. Friedman, "What might the psychobiology of posttraumatic stress disorder teach us about future approaches to pharmacotherapy?" *Journal of Clinical Psychiatry*, vol. 61, no. 7, pp. 44–51, 2000.

[134] A. Garakani, S. J. Mathew, and D. S. Charney, "Neurobiology of anxiety disorders and implications for treatment," *Mount Sinai Journal of Medicine*, vol. 73, no. 7, pp. 941–949, 2006.

[135] D. J. Nutt, "The psychobiology of posttraumatic stress disorder," *Journal of Clinical Psychiatry*, vol. 61, no. 5, pp. 24–32, 2000.

[136] U. Heresco-Levy, A. Vass, B. Bloch et al., "Pilot controlled trial of d-serine for the treatment of post-traumatic stress disorder," *International Journal of Neuropsychopharmacology*, vol. 12, no. 9, pp. 1275–1282, 2009.

[137] M. A. Grados, M. W. Specht, H. M. Sung, and D. Fortune, "Glutamate drugs and pharmacogenetics of OCD: a pathway-based exploratory approach," *Expert Opinion on Drug Discovery*, vol. 8, no. 12, pp. 1515–1527, 2013.

[138] W. L. Cleveland, R. L. DeLaPaz, R. A. Fawwaz, and R. S. Challop, "High-dose glycine treatment of refractory obsessive-compulsive disorder and body dysmorphic disorder in a 5-year period," *Neural Plasticity*, vol. 2009, Article ID 768398, 25 pages, 2009.

[139] W. M. Greenberg, M. M. Benedict, J. Doerfer et al., "Adjunctive glycine in the treatment of obsessive-compulsive disorder in adults," *Journal of Psychiatric Research*, vol. 43, no. 6, pp. 664–670, 2009.

[140] Hoffmann-La Roche, "A study of bitopertin (RO4917838) in combination with selective serotonin reuptake inhibitors in patients with obsessive-compulsive disorder," National Library of Medicine (US), Bethesda, Md, USA, 2013, NLM Identifier: NCT01674361, http://clinicaltrials.gov/show/NCT01674361.

[141] N. B. Farber, J. W. Newcomer, and J. W. Olney, "The glutamate synapse in neuropsychiatric disorders: focus on schizophrenia and Alzheimer's disease," *Progress in Brain Research*, vol. 116, pp. 421–437, 1998.

[142] H. W. Querfurth and F. M. LaFerla, "Alzheimer's disease," *The New England Journal of Medicine*, vol. 362, no. 4, pp. 329–344, 2010.

[143] C. G. Parsons, A. Stöffler, and W. Danysz, "Memantine: a NMDA receptor antagonist that improves memory by restoration of homeostasis in the glutamatergic system—too little activation is bad, too much is even worse," *Neuropharmacology*, vol. 53, no. 6, pp. 699–723, 2007.

[144] G. J. Uhász, B. Barkóczi, G. Vass et al., "Fibrillar Aβ1-42 enhances NMDA receptor sensitivity via the integrin signaling pathway," *Journal of Alzheimer's Disease*, vol. 19, no. 3, pp. 1055–1067, 2010.

[145] E. Alberdi, M. V. Sánchez-Gómez, F. Cavaliere et al., "Amyloid β oligomers induce Ca^{2+} dysregulation and neuronal death through activation of ionotropic glutamate receptors," *Cell Calcium*, vol. 47, no. 3, pp. 264–272, 2010.

[146] D. A. Butterfield and C. B. Pocernich, "The glutamatergic system and Alzheimer's disease: therapeutic implications," *CNS Drugs*, vol. 17, no. 9, pp. 641–652, 2003.

[147] S. Lesné, C. Ali, C. Gabriel et al., "NMDA receptor activation inhibits α-secretase and promotes neuronal amyloid-β production," *The Journal of Neuroscience*, vol. 25, no. 41, pp. 9367–9377, 2005.

[148] W. Gordon-Krajcer, E. Salińska, and J. W. Łazarewicz, "N-methyl-d-aspartate receptor-mediated processing of β-amyloid precursor protein in rat hippocampal slices: in vitro-superfusion study," *Folia Neuropathologica*, vol. 40, no. 1, pp. 13–17, 2002.

[149] K. Ando, K. Uemura, A. Kuzuya et al., "N-cadherin regulates p38 MAPK signaling via association with JNK-associated leucine zipper protein: implications for neurodegeneration in Alzheimer disease," *The Journal of Biological Chemistry*, vol. 286, no. 9, pp. 7619–7628, 2011.

[150] K. Yamada and T. Nabeshima, "Changes in NMDA receptor/nitric oxide signaling pathway in the brain with aging," *Microscopy Research and Technique*, vol. 43, no. 1, pp. 68–74, 1998.

[151] C. Ikonomidou, V. Stefovska, and L. Turski, "Neuronal death enhanced by N-methyl-D-aspartate antagonists," *Proceedings of the National Academy of Sciences of the United States of America*, vol. 97, no. 23, pp. 12885–12890, 2000.

[152] S. M. Adams, J. C. De Rivero Vaccari, and R. A. Corriveau, "Pronounced cell death in the absence of NMDA receptors in the developing somatosensory thalamus," *The Journal of Neuroscience*, vol. 24, no. 42, pp. 9441–9450, 2004.

[153] J. W. Olney, D. F. Wozniak, and N. B. Farber, "Excitotoxic neurodegeneration in Alzheimer disease: new hypothesis and new therapeutic strategies," *Archives of Neurology*, vol. 54, no. 10, pp. 1234–1240, 1997.

[154] D. F. Wozniak, K. Dikranian, M. J. Ishimaru et al., "Disseminated corticolimbic neuronal degeneration induced in rat brain by MK-801: potential relevance to Alzheimer's disease," *Neurobiology of Disease*, vol. 5, no. 5, pp. 305–322, 1998.

[155] Y.-J. Huang, C.-H. Lin, H.-Y. Lane, and G. E. Tsai, "NMDA neurotransmission dysfunction in behavioral and psychological symptoms of Alzheimer's disease," *Current Neuropharmacology*, vol. 10, no. 3, pp. 272–285, 2012.

[156] A. W. Procter, E. H. F. Wong, G. C. Stratmann, S. L. Lowe, and D. M. Bowen, "Reduced glycine stimulation of [3H]MK-801 binding in Alzheimer's disease," *Journal of Neurochemistry*, vol. 53, no. 3, pp. 698–704, 1989.

[157] E. L. Schaeffer and W. F. Gattaz, "Cholinergic and glutamatergic alterations beginning at the early stages of Alzheimer disease: participation of the phospholipase A2 enzyme," *Psychopharmacology*, vol. 198, no. 1, pp. 1–27, 2008.

[158] E. M. Snyder, Y. Nong, C. G. Almeida et al., "Regulation of NMDA receptor trafficking by amyloid-β," *Nature Neuroscience*, vol. 8, no. 8, pp. 1051–1058, 2005.

[159] A. Auffret, V. Gautheron, M. Repici et al., "Age-dependent impairment of spine morphology and synaptic plasticity in hippocampal CA1 neurons of a presenilin 1 transgenic mouse model of Alzheimer's disease," *The Journal of Neuroscience*, vol. 29, no. 32, pp. 10144–10152, 2009.

[160] A. Auffret, V. Gautheron, M. P. Mattson, J. Mariani, and C. Rovira, "Progressive age-related impairment of the late long-term potentiation in Alzheimer's disease presenilin-1 mutant knock-in mice," *Journal of Alzheimer's Disease*, vol. 19, no. 3, pp. 1021–1033, 2010.

[161] M. Martinez, A. Frank, E. Diez-Tejedor, and A. Hernanz, "Amino acid concentrations in cerebrospinal fluid and serum in Alzheimer's disease and vascular dementia," *Journal of Neural Transmission—Parkinson's Disease and Dementia Section*, vol. 6, no. 1, pp. 1–9, 1993.

[162] K. Hashimoto, T. Fukushima, E. Shimizu et al., "Possible role of D-serine in the pathophysiology of Alzheimer's disease," *Progress in Neuro-Psychopharmacology and Biological Psychiatry*, vol. 28, no. 2, pp. 385–388, 2004.

[163] S. L. Lowe and D. M. Bowen, "Glutamic acid concentration in brains of patients with Alzheimer's disease," *Biochemical Society Transactions*, vol. 18, no. 3, pp. 443–444, 1990.

[164] X. Ye and T. J. Carew, "Small G protein signaling in neuronal plasticity and memory formation: the specific role of ras family proteins," *Neuron*, vol. 68, no. 3, pp. 340–361, 2010.

[165] L. V. Kalia, S. K. Kalia, and M. W. Salter, "NMDA receptors in clinical neurology: excitatory times ahead," *The Lancet Neurology*, vol. 7, no. 8, pp. 742–755, 2008.

[166] E. Scarpini, P. Scheltens, and H. Feldman, "Treatment of Alzheimer's disease: current status and new perspectives," *Lancet Neurology*, vol. 2, no. 9, pp. 539–547, 2003.

[167] F. Gardoni and M. Di Luca, "New targets for pharmacological intervention in the glutamatergic synapse," *European Journal of Pharmacology*, vol. 545, no. 1, pp. 2–10, 2006.

[168] L. Morè, A. Gravius, J. Nagel, B. Valastro, S. Greco, and W. Danysz, "Therapeutically relevant plasma concentrations of memantine produce significant L-N-methyl-D-aspartate receptor occupation and do not impair learning in rats," *Behavioural Pharmacology*, vol. 19, no. 7, pp. 724–734, 2008.

[169] T. M. Ballard, M. Pauly-Evers, G. A. Higgins et al., "Severe impairment of NMDA receptor function in mice carrying targeted point mutations in the glycine binding site results in drug-resistant nonhabituating hyperactivity," *The Journal of Neuroscience*, vol. 22, no. 15, pp. 6713–6723, 2002.

[170] J. N. C. Kew, A. Koester, J.-L. Moreau et al., "Functional consequences of reduction in NMDA receptor glycine affinity in mice carrying targeted point mutations in the glycine binding site," *The Journal of Neuroscience*, vol. 20, no. 11, pp. 4037–4049, 2000.

[171] J. F. Flood, J. E. Morley, and T. H. Lanthorn, "Effect on memory processing by D-cycloserine, an agonist of the NMDA/glycine receptor," *European Journal of Pharmacology*, vol. 221, no. 2-3, pp. 249–254, 1992.

[172] G. M. Schuster and W. J. Schmidt, "D-Cycloserine reverses the working memory impairment of hippocampal-lesioned rats in a spatial learning task," *European Journal of Pharmacology*, vol. 224, no. 1, pp. 97–98, 1992.

[173] C. Randolph, J. W. Roberts, M. C. Tierney, D. Bravi, M. M. Mouradian, and T. N. Chase, "D-Cycloserine treatment of Alzheimer disease," *Alzheimer Disease and Associated Disorders*, vol. 8, no. 3, pp. 198–205, 1994.

[174] G. E. Tsai, W. E. Falk, and J. Gunther, "A preliminary study of D-cycloserine treatment in Alzheimer's disease," *Journal of Neuropsychiatry and Clinical Neurosciences*, vol. 10, no. 2, pp. 224–226, 1998.

[175] T. D. Fakouhi, S. S. Jhee, J. J. Sramek et al., "Evaluation of cycloserine in the treatment of Alzheimer's disease," *Journal of Geriatric Psychiatry and Neurology*, vol. 8, no. 4, pp. 226–230, 1995.

[176] P. Bado, C. Madeira, C. Vargas-Lopes et al., "Effects of low-dose d-serine on recognition and working memory in mice," *Psychopharmacology*, vol. 218, no. 3, pp. 461–470, 2011.

[177] C. H. Lin, P. K. Chen, Y. C. Chang et al., "Benzoate, a D-amino acid oxidase inhibitor, for the treatment of early-phase Alzheimer disease: a randomized, double-blind, placebo-controlled trial," *Biological Psychiatry*, vol. 75, no. 9, pp. 678–685, 2014.

[178] B. Reisberg, R. Doody, A. Stöffler, F. Schmitt, S. Ferris, and H. J. Möbius, "Memantine in moderate-to-severe Alzheimer's disease," *The New England Journal of Medicine*, vol. 348, no. 14, pp. 1333–1341, 2003.

[179] L. S. Schneider, K. S. Dagerman, J. P. T. Higgins, and R. McShane, "Lack of evidence for the efficacy of memantine in mild Alzheimer disease," *Archives of Neurology*, vol. 68, no. 8, pp. 991–998, 2011.

[180] A. C. Ludolph, J. Brettschneider, and J. H. Weishaupt, "Amyotrophic lateral sclerosis," *Current Opinion in Neurology*, vol. 25, no. 5, pp. 530–535, 2012.

[181] P. Paul and J. De Belleroche, "The role of D-amino acids in amyotrophic lateral sclerosis pathogenesis: a review," *Amino Acids*, vol. 43, no. 5, pp. 1823–1831, 2012.

[182] J. Sasabe, Y. Miyoshi, M. Suzuki et al., "D-Amino acid oxidase controls motoneuron degeneration through D-serine," *Proceedings of the National Academy of Sciences of the United States of America*, vol. 109, no. 2, pp. 627–632, 2012.

[183] J. Mitchell, P. Paul, H.-J. Chen et al., "Familial amyotrophic lateral sclerosis is associated with a mutation in D-amino acid oxidase," *Proceedings of the National Academy of Sciences of the United States of America*, vol. 107, no. 16, pp. 7556–7561, 2010.

[184] V. I. Tishkov and S. V. Khoronenkova, "D-Amino acid oxidase: structure, catalytic mechanism, and practical application," *Biochemistry*, vol. 70, no. 1, pp. 40–54, 2005.

[185] H. Hasegawa, T. Matsukawa, Y. Shinohara, R. Konno, and T. Hashimoto, "Role of renal D-amino-acid oxidase in pharmacokinetics of D-leucine," *The American Journal of Physiology—Endocrinology and Metabolism*, vol. 287, no. 1, pp. E160–E165, 2004.

[186] S. M. Smith, J. M. Uslaner, and P. H. Hutson, "The therapeutic potential of D-amino acid oxidase (DAAO) inhibitors," *Open Medicinal Chemistry Journal*, vol. 4, no. 1, pp. 3–9, 2010.

[187] D. Ferraris, B. Duvall, Y.-S. Ko et al., "Synthesis and biological evaluation of D-amino acid oxidase inhibitors," *Journal of Medicinal Chemistry*, vol. 51, no. 12, pp. 3357–3359, 2008.

[188] K. Hashimoto, Y. Fujita, M. Horio et al., "Co-administration of a D-amino acid oxidase inhibitor potentiates the efficacy of D-serine in attenuating prepulse inhibition deficits after administration of dizocilpine," *Biological Psychiatry*, vol. 65, no. 12, pp. 1103–1106, 2009.

[189] A. W. Krug, K. Völker, W. H. Dantzler, and S. Silbernagl, "Why is D-serine nephrotoxic and α-aminoisobutyric acid protective?" *The American Journal of Physiology—Renal Physiology*, vol. 293, no. 1, pp. F382–F390, 2007.

[190] World Health Organization, "Concise International Chemical Assessment, Document 26. Benzoic Acid and Sodium Benzoate," World Health Organization, Geneva, Switzerland, 2000, http://www.who.int/ipcs/publications/cicad/cicad26_rev_1.pdf.

[191] W.-J. Zhao, Z.-Y. Gao, H. Wei et al., "Spinal D-amino acid oxidase contributes to neuropathic pain in rats," *Journal of Pharmacology and Experimental Therapeutics*, vol. 332, no. 1, pp. 248–254, 2010.

[192] N. Gong, Z.-Y. Gao, Y.-C. Wang et al., "A series of d-amino acid oxidase inhibitors specifically prevents and reverses formalin-induced tonic pain in rats," *Journal of Pharmacology and Experimental Therapeutics*, vol. 336, no. 1, pp. 282–293, 2011.

[193] H. K. Park, Y. Shishido, S. Ichise-Shishido et al., "Potential role for astroglial D-amino acid oxidase in extracellular D-serine metabolism and cytotoxicity," *Journal of Biochemistry*, vol. 139, no. 2, pp. 295–304, 2006.

[194] A. Jana, K. K. Modi, A. Roy, J. A. Anderson, R. B. Van Breemen, and K. Pahan, "Up-regulation of neurotrophic factors by cinnamon and its metabolite sodium benzoate: therapeutic implications for neurodegenerative disorders," *Journal of Neuroimmune Pharmacology*, vol. 8, no. 3, pp. 739–755, 2013.

[195] H. Y. Lane, C. H. Lin, M. F. Green et al., "Add-on treatment of benzoate for schizophrenia: a randomized, double-blind, placebo-controlled trial of D-amino acid oxidase inhibitor," *JAMA Psychiatry*, vol. 70, no. 12, pp. 1267–1275, 2013.

20

Temperament and Eating Attitudes in an Adolescent Community Sample: A Brief Report

Enrica Marzola, Secondo Fassino, Federico Amianto, and Giovanni Abbate-Daga

Eating Disorders Center, Department of Neuroscience, University of Turin, Via Cherasco 15, 10126 Turin, Italy

Correspondence should be addressed to Giovanni Abbate-Daga; giovanni.abbatedaga@unito.it

Academic Editor: Xingguang Luo

Objective. Temperament traits like high harm avoidance (HA) have been proposed as putative risk factors for the development of eating disorders (EDs). We aimed at studying the relationship between temperament and eating attitudes on a large community sample of adolescents. *Method.* We recruited 992 high school students aged 14–18. In addition to measuring body mass index (BMI), participants were asked to complete the temperament and character inventory and the food frequency questionnaire. *Results.* Sixty-two percent of the sample reported overeating, 22.8% reported normal eating, and 15.2% reported under eating. Under and normal eaters had higher BMI than that of over eaters. Harm avoidance was found to be significantly higher in those participants with lower eating intakes whilst novelty seeking was found to be higher in over eaters. *Conclusion.* An interesting association between temperament (high HA) and food approach (under eating) emerged. Longitudinal studies are needed to evaluate whether these traits represent a risk factor for the development of EDs.

1. Introduction

Eating disorders (EDs) are serious illnesses characterized by high comorbidity and mortality, life-threatening sequelae, and low quality of life. Notwithstanding the recent insights into the mechanisms underpinning and maintaining such disorders, to date their aetiology remains unknown and uncertainty persists on what to consider as vulnerability factors.

Among various other posited factors, personality has been called into question as regards ED developmental trajectories. According to the widely used instrument temperament and character inventory (TCI) [1], high scores on the temperament dimension of harm avoidance (HA) are shared by both actively ill and recovered individuals [2]; although its role is not univocal, these lines of research seem to propose it as candidate risk factor for the development of EDs [3].

More in detail, the rationale for considering personality as risk factor could be represented by its role in modulating coping abilities, namely, those responses based on personal vulnerability to stressors that are shared by many individuals. Earlier studies showed how the combination of high HA and low self-directedness may impair the ability to face distress [4] and recent research proposed that personality traits may indirectly influence eating attitudes and food approach through thin-ideal internalization [5].

In addition to an earlier study [6] focusing on disordered eating in adolescents, with the present report we aimed to assess the relationship between temperament traits and eating attitudes on a large community sample of adolescents. In line with the pattern of personality traits—as measured by the TCI—characterizing patients affected by EDs (i.e., particularly high HA) [4, 7] our a priori hypothesis was to find an association between a highly avoidant temperament and food approach.

2. Methods

2.1. Participants. Methods are described in detail elsewhere [6]. Ten high schools in Turin were randomly selected and asked to participate in this study; of these, six agreed on being involved. We finally enrolled 992 students ($N = 247$ males; $N = 745$ females), aged 14–18 years old. No exclusion/inclusion criteria were adopted. All students were Caucasian and assessed while being at school.

TABLE 1: Comparison of personality characteristics as measured with the TCI among caloric intake groups according to the food frequency questionnaire.

	Under eaters (UE)	Normal eaters (NE)	Over eaters (OE)	P	Test statistics Bonferroni post hoc
Body mass index	21.8 ± 3.5	21.9 ± 3.6	20.9 ± 3.2	<0.001	OE < NE, UE
Harm avoidance	19.4 ± 6.1	17.6 ± 6.7	16.7 ± 6.7	<0.001	UE > OE, NE NE > OE
Novelty seeking	19.1 ± 6.0	19.9 ± 6.1	21.2 ± 5.9	<0.001	OE > NE, UE

All participants over the age of 18 gave their written informed consent; those under the age of 18 provided written informed assent in addition to their parents' written informed consent and permission. All consent/assent procedures were conducted according to the ethical committee of the Department of Neuroscience of the University of Turin.

2.2. Measures. All participants' weight and height were measured by a registered dietician and body mass index (BMI) was then calculated. All students were asked to provide their personal information and to complete the following self-reported questionnaires: (1) temperament and character inventory (TCI) [1] to evaluate personality according to seven dimensions (temperament: novelty seeking [NS], harm avoidance [HA], reward dependence [RD], and persistence [P]; and character: self-directedness [SD], cooperativeness [C], and self-transcendence [ST]); and (2) food frequency questionnaire (FFQ) [8] to measure individuals' usual food and caloric intake. Norms are based on the nutritional recommendations (adjusted for age and gender) for the Italian population described by the Italian Society of Human Nutrition [9]. According to such recommendations, subjects can be divided into 3 groups: under eaters (UE), normal eaters (NE), and over eaters (OE).

2.3. Statistical Analysis. The SPSS statistical software package was used for data analysis. Descriptive statistics were computed. A one-way analysis of variance (ANOVA) with Bonferroni post hoc was calculated to assess personality dimensions by eating attitudes.

3. Results

Details on data collection have been described elsewhere [6]; 992 adolescents were contacted, 972 were enrolled, and 967 returned the questionnaires; of these, 860 completed all the assessments. Participants' mean age was 16.2 ± 1.5 years.

As regards food intake, the majority of the sample (62%) reported overeating, 22.8% normal eating, and 15.2% under eating whilst with respect to BMI, UE, and NE groups were found to have a significantly higher BMI than OE.

With respect to personality, harm avoidance (HA) was significantly higher (*P* < 0.001) in those participants with lower eating intakes when compared to other groups whilst novelty seeking (NS) was found to be higher in over eaters (*P* < 0.001) than that in the other groups (see Table 1).

4. Discussion

Interestingly, under eaters showed a temperament profile similar to individuals affected by EDs, scoring higher on the harm avoidance scale when compared to normal and over eaters. Harm avoidance is a temperament dimension related to behavioral inhibition, anxiety, fearfulness, pessimism, and inflexibility and it has been widely demonstrated to be high in patients affected by EDs [2, 4]. As extensively reported in literature [7], HA levels are connected to the serotonin system in the brain, namely, the neurobiological substratum that is strictly related to mood, impulse control, and satiety.

Individuals affected by anorexia nervosa starve themselves to death and robust evidence has now accumulated suggesting that starvation per se could contribute to modulate dysphoric mood potentially generated by an increased activity of brain serotonin systems [7]. The association we found between high HA and under eating in healthy adolescents raises the intriguing hypothesis that also for certain individuals from the community lower caloric intakes may represent an attempt to attenuate aversive anxious and dysphoric states related to a highly avoidant temperament.

Moreover, a mismatch between self-reported eating attitudes and BMI emerged since under eaters reported low caloric intakes although their BMI was found to be higher than that of over eaters. On one hand this finding may be due to young participants' lack of accuracy in self-evaluation or age-related different metabolic requirements but on the other hand it could describe instead under eaters' peculiar food approach. In fact, it could be speculated that such tendency to underestimate energy intakes may be explained by factors like thin-ideal internalization and body dissatisfaction. Such factors have been suggested to promote the ED onset [10] and also recently they have been proposed as mediators between personality and food approach [5].

As regards novelty seeking, higher levels on this dimension corresponded to larger food intakes. Also this datum is in line with the ED literature with lower NS scores in individuals who restrict their eating rather than in those who engage in binge-purging behaviors [4].

This report suffers from several limitations: participants were not screened for psychiatric comorbidities potentially biasing HA levels and disordered eating could have been assessed with more powerful tools. Moreover, food intake can be influenced by multiple factors including stress, mood, and general health which should be controlled for. However, the match we found between temperament traits of clinical and community samples is of interest in the context of the ongoing debate on developmental risk factors for EDs. Further studies with a longitudinal design may want to ascertain as to whether some temperament traits may constitute a slippery slope for predisposed individuals towards full-blown EDs through the impairment of coping abilities. Still, larger studies are warranted to shed light on the mismatch we found between self-report food intake and BMI.

Prompted by the need of distress modulation, a whole spectrum of food approaches ranging from avoidance (high HA) to urgency (high NS) may rely on different temperament profiles.

5. Conclusions

An intriguing association between temperament, namely, high HA, and food approach (under eating) emerged. Longitudinal studies may want to evaluate whether these traits represent a risk factor for the development of EDs.

Conflict of Interests

The authors declare that there is no conflict of interests regarding the publication of this paper.

References

[1] C. R. Cloninger, D. M. Svrakic, and T. R. Przybeck, "A psychobiological model of temperament and character," *Archives of General Psychiatry*, vol. 50, no. 12, pp. 975–990, 1993.

[2] K. L. Klump, M. Strober, C. M. Bulik et al., "Personality characteristics of women before and after recovery from an eating disorder," *Psychological Medicine*, vol. 34, no. 8, pp. 1407–1418, 2004.

[3] L. R. R. Lilenfeld, "Personality and temperament," *Current Topics in Behavioral Neurosciences*, vol. 6, pp. 3–16, 2011.

[4] S. Fassino, G. Abbate-Daga, F. Amianto, P. Leombruni, S. Boggio, and G. G. Rovera, "Temperament and character profile of eating disorders: A controlled study with the temperament and character inventory," *International Journal of Eating Disorders*, vol. 32, no. 4, pp. 412–425, 2002.

[5] P. K. Keel and K. J. Forney, "Psychosocial risk factors for eating disorders," *International Journal of Eating Disorders*, vol. 46, no. 5, pp. 433–439, 2013.

[6] G. Abbate-Daga, C. Gramaglia, G. Malfi, A. Pierò, and S. Fassino, "Eating problems and personality traits. An Italian pilot study among 992 high school students," *European Eating Disorders Review*, vol. 15, no. 6, pp. 471–478, 2007.

[7] W. H. Kaye, J. L. Fudge, and M. Paulus, "New insights into symptoms and neurocircuit function of anorexia nervosa," *Nature Reviews Neuroscience*, vol. 10, no. 8, pp. 573–584, 2009.

[8] P. Pisani, F. Faggiano, V. Krogh, D. Palli, P. Vineis, and F. Berrino, "Relative validity and reproducibility of a food frequency questionnaire for use in the Italian EPIC centres," *International Journal of Epidemiology*, vol. 26, supplement 1, pp. S152–S160, 1997.

[9] Società Italiana di Nutrizione Umana, "Livelli di assunzione raccomandati di energia e nutrienti per la popolazione Italiana," in *Proceedings of the Acts of 25th National Meeting*, 2012.

[10] E. Stice, J. Ng, and H. Shaw, "Risk factors and prodromal eating pathology," *Journal of Child Psychology and Psychiatry and Allied Disciplines*, vol. 51, no. 4, pp. 518–525, 2010.

21

The Dimensional Structure of the Schizotypal Personality Questionnaire Adapted for Children (SPQ-C-D): An Evaluation in the Dutch Population and a Comparison to Adult Populations

Sophie van Rijn,[1,2] **Pieter Kroonenberg,**[3] **Tim Ziermans,**[1,2] **and Hanna Swaab**[1,2]

[1]*Clinical Child and Adolescent Studies, Leiden University, Wassenaarseweg 52, 2333 AK Leiden, Netherlands*
[2]*Leiden Institute for Brain and Cognition, P.O. Box 9600, 2300 RC Leiden, Netherlands*
[3]*Family Studies, Leiden University, Wassenaarseweg 52, 2333 AK Leiden, Netherlands*

Correspondence should be addressed to Sophie van Rijn; srijn@fsw.leidenuniv.nl

Academic Editor: Takahiro Nemoto

The increasing interest in dimensional approaches towards schizophrenia spectrum pathology calls for instruments that can be used to study developmental markers conveying risk for psychopathology prior to onset of the disorder. In this study we evaluated the Dutch child version (SPQ-C-D) of the Schizotypal Personality Questionnaire (SPQ) developed by Raine, in terms of reliability and factorial structure in comparison to SPQ data from two studies with adults. The 74-item SPQ-C-D was completed by 219 children and adolescents aged 9 to 18 years. Internal consistency was assessed and the factorial structure was analyzed using principal component analysis (PCA) and confirmatory factor analysis. Results showed that most of the subscales had high Cronbach's alphas, indicating good internal consistency. PCA resulted in three components, similar to the adult studies: Cognitive-Perceptual, Interpersonal, and Disorganization. The pattern of individual subscales loading on each of the components was identical to the original Raine study, except for one additional subscale loading on the Disorganization component. In addition, forcing Raine's factorial structure on our data with confirmatory factor analysis resulted in an overall adequate model fit. In conclusion, the SPQ-C-D appears to be a suitable dimensional measure of schizotypal traits in populations aged 9 to 18 years.

1. Introduction

The introduction of the fifth edition of the Diagnostic Statistical Manual of Mental Disorders (DMS-5) and the Research Domain Criteria (RDoC) project constitutes a major shift in schizophrenia research, which urges the use of dimensional approaches of psychotic-like phenomena. Phenomena that are part of the clinical phenotype of schizophrenia spectrum disorders are quantitatively distributed along a continuum, rather than or in addition to being categorical disease entities [1, 2]. Such subclinical experiences which do not meet the clinical threshold or criteria for schizophrenia spectrum disorders are known as "psychosis proneness," "at-risk mental states," or "schizotypal personality traits" [3–7]. In this paper we will refer to these characteristics as "schizotypal traits," which can be measured using self-report questionnaires, such

as the Schizotypal Personality Questionnaire (SPQ), which exists as an extended, 74-item version [8] and an abbreviated 22-item version, that is, the SPQ-B [9].

Most studies on schizotypal traits have concentrated on adult samples, specifically on individuals with schizophrenia spectrum disorder or schizotypal disorder and their relatives. However, there is compelling evidence suggesting that, already many years before the onset of the illness, deviant behavioural and cognitive development is present in children who are later diagnosed with schizotypal personality disorder or schizophrenia spectrum disorders [10–12]. It is important to be able to measure schizotypal traits, preferably in childhood and adolescence, as it is necessary to focus on development before and during adolescence in order to gain insight into the processes of aberrant (neuro-)development that indicates risk for severe outcome in adulthood [13].

Self-report questionnaires assessing schizotypal traits have good long-term predictive validity as empirical evidence shows that individuals with high scores on self-reports of schizotypal traits are at increased risk for later development of schizophrenia spectrum disorders in both community [14–17] and clinical samples [18, 19]. The use of psychometric inventories for assessing levels of schizotypal traits (the so-called psychometric high-risk method) has advanced considerably in the last three decades and is considered a feasible, valid, inexpensive, and noninvasive technique for identifying schizotypal traits [20].

Scales measuring schizotypal traits have been shown to have a highly similar factorial structure in the general population, with latent factors resembling the classical schizophrenia positive, negative, and disorganization symptom dimensions [8, 21–23]. Much research has been done on the number of factors as well as the extent to which they are correlated. The consensus from primarily US studies centers around both a three-factor structure [22] and a four-factor structure [24, 25]. The few studies examining a four-factor structure [24–26] support Stefanis et al. model with the factors Paranoid, Interpersonal, Cognitive-Perceptual, and Disorganization. For the three-factor models, the most commonly used factor labels are Cognitive-Perceptual, Interpersonal-Affective, and Disorganization (or Positive Schizotypy, Negative Schizotypy, and Disorganization). Ericson et al. [27] state that a three-factor structure has been replicated in at least 14 independent adult samples, across several populations, and in samples of both schizophrenic in patients and outpatients; for an overview of different type of models, see [26]. This indicates that a three-factor structure is a dominant and leading model for the clustering of schizotypal traits.

Considering the potential contribution in understanding neurodevelopmental mechanisms underlying schizotypal traits over the course of development (preceding the typical age of onset of schizophrenia spectrum disorders), there is a need for developing instruments measuring schizotypal traits in children and adolescents. Regarding the SPQ, there is a brief 22-item version for children 11 years and older (SPQ-C) [27], of which the factorial structure parallels those found in older and clinical groups. However, there is no full 74-item version of the SPQ for children and adolescents, which would allow the measurement of specific schizotypal traits on subscale level.

Given the need for early identification of specific schizotypal traits in children, a children's version of the Schizotypal Personality Questionnaire was developed by adapting the original full 74-item adult SPQ [28]. As part of the validation of psychometric instruments assessing schizotypal traits comes from the dimensional structure of schizotypal traits, the aim of the present study was to evaluate the SPQ-C-D in Dutch children between 9 and 18 years old in terms of reliability and factor structure and to compare it with similar information from the original SPQ data by [8] and SPQ data from young adult participants in a study by Compton et al. [24].

2. Materials and Methods

2.1. Participants. The SPQ was completed by 219 children and adolescents (106 girls and 113 boys). Age ranged from 9 to 18 years, with a mean age of 11.8 years (sd 2.4). The period of data collection was between 2003 and 2011. Children were recruited from ten mainstream schools distributed across the western half of Netherlands. All children were screened for psychopathology, with none of the included participants scoring in the clinical range (>70) on the Childhood Behavior Checklist (CBCL) [29]. After providing a complete description of the study to the subjects and to their parents, we obtained written informed consent according to the Declaration of Helsinki. The study was approved by the ethical committees of Leiden University Medical Center and the University Medical Center Utrecht.

2.2. Instruments. All subjects completed the children's version of the Schizotypal Personality Questionnaire (SPQ) [8], originally translated into Dutch and validated for adults by Vollema et al. [23, 28, 30]. Adaptations to the Dutch SPQ version for children were done (in consensus) by the authors who are working in the field of developmental neuropsychology. Such an expert committee is needed to "achieve four types of equivalence: semantic (i.e., equivalence in meaning of words), idiomatic (i.e., equivalent expressions have to be found or items have to be substituted), experiential (i.e., the situation evoked or depicted in the source version should fit the target cultural context), and conceptual (i.e., is the concept explored valid in the target culture?)" [31]. The expert committee made such minor adaptations, which involved a change in using simpler expressions rather than complex expressions to accommodate a younger age group. In some of the questions developmentally specific words such as "work" were replaced with "school" and "writing letters" was changed to "texting and sending emails" to place the questions in an appropriate context. For all items. The SPQ-C-D is a 74-item questionnaire with a dichotomous response format (applies to me, does not apply to me), with a total score ranging from 0 to 74.

2.3. Statistical Methods

2.3.1. Reliability: Internal Consistency. Given that previous studies used Cronbach's alpha to establish the internal consistency of the subscales, we compared Cronbach's alphas of the subscales of the SPQ-C-D with those of the subscales published by Raine [32] and Compton et al. [24].

2.3.2. Factorial Structure. The analyses on our data and those by Compton et al. [24] were carried out with SPSS19 using an oblimin rotation. Unfortunately no other principal component outcomes were available for comparison with the literature.

Most published analyses of the SPQ are carried out via a confirmatory factor analysis but we decided to first perform a principal component analysis with an oblique rotation in order not to prejudice the solution of the three factors towards already existing solutions. The results were compared with the outcomes of data from Compton et al. [24] who kindly supplied us with their data set on undergraduates filling out Raine's standard SPQ. Subsequently, we compared our EQS

TABLE 1: Internal consistencies of SPQ-C-D, Compton et al. [24] sample and Raine's [8] samples.

Subscale names	Items in subscales	SPQ-C-D α	Compton α	Raine α	N items
Interpersonal					
Social Anxiety	Item 2, item 11, item 20, item 29, item 38, item 46, item 54, item 71	.73	.79	.72, .88	8
Constricted Affect	Item 8, item 17, item 26, item 35, item 43, item 51, item 68, item 73	.56	.71	.66, .65	8
No Close Friends	Item 6, item 15, item 24, item 33, item 41, item 49, item 57, item 62, item 66	.48	.75	.67, .74	9
Cognitive/Perceptual					
Unusual Perceptual (Experiences)	Item 4, item 13, item 22, item 31, item 40, item 48, item 56, item 61, item 64	.78	.73	.71, .73	9
(Suspiciousness/Paranoid Ideation) Paranoia	Item 9, item 18, item 27, item 36, item 44, item 52, item 59, item 6	.73	.75	.78, .73	8
Ideas of Reference	Item 1, item 10, item 19, item 28, item 37, item 45, item 53, item 60, item 63	.72	.74	.71, .71	9
(Odd Beliefs/)Magical Thinking	Item 3, item 12, item 21, item 30, item 39, item 47, item 55	.67	.70	.81, .75	7
Disorganization					
Eccentric(/Odd) Behaviour	Item 5, item 14, item 23, item 32, item 67, item 70, item 74	.77	.83	.78, .74	7
Odd Speech	Item 7, item 16, item 25, item 34, item 42, item 50, item 58, item 69, item 72	.74	.77	.70, .74	9
Interpersonal		.84	.89		25
Cognitive/Perceptual		.89	.88		33
Disorganization		.82	.86		16
Total scale (based on 9 subscales)		.85	.87		9
Total scale (based on 74 items)		.92	.94	.91, .90	74

confirmatory factor analysis results with those analyses available from the literature.

2.3.3. Effects of Age and Sex. Based on the reliabilities and factorial analyses that are part of this study, we analyzed the effects of age and sex for three SPQ domains as well as the total SPQ score. The age distribution of our sample is such that in order to get sufficient persons in a group for reliable estimates we grouped the 13- and 14-year-olds, and the 15-, 16-, 17+-year-olds. Only cases with scores on all items were included.

3. Results

3.1. Reliability: Internal Consistency. First, with respect to the three domain scores and the total score, all reliabilities were larger than .82. They were very similar to the Compton et al. ones (Raine's domain score reliabilities were not available). The subscale reliability analysis showed that the subscales have comparable Cronbach's α's to Raine's and Compton et al. samples, except for relatively low α's for the Interpersonal subscales, No Close Friends ($\alpha = .47$), and Constricted Affect ($\alpha = .56$) as well as Magical Thinking ($\alpha = .67$) in our study. Note that the No Close Friends and Constricted Affect were

also borderline in the Raine samples but fully acceptable for the Compton et al. sample. See Table 1 for all Cronbach's α's.

3.2. Factorial Structure

3.2.1. Principal Component Analysis. In our evaluation of the SPQ-C-D we restricted analysis to a three-factor structure with an oblique rotation. The comparison between the SPQ-C-D and the Compton et al. results shows both agreement and some differences with respect to which subscale belongs to which component. All results are presented in Table 2 and the items in the outlined text boxes indicate Raine's structure of the original SPQ. Results show that the pattern of subscales loading on the three components of the SPQ-C-D resembles closely the pattern of Raine's confirmatory factor analyses. Different from Raine's original construction, in our study Constricted Affect loaded on two components, that is, Interpersonal and Disorganization. Dissimilarities with Raine's solution were also emphasised by Compton et al. who concluded after carrying out a confirmatory factor analysis that their data conformed more with the Stefanis et al. four-factor model than with Raine's three-factor model. It is interesting to note that the correlations between the components were very similar in both studies.

TABLE 2: Factorial structure of the SPQ-C-D and Compton et al. [24] sample: three-component solution based on subscales.

(a) Pattern matrix SPQ-C-D

	Component		
	Cognitive/ Perceptual	Interpersonal	Disorganization
Ideas of Reference	.66*		.21
Magical Thinking	.95*		−.15
Unusual Perceptual Experiences	.79*		.18
Paranoid Ideation	.47*	.34*	.29
Social Anxiety	.16	.89*	−.22
No Close Friends		.75*	.27
Constricted Affect		.47*	.53
Eccentric Behaviour	.15		.78*
Odd Speech			.77*

Component correlation matrix

Component	CP	IP	DO
CP	1.00	.38	.38
IP	.38	1.00	.31
DO	.38	.31	1.00

Rotation method: oblimin with Kaiser normalization.
Alphas <.15 are not presented. Bold: subscale loads on component. Data with "*": factorial structure Raine.
CP: Cognitive Perceptual, IP: Interpersonal, and DO: Disorganization.

(b) Pattern matrix Compton et al. study

	Component		
	Cognitive/ Perceptual	Interpersonal	Disorganization
Ideas of Reference	.82*		.20
Magical Thinking	.18*	−.21	.79
Unusual Perceptual Experiences	.29*		.72
Paranoid Ideation	.68*	.37*	
No Close Friends		.85*	
Social Anxiety	−.26	.75*	
Constricted Affect		.82*	.17
Eccentric Behaviour	−.17	.29	.75*
Odd Speech		.41	.58*

Component correlation matrix

Component	CP	IP	DO
CP	1.00	.29	.36
IP	.29	1.00	.33
DO	.36	.33	1.00

Rotation Method: Oblimin with Kaiser normalization.
Alphas <.15 are not presented. Bold: subscale loads on component.
CP: Cognitive Perceptual, IP: Interpersonal, and DO: Disorganization.

3.3. Confirmatory Factor Analysis.

To compare the structure of our questionnaire in more detail with that of Raine et al.'s [22] US sample we performed a confirmatory factor analysis on our data taking as our starting point Raine et al.'s [22] solutions for their undergraduate and their community samples (see right-hand panel of Table 3). Given the large coefficient for Constricted Affect on the Disorganization component solution we tested whether it was necessary to include this regression coefficient in the basic confirmatory factor analysis, but this turned out not to be necessary. In Table 3 we have given an overview of several models fitted, including Compton et al.'s favoured three-factor model. In sum, a three-factor model with an additional path from the Disorganization factor to Unusual Perceptual Experiences but especially a correlated error term between Unusual Perceptual Experiences and Magical Thinking was needed to get an adequate model fit. Moreover, for the SPQ-C-D, Compton et al.'s adaption was not necessary. For an overview of the factor loadings see Table 4.

3.4. Properties of the Total Score and Three Domain Scores

3.4.1. Distribution. The distributions of the total score and three dimensions showed a positive skew with a lower bound of 0, indicating that high scores are relatively rare. Furthermore, there were several subjects with outlying score on two of the domains, but none of them on all three domains. Although there were some outliers for all variables, there were virtually no extreme scores.

3.4.2. Effects of Age and Sex. We found no significant differences in mean scores between boys and girls, and there were no significant differences in mean scores between the age groups; see Table 5 for means and standard deviations. Average total score in our 9–18-year-old sample (16.3) was significantly lower than the average total score in the young adult sample in the Compton et al. study (23.2), $t = 6.8$, df = 974; $P < .001$; Cohen's $d = 54$ (see Table 5).

4. Conclusion

The aim of the present study was to evaluate the 74-item Schizotypal Personality Questionnaire adapted for Dutch children between 9 and 18 years old (SPQ-C-D). It was evaluated in terms of reliability, factor structure, and distribution of scores and compared to the original SPQ data by Raine [8] and another study with young adult participants.

First, reliability in terms of internal consistency was assessed. As for the total score and the three domain scores (Interpersonal, Cognitive-Perceptual, and Disorganization) reliabilities were between 0.82 and 0.92. Therefore, the SPQ-C-D is a reliable instrument for assessing schizotypal traits in children using these dimensions. The three domains were correlated, similar to what is found in other studies, which may point to one single underlying factor conveying overall level of schizotypal traits. Regarding reliability of the nine individual subscales, most showed good reliability with α ranging from 0.72 to 0.78. Similar to the other studies on adult

TABLE 3: Model fit of Raine et al. and Compton et al. based on confirmatory factor analyses.

Models	χ^2	df	χ^2/df	Comparative fit index (CFI)	RMSEA	RMSEA interval	AIC
Raine et al. [22], three-factor model							
Base	81.9	23	3.56	.92	.11	.08–.14	35.9
+r(MT, UPE)	48.7	22	2.21	.96	.08	.05–.10	4.7
+(DO → UPE) and r(MT, UPE)	26.7	21	1.27	.99	.04	.00–.07	−15.3
Compton et al. [24], three-factor model							
Base	46.9	20	2.35	.96	.08	.05–.11	6.9
−CP → SocAnx	48.1	21	2.29	.96	.08	.05–.11	6.2

Note: for the confirmatory factor analysis 6 children were excluded because of their large contribution to the multivariate kurtosis, while five children were excluded because they did not have complete data on all of the subscales. RMSEA = root mean square error of approximation; AIC = Akaike information criterion, and df = degrees of freedom. r(MT, UPE) = correlated error between Magical Thinking and Unusual Perceptual Experiences; DO → UPE = path between the Disorganization component and Unusual Perceptual Experiences. CP → Social Anxiety = path between the Cognitive/Perceptual Component and Social Anxiety.

populations, there were relatively low α's for the subscales "No Close Friends" ($\alpha = .47$), "Constricted Affect" ($\alpha = .56$), and "Magical Thinking" ($\alpha = .67$). Overall, given the differences in samples and the translation steps, there is a high degree of agreement in reliabilities between the SPQ-C-D and the other two studies, that is, samples of Raine et al. [22] and Compton et al. [24]. Thus, the SPQ-C-D can also be reliably used for assessing specific types of schizotypal traits.

Second, we explored the factorial structure of the SPQ-C-D by using principal component analysis (PCA). PCA showed that "Ideas of Reference," "Magical Thinking," "Unusual Perceptual Experiences," and "Paranoid Ideation" loaded on one component, identical to the Cognitive-Perceptual component in the original study by Raine. Furthermore, "Paranoid Ideation," "Social Anxiety," "No Close Friends," and "Constricted Affect" loaded on one component, identical to the Interpersonal component in the original study by Raine. Finally, again similar to the Raine study, "Eccentric Behavior" and "Odd Speech" contributed to one component, that is, Disorganization. Here, one difference with the original Raine study was that Constricted Affect also loaded on this component in our study. The components in our study also resembled those of the Compton et al. study, except for some small variations. Two out of four subscales that load on Cognitive-Perceptual component in the Raine study loaded on Disorganization in the Compton et al. study. In addition, Odd Speech loaded not only on Disorganization, but also on the Interpersonal component in the Compton et al. study. Thus, slight variations in loading of subscales to components have been found in several other studies with the original instrument and are not specific to our study. Nonetheless, the high loading of "Constricted Affect" on the Disorganization component in our study needs replication in future studies.

Third, in order to more thoroughly test if data collected with the SPQ-C-D fit the factorial structure of the original study by Raine et al. [22], we used confirmatory factor analysis. Forcing Raine's factorial structure on our data resulted in an adequate model fit with the presence of a correlated error term between Unusual Perceptual Experiences and Magical Thinking and an additional path from the Disorganization factor to Unusual Perceptual Experiences. Taken together,

comparing factorial structure using both explorative techniques, that is, principal component analysis, and model fit techniques, that is, confirmatory factor analyses, showed that the factorial structure of the SPQ-C-D is very similar to that in the original Raine study and that the degree of variation was similar to the degree of variation found in other samples using Raine's original version of the SPQ.

5. Discussion

Although analysis of the factorial structure indicated adequate properties of the SPQ-C-D, it is important to discuss factors that should be taken into account. In terms of distribution of the mean SPQ-C-D scores, this was somewhat skewed with most scores on the lower end as could be expected in a nonclinical sample. However, considering the large sample size, this did not have a negative effect on analyses of the reliability and factorial structure of the SPQ-C-D. There were no differences between boys and girls, and there was no effect of age on mean scores. The mean number of affirmative responses ("applies to me") on item level was overall lower in our study as compared to the Compton et al. [24] undergraduate study, particularly for items in the Cognitive-Perceptual domain. This may have several implications. First, if there are any effects of variation in interpretation of the questions and level of self-reflection in this relatively young group, that is, 9 to 18 years old, any bias that would result from this would be in the direction of underreporting rather than overreporting schizotypal traits according to our findings. Second, although differences in number of affirmative responses might be due to interpretation factors, it could also be related to developmental effects, with the younger group (9 to 18 years old) in our study having significantly lower levels of schizotypal traits as compared to the young adult group in the study by Compton et al. [24], who are more close to the typical peak age of onset of psychotic disorders [33]. However, this is in contrast to findings from meta-analysis of developmental dynamics of psychotic symptoms, which has shown higher rates in children as compared to adolescents and adults and a decline of the incidence of psychotic symptoms over

TABLE 4: Confirmatory factor analysis: the three-factor solution based on subscales for the SPQ-C-D and Raine's samples.

(a) SPQ-C-D study

	Component		
	Cognitive/ Perceptual	Interpersonal	Disorganization
Ideas of Reference	.87*		
Magical Thinking	.60*		
Unusual Perceptual Experiences	.32*		.43
Paranoid Ideation	.58*	.38*	
Social Anxiety		.54*	
No Close Friends		.81*	
Constricted Affect		.74*	
Odd Behaviour			.71*
Odd Speech			.68*

Component correlation matrix			
Component	CP	IP	DO
CP	**1.00**	.45	.64
IP	.45	**1.00**	.70
DO	.64	.70	**1.00**
R(UPE, MT)		.55	

Alphas <.15 are not presented. Bold: subscale loads on component. Data with "*": factorial structure Raine. CP: Cognitive Perceptual, IP: Interpersonal, and DO: Disorganization.

(b) Raine et al. [22]: undergraduate sample (left); community sample (right)

	Component		
	Cognitive/ Perceptual	Interpersonal	Disorganization
Ideas of Reference	.75/.83*		
Magical Thinking	.62/.53*		
Unusual Perceptual Experiences	.78/.74*		
Paranoid Ideation	.47/.56*	.45/.41*	
Social Anxiety		.58/.66*	
No Close Friends		.77/.89*	
Constricted Affect		.76/.81*	
Odd Behaviour			.62/.49*
Odd Speech			.74/.88*

Component correlation matrix			
Component	CP	IP	DO
CP	**1.00**	.20/.37	.71/.75
IP	.20/.37	**1.00**	.44/.60
DO	.71/.75	.44/.60	**1.00**

Alphas <.15 are not presented. Bold: subscale loads on component. Data with "*": factorial structure Raine. CP: Cognitive Perceptual, IP: Interpersonal, and DO: Disorganization.

time [6, 33, 34]. This has led some to speculate that "early adult neurodevelopmental processes (e.g., increased myelination of white matter, gray matter loss) or changes in social circumstances (e.g., marriage, transition from school to employment) may give clues as to factors that ameliorate and even protect against schizotypal personality disorder" [33]. Unfortunately, the cross-sectional comparisons in our study do not allow drawing firm conclusions about developmental dynamics of schizotypal traits as measured with the SPQ.

There are some limitations of this study that should be noted. First, we only assessed reliability and factorial structure of the SPQ-C-D in a nonclinical sample. Inclusion of clinical groups would have provided stronger empirical support and would have allowed us to investigate if and how the SPQ-C-D could be used in clinical context. Second, we did not have a longitudinal design. This prevented us from assessing test-retest reliability. This also did not allow us to test to what degree scores on the SPQ-C-D are predictive of psychopathology later in development. Third, as some of the subscales showed relatively low reliability, interpretation of these subscales should occur with caution, especially on the level of individual assessment. Fourth, we cannot exclude that translation issues and age differences between our study and others may have added "noise" to the data. However, in spite of this added variation, a factorial structure that is very similar to the original SPQ was found, implying that the SPQ-C-D is valid in spite of these potential issues.

In the future, it would be interesting to consider Likert rating scales with five scale points ranging from 0 (strong disagree) to 4 (strongly agree), as has been done in other studies, for example, Wuthrich and Bates [26], to add an even more robust and sensitive evaluation of levels of traits. Notwithstanding we have decided to follow the original questionnaire and use binary items to stay in line with previous research; a detailed study of comparing the effectiveness of both types of items is warranted. Also, it would be interesting to use the SPQ-C-D in a longitudinal design, such as a ten-year follow-up of the sample in this study, which allows assessment of the predictive value of schizotypy scores for level of psychopathology in early adulthood.

Conflict of Interests

The authors declare that there is no conflict of interests regarding the publication of this paper.

Acknowledgments

The authors are very grateful to Michael Compton and Erin Brooke Tone for providing them with their data, which enabled them to carry out the comparisons reported in this paper. They thank Marit Bierman for help with adapting the SPQ questionnaire. This work was supported by a personal grant (Grant no. 016.095.060) to Sophie van Rijn from the Netherlands Organization for Scientific Research (NWO).

TABLE 5: Total score and domain scores for the different age groups.

Age group		Total Score		Interpersonal		Cognitive/Perceptual		Disorganization	
	N	M	sd	M	sd	M	sd	M	sd
9	39	**16.7**	9.2	**8.3**	4.2	**6.5**	5.4	**3.4**	3.1
10	45	**19.2**	12.9	**8.6**	6.2	**7.6**	7.3	**4.7**	3.5
11	39	**16.6**	12.1	**7.5**	5.0	**6.2**	6.6	**4.3**	3.6
12	36	**15.5**	11.6	**6.5**	5.2	**5.6**	5.7	**4.7**	3.7
13 + 14	27	**15.2**	11.0	**6.6**	5.5	**6.4**	5.3	**3.9**	3.7
15–18	33	**13.2**	10.2	**5.3**	4.9	**5.5**	5.6	**3.6**	3.6
Total	219	**16.3**	11.4	**7.3**	5.3	**6.4**	6.1	**4.2**	3.5
Compton et al. [24]	757	**23.2**	13.7	**10.2**	7.0	**10.5**	6.7	**5.3**	4.1
t-value		6.8		5.7		8.1		3.6	
Effect size (d)		.54		.46		.64		.29	

Notes: df = 974; all P values <.001.

References

[1] R. J. Linscott and J. van Os, "Systematic reviews of categorical versus continuum models in psychosis: evidence for discontinuous subpopulations underlying a psychometric continuum. Implications for DSM-V, DSM-VI, and DSM-VII," in *Annual Review of Clinical Psychology*, S. Nolen-Hoeksema, T. D. Cannon, and T. Widiger, Eds., vol. 6, pp. 391–419, Annual Reviews, Palo Alto, Calif, USA, 2010.

[2] R. Mullen, "Delusions: the continuum versus category debate," *Australian and New Zealand Journal of Psychiatry*, vol. 37, no. 5, pp. 505–511, 2003.

[3] J. P. Chapman, L. J. Chapman, and T. R. Kwapil, "Scales for the measurement of schizotypy," in *Schizotypal Personality*, A. Raine, T. Lencz, and S. A. Mednick, Eds., Cambridge University Press, New York, NY, USA, 1995.

[4] G. Claridge, *Schizotypy: Implications for Illness and Health*, Oxford University Press, Oxford, UK, 1997.

[5] P. E. Meehl, "Schizotaxia revisited," *Archives of General Psychiatry*, vol. 46, no. 10, pp. 935–944, 1989.

[6] J. van Os, R. J. Linscott, I. Myin-Germeys, P. Delespaul, and L. Krabbendam, "A systematic review and meta-analysis of the psychosis continuum: evidence for a psychosis proneness-persistence-impairment model of psychotic disorder," *Psychological Medicine*, vol. 39, no. 2, pp. 179–195, 2009.

[7] A. R. Yung, H. P. Yuen, L. J. Phillips, S. Francey, and P. D. McGorry, "Mapping the onset of psychosis: the comprehensive assessment of at risk mental states (CAARMS)," *Schizophrenia Research*, vol. 60, no. 1, pp. 30–31, 2003.

[8] A. Raine, "The SPQ: a scale for the assessment of schizotypal personality based on DSM-III-R criteria," *Schizophrenia Bulletin*, vol. 17, no. 4, pp. 555–564, 1991.

[9] A. Raine and D. Benishay, "The SPQ-B: a brief screening instrument for schizotypal personality disorder," *Journal of Personality Disorders*, vol. 9, no. 4, pp. 346–355, 1995.

[10] T. J. Crow, D. J. Done, and A. Sacker, "Childhood precursors of psychosis as clues to its evolutionary origins," *European Archives of Psychiatry and Clinical Neuroscience*, vol. 245, no. 2, pp. 61–69, 1995.

[11] M. Isohanni, P. Jones, L. Kemppainen et al., "Childhood and adolescent predictors of schizophrenia in the Northern Finland

1966 Birth Cohort—a descriptive life-span model," *European Archives of Psychiatry and Clinical Neuroscience*, vol. 250, no. 6, pp. 311–319, 2000.

[12] A. Reichenberg, A. Caspi, H. Harrington et al., "Static and dynamic cognitive deficits in childhood preceding adult schizophrenia: a 30-year study," *The American Journal of Psychiatry*, vol. 167, no. 2, pp. 160–169, 2010.

[13] E. Walker and A. M. Bollini, "Pubertal neurodevelopment and the emergence of psychotic symptoms," *Schizophrenia Research*, vol. 54, no. 1-2, pp. 17–23, 2002.

[14] N. Kaymaz, M. Drukker, R. Lieb et al., "Do subthreshold psychotic experiences predict clinical outcomes in unselected non-help-seeking population-based samples? A systematic review and meta-analysis, enriched with new results," *Psychological Medicine*, vol. 42, no. 11, pp. 2239–2253, 2012.

[15] T. R. Kwapil, "Social anhedonia as a predictor of the development of schizophrenia-spectrum disorders," *Journal of Abnormal Psychology*, vol. 107, no. 4, pp. 558–565, 1998.

[16] R. Poulton, A. Caspi, T. E. Moffitt, M. Cannon, R. Murray, and H. Harrington, "Children's self-reported psychotic symptoms and adult schizophreniform disorder: a 15-year longitudinal study," *Archives of General Psychiatry*, vol. 57, no. 11, pp. 1053–1058, 2000.

[17] W. Rössler, A. Riecher-Rössler, J. Angst et al., "Psychotic experiences in the general population: a twenty-year prospective community study," *Schizophrenia Research*, vol. 92, no. 1–3, pp. 1–14, 2007.

[18] L. J. Chapman, J. P. Chapman, T. R. Kwapil, M. Eckblad, and M. C. Zinser, "Putatively psychosis-prone subjects 10 years later," *Journal of Abnormal Psychology*, vol. 103, no. 2, pp. 171–183, 1994.

[19] D. C. Gooding, K. A. Tallent, and C. W. Matts, "Clinical status of at-risk individuals 5 years later: further validation of the psychometric high-risk strategy," *Journal of Abnormal Psychology*, vol. 114, no. 1, pp. 170–175, 2005.

[20] M. F. Lenzenweger, "Psychometric high-risk paradigm, perceptual aberrations, and schizotypy: an update," *Schizophrenia Bulletin*, vol. 20, no. 1, pp. 121–135, 1994.

[21] G. Claridge, C. McCreery, O. Mason et al., "The factor structure of 'schizotypal' traits: a large replication study," *British Journal of Clinical Psychology*, vol. 35, no. 1, pp. 103–115, 1996.

[22] A. Raine, C. Reynolds, T. Lencz, A. Scerbo, N. Triphon, and D. Kim, "Cognitive-perceptual, interpersonal, and disorganized features of schizotypal personality," *Schizophrenia Bulletin*, vol. 20, no. 1, pp. 191–201, 1994.

[23] M. G. Vollema and R. J. van den Bosch, "The multidimensionality of schizotypy," *Schizophrenia Bulletin*, vol. 21, no. 1, pp. 19–31, 1995.

[24] M. T. Compton, S. M. Goulding, R. Bakeman, and E. B. McClure-Tone, "Confirmation of a four-factor structure of the Schizotypal Personality Questionnaire among undergraduate students," *Schizophrenia Research*, vol. 111, no. 1–3, pp. 46–52, 2009.

[25] N. C. Stefanis, N. Smyrnis, D. Avramopoulos, I. Evdokimidis, I. Ntzoufras, and C. N. Stefanis, "Factorial composition of self-rated schizotypal traits among young males undergoing military training," *Schizophrenia Bulletin*, vol. 30, no. 2, pp. 335–350, 2004.

[26] V. M. Wuthrich and T. C. Bates, "Confirmatory factor analysis of the three-factor structure of the Schizotypal Personality Questionnaire and Chapman schizotypy scales," *Journal of Personality Assessment*, vol. 87, no. 3, pp. 292–304, 2006.

[27] M. Ericson, C. Tuvblad, A. Raine, K. Young-Wolff, and L. A. Baker, "Heritability and longitudinal stability of schizotypal traits during adolescence," *Behavior Genetics*, vol. 41, no. 4, pp. 499–511, 2011.

[28] M. G. Vollema and H. Hoijtink, "The multidimensionality of self-report schizotypy in a psychiatric population: an analysis using multidimensional Rasch models," *Schizophrenia Bulletin*, vol. 26, no. 3, pp. 565–575, 2000.

[29] T. M. Achenbach, *Manual for the Child Behaviour Checklist/4–18 and 1991 Profile*, Department of Psychiatry, The University of Vermont, Burlington, Vt, USA, 1991.

[30] M. G. Vollema, M. M. Sitskoorn, M. C. M. Appels, and R. S. Kahn, "Does the Schizotypal Personality Questionnaire reflect the biological-genetic vulnerability to schizophrenia?" *Schizophrenia Research*, vol. 54, no. 1-2, pp. 39–45, 2002.

[31] C. Acquadro, K. Conway, A. Hareendran, and N. Aaronson, "Literature review of methods to translate health-related quality of life questionnaires for use in multinational clinical trials," *Value in Health*, vol. 11, no. 3, pp. 509–521, 2008.

[32] A. Raine, "The SPQ: a scale for the assessment of schizotypal personality based on DSM-III-R criteria," *Schizophrenia Bulletin*, vol. 17, no. 4, pp. 555–564, 1991.

[33] A. Raine, "Schizotypal personality: neurodevelopmental and psychosocial trajectories," *Annual Review of Clinical Psychology*, vol. 2, pp. 291–326, 2006.

[34] I. Kelleher, D. Connor, M. C. Clarke, N. Devlin, M. Harley, and M. Cannon, "Prevalence of psychotic symptoms in childhood and adolescence: a systematic review and meta-analysis of population-based studies," *Psychological Medicine*, vol. 42, no. 9, pp. 1857–1863, 2012.

22

The Concept of Schizophrenia: From Unity to Diversity

Heinz Häfner

Schizophrenia Research Group, Central Institute of Mental Health, Mannheim Faculty of Medicine, University of Heidelberg, J5, 68159 Mannheim, Germany

Correspondence should be addressed to Heinz Häfner; heinz.haefner@zi-mannheim.de

Academic Editor: Joseph M. Pierre

After over 100 years of research without clarifying the aetiology of schizophrenia, a look at the current state of knowledge in epidemiology, genetics, precursors, psychopathology, and outcome seems worthwhile. The disease concept, created by Kraepelin and modified by Bleuler, has a varied history. Today, schizophrenia is considered a polygenic disorder with onset in early adulthood, characterized by irregular psychotic episodes and functional impairment, but incident cases occur at all ages with marked differences in symptoms and social outcome. Men's and women's lifetime risk is nearly the same. At young age, women fall ill a few years later and less severely than men, men more rarely and less severely later in life. The underlying protective effect of oestrogen is antagonized by genetic load. The illness course is heterogeneous and depressive mood the most frequent symptom. Depression and schizophrenia are functionally associated, and affective and nonaffective psychoses do not split neatly. Most social consequences occur at the prodromal stage. Neither schizophrenia as such nor its main symptom dimensions regularly show pronounced deterioration over time. Schizophrenia is neither a residual state of a neurodevelopmental disorder nor a progressing neurodegenerative process. It reflects multifactorial CNS instability, which leads to cognitive deficits and symptom exacerbations.

1. Introduction

For more than a century, there has been research into the question of what schizophrenia really is. We have developed an array of fascinating new research techniques and amassed a wealth of detailed knowledge, but we are still lacking a comprehensive answer to that question. Since its early days, the disease concept of schizophrenia [1, 2] has undergone several modifications. The aim of the present article is to describe, in broad sketches, how the understanding of the disorder has evolved to what it is now.

Comparable reviews have appeared in great numbers before, for example, by Tsuang and Faraone [3], Weinberger and Harrison [4], Andreasen [5] and the series of articles published on the occasion of the founding and the 10th and the 20th anniversaries of the journal "Schizophrenia Research." The first of the latter articles, authored by the journal's cofounder Wyatt together with Alexander, Egan, and Kirch, was entitled "Schizophrenia, Just the Facts" and appeared in 1988 [6]. Further articles carrying that title were to follow [7–11], until the series finally closed with the conclusion "*The current construct…is in need of reconceptualization*" [12].

The ensuing debate, however, prompted the authors to take a conservative stance.

> "*Giving a new name to a common and well known disease cannot be taken lightly, as it has momentous clinical, legal, societal, connotative and economic implications*" [13].

This explains the authors' reluctance to reform the concept. But there is more into the issue than just finding a new name, because the fundamentals of the diagnosis itself are caught in an "intellectual crisis" [14]. We should, therefore, once more take a look at the disease concept.

In our analysis, we will concentrate on research perspectives [15–20], focusing on the epidemiological and psychopathological aspects involved in the genesis and course of the disorder and leaving therapy and neurobiological issues aside.

2. Disease Concept and Diagnosis

In his comprehensive description of the disorder, Emil Kraepelin termed it "dementia praecox" [1]. The Swiss psychiatrist

Eugen Bleuler changed that name into "schizophrenia" [2], because the disorder does not have its onset exclusively early in life, nor does it invariably lead to dementia. Bleuler also rejected Kraepelin's natural-scientific disease concept, which proceeded from "natural disease entities" [21, 22].

Kraepelin's hope that psychiatric nosology could be placed on a neurobiological footing is still very much alive [23]. In the course of the preparations for the revision of the DSM-IV into the DSM-V, Hyman, prior director of the NIMH, declared that

> "Mental disorders are a diverse group of brain disorders. The boundary between mental and neurological disorders is arbitrary" [24].

Growing disillusionment in the run-up to the DSM-V prompted the NIMH in 2008 to set up a plan to "develop, for research purposes, new ways of classifying mental disorders" [25]. The thus initiated RDoC (research domain criteria) project [25] is looking for a new nosology based on neuroscience and behavioral science rather than descriptive phenomenology. In the face of the reductionism informing this endeavor, several authors have criticized the neglect of psychopathology and the deviation from the long-standing clinical tradition in the field of schizophrenia [17, 19, 20, 26–28].

Unlike Kraepelin, Eugen Bleuler ushered in psychoanalytic influences, changing the schizophrenia concept in a fundamental way. He identified ambivalence, autism, affective incongruity, and association disturbances, the "four A's," as "basic symptoms" (Grundsymptome). Delusions and hallucinations, which occur in other disorders, too, he regarded as resulting from adaptive and defensive reactions, classifying them as "accessory symptoms." Bleuler also assumed continuity between psychosis and normality (for a review see [29]). The continuity hypothesis was to play a key role in the constitution typology proposed by the German psychiatrist Kretschmer [30]. He postulated a continuum ranging from schizophrenic psychosis to schizoid personality and schizothymic character.

The early chasm between Kraepelin's categorical and Bleuler's dimensional diagnostic concepts, boiling down to the question whether they can be "clearly separated from one another or from normality" [31, 32], has accompanied the debate about the schizophrenia concept until the present day.

In the 6th edition of his textbook, Kraepelin [33] introduced a new principle to the nosology of functional psychoses. He distinguished dementia praecox, because of its tendency to progressive deterioration, from manic-depressive insanity of a benign illness course leading neither to a defect state nor dementia. Even the misgivings Kraepelin [22] himself later developed about a clear-cut separability of these disorders have been unable to fully unhinge the dichotomy model [34].

In European psychiatry, Jaspers [35] distinguished two levels of gaining insight in psychiatry: the natural-scientific level of causal explaining of neurobiological processes and the psychological level of hermeneutic understanding of meaningful associations [36–38].

The phenomenology Jaspers developed following the German philosopher Edmund Husserl (1859–1938) required a pure perception of conscious phenomena. In psychopathology, that meant getting rid of any kind of personal or theoretical prejudice. A simplified version of that phenomenology, the so-called "descriptive method," became the standard approach to accessing psychopathological phenomena worldwide and has remained so until today [35, 38–40].

Jaspers [35] criticized Meynert's and Wernicke's theories, according to which all mental disorders were brain disorders, as one-sided generalizations, and called them brain mythologies. Kraepelin, who, over the course of his life, kept updating his theories from growing experience and new evidence, first regarded mental disorders, which he believed were caused by known or still unknown neuropathology, as natural disease entities—similar to Carl von Linnè's botanical species. Jaspers criticized Kraepelin's disease concept, too, because in his opinion it was biased and lacked an empirical foundation. In that respect, Kraepelin's theory was just another brain mythology. However, in order to be able to classify psychiatric disorders on the basis of precisely defined diagnoses, Kraepelin came up with a system of syndrome-course units (Syndromverlaufseinheiten) for mental disorders of unknown aetiology. It was a pragmatic way of defining disease constructs and related diagnoses. Originally, he regarded them as a temporary solution, believing that the underlying neuropathological causes would ultimately be detected. In his later works (e.g., [22]), however, he modified the theoretical foundations of his classification system.

Adolf Hitler's antisemitism forced numerous leading German and Austrian psychiatrists to emigrate. Psychoanalysts moved primarily to the USA, spreading there Sigmund Freud's theory. Wilhelm Mayer-Gross, a colleague of Karl Jaspers' at the University of Heidelberg Psychiatric Department, emigrated to Great Britain in 1933. The textbook on "Clinical Psychiatry" (1954; 2nd edn. 1960, 3rd edn. 1969) [41], which he coauthored with the psychiatrist Martin Roth and the geneticist Elliott Slater, introduced Karl Jaspers' "General Psychopathology" to British psychiatrists [42].

It was under this influence that John Wing, head of the Department of Social Psychiatry at the Institute of Psychiatry in London, and Norman Sartorius, director of the World Health Organization (WHO) Mental Health Division, laid the foundation for the WHO's international studies of schizophrenia. On the initiative of these two men, the "Present State Examination" (PSE), including CATEGO, an evaluation programme, was created as a semistandardized instrument for symptom assessment [43]. The instrument permits symptom assessment in different cultures. The PSE has now been superseded by the "Schedules for Clinical Assessment in Neuropsychiatry" (SCAN), including the CATEGO-V system, as a comprehensive tool for assessing and measuring mental illness [44].

The PSE was greatly influenced by "Clinical Psychopathology," a book authored by Jaspers' student Kurt Schneider [45]. In that book, Schneider had attempted to sharpen the schizophrenia diagnosis by discriminating between symptoms of first and second rank. He regarded the presence of one or more of the following 11 first-rank symptoms he had identified purely on the basis of clinical experience as pathogenomic for schizophrenia [46]: delusional perception, audible thoughts, voices arguing or discussing, voices commenting on the patient's action, thought withdrawal, thought insertion, thought broadcasting (diffusion of thought), passivity of affect, passivity of impulse, passivity of volition, and somatic passivity [45, 47]. In contrast, only a multiple presence of second-rank symptoms would permit a diagnosis of schizophrenia.

The frequency of first-rank symptoms varies in patients with schizophrenia. In a review of 13 studies, Fenton et al. [48] reported it ranging from 24% to 72%. In the WHO determinants of outcome of severe mental disorders (DOSMeD) study [49], 96% of the probands diagnosed with the PSE-CATEGO instrument showed one or more symptoms of first rank. First-rank symptoms have been observed in other mental disorders, too, particularly frequently in psychotic depression [50–52].

As the first-rank symptoms included neither negative symptoms nor any course-related criteria, the schizophrenia diagnosis became restricted to psychotic illness and, hence, considerably more narrow in scope. That increased its reliability and benefited transcultural epidemiological studies and therapy research.

While in the DSM-IV and DSM-IV-TR, used by American psychiatrists, the persistence of just one first-rank symptom for more than a month was sufficient to justify a diagnosis of schizophrenia, this special significance of these symptoms has been eliminated in the DSM-V, because it has not been possible to prove their diagnostic specificity. In the DSM-V, they are treated just like other positive symptoms.

In the Kraepelinian tradition, Kurt Schneider regarded symptoms merely as preliminary signs of an as yet undetected somatic process. He adopted "endogeneity," coined by Möbius [53], as a generic term to denote the category of disorders of unknown biological origin as represented by schizophrenia. This differed considerably from the broader and less precise psychodynamic diagnoses in use in the USA.

Over the course of time, the exclusivity of categorical diagnoses became replaced by an assumption of continuity to normality and to related diagnostic groups [54–56]. Nevertheless, the categorical diagnoses continue to be used in clinical practice and are maintained in the two international classification systems. Separate categories have been introduced to denote the intermediate forms of pathology between schizophrenia and affective psychosis—for example, schizoaffective psychoses—and between psychosis and normality—for example, schizotypy and schizophreniform disorder in the International Classification of Diseases, ICD-10 [57, 58], and the Diagnostic and Statistical Manual, DSM-IV [59, 60]. These intermediate forms have permitted taking an aspect of continuity into account without having to give up the categorical nature of the diagnoses.

Several studies have demonstrated the great influence diagnostic definitions have on the incidence of schizophrenia (e.g., [61–64]).

In den USA, the birth of a psychodynamic strand of psychiatry was promoted by Hans Wolfgang Maier (1882–1945), a Swiss emigrant, and immigrant German psychiatrists, who helped spread psychoanalysis [46]. The differences to the psychopathology practised in Europe grew increasingly

visible [65–68]. On the initiative of Zubin [69] and Kramer [65] (USA), the US-UK Study, a comparison of psychiatric diagnoses was launched. First, Gurland et al. [70] compared the diagnoses of patients who had been admitted to the Institute of Psychiatry in London and to New York State Psychiatric Institute. The proportion of patients receiving a diagnosis of schizophrenia was significantly higher in New York [46, 71]. Then, eight conservative psychiatric interviews were rated by a group of British and a group of U.S. psychiatrists, and the result was the same [72, 73]: the diagnostic definition of schizophrenia applied by the U.S. psychiatrists was considerably broader than that used by their British colleagues [71, 73].

The "neo-Kraepelinian" transition in North-American psychiatry fell in the period of the US-UK study [74–80]. In a paper entitled "Establishment of diagnostic validity in psychiatric illness: its application to schizophrenia," Robins and Guze [81] published their critique of the ambiguous psychodynamic method of diagnosing. They introduced a "descriptive" approach to diagnosing psychopathological phenomena.

It was strictly on this descriptive basis that the DSM-III [82] was developed as a classification system. Although designed to be free of any theory, it, in fact, proceeded from Kurt Schneider's conservative view of psychopathology [46, 83] and from Kraepelin's speculative assumption "*that all disorders are brain biological disorders*" [84–86]. A few authors, for example, McHugh and Slavney [87, 88], continued to defend the plurality of methods professed by Jaspers in his "General Psychopathology," but with a modest success [71].

With the introduction of the restrictive diagnosis, the annual rate of first admissions with a diagnosis of schizophrenia to a university hospital in the USA fell from 25% ($N = 5143$) in 1975–1979 to 13% ($N = 5771$) in 1981–1985 [67] and at six North-American psychiatric hospitals from 27% in 1976 to 9% in 1989 [89]. Simultaneously, the figures for diagnoses from the category of affective disorders rose steeply.

3. Epidemiology

3.1. General Epidemiology. Schizophrenic psychosis, characterized by positive symptoms such as hallucinations, delusions, and thought disorders, is encountered in all ethnic groups, cultures, political systems, and socioeconomic classes at frequencies that show only moderate variation when based on a sufficiently reliable and culture-independent diagnosis (e.g., PSE-CATEGO).

The WHO has reported annual incidence rates for schizophrenia from different parts of the world. Figure 1 shows the results from eight study centres for a narrow (CATEGO S+) and a broad definition of the diagnosis (clinical/CATEGO S, P, O) for populations aged 15 to 54 years. The age-corrected rates based on a restrictive diagnosis, which range from 0.07 to 0.14 per 1000 population, and the much higher rates based on a broad diagnosis, which vary from 0.16 to 0.42 per 1000 population, speak for themselves [46]. The incidence data on schizophrenia collected in the ECA (Epidemiologic Catchment Area) Program in the USA by lay interviewers

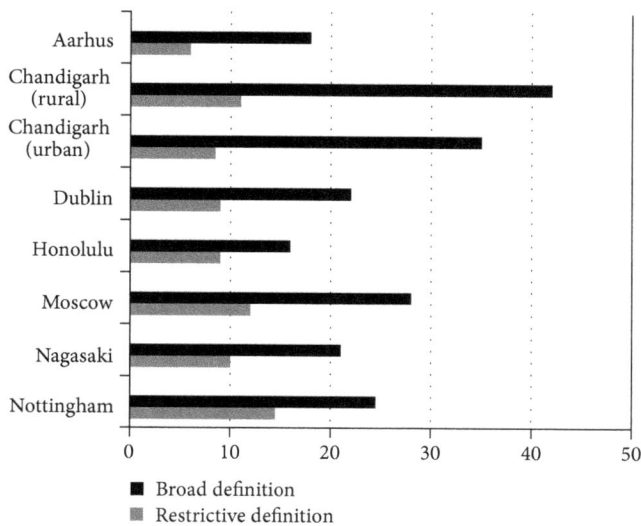

FIGURE 1: Annual incidence of schizophrenia per 100 000 population aged 15–54 (both sexes) for the broad and restrictive definitions. Source: [46].

using the DIS (Diagnostic Interview Schedule) [90] yielded considerably higher age-corrected rates, which ranged from 1.0 to 1.7/1000 [91]. Copeland et al. [92] have shown the weaknesses of such an approach.

Tandon et al. [9] calculated an annual incidence of 15/100,000, comparable in size to the WHO rates, a point prevalence of 4.5/1000 and a lifetime risk of 0.7% as—worldwide—modal rates for both sexes across all age groups.

According to McGrath & Murray [93], Messias et al. [94], and Eaton [95], the incidence of schizophrenia has fallen considerably over time. But changes in incidence rates over lengthy periods of time are difficult to assess. Fairly comprehensive data would be needed on all new cases based on identical diagnostic definitions from sufficiently large populations not subject to any dramatic upheavals (e.g., wars). National psychiatric case registers—such as those in Denmark, Norway, and Sweden—or national health services that keep records of all persons seeking medical help—such as those in Finland, Israel, or Australia—are fairly recent creations and in place only in few countries [46]. For this reason only trends can be reported, calculated over a maximum of 150 years on the basis of the case records of individual hospitals serving defined populations over long periods of time or on data from other national registers [96–98]. No robust indication of either an increase or a decrease of any considerable size has been found [99].

In the early 1980s, some authors [100, 101] thought to have found signs of a marked increase in the incidence of schizophrenia occurring with growing civilization after the mid 19th century. But no reliable data to prove this assumption have yet emerged. In 1990, some British researchers considered it likely that schizophrenia might be dying out altogether, because schizophrenia admissions to mental hospitals in England and Wales had fallen by about 50% in the period from 1965 to 1986 [102, 103]. In that same period,

however, the number of available mental-hospital beds had decreased by the same magnitude [104–106]. Demonstrating that there had been a shift to diagnoses from the affective spectrum, Kendell et al. [107] called the alleged fall in schizophrenia incidence an artefact.

3.2. Analytical Epidemiology

3.2.1. Geographic, Ecological, and Social Patterns of Distribution of Schizophrenia Incidence.
Researchers have long been hoping to gain insight into the causes underlying schizophrenia and new approaches to its prevention and therapy by studying ecological and socioeconomic factors associated with the disorder. The first seminal project in this field was the "Ecological study of schizophrenia and other psychoses," conducted by Faris & Dunham [108–111] and inspired by the urban sociology influential at that time in the USA (Earnest W. Burgess, Albion Woodbury-Small). The authors recorded the residential addresses of all first admissions with a diagnosis of schizophrenia or manic-depressive disorder in the period of 1922 to 1934 by means of ecological mapping in the city of Chicago. They found a close relationship between schizophrenia—clustering in almost concentric circles around the city centre—and the ecological structure of the city. The prevalence rates for schizophrenia ranged from 362/100,000 population in disorganized areas near the centre of the city to 55.4/100,000 population in residential areas at the outskirts. The rates for manic-depressive insanity were randomly distributed.

Further studies conducted in other large cities in the USA (e.g., [112–115]) and Europe [116–124] yielded similar results. Twenty-five years after Faris and Dunham, Levy and Rowitz [125, 126] again studied the ecological distribution of schizophrenia in Chicago. They found a concentric pattern of distribution for readmissions only, while first admissions with schizophrenia showed a random distribution. Accounting for this difference were structural changes undertaken in the city, for example, urban development programmes. In Detroit, Dunham [115] found a distribution pattern stable for over 20 years and very similar to that revealed by the first Chicago study. Giggs and Cooper [127] reported a concentric distribution stable over 15 years in the British city of Nottingham.

Changes in the distribution patterns of schizophrenia were also studied in a fairly large German city (Mannheim) with a population of about 330,000 in three waves over a period of 25 years [116, 117, 119, 128]. The result of the first wave (1965) was almost the same concentric distribution as in Chicago [116, 128]. The stability of that pattern was confirmed, more or less, by the second (1975–81) [117] and the third waves (1989-90) [119]. Smaller changes across municipal districts were attributable to urban renewal programmes.

Only few investigators have found no excess rates for first admissions for schizophrenia from the centres of the cities they have studied: Clausen and Kohn [128–131] in the USA and Stein [132] and Klusmann and Angermeyer [133] in Germany.

The explanations offered for the concentric distribution patterns range from sociogenic hypotheses (e.g., [108, 134–137]) to behaviour-genetic and economic forces operating through selective mobility (e.g., [111, 138–140]). In the city of Nottingham, Dauncey et al. [141] found that individuals with schizophrenia, as a result of their disorder, tended to remain in neighbourhoods characterized by growing poverty and a deteriorating quality of housing, while the economically more successful individuals preferred to move to better residential areas. Ödegård [142, 143] demonstrated that persons later falling ill with schizophrenia showed selective migration, in both geographic and occupational terms, to less attractive neighbourhoods and dying occupations, even before the onset of psychosis.

From fairly early on, research into geographical risk differences has focused on *urban-rural differences*. Most of these studies have reported lower incidence rates for schizophrenia in rural than urban areas, for example, from the USA, the Netherlands, Ireland, England, and Denmark [118, 143–147]. Using data from the national Danish case register, Mortensen et al. [120] and Eaton et al. [148] found a relative risk for developing schizophrenia of 2.4 and 4.2, respectively, for those born in the capital city (Copenhagen) versus rural areas. The population attributable risk of schizophrenia was 34.6% for urban birth, whereas the "genetic" population attributable risk for schizophrenia (at least one first-degree relative with a history of schizophrenia) was a mere 5.5% because of the low number of risk gene carriers [120]. When urbanicity was broken down to five levels [121, 147]: (1) capital city (Copenhagen), (2) capital suburb, (3) provincial city, (4) provincial town, and (5) rural area, a dose-response relationship emerged: the larger the size of population of the place of birth, the higher the relative risk of falling ill with schizophrenia (1.0–2.30) [147]. The authors further demonstrated that, besides the place of birth, also the place of upbringing played a decisive role [122].

A comparison of the influence of urban and rural environment (Southeast London as an urban area and Nottinghamshire as a rural area) on five-symptom dimensions showed that, unlike negative, manic, and disorganisation symptoms, hallucinations (effect size: 0.15) and depression (effect size 0.21) were significantly more frequent in more densely populated environments [149]. In the Netherlands, according to the Netherlands Mental Health Survey and Incidence Study (NEMESIS), even mentally healthy people with subclinical psychosis-like symptoms (delusions and hallucinations) clearly experienced more of them if they had been brought up in an urban environment (either delusions or hallucinations or both: 18.6%) compared with individuals growing up in a rural environment (14.7%) [150].

A recently published nationwide investigation of psychiatric morbidity in Germany [151], based on four levels of urbanicity defined by population size (<20,000, ≤100,000, ≤500,000, >500,000), showed equal annual prevalence rates for psychosis in all big cities with a population of <500,000 (levels 1 to 3) (total = 2.6%). In the cities of the highest degree of urbanicity (>500,000 inhabitants), the rate for psychotic disorder, at 5.2%, was significantly elevated, compared with 2.5% for the lowest degree of urbanicity. Remarkably, the prevalence of mood disorders, too, was equally elevated in the highest category of urbanicity: 13.9% as against 7.8% in the lowest category [151].

Unlike the first Chicago study [108], more recent urban-ecological and geographical studies have also found comparable distribution patterns for affective psychoses [151, 152] and major depression [153, 154].

To explain the variation in the risk of schizophrenia in different living environments, two hypotheses have been proposed: (1) life in big cities is more distressing and, hence, associated with a greater risk for mental illness and (2) individuals with an excess genetic risk for psychosis—for example, "schizoid" personalities with bonding problems—are more inclined to leave their families and small neighbourhoods in search for more independent and anonymous life in the city [155–159].

The increasing drift of population to urban areas in the 19th and the 20th centuries in the wake of the Industrial Revolution may have led to a slight overrepresentation of genetically vulnerable individuals among city-dwellers. The proportion of individuals with schizophrenia who have first-degree relatives with a history of schizophrenia has been found to be slightly elevated in big cities [122, 157, 160]. Van Os et al. [157, 160] estimate the genetic contribution at 20% to 30%.

It is not quite clear yet whether the contribution of urbanicity to schizophrenia risk [160, 161] is valid worldwide, because human settlements vary a lot across cultures [162].

Recently, a new approach was adopted to explain the causality. Lederbogen et al. [163] proceeded from the assumption that growing up in a city might be associated with a higher level of stress from early on compared with rural environments. In a controlled morphological and functional MRI study, the authors found that current city dwelling was associated with a significantly increased amygdala activity compared with living in a rural environment. They write that "*urban upbringing affected the perigenual anterior cingulate cortex, a key region for regulation of amygdala activity, negative affect and stress.*" The findings were specific both regionally and behaviourally: none of the other brain structures showed comparable effects. In a control experiment involving cognitive processing without stress in solving arithmetic tasks, no such activation of the amygdala region was observed. The authors presume that vulnerability to social stress associated with urbanicity is reduced later in life. This approach to explaining the elevated rates of schizophrenia associated with urban birth and upbringing is interesting, but it needs replication.

3.2.2. Schizophrenia and Emigration.
Results from the innumerable studies into the risk of schizophrenia in immigrant populations are not easy to sum up, because the populations studied and their situations in the countries of immigration vary a great deal. The reasons for immigration range from purely economic motives to severe traumatic experiences. Culturally and economically fairly well-adapted long-term immigrants differ a lot from recent refugees who have suffered traumatic experiences and losses shortly before leaving their countries of origin and are still grappling with economic hardship and acculturation in the host country.

Ödegård's study [155] was of paradigmatic importance. He found a twofold risk for first admission for schizophrenia among Norwegian immigrants to Minnesota (USA) compared with their Norwegian countrymen. He explained it by the genetic drift hypothesis. Weiser et al. [164], who compared data for 660,000 adolescents from the Israeli National Draft Board Register and the Israeli National Hospitalization Psychiatric Case Registry, calculated a surplus rate for schizophrenia, independent of socioeconomic status, of 60% for Russian immigrants and of 300% for culturally more diverse Ethiopian immigrants. Corcoran et al. [165] studied second-generation immigrants from western Asia and North Africa as well as Europe and other industrialized countries to Israel, but could not find a significant increase in their risk for schizophrenia.

Turkish migrant workers, who had moved from Anatolia/Turkey to Germany for economic reasons, showed significantly lower incidence rates of schizophrenia, whereas their spouses and also their children showed rates that were equally high as those for the population of the host country [166, 167]. Selection factors were presumed to be the cause: a positive self-selection of those men courageous enough to go to work in a foreign country with a foreign culture as well as a mandatory premigration health screeing at German diplomatic missions in Turkey.

The highly elevated incidence rates for schizophrenia among Afro-Caribbean immigrants to Great Britain [168–176], among Surinamese immigrants to the Netherlands [177–179] and among mostly Asian and African immigrants to Denmark [180] and Sweden [181], are outliers. Most of these immigrants have left their home countries for economic reasons. Reports of an even more markedly elevated incidence of schizophrenia among second- than first-generation immigrants [170, 182, 183] make the phenomenon even more puzzling. The effects have been found to be in part sex-specific: higher rates for women immigrating from Pakistan and Bangladesh, but not for Indian women. No evidence has emerged in support of the assumption that immigrants' lower socioeconomic status in their home countries would explain their elevated schizophrenia incidence [184–186].

Studies of the incidence of schizophrenia in the immigrants' home countries, for example, in Jamaica [187], Barbados [188], Trinidad [189], and Surinam [178, 190], have yielded rates similar to those of the British or Dutch population.

Evidence has also refused to emerge for the hypotheses that traumatic childhood experiences, a more frequent substance misuse, or a greater inclination to magical thinking would explain the elevated rates of schizophrenia in immigrant populations. Social disintegration, social adversity, and neighbourhood factors have also been proposed [154, 191]. Immigrant groups living as ethnic minorities in neighbourhoods with a predominantly native population tend to have elevated incidence rates for schizophrenia [192–197]. This also applies to second-generation immigrants. More research is needed to fully understand these phenomena.

3.2.3. Reduced Fertility of People with Schizophrenia. Since the reproductive rates of men and women with schizophrenia are consistently lower than those for the population in general, the incidence of schizophrenia should actually keep falling from generation to generation [198–210]. The lack of such intergenerational decline has been explained by a higher reproductive fitness of the affected persons' siblings [211–213]. The hypothesis has been proven wrong in large northern-European population and birth cohort studies, which have failed to produce any evidence in support of significantly higher fertility rates for nonaffected twins or siblings [206, 207, 209].

Modern genetic research helps understand why the reduced fertility rates do not have any effect on incidence. Schizophrenia, for the overwhelming part, is transmitted by genes that account merely for a small share, mostly less than 1.3%, in the overall risk for the disorder [214]. The reproductive failure of affected persons is probably negligible in comparison with the large number of healthy individuals also carrying those risk genes.

4. Genetics

Schizophrenia is a heterogeneous and complex neuropsychiatric disorder, whose etiology involves both environmental and genetic factors. In individual cases, the relative contribution of genetic and environmental factors is impossible to ascertain.

Numerous studies have investigated the role of environmental factors in schizophrenia. Established environmental risk factors include pre-, peri-, and early postnatal complications [215–217]; viral infections in childhood [218]; childhood meningitis [219, 220]; being born and growing up in an urban environment [120–122, 179]; immigrant status [170, 173, 221]; substance misuse; and other determinants of mild cerebral dysfunction. Other possible, but still contentious, environmental risk factors are winter birth, prenatal exposure to influenza epidemics, and maternal malnutrition during the second trimester of pregnancy. To date, however, research has failed to identify any environmental factors that increase the risk of schizophrenia by more than a few percentage points.

Multiple formal genetic studies have demonstrated the contribution of genetic factors to schizophrenia risk. These investigations have applied twin (e.g., [222–229]), family (e.g., [230–236]), and adoption approaches [237, 238]. Estimated heritability (i.e., the proportion of variance due to genetic factors) is around 0.8 [234]. The lifetime schizophrenia risk of first degree relatives shows a 5–10-fold increase compared to that observed in the general population (lifetime prevalence 1%). However, although some clinical features of schizophrenia (e.g., age at onset, disease course, and degree of impairment) display high familiality (e.g., [239]), the relatives of individuals with schizophrenia also show elevated rates of schizoaffective psychosis, bipolar affective disorder, and major depressive disorder [232, 240, 241]. This indicates that schizophrenia cannot be conceptualized as a homogeneously-transmitted clinical entity [242].

Over the past decade, advances in genomic technology, in particular the advent of genome-wide association studies (GWAS), have led to the identification of a substantial number of genetic risk variants for schizophrenia [243]. The number of identified independent risk loci, which is already above 100 [244], continues to increase. At the time of writing, research has implicated around 6,000 to 10,000 common variants in the aetiology of schizophrenia [243]. GWAS have identified long known candidate genes such as genes with an involvement in glutamatergic and dopaminergic neurotransmission, thus, providing independent support for the long-standing hypothesis that these pathways are involved in schizophrenia development. The most consistently implicated locus is the HLA region. This finding is consistent with the hypothesis that infectious/immunological mechanisms underlie a proportion of schizophrenia cases. However, most of the loci identified in molecular-genetic studies to date are novel, and these findings will guide further multidisciplinary research into neuronal pathology.

GWAS are designed to identify common risk variants with allele frequencies of >1%. They involve the use of genomic markers, that is, several-hundred-thousand to millions of single nucleotide polymorphisms (SNPs). These nucleotides are evenly dispersed across the genome, and show interindividual variation. As in other complex disorders large samples are necessary to achieve genome-wide significance, and the most recent GWAS meta-analysis for schizophrenia involved more than 35,000 patients [244]. Given the large amount of markers tested, the significance threshold is very low (5×10^{-8}), and it has been shown that many more SNPs not reaching the threshold level contribute to the disorder. The identified risk SNPs are also quite common in the general population, and each accounts for only a small proportion (normally below 1.3%) of the risk for schizophrenia [214].

An approach to refine such association findings is the investigation of genotype-endophenotype correlations. Research suggests that association with an endophenotype is stronger than with a heterogeneous entity, such as a categorical diagnosis [245]. A host of successful reverse genetic studies have been published, in particular imaging genetic studies, which explore the correlation between the identified risk variant and endophenotypes that have been assessed through neuropsychological and fMRI examination. A review of the results of these studies is beyond the scope of the present chapter. However, an example may serve to illustrate the reverse genetic approach. For the first genome-wide significant variant identified for schizophrenia, that is, in the gene *ZNF804A*, an imaging genetic study demonstrated alterations in the functional coupling of the dorsolateral prefrontal cortex (DLPFC) across hemispheres in risk-variant carriers [246]. This finding attracted much attention and led to the performance of numerous follow-up studies. While this effect was replicated in subsequent studies, others found associations with further endophenotpyes [247]. Until they are replicated, researchers cannot be sure whether the latter indicate pleiotropy (i.e., the phenomenon whereby one variant causes diverse phenotypic effects) or whether they represent chance findings. Meanwhile, large international research consortia merge their GWAS and imaging data, and these genotype-endophenotype data are made available to the public (http://www.brainmapping.org/NITP/images/Summer2012Slides/ENIGMA-Thompson.pdf), an approach which will facilitate multidisciplinary research into schizophrenia and other neuropsychiatric disorders.

To optimize exploitation of GWAS data and improve upon the "single phenotype-single variant" analysis approach, researchers have developed a range of more sophisticated biostatistical methods. Two examples, both of which examine the joint effect of SNPs, are (i) polygenic score analysis [248] and (ii) genome complex trait analysis (GCTA) [249]. Polygenic score analysis uses sets of top risk, SNPs (above and below the threshold for genome wide significance), from a "discovery" GWAS in order to generate risk-scores in individuals from independent "target" samples. This allows testing whether individuals with higher risk scores differ from those with lower risk scores and, if so, in which particular phenotypic dimensions. The GCTA approach estimates the variance for a complex trait, as explained by all SNPs. Since it is based on the assumption of an additive model, GCTA does not account for gene-gene interactions. The GCTA approach is used to investigate SNP-based genetic overlap between phenotypes/disorders.

In accordance with the hypothesis that schizophrenia is a polygenic disorder, the novel biostatistical approaches have shown that common, yet unidentified, SNPs explain approximately 30% of the total variation in schizophrenia susceptibility. These methods have generated a multitude of other interesting results. These findings include evidence, for example: (i) a significant enrichment of risk variants in brain genes; (ii) distribution of the risk variants across the entire genome [243, 250]; (iii) no major differences between men and women in the genetic variance for schizophrenia [250]; (iv) a high correlation between schizophrenia and bipolar disorder, a moderate correlation between schizophrenia and major depression, and a low correlation between schizophrenia and autism spectrum disorders [251]; and (v) a correlation in schizophrenia patients between a higher schizophrenia risk score and a more severe disease course [252]. Furthermore, these approaches have demonstrated that individuals from the general population with higher schizophrenia risk scores had lower cognitive abilities and that schizophrenia patients had higher "poor cognitive performance" scores, as based on GWAS data on cognitive performance [253].

The heritability estimate from formal genetic studies is more than twice as high as the variance explained by common variants. This raises the issue of how the "missing" heritability can be explained. One possibility is that since the methods do not consider gene-gene interactions, this approach underestimates the genetic contribution. A further likely possibility is that many rare variants with moderate-to-large effects still await identification. The first genome-wide exome sequencing studies have already been published, and this approach may uncover many more of these rare variants [254].

Some rare variants with larger effects have already been identified. These are mainly structural variants, so-called copy number variants (CNVs) (microdeletions and/or duplications of thousands to millions of DNA bases).

Although these are relatively potent risk factors for schizophrenia, they are not specific to schizophrenia; they also enhance the risk for other mental disorders, such as autism, bipolar affective psychosis, major depression, and personality disorder. Despite being extremely rare, the implicated single CNVs are found in 4% to 5% of individuals with schizophrenia. Hence, their aggregate contribution to schizophrenia is substantial [255, 256].

In a recent genetic-epidemiological study [257] investigated 26 CNVs with a reported association with schizophrenia or autism in order to determine whether cognitive deficits and brain morphological changes were also present in mentally healthy carriers. The investigated variants were relatively rare. They occurred at frequencies of 0.002% to 0.2% and showed a combined prevalence of 1.6% in the investigated population, and some of the CNVs were associated with reduced fecundity. The authors demonstrated an association between the investigated CNVs and cognitive test outcomes that ranked between those for schizophrenia cases and healthy population controls. Different CNVs were associated with different cognitive domains. Non-mentally ill carriers of the 15q11.2 (BP1-BP2) showed a history of dyslexia and dyscalculia rather than any other discernible cognitive autonomous.

In conclusion, GWAS of schizophrenia have generated important findings, and these have opened up a diversity of novel avenues for multidisciplinary research. Experts in the field are hopeful that increasing biostatistical sophistication, refinement of neuropsychiatric phenotypes, and the application of convergent approaches (integrating results from expression, pathway, epigenetic, and animal studies) will lead to genuine breakthroughs in our understanding of the molecular-genetic background of this devastating disorder. Important goals for future schizophrenia research are the establishment of a verifiable genetic model and the identification of robust biomarkers. The array of results generated through molecular-genetic research to date thus represents a complex and intriguing puzzle which still awaits resolution in order to translate findings to the benefit of patients.

5. From Predisposition to Manifest Illness

5.1. Risk Factors, Precursors, and Precipitants of Psychosis. Factors at work before the onset of schizophrenia enhance the risk for it. The most frequent risk factor predisposing for schizophrenia is genetic in nature, but environmental factors, too, as discussed above, play a role [93, 94, 258–260]. Such factors are pre- or perinatal brain injury, mostly due to anoxia [217, 261], viral childhood encephalitis [218], infant bacterial meningitis [219], and, to a lesser extent, other factors impacting the development of the central nervous system. Most of these factors, however, have been found to increase the risk not only for schizophrenia, but also for other mental disorders: affective psychosis, autism, intellectual deficits, neurological symptoms, and epilepsy [217–220, 262, 263].

Probands with a predisposition for schizophrenia, for example, offspring of women with schizophrenia or carriers of risk genes [264], have elevated rates of neurointegrative deficits and cognitive [265] and social impairment as well as an earlier onset of schizophrenia [233, 266–280]. An

increased genetic vulnerability has frequently been found to be a precondition for the risk-enhancing effect of environmental factors [93, 281].

Predisposition factors increase the lifetime risk. They must be distinguished from exogenous precipitants capable of triggering the onset of manifest episodes. One such precipitant of health-policy relevance is the misuse of cannabis and other psychoactive substances, for example, amphetamine combinations [282, 283], cocaine and psychomimetics such as phencyclidine [284], psilocybine, and LSD. These substances can provoke a short-term intoxication psychosis, which usually remits as soon as the substance in question is excreted from the body. But they may also trigger an autonomous course of schizophrenia [285–293]. A long-term use of cannabis may also have adverse effects, as shown in a study with the longest observation period yet, 34 years (1973–2007), in a sample of 50,087 Swedish conscripts with data on cannabis use at the ages of 18 to 20 years [293]. The authors identified 357 cases of schizophrenia from in-patient care and followed them up from 1973 to 2007. Patients with a history of cannabis use at baseline had a more unfavourable illness course compared with nonusers in terms of a significantly higher frequency of both readmissions to hospital and hospital stays lasting for 2 years or more.

5.2. Individual Development from Birth to Psychosis. Progression from birth to psychosis onset has been studied intensively. In two British studies—the National Survey of Health and Development (NSHD) study ($N = 5362$) [294–296] and the National Child Development Study (NCDS) ($N = 15.398$) [297]—persons later developing schizophrenia were followed up from birth to adult age. The same was done in the New-Zealand Dunedin Study [217, 298, 299] and the northern-Finland birth cohort study [262, 263, 300–302]. Compared with controls, the probands in these and comparable studies consistently showed mild developmental delays in their first years of life [217, 269, 270, 295, 303, 304], mild deficits in cognitive and social functioning, and minor neuromotor deficits in infancy, childhood, and adolescence [275, 299]. Like genetic vulnerability, these early antecedents also enhanced the risk for affective and other mental disorders [305–307].

Studies based on male Swedish adolescent conscripts (aged 18–20 years) [308, 309] and Israeli conscripts, both male and female (aged 16-17 years) [310, 311], have identified further risk factors. All inpatient admissions for schizophrenia during the period of risk were counted on data from the national psychiatric case registers at 15-year follow-up in the Swedish study and at 4- to 15-year follow-up in the Israeli study.

The Swedish conscripts who later developed schizophrenia showed, on average, a slightly lower IQ and a significantly higher frequency of four behavioural items: "having fewer than two friends," "preference for socializing in small groups," "feeling more sensitive than others," and "not having a steady girlfriend." 3% of the conscripts who endorsed all four items went on to develop schizophrenia in the 15-year period [309]. Because these behavioural items were also quite prevalent in the same-age Swedish male population who did not develop schizophrenia, their population-based predictive power was not very high. In the Israeli study, mild cognitive deficits—about 0.5 standard deviation—and indicators of social autonoimpairment turned out to predict schizophrenia incidence [310], but interindividual variance was considerable. There have also been reports of schizophrenia being associated with above-average intelligence [263, 312].

A further risk factor for schizophrenia as well as for bipolar disorder, mental retardation and autism spectrum disorder, is a *higher paternal age* (≥30 years) [313–318], confirmed in several birth cohort studies, record-linkage analyses, and large collectives [314, 319]. In a meta-analysis, Miller et al. [320] estimated a 3.1-fold excess risk up to a paternal age of 55 years. The factor accounting for this phenomenon is presumed to be an age-related increase in de novo mutations in paternal sperm [321]. But a low paternal age (below 18 years), too, seems to increase the risk for schizophrenia in the offspring [318].

In a recent study, Jaffe et al. [319] studied 371 families with at least two children, of whom at least one had developed schizophrenia. The authors found that an increase in schizophrenia risk was associated with a significantly higher paternal age at the time when the first child was born—a similar finding had previously been reported by Petersen et al. [322] on data from the Danish case register. A higher maternal age was associated with a higher rate of pre- and perinatal complications in the offspring diagnosed with schizophrenia. This finding slightly weakens the etiological relevance of paternal de novo mutations.

To sum up, like the genetic risk factors, each of the exogenous factors discussed accounts only for a small share in the risk for schizophrenia and other mental disorders, such as affective psychosis, autism, and learning disability.

5.3. Subclinical Symptoms as Precursors of Psychosis. In about 2/3 of cases, transition from mental health to psychosis takes more than a year. It is characterized by the onset of symptoms and aberrant behaviour, eventually culminating in the climax of the first illness episode [323]. Highly acute transitions, within four weeks or less, are much rarer; in the sample of the German Age Beginning Course (ABC) Schizophrenia Study it was the case only in 18% [323].

Isolated subclinical psychosis-like symptoms frequently occur as precursors at the beginning of the prodromal stage. Subclinical psychotic-like symptoms (delusions and hallucinations), affective and negative symptoms and signs of cognitive impairment are also prevalent in individuals without a history of psychotic illness in the general population [161, 324–328]. In the population-based Netherlands Mental Health Survey and Incidence Study (NEMESIS) the prevalence of isolated psychotic symptoms in the population aged 18 to 64 years was 4.2% for definite delusions and hallucinations and 17.5% for all such, including uncertain, symptoms [329, 330]. In the German population-based Early Developmental Stages of Psychopathology (EDSP) study of young adults (age 14 to 24 years), the prevalence of hallucinations was 4.6% and that of delusions was 15.7% (definite or probable) [331].

In a New-Zealand birth cohort study, 25% of the children who, at age 9 to 11 years, had experienced hallucinatory symptoms had a 16-fold excess risk of developing psychotic illness by age 26 years [298]. In the Dutch NEMESIS study, 8% of the adults (aged 18–64 years) who had experienced subclinical hallucinations developed clinical psychosis within two years, which corresponded to an excess risk of about 60% compared with symptom-free controls [161, 332, 333]. In the German EDSP study, in which probands initially aged 14 to 17 years were assessed four times over a period of 8.4 years, transitions to psychosis depended, in a dose-response relationship, on the persistence of subclinical psychotic symptoms at the follow-up assessments over the first five years: persistence at one measurement was associated with an odds ratio (OR) of 1.5, at two measurements with an OR of 5.0 and at all three measurements with an OR of 9.9 [334].

Multiple subclinical symptoms increase the risk for clinical psychosis: in the Dutch study, 3% of the probands who had experienced a single psychotic symptom developed clinical psychosis within two years, whereas 14% of those with two symptoms and 20% of those with three symptoms did so [335].

Several studies have addressed the question of how long the risk of transiting to psychosis persists, after characteristic subclinical symptoms have manifested themselves [328, 336, 337]. Most studies on the topic have looked at risk periods of one year [328] and only few studies at periods of two or more years [336]. In a systematic review of 35 cohort studies with follow-up periods of up to 20 years, van Os et al. [161] found that, after the first year, the frequency of transitions decreased by 10% and after 20 years by a total of 25% (cumulatively). The overwhelming majority of the subclinical symptoms either remitted or persisted without progressing to psychosis [161, 325].

The risks associated with the different symptom dimensions of schizophrenia have recently been placed at the centre of interest. Lyne et al. [338] studied the predictive specificity of prodromal negative symptoms. The authors found a significant increase in these symptoms after first admission, while the symptoms of the other dimensions showed no increase. Other studies have indicated that a decrease or an increase in subclinical affective symptoms and anxiety at the prodromal stage in persons also experiencing subclinical hallucinatory symptoms is associated with a significant decrease or increase in transitions to clinical psychosis [326, 339, 340]. Obviously, there is a functional association between the affective and the psychotic symptom dimension at the prodromal stage.

A different picture emerges when, instead of representative population samples, probands at ultra-high risk for schizophrenia are studied. Klosterkötter et al. [341, 342], using the Bonn Scale for the Assessment of Basic Symptoms (BSABS) [343], assessed the presence of "basic symptoms" in 160 hospitalized patients suspected of suffering from schizophrenia and checked their diagnoses in their medical records at follow-up an average of 9.6 years later. The basic symptoms yielded correct predictions in 78.1% and false-positive predictions in 20.6% of the cases. In this study, too, risk assessment was done fairly close to the timepoint of maximum risk.

As part of the North-American Prodrome Longitudinal Study (NAPLS) [344], 291 help-seeking persons were identified as high-risk cases by means of an early-recognition instrument [337]. At follow-up 6 months later 12.7%, at 12 months 21.7% (cumulative), at 18 months 26.8%, and at 24 months 35.3% of the patients had developed a psychosis. Over the 30-month follow-up period, the transition rate decelerated continuously by 13%, 9%, 5%, 5%, and 2.7%. No transitions to psychosis occurred among healthy controls [337].

The cumulative transition rates calculated in a recent meta-analysis [345] based on 2502 (clinical) high-risk and ultra-high-risk [346] individuals from 27 studies from different countries were 18% at 6-month follow-up, 22% at 1 year, 29% at 2 years, 32% at 3 years, and 36% after 3 years [346, 347]. This meta-analysis, however, has considerable weaknesses. Because the transition rates calculated in the studies included in the analysis varied a great deal (from 0.09% to 79%), as did the study populations in size (from 9 to 365 persons) and the baseline risk status of the probands examined (randomly selected population cohorts versus inpatient admissions for suspected schizophrenia), the results should be taken with caution.

To conclude, the research discussed indicates that a maximum of transitions occurs quite soon after a high-risk status has been established and that, with increasing time, transitions become rarer. In most cases, subclinical psychosis-like symptoms either remit fully or continue to persist without further progression.

6. The Clinical Symptoms of Schizophrenia

The three characteristic syndromes of schizophrenia, which, though in different degrees, manifest themselves in the prodromal phase and sometimes even before that, comprise psychotic or positive symptoms, a variety of negative symptoms, and a repertoire of subjectively experienced and objectively identifiable thought disorders. Further symptoms are cognitive disturbances in a stricter sense, disintegrative symptoms, and affective disturbances, depression in particular—the latter were ignored in the past and sometimes still are today—and an array of individually heterogeneous forms of aberrant experiences and behaviours.

Numerous attempts have been made to establish the empirical symptom structure of schizophrenia [348–354]. Factor-analytical approaches have yielded only partly comparable results, for example, five-factor solutions resembling the five sections of the Scale for the Assessment of Negative Symptoms (SANS) [355, 356]. Two- and three-factor solutions, too, have been proposed [354, 357–359]. The three-factor model presented by Liddle and Barnes [348] enjoys wide acceptance: "*reality distortion*" is more or less equivalent to positive symptoms and "*psychomotor poverty*" to negative symptoms, whereas "*disintegration*" includes an overload of acute and chronic symptoms [360]. A depression factor was not detected until the assessment tools were expanded to permit screening for other than positive and negative symptoms [361–366].

6.1. Negative Symptoms and Cognitive Impairment. The negative symptoms of psychosis reflect deficits in cognitive functioning, in experience of pleasure and interest, in motivation and engagement in the world [367–369]. A broad definition like that makes it difficult to distinguish between a negative syndrome and cognitive deficits, although, according to Harvey et al. [370], Nuechterlein et al. [371], and Blanchard et al. [368], they are "separable domains of illness." According to Goldberg et al. [372] and Nuechterlein et al. [371], "cognitive factors are core features of schizophrenia" [371]. They consider schizophrenia a cognitive disorder. Keefe [373] even suggested including cognitive impairment as a diagnostic criterion for schizophrenia in the DSM-V [374]. The suggestion triggered a lively debate [375], because comparable cognitive deficits are also encountered in other mental disorders [274, 376].

A fact common to both syndromes is that despite more than a century of schizophrenia research there are very few treatments, if any, that have proven efficacious [377]. Since both involve functional impairment in course and outcome [377] and deficits in social cognition play a crucial role in everyday functioning [371], negative symptoms and cognitive impairment have been placed at the centre of interest in therapy research and efforts to develop new treatments, though without much success yet [371, 378–385].

Cognitive deficits and negative symptoms can be operationally distinguished from one another by neuropsychological tests that measure cognitive functioning. Reduced to a lack of pleasure and motivation, the negative syndrome can be ascertained primarily by the observation of behaviour and by self-rating [367, 369].

Since both phenomena are characterized mainly by diminution or lack of normal functions and are difficult to distinguish clearly in phenomenological terms, they are usually treated as one category in clinical practice, which is a drawback both to research and therapy trials and to targeted training measures.

Prevalence rates for negative symptoms ranging from 50% to 90% at the climax of the first episode and at first admission have been reported [386–389]. With the remission of the first episode, negative symptoms, too, decrease to rates varying from 35% to 70% [389–392]. Depending on the initial diagnosis, some 15% to 40% of patients with schizophrenia never develop any negative symptoms [393].

It is an established fact that both cognitive deficits and negative symptoms run a stable course after the first psychotic episode [274, 371, 378, 382, 394–396].

In the 2010 Australian National Psychosis Survey, which included all persons ever diagnosed with and treated for schizophrenia, patients' mean IQ was, regardless of their duration of illness, 0.5 standard deviation below that of the general population [397]. Comparisons of cognitive function profiles between patients and healthy controls have shown that only few deficits, that is, impairment in attention, memory, and executive functioning, are clearly attributable to schizophrenia [354, 377, 398, 399].

Elevated rates of cognitive deficits have also been observed in first-degree relatives of people with schizophrenia [400–402]. As the population-cohort and the conscript studies cited showed, they are measurable already at the prodromal stage [308, 309, 333, 371, 403, 404]. The birth cohort studies [273, 299, 301, 302, 391, 394] and the Israeli [311, 404, 405] and the Swedish [308, 309] conscript studies have demonstrated that minor delays in cognitive development and/or deficits in academic attainment and verbal skills are already manifest in childhood and adolescence in individuals later developing schizophrenia.

No reliable body of evidence has turned up either from methodologically sound cross-sectional comparisons of patients at first admission and after long histories of illness or from longitudinal studies for the notion that cognitive deficits progress during the illness course [371, 403, 406]. Negative symptoms clearly increase in prevalence and severity only in the prodromal phase [323, 407]. In the further course of the disorder they have been found to increase only in a small proportion of patients [408, 409].

During the run-up to the revision of the DSM-IV to DSM-V, it was intensively debated whether cognitive impairment should be included as a diagnostic criterion for schizophrenia [410]. It was decided not to do so, because cognitive deficits have not been found to sufficiently distinguish between schizophrenia and several other "boundary" disorders. In the course of that revision, the subtypes of schizophrenia dating back to Kraepelin were removed from the DSM-V and replaced by empirically founded psychopathological dimensions with cognitive impairment included as one such dimension [410].

6.1.1. Types of Negative Symptoms.

A distinction has been drawn between primary and secondary negative symptoms [411]. The secondary negative syndrome [412] has been explained as representing a corollary of depression, substance abuse, and side-effects of neuroleptic medications [413, 414]. The primary or "deficit" syndrome has been presumed to originate in the disease process itself, to be independent of environmental factors, to have a persistent course, and not to be amenable to therapy [385, 415]. The deficit syndrome described by Wing & Brown [416] as secondary impairment is caused by social and cognitive deprivation during long hospital stays.

In the long-term illness course, the symptom complexes of abulia-apathy and anhedonia-asociality have proven to be the most stable components of the negative syndrome [407, 417, 418].

The increased risk of schizophrenia associated with minor early brain lesions, the lifelong persistence of cognitive impairment, and findings from morphological MRI studies have prompted some authors to conclude that schizophrenia is a neurodevelopmental disorder [419–423]. According to Crow [424], the hypothesis applied only to one of the two subtypes of schizophrenia he postulated. Type I, characterized by positive symptoms, an acute and benign illness course, he presumed, was attributable to dopamine dysfunction. Type 2, characterized by negative symptoms, cognitive impairment, and a poor, often chronic illness course, he saw as a neurodevelopmental disorder exogenously caused by pre- and/or perinatal brain damage. However, the hypothesis could not be verified [425].

6.1.2. The Assessment of Negative Symptoms.

The Scale for the Assessment of Negative Symptoms (SANS), developed by Andreasen [355], comprises the following five sections:

(1) Affective Flattening or Blunting
(2) Alogia
(3) Avolition-Apathy
(4) Anhedonia-Asociality
(5) Attention.

It is used worldwide for measuring negative symptoms. It is included in the Positive and Negative Symptom Scale for Schizophrenia (PANSS) [426], which permits the assessment of other symptoms, too.

In 2006, a conference at the National Institute of Mental Health (NIMH) adopted a "Consensus Statement on Negative Symptoms" [427] and initiated the development of a "next-generation negative symptoms scale," the Clinical Assessment Instrument for Negative Symptoms (CAINS) [428, 429] as an NIMH project. The CAINS, now completed, has been designed to ensure a reliable assessment of negative symptoms. Included in it are the following five domains: asociality, avolition, anhedonia, blunted affect, and alogia, and, thus, most of the SANS items.

First trials have been run with satisfactory results. They have shown "*that amotivation and avolition—and, thus, negative symptoms—constitute the core deficits in schizophrenia*" [398]. Conclusive evidence is still lacking that the CAINS permits more valid measurements of negative symptoms to replace the SANS.

In rare studies, negative symptoms have been found to be weakly correlated with positive symptoms. There is no consistent evidence showing that cognitive impairment and psychotic symptoms are associated with each other. Psychosis frequently involves cognitive deficits, but the two symptom dimensions evolve independently over time [360, 403, 430–432]. Cognitive deficits are not specific for schizophrenia. They also occur in other mental disorders, for example, severe mood disorders [433], and in mild psychoorganic syndromes.

7. The Prodromal Stage of Psychosis

With the aim of creating the preconditions for therapeutic early intervention, Sullivan [434] and Cameron [435] attempted a systematic analysis of the prodromal stage of schizophrenia, but with little success. Conrad [436] later proposed a stage model based on gestaltpsychologie and Docherty et al. [437] a psychodynamically influenced stage model of incipient schizophrenia. Neither Docherty et al.'s nor Conrad's model has been confirmed on empirical data, apart from a prepsychotic stage (trema) turning out to be distinguishable from a psychotic (apopheny) prodromal stage [350, 438, 439].

An array of studies have recently investigated the prodromal phase of schizophrenia with regard to both the time involved (course) and its nature (symptoms) (e.g., [323, 327, 341, 342, 350, 440–452]). The first symptoms to appear—apart from mild cognitive deficits frequently preceding them—are mostly depression and anxiety, followed by negative symptoms and, finally, by rapidly accumulating positive symptoms [323]. The so-called prepsychotic prodrome, from the onset of the first symptom to the onset of the first psychotic symptom, takes, on average, several years to unfold. In the ABC Schizophrenia Study, its mean duration was 4.8 years (median 2.3) [323]. A psychotic prodromal stage, counted from the onset of the first (new) psychotic symptom to the climax of the first episode, defined by maximum symptom prevalence, had a mean duration of 1.1 years (median 0.6 years) and, when the 0.2 months until first admission were included, a total duration of 1.3 years (median 0.8 years) [323].

Type and temporal sequence of prodromal symptom manifestation are very similar in major depressive disorder and schizophrenia. The two disorders become diagnostically distinguishable only with the onset of and a steep increase in psychotic symptoms in the cases transiting to psychosis [453].

This finding has theoretical implications for the disease concept of schizophrenia. It is conceivable to assume a preformed sequence of the two syndromes, in which the affective syndrome represents the expression of milder neural dysfunction and the psychotic syndrome considerably more severe dysfunction [60, 453].

Prodromal depression has consequences. Patients experiencing prodromal depression develop more positive and depressive symptoms in the first psychotic episode, but this excess symptomatology soon levels off in the further (1- to 2-year) illness course [444]. Patients without prodromal depression tend to develop significantly more negative symptoms, almost exclusively affective blunting, in the first episode and medium-term (5-year) course, [444]. The reason could be reduced emotional responsiveness either caused by the disorder or representing a personality trait.

The duration of untreated psychosis (DUP) [454, 455] has turned out be a predictor of the illness course. A lengthy DUP is associated with a more severe first episode, with a greater amount of adverse social consequences, more inpatient days and higher costs, and so forth [440, 454–461]. Whether it is also associated with a greater number of relapses, as presumed by Altamura et al. [462], is not yet clear. More longitudinal studies on the topic are needed.

An extended duration of untreated illness (DUI), characterized primarily by depressive and negative symptoms and functional impairment, is mainly associated with more negative symptoms and social impairment in the further illness course [461].

DUP and DUI are determined by the availability of mental health services and by patients' help-seeking behaviour [459, 463]. Cognitive deficits, which can be ascertained by neuropsychological tests, are independent of the prodromal symptoms of psychosis and, thus, not affected by DUP [464].

Some of these findings lie behind the speculative theory that psychotic symptoms might exert a toxic impact on the brain and that that effect can be warded off by antipsychotic medication, for example, olanzapine, if administered early enough [465–469]. The toxicity hypothesis has not been confirmed, but the insight is still prevailing that early intervention is worthwhile pursuing.

Given the chances offered by early intervention to benignly influence the onset and course of schizophrenia, the idea was entertained during the revision of the DSM-IV to include an "attenuated psychosis syndrome" as an indicator of the schizophrenia prodrome in the diagnosis of schizophrenia in Section 1 of the DSM-V [470]. After an intensive discussion, the idea was dismissed because of the fairly low rates of transition to psychosis, the high risk of transition to other types of mental disorder, and the fairly high rates of remission. Instead, attenuated psychosis syndrome has been integrated as a diagnostic category in Section 3 (Appendix) of the DSM-V [471].

7.1. Early Intervention. Early intervention at the psychotic prodromal stage should be targeted not only at the persisting prepsychotic symptoms, but also at functional impairment and newly appearing positive symptoms. Most early-intervention trials [442, 472–477] have tested combinations of psychological treatment, mostly cognitive behavioural therapy [478–483], and a low-dose neuroleptic medication [474, 475]. Compared with controls, significantly fewer probands have been found to transit to full-blown psychosis over one or two years. Psychological intervention without neuroleptic medication, tested on high-risk probands, has also turned out to be effective in significantly postponing transition to psychosis [479, 484].

8. Schizophrenia and Depression

In a review of literature, Bartels & Drake [485] reported prevalence rates for depressive symptoms in manifest schizophrenia ranging from 20% to 70%. According to another review, the rates vary from 6% to 75% [486]. Reasons for the great discrepancy are differences in study designs, for example, whether single depressive symptoms, syndromes, or diagnoses are used for calculating point or period prevalences.

As mentioned, Emil Kraepelin himself ultimately came to question the validity of the dichotomy hypothesis [22]. And indeed there is reason for doubt. Kendell and Brockington [54] showed that continuity exists and no "point of rarity" can be found between schizophrenia and mood disorders at the symptom level. Anxiety, depressive mood, and excessive worrying are the most frequent initial symptoms in schizophrenic psychosis [450, 453]. In the ABC Schizophrenia study, around 85% of the probands experienced one or more episodes of depressive mood for at least two weeks [453, 487]. Furthermore, depressive mood is the most frequent symptom in the entire course of schizophrenia [453, 487].

9. The Influence of Age and Sex on Symptom Manifestation

9.1. Sex Difference in Age at Onset. Schizophrenia, as based on the ICD-10 or DSM-IV diagnosis, manifests itself primarily in adolescence and at early adult age. Kraepelin had already observed an age difference of several years between men and women at first admission for dementia praecox [488, 489]. This also applies to age at first-ever onset, as confirmed in

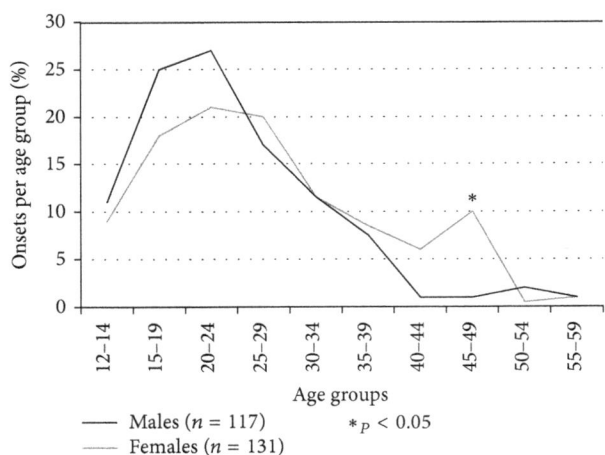

Figure 2: Age distribution of schizophrenia onsets of a broad diagnostic definition (ICD-9: 295, 297, 298.3, 298.4) for men and women. Source: [494].

numerous studies [490–492] and described by Castle [493] as "universally accepted."

In the ABC study sample of patients with first-ever admission with schizophrenia of either a broad or restricted diagnostic definition (ICD-9), the patients were compared with age- and sex-matched healthy controls from the same catchment area—male patients showed a peak of illness onsets at age 15 to 24 years and, hence, earlier than female patients did [494]. After that peak the rates fell to a low plateau. The first peak of female onsets was lower and occurred somewhat later, at age 15 to 29 years. After a decline similar to that in the male rates, a second peak, narrower and lower than the first one, occurred at age 45 to 49 years, again followed by a decline [494] (Figure 2).

The mean age difference, calculated both for a restricted and broad diagnosis, was 3 to 4 years [323, 495]. Data from the national Danish case register, analysed using the same study design, yielded almost identical values, thus, confirming the finding [495, 496].

A recent meta-analysis looked into the sex difference on the basis of 46 studies published in English-language journals between 1987 and 2009 [497]. The definitions of onset used in the studies differed. The diagnoses were based on the ICD-9 and its later versions or the DSM-III and its later versions. The age differences found were considerably smaller: women's mean age was 1.63 years higher at first-ever sign of schizophrenia, 1.48 years higher at first psychotic symptom, 1.22 years higher at first contact, and 1.07 years higher at first admission to inpatient care. The DSM-based diagnoses yielded slightly higher age differences compared to the ICD diagnoses. The age difference attained significance only in developed countries, whereas in developing (Asian) countries women's age at first admission was 1.54 lower than men's.

This deviating result concerning a "universally accepted" phenomenon requires a closer look. And indeed the meta-analysis has weaknesses. Because of the small number of studies included, single values from developing countries have

influenced the means: for example, the study conducted by Gangadhar et al. [498] in India—published only as a short communication—reported a 4.2-year higher mean age for men. The study was based on the case records of two samples (N = 70 each) admitted with a clinical diagnosis of schizophrenia to the Department of Psychiatry of the National Institute of Mental Health and Neuroscience (NIMHANS) in Bangalore. One sample came from the Indian state of Karnataka and the other from the southern Indian state of Kerala. In a previous study [499] from the same institute, coauthored by Gangadhar, such a design was described as a "limited approach." Gangadhar et al. do not tell why patients from two different states were admitted for inpatient care at the Bangalore institute. Unlike the Karnataka sample with a sex difference of 4.2 years in age of onset, the Kerala sample did not show any significant difference. The number of probands (32 women and 38 men from the state of Karnataka), on the basis of which the means were calculated, was unusually small to ensure valid results across the total age range.

The previous study [499] avoided some of the weaknesses of the Gangadhar study. 100 male and 100 female patients with a DSM-IV diagnosis of schizophrenia consecutively admitted to a hospital were examined individually. Whether the sample was representative of the population is not quite clear. In about half the sample, patients' date of birth was not officially documented, so it had to be estimated. This was probably the case in Ghangadhar's study, too, but was not mentioned by the authors. Murthy et al. [499] could not find any significant age difference between male and female patients.

The study by Stöber et al. [500], also included in the meta-anaylsis, is questionable, too. It focused only on two rare syndromes, systematic catatonia and periodic catatonia, using the internationally little known classification by Leonhard [501]. Age at onset was lower for males in one group and higher in the other compared with females.

These examples suffice to illustrate the quality of the meta-analysis by Eranti et al. [497].

Good epidemiological studies looking into age at onset of schizophrenia in developing countries are rare and difficult to conduct for various reasons. The WHO 10-country study covering the same age range (15 to 54 years) and using culture-independent techniques of measuring symptoms reported a higher age of onset for women from all the three developing countries participating: Columbia (Cali): 3.0, Nigeria (Ibadan): 2.9, India (Agra): 0.4, (Chandigarh): 1.0 years [49, 502].

The finding that women are several years older than men at the onset of the first symptom of schizophrenia, at the onset of the first positive symptom and also at first admission in countries with well-developed mental-health care systems, has been confirmed in numerous studies and included in the ICD-10 [502, 503]: "This gender difference is currently assumed to be among the few robust, well replicated findings in the entire field of schizophrenia research" [504, p.171]. It cannot be explained by men's higher mortality or shorter life-expectancy [505].

Since social hypotheses have failed to explain this sex-difference [496, 505], biological explanations have been sought: women's second peak of onsets at menopausal age (cf. Figure 2) makes one think of the age curve of oestrogen secretion. Animal experiments have shown that oestrogen applications are capable of attenuating dopaminergic behaviour by downregulating D_2-receptor sensitivity [506, 507]. Testosterone has no such effect [506].

It must be assumed that oestrogen secretion downregulates D_2 receptor function at young age [508–514]. As a consequence, either the onset of schizophrenia is delayed or the disorder produces less severe symptoms in part of the women at risk for developing the disorder. With diminishing oestrogen secretion in menopause, some of the at-risk women finally fall ill, thus, producing the second peak of onsets [506, 507, 515]. The oestrogen hypothesis has been confirmed in studies demonstrating the efficacy of adjunctive oestrogen treatment in patients with schizophrenia [516–518].

The sex difference in age of onset has turned out to be smaller or nonexistent in twins and siblings with schizophrenia [519–522]. Hence, it has been presumed that the risk-reducing hormonal effect of oestrogen might be antagonized by a risk-increasing effect of genetic vulnerability [60, 522]. The hypothesis was confirmed in the ABC Schizophrenia Study, in which first-onset patients with schizophrenia and equally affected first-degree relatives were compared with patients without familial schizophrenia [60, 522].

9.2. Late-Onset Psychosis. As schizophrenia is regarded primarily as a disorder of the first half of life, the upper age limits are remarkably low in several diagnostic classification systems: 40 years in the Research Diagnostic Criteria [523], 45 years in the Feighner criteria [74] and the DSM-III [82]. As a result, schizophrenias manifesting themselves at higher ages have been neglected in most large-scale incidence studies. The few studies covering the entire age range have revealed that new cases, mainly based on the schizophrenia spectrum diagnoses, occur at considerable frequencies at higher age, too [494, 524, 525]. The main symptoms presented by these late-onset cases are the first-rank symptoms defined by Schneider.

In the first half of the life span, incident cases tend to be more frequent and more severe in men than women [526]. Beyond age 60 years, however, there is a *"massive female preponderance in very-late schizophrenia (late paraphrenia, usually with an onset after the age of 60)"* [527], a fact often ignored.

At ages after 60 years, incident schizophrenia is associated with more severe symptoms in women than men [493, 528–531]. In practice, patients with late-onset psychoses are often given a diagnosis of late paraphrenia [532–534] or of a similar disorder rather than schizophrenia. This leaves one wondering whether the symptoms of schizophrenia might vary with age, especially since paranoid symptoms tend to be very prevalent in old age [531, 532, 534].

A comparison of the most frequent syndromes across 5-year age groups over the entire age range in a sample of consecutive first admissions for schizophrenia spectrum disorder (ICD-9) from a catchment area in Germany ($N = 1109$) revealed that most of the syndromes studied showed no significant age differences [531, 535]. There were only two exceptions: paranoid and systematized delusions in incident schizophrenia showed linear and significant increases with age: delusions of persecution from $\leq 10\%$ (for males and females) at young age to over 20% (males) and over 45% (females) at age 75+; systematized delusions from just over 30% (for males and females) to 65% (females) and 50% (males) in old age. The age-related rates for patients presenting incoherence of thought and disorders of self sank almost inversely from maximum values of just over 30% (females) and 55% (males) for the former to below 10% (both sexes) in old age and from just over 45% (both sexes) for the latter to about 20% (females) and almost zero (males) [531, 535]. These significant inverse trends could not be explained by an age-related decrease in the influence of genetic and environmental risk factors.

The authors proposed a heuristic explanation [60, 531]: the onset of psychosis at a very early age interferes with basic mental functions, causing severe anxiety, inappropriate affect, thought disorder, and a disordered sense of self and perception of the world [536–538]. At an early age, when the developing brain and personality are still malleable, psychosis onset can easily cause severe mental disturbance. At an advanced age, when psychological reaction patterns have grown stable over the course of life, basic mental functions are not easily disturbed and severe psychotic disintegration is, thus, less likely to occur. Both brain and personality have developed defense mechanisms protecting them against the destructive influences of the disease process. Rather than mental disintegration, elderly persons develop paranoid and systematized delusions as a rational way of coping with neural dysfunction [539].

9.3. Early Social Course. The early social course, too, depends on age. Social consequences become manifest primarily in the prodromal phase and early illness course. The peak of illness onsets falls in the period of life in which major socioeconomic development takes place. Equal proportions of high-risk individuals and controls, in the mean, are capable of finishing basic school education, but the former frequently drop out of lengthy further education, for example, university. In terms of marriage, patients do not differ from controls at illness onset, but they fall behind their healthy peers during the prodromal phase. This also applies to their occupational career (e.g., having a regular job and earning one's living) [526]. Due to their lower age at illness onset, male patients suffer a greater number of and more pronounced social deficits at illness onset compared with women.

Men's more unfavourable socioeconomic starting conditions at illness onset—despite a stable course of the core symptoms—are the reason for their more unfavourable medium-term social course. Another factor influencing the social course—mediated by therapy adherence and coping behaviour—is the adverse social behaviour exhibited by young men falling ill with schizophrenia: self-neglect, lack of hygiene, lack of interest in finding or keeping a job, and lack of interest in leisure activities and social contacts [540]. In contrast, women with schizophrenia tend to exhibit

TABLE 1: Five selected (older) European studies on the long-term outcome of schizophrenia.

Author(s)	N	Sample	Length of illness up to follow-up	Outcome Good	Outcome Poor
Bleuler 1972/Zurich [555]	208	First-/readmitted patients treated by the author	>20 years	20%	24%
Hinterhuber 1973/Innsbruck [556]	157	First admissions	30–40 years	29%	31%
Ciompi and Müller 1976/Lausanne [557]	289	First admissions	Ø 37 years (Range 10–65)	27%	27%
Huber et al. 1979/Bonn [558]	502	First-/readmissions	Ø 22 years (Range 9–59)	22%	35%
Marneros et al. 1991/Cologne [554]	148	First admissions	Ø 25 years (Range 10–50)	7%	42%

Source: [559], modified.

socially positive behaviour, for example, over-adaptiveness and conformity [526].

All these conclusions apply only to the age range studied (12 to 59 years) [526]. The situation is different after 60 years of age when working life comes to an end and certain risk factors and the living conditions change. Males' adverse social behaviour becomes less frequent at later age. In countries with well-developed social safety nets, pension systems guarantee the socioeconomic status of the elderly. Long-standing partnerships tend to reduce losses in this domain. A stable matrix of psychological reaction patterns reduces the risk of extremely severe symptoms appearing at illness onset. As a consequence, the risk of experiencing adverse effects in the socioeconomic and personal domains is also reduced. Although the features of mental disintegration and social deterioration are lacking, late-onset psychoses must be classified as part of the disease construct currently called schizophrenia.

10. Course and Outcome of Full-Blown Disorder

Unlike in the prodromal phase, it is the treated rather than the natural course of schizophrenia that can be studied after first admission, because it would be unethical to withhold treatment for research purposes.

Like incidence and prevalence, the results of follow-up studies, too, depend on the underlying diagnosis. The requirement for a diagnosis of schizophrenia according to the DSM-III to -V that functional impairment has persisted for at least six months and positive symptoms for at least four weeks prior to initial assessment yields an excess of poor illness courses. In contrast, the criteria of the ICD-9 and -10 (four weeks of symptoms without an indication of functional impairment) lead to a selection of more acute and benign illness courses. This has prognostic implications for course and outcome.

In studies proceeding from population-based cohorts of first-episode cases of ICD-9 or -10 schizophrenia, the psychotic symptom dimension, as based on mean scores for males and females, displays neither significant deterioration nor significant amelioration over the medium-term course

(5 years or so) following the remission of the first episode [60, 444].

There is an important distinction to make between outcome studies and longitudinal studies. Outcome studies compare findings between an initial and a follow-up assessment (pre-post comparisons). The illness course between these timepoints has to be reconstructed: the longer the period in question, the higher the risk of misinterpretation. More assessments done over the period covered yield a more realistic picture of the illness course [392].

According to the results of a wealth of longitudinal studies, the proportions of patients with a good outcome vary from 0 to 68% [392, 541–553]. Reasons for this variation are differences in the definitions of good/poor outcome, in the inclusion criteria of the cohorts studied, for example, first admissions versus hospitalized patients in general, and in the lengths of illness [546]. Allardyce & van Os [333] have listed the possible confounders and biases involved.

In the 1970s, a few European longitudinal studies covering histories of illness of 20 years or more were published (Table 1). Although the information provided on the inclusion criteria, histories of illness (20 to 40 years), and the assessment and evaluation methods used was in part incomplete or lacking and these parameters varied a lot across the studies, the simple outcome rates were fairly similar in size, except for the study listed at the bottom of Table 1 [554]. These surprisingly favourable results attracted a lot of interest in the USA, especially since they fell in the period when convergence to European diagnostic definitions was under way in the USA [72, 73, 77].

Examples of more recent longitudinal investigations are the long-term follow-ups of samples from the former WHO schizophrenia studies: ISoS [549–551, 560–562] and DOSMeD [49, 563, 564]. The DOSMeD Study reported higher proportions of acute psychosis showing rapid remissions in developing countries compared with industrialized countries. This transcultural difference has not yet been explained conclusively despite several attempts.

Two recent longitudinal studies from a high-income country (Germany) are worth mentioning: the one assessed first-admission patients with schizophrenia (Schneiderian first-rank symptoms) in age range 15 to 44 years at nine cross-sections ($N = 70$ initial; $N = 51$ follow-up) over a period of 15.6 years [548–550], the other was a population-based study of a sample of first-episode patients with schizophrenia (ICD-9) (N = 232) aged 12 to 59 years—including healthy individuals and patients diagnosed with moderately severe or major depression as controls matched for age and sex—from illness onset to final follow-up an average of 12.3 years after first admission [60, 388, 396]. Seven cross-sectional assessments were done with half of the sample (n = 115) and only one follow-up assessment was conducted with the rest (n = 117). Both studies showed that, compared with healthy controls, the majority of patients with schizophrenia are considerably worse off in socioeconomic terms after a 12-year history of illness: for example, 33% of the patients had a regular job compared with 70% of the healthy controls from the same catchment area [396]. But, as already mentioned, the bulk of social impairment is suffered in the prodromal phase.

At final follow-up, sex differences were visible in patients' marital status and living situation: fewer female patients were living alone, as had been the case at first admission. More female than male patients were married, but their number was lower than that for married healthy controls. Both male and female patients showed a high rate of divorce, but it was almost exclusively female patients that had remarried after illness onset. Large proportions of male patients, but very few women with schizophrenia, were living in residential homes or supervised apartments [396].

More or less similar results have been reported from the follow-up assessments of samples from the WHO longitudinal studies of schizophrenia, comparable in their methods and designs—done, besides in Mannheim (Germany) [548–550], in Nottingham (UK) [564], and in Groningen (NL) [562].

Both the medium and the long-term course of schizophrenia are influenced by age. Illness onset in youth and adolescence is associated with social stagnation rather than social decline, because illness at this early age impedes typical social ascent. Late-onset illness, after a long period of life lived in health, usually permits patients to experience normal social ascent. This is why these patients tend to suffer considerable social decline. Patients with illness onset at an intermediate age occupy an intermediate position between these two groups [396]. In sum, the risk of social decline is first and foremost determined by patients' social status at illness onset.

Modal values for the overall course of schizophrenia that would be valid worldwide are impossible to calculate due to the heterogeneity of sociocultural environments, due to differences in the proportions of acute, rapidly remitting cases and due to the variation in the quality of the studies on the topic. This has not deterred Allardyce and van Os [333] from estimating good outcome at 42%, intermediate outcome at 35%, and poor outcome at 27% on the basis of a review of 37 studies published between 1966 and 2003 [565].

A finding that has implications for our understanding of schizophrenia is the missing or only modest deterioration in both the symptom-related and social course, as based on mean values, in the period starting some time after the remission of the first episode (on average about 2 years), while individual illness courses vary a lot. The way Kraepelin

understood the disease concept, that is, as a progressive process leading to increasing deficits, is applicable only to a tiny proportion of cases.

Typical of the symptom-related course of schizophrenia are irregular relapse episodes with intervals occurring in between with only few, if any, symptoms present [388, 391]. The number of episodes depends on their definition.

To ensure comparability of the results, the authors of the ABC Schizophrenia Study [60, 388, 391] right censored history of illness (mean 12.3 years) by the earliest follow-up assessment of a patient (11.2 years after initial assessment) on the basis of IRAOS data (Interview for the Retrospective Assessment of the Onset and Course of Schizophrenia and Other Psychoses) [566, 567]. To compensate for this error-prone approach, a subsample (n = 130) of the initial sample (N = 232) was assessed at seven cross sections using another instrument (PSE-CATEGO). Over the period of 134 months, the authors counted a total of 333 psychotic relapse episodes, operationalized by an at least 14-day period of increasing symptoms between two at least 4-week intervals of decreasing symptoms. The fact that the number of episodes varied from 0 to 29 with a mean of three per patient reflects the heterogeneity of the illness course [388, 396].

Besides the psychotic relapse episodes, a total of 73 (=18%) purely depressive episodes without psychotic symptoms were counted [388, 391, 487]. Depressive relapse episodes free of psychotic symptoms in patients with schizophrenia were also found by Jablensky [568] in 16% of a cohort of the WHO 10-country study over a period of two years and by Bressan et al. [569] in an identical proportion of a cohort of first-admission patients prospectively studied over 1.5 years (as based on the DSM-IV definition of major depressive episodes).

10.1. Types of Illness Course. The great variation observed in the illness courses was one of the reasons why attempts have been made to identify simple course types that would be of prognostic relevance in clinical practice.

Harding [570] compared longitudinal studies, two from Switzerland and one from the USA, on the basis of eight course types. We have added in that comparison another US study and a WHO study. The criteria Harding used for defining the course types and estimating the proportions of patients exhibiting them are not precise enough, so the results are not really comparable (Figure 3).

For this reason, British authors [572] limited the number of course types to four and defined them by simple criteria—number of episodes, presence of functional impairment, and persistence of versus increase in symptoms and impairment (Figure 4). Simple models like this are more useful in clinical practice.

As stated, individual illness courses differ a great deal. Around 20% of persons affected experience only one psychotic episode without further relapses and any discernible social consequences [392]. In a small proportion—about equal in size—the disorder has a progressive course sometimes leading to need for residential care.

	Onset	Course type	End state	Lausanne study	Burghölzli study	Vermont study	Chicago study	ISoS study[1]
(1)	Acute	Undulating	Recovery/mild	25.4	30–40 25–35	7	10.8	29.4
(2)	Chronic	Simple	Moderate/severe	24.1	10–20	4	36.5	14.4
(3)	Acute	Undulating	Moderate/severe	11.9	5	4	9.5	4.9
(4)	Chronic	Simple	Recovery/mild	10.1	5–10	12	4.1	10.4
(5)	Chronic	Undulating	Recovery/mild	9.6	—	38	6.8	22.6
(6)	Acute	Simple	Moderate/severe	8.3	5–15	3	13.5	9.1
(7)	Chronic	Undulating	Moderate/severe	5.3	—	27	12.2	4
(8)	Acute	Simple	Recovery/mild	5.3	5	5	6.8	5.3

[1]Incidence studies only
Lausanne study: Ciompi and Muller [557]
Burghölzli study: Bleuler [555]
Vermont study: Harding et al. [543, 544]
Chicago study: Marengo et al. [553]
ISoS study: Harrison et al. [564]

FIGURE 3: Course types in schizophrenia. On the right, each of the five columns represents a study. The numbers indicate the percentage of patients with the course type depicted on the left; for example, 7% of the patients in the Vermont Study demonstrated an acute onset, an undulating course, and a recovered/mild end state (type 1), in contrast to the ISoS Study, where 29.4% of the patients belong to this course type. Based on [570] data from the Chicago and the ISoS study were added by the authors. Source: [571].

11. Reduced Life-Expectancy

The life-expectancy of patients with schizophrenia is considerably reduced compared with that of general populations [392, 573]. The figures vary. A meta-analysis of 37 studies calculated a median standard mortality rate of 2.6 for individuals with schizophrenia [574]. It means that the risk of dying in the following year is 2.6 times higher for people with schizophrenia than for the population in general. Brown et al. [575] found a two to three times higher mortality risk for people with schizophrenia in Southampton/UK. According to Seeman [576], the life-expectancy of persons with schizophrenia was 61 years compared with 76 years for the general population. Controlling for age, Colton and Manderscheid [577] found a median of lost years of life varying from 25 to 30 years in several US states, a surprisingly high figure.

22%	One episode only — no impairment	
35%	Several episodes with no or minimal impairment	
8%	Impairment after the first episode with subsequent exacerbation and no return to normality	
38%	Impairment increasing with each of several episodes and no return to normality	

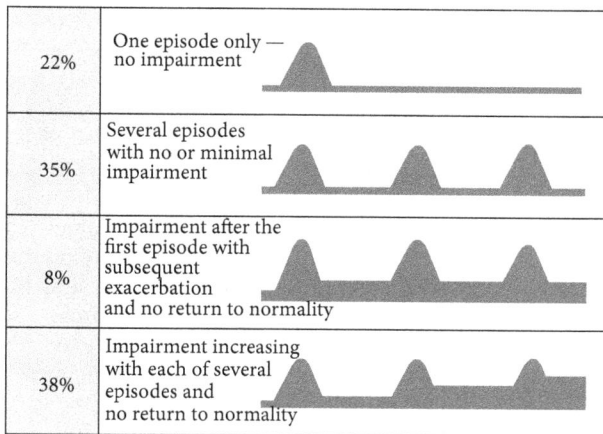

FIGURE 4: Graded course of illness in first-admission patients with schizophrenia as indicated by episodes of illness, symptomatology, and social impairment at assessment during 5 years (N = 49). Source: [572], modified.

A direct comparison of age at death for persons with schizophrenia on data from the national psychiatric case register in Denmark and for the Danish general population revealed considerable differences [578]. Men with schizophrenia had a mean of 18.7 years and women had a mean of 16.3 years shorter lives than their peers in the general population. An excess mortality risk for patients with schizophrenia can, thus, be regarded as established.

11.1. The Causes of Premature Death. Schizophrenia as such is not a deadly disease. Only the extremely severe subtype of "pernicious catatonia" can lead to death as a result of severe cardiovascular crises and electrolyte disorders. Nowadays, when the risk of death can be successfully warded off by timely recognition and appropriate treatment, it is nearly exclusively from countries with inadequate health care systems that fatal outcomes of pernicious catatonia are reported [579, 580].

As long as patients with schizophrenia used to be hospitalized under poor hygienic conditions over extended periods of time, infectious diseases, tuberculosis in particular, were the main cause of premature death [581–583]. Today, long hospital stays are an exception in industrialized countries and, if necessary, they take place under adequate hygienic conditions. In addition, most infectious diseases can nowadays be cured.

Contributing to the excess risk of death in schizophrenia used to be suicide and other unnatural causes (accidents, etc.), and this is still the case today. Recent reports are consistent in indicating that cardiovascular disorders have overtaken the other causes of extra deaths in schizophrenia [575, 577, 582, 584–587]. According to Laursen et al. [585], death from heart disease is now nearly three times more common in people with severe mental illness. In a review of the topic, Leucht et al. [584] found elevated rates of neoplasms (cancer) and capillary-vascular disease (CVD). Since this spectrum of

causes of death was, more or less, similar to that of the general population, it was only natural to see whether the same risk factors showed excess frequencies in schizophrenia, too, and indeed, the rates for nearly all relevant risk factors were found to be elevated [573, 588].

The prevalence of risk behaviour is illustrated by the results of the 2010 Australian National Psychosis Survey conducted among persons with psychotic disorder (ICD-10 schizophrenia) aged 18 to 64 years: 65% were current smokers, 49.8% had a lifetime history of alcohol abuse or dependence, and 50.8% abused cannabis [397]. Responsible for these elevated prevalences were, in part, an unhealthy way of life and lack of prevention, in part also addiction [573, 588].

Obesity plays a key role as a risk factor for cardiovascular disease [589–591]: it is up to twice as frequent in patients with schizophrenia as in the general population [592–595]. Obesity and weight gain increase the risk for hypertension, elevated blood fat levels, and type-2 diabetes. These factors lead to a metabolic syndrome, which in the Australian study was the case in 68% of the patients with psychotic illness [397], and also contribute to the risk for cardiovascular disease [589, 590].

These metabolic risks can also be associated with neuroleptic medications, which is a severe problem. Various neuroleptics, especially the new ones, have adverse metabolic effects in different degrees, so research results in this field urgently need to be translated into preventive action.

The elevated risk of suicide in patients with schizophrenia is associated with the same demographic risk factors as in the general population: male sex, social isolation, being single, and recent loss [596]. They are compounded by illness-related factors, depressive mood in particular in the early course of the disorder [392, 596–600], and preserved insight [601–603], which, on the other hand, is an indicator of good outcome.

12. Dimensional Models of Schizophrenia

Recently, the question was raised again whether the disease construct of schizophrenia should be continued to be defined categorically or better broken down to dimensions. A dimensional understanding of the disease process was intensively debated during the preliminary consultations for the 5th edition of the DSM [410, 604–606]. However, it was finally decided not to adopt the dimensional approach in the interest of a more than 100-year history of the disease concept, its worldwide use, and the role it plays in clinical practice. For research purposes, however, dimensional models are preferred.

The empirical course of symptom dimensions, for example, of the factors proposed by Liddle and Barnes [348]: *"reality distortion," "psychomotor poverty,"* and *"disintegration,"* was studied by Arndt et al. [607] over two years and by Salokangas [364] and Löffler and Häfner [360] over five years in first-episode patients of schizophrenia. The negative dimension turned out to be the most stable one and fairly independent of the other symptom dimensions.

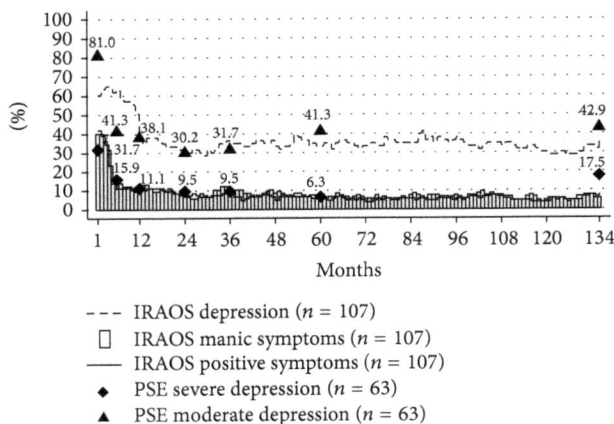

FIGURE 5: Long-term course of three-symptom dimensions of schizophrenia—percentages of patients with core symptoms of each dimension. Source: [487].

In the ABC long-term follow-up study, the authors defined four clinical symptom dimensions phenomenologically: a psychotic, negative, depressive, and manic dimension. Since many of the symptoms belonged to multiple dimensions, the four most prevalent symptoms with the least overlap with the other dimensions were chosen on each dimension as constituting a core dimension. The course of these core dimensions (as based on the prevalence of symptoms present at least for 50% of the time in each month) was mapped in monthly intervals over 11.2 years [60, 388, 396].

The depression rates depicted in Figure 5 were assessed both retrospectively in the total sample using the IRAOS (dotted line) and prospectively for validation purposes in the half-split subsample using the PSE (black triangles = CATEGO moderately severe depression, black rhombuses = major depression). As the figure illustrates, the rates for depressive, positive, and manic symptoms exhibit plateau-like trajectories after 1 to 2 years following first admission without any change in their frequencies relative to each other. The pronounced decrease in symptoms on all three symptom dimensions after the first psychotic episode is accounted for by treatment effects and spontaneous remissions, but it is partially also attributable to an artefact: because first psychotic episode was used as the inclusion criterion, the patients studied all had maximum symptom scores at entry in the study. Afterwards, they showed the usual sequence of episodes and intervals.

The trajectories depicted only confirm what the medium-term course had already indicated, namely, that, under the study conditions described, the core dimensions of schizophrenia show no clear-cut trend of either improvement or deterioration after the remission of the first psychotic episode (1 to 2 years after first admission). And the same was true for the overall symptomatology [60, 388, 396].

12.1. Duration and Frequency of Symptom Exacerbations. To find out whether there are factors at work on the individual

level that influence the seemingly uniform, but interindividually heterogeneous illness course the investigators in the ABC Schizophrenia study ascertained the individual durations of all symptom exacerbations on the psychosis and the depression dimension over the 134-month period—instead of just counting the number of relapse episodes operationally limited in their duration [60, 391, 392, 396, 487, 608]. The manic dimension could not be included because of low values. The median duration of symptom exacerbations was five months (mean: 20 months) on the depression dimension and two months (mean: 6.3 months) on the psychosis dimension. Symptoms persisting over the entire illness course—the purest form of chronicity—were very rare, occurring only in 6% on the depression and in 1% on the psychotic dimension.

Negative symptomatology, not yet broken down to dimensions, was assessed on the basis of a sum score of 19 IRAOS items. After the remission of the first episode the prevalence of negative symptoms decreased markedly, showing a plateau-like course after five years of initial assessment in male patients and after three years in female patients. An explanation for this unexpected finding has not yet been found.

13. Stigma and Discrimination

In the past, persons who fell ill with schizophrenia and sought help at mental-health services used to be—and still are today—subject to social isolation in many countries. In part, they are also discriminated against in the family, at workplace, and in public [609–613]. The consequences are an increased psychological strain on the patients and their families, reduced help-seeking and shortcomings in mental-health care and therapy. It was for these reasons that the WHO and the World Psychiatric Association launched the WPA "Open the doors" Programme "Against Stigma and Discrimination Because of Schizophrenia" (http://www.wpanet.org/detail.php?section_id=8&content_id=397) and initiatives and programmes combating stigma and discrimination have sprung up in many countries. In Japan, psychiatrists have gone as far as introducing "integration disorder" as a diagnosis to reduce stigma, but with limited success [614, 615].

How public opinion can be influenced by national initiatives is reflected in people's attitudes towards schizophrenia, depression, and alcohol dependence surveyed between 1990 and 2011 in Germany (former West-Germany) [616]. By 2011, people had become more open-minded towards individuals suffering from these disorders, knowledge on mental disorders had increased, and mental health care had considerably improved. Although more people than 20 years earlier regarded schizophrenia as a biological disorder and willingness to seek help at mental health services, if need be, had considerably increased, individual attitudes towards persons with schizophrenia had even worsened. An investigation of attitudes in the aftermath of an antistigma and antidiscrimination campaign in New Zealand yielded a similar result [617].

These are just two examples for an issue still of current relevance worldwide.

14. Conclusions

The diagnosis of schizophrenia and the underlying disease concept have recently been subject of debate, and not for the first time. Today, it can be considered established that there is a continuum ranging from the spectrum of schizophrenia symptoms to related syndromes, affective psychosis in particular, to mild schizophrenia-like disorders and normality. The continuity also seems to be reflected on the neurobiological and genetic level. This multilevel picture of a continuum is better compatible with a dimensional than a categorical disease model. However, bidding farewell to the categorical diagnosis of schizophrenia would have far-reaching consequences, so it has been deferred for the time being.

Approaching an answer to the question of what schizophrenia is, we must start by accepting the fact that, contrary to a widespread belief, it is not just a disorder of the young, but can strike at any age. Age at onset, severity of illness, some of the symptoms, and the social consequences involved are influenced by genetic factors, environmental risk factors, hormones (oestrogen secretion), and sociocultural factors, depending on age. As a consequence, symptoms, illness course, and social outcome vary a great deal between the sexes and between young, medium, and old age. Men fall ill with schizophrenia more frequently and more severely in the first half of life, women more frequently and more severely in the second.

Late- and very-late-onset "schizophrenic" psychoses are characterized by rational delusions rather than a severe psychotic breakdown, and mostly no social decline occurs. In spite of this, mild late- and very-late-onset psychoses should be classified as representing the disease process currently called schizophrenia. When this is done, the sex difference in schizophrenia incidence disappears almost completely over the entire age range.

Among the most important recent (re)discoveries are the findings on the precursors and the prodromal phase of psychosis and the underlying psychopathological, neurophysiological, and functional-morphological associations. Thanks to these advances, early recognition and early intervention are now possible and capable of delaying psychosis onset and reducing the adverse effects psychosis typically has on patients' personal lives and socioeconomic situations.

The discovery that oestrogen secretion, probably by reducing the sensitivity of D_2 receptors, is capable of postponing psychosis onset and reducing symptom severity has opened up new avenues of therapy. Although their efficacy has already been confirmed, they are not yet in widespread use because of the risk of unwanted side-effects.

Genetic vulnerability reduces or eliminates altogether the sex difference in age of onset by reducing women's age at onset, thus, indicating that the genetic penetrance of schizophrenia antagonizes the hormonal protection against psychosis.

Based on the ICD-9 or -10 diagnosis with emphasis on the psychotic symptomatology, the schizophrenia syndrome seems to be encountered and to be fairly evenly distributed in all cultures and ethnicities. This is at least what the results of the WHO 10-country study of schizophrenia (DOSMeD) indicate. In that multisite study conducted with fairly similar designs and culture-independent assessment techniques, annual incidence rates for (ICD-9) schizophrenia were calculated for populations aged 15 to 54 years in ten countries—four centres in three developing countries and six in industrialized countries. A restrictively defined, precise diagnostic definition produced annual incidence rates showing fairly little variation, while the incidence based on a broader, less precise diagnostic definition varied more markedly across the centres. None of the later transnational and transcultural studies have provided more reliable incidence data, although, strictly speaking, in the WHO study, too, the number of countries adequately researched was too small.

The course of schizophrenia is characterized by irregularly alternating episodes of exacerbation and remission of psychotic, partly also of depressive symptoms. If all exacerbations on the positive, negative, and depressive symptom dimensions are counted irrespective of their duration, differences will emerge in their frequency, with the exacerbations on the positive dimension showing the highest frequency and the shortest duration and those on the depression dimension a considerably lower frequency and longer duration. Negative symptom exacerbations, not yet analysed as a dimension, are even less frequent and of a longer duration than the depressive ones. But negative symptoms, too, show an episodic course over time despite stable mean values.

The construct of a disease entity, the way the early Kraepelin understood dementia praecox or schizophrenia, has become untenable, no matter which way we look at it, and the Kraepelinian dichotomy of affective and schizophrenic psychosis is now questionable.

Schizophrenia is very unlikely to have a uniform aetiology. It rather represents the expression of recurring functional vulnerability of various neural networks in the human brain caused by different types of neurobiological disorder. It is the resulting neural dysfunction that brings forth the exacerbations described and their combinations, thus, leading to schizophrenia, which, hence, is nothing else than the final common pathway of various influences. Quite frequently neuroreparative mechanisms seem to be capable of bringing that dysfunction to remission, partly or completely.

In sum, we still do not really know what schizophrenia is, but at least we have a better idea of what it is not. And it is uncertain whether we will ever know its real cause, because single causation does not exist and, given the diversity of the aetiological factors involved, it is difficult to single out those ultimately responsible for it.

Conflict of Interests

The author declares that, concerning this paper, there is no conflict of interests.

Acknowledgments

The author wishes to thank Professor Marcella Rietschel, head of the Department of Genetic Epidemiology in Psychiatry, Central Institute of Mental Health, for the intensive discussions and her active support in writing the Genetics chapter. The author also thanks his research assistant Auli Komulainen-Tremmel for her help in preparing the various drafts of the paper and for compiling the References section.

References

[1] E. Kraepelin, *Psychiatrie. Ein Lehrbuch für Studierende und Aerzte*, Barth, Leipzig, Germany, 4th edition, 1893, (German).

[2] E. Bleuler, "Dementia praecox oder Gruppe der Schizophrenien," in *Handbuch der Psychiatrie*, G. Aschaffenburg, Ed., pp. 1–420, Deuticke, Leipzig, Germany, 1911, (German).

[3] M. T. Tsuang and S. V. Faraone, *Schizophrenia*, Oxford University Press, New York, NY, USA, 2nd edition, 2005.

[4] D. R. Weinberger and P. J. Harrison, *Schizophrenia*, Wiley-Blackwell, Oxford, UK, 3rd edition, 2011.

[5] N. C. Andreasen, "Concept of schizophrenia: past, present, and future," in *Schizophrenia*, D. R. Weinberger and P. J. Harrison, Eds., pp. 3–8, Wiley-Blackwell, Oxford, UK, 3rd edition, 2011.

[6] R. J. Wyatt, R. C. Alexander, M. F. Egan, and D. G. Kirch, "Schizophrenia, just the facts. What do we know, how well do we know it?" *Schizophrenia Research*, vol. 1, no. 1, pp. 3–18, 1988.

[7] M. S. Keshavan, R. Tandon, N. N. Boutros, and H. A. Nasrallah, "Schizophrenia, "just the facts": What we know in 2008. Part 3: neurobiology," *Schizophrenia Research*, vol. 106, no. 2-3, pp. 89–107, 2008.

[8] R. Tandon, M. S. Keshavan, and H. A. Nasrallah, "Schizophrenia, "Just the Facts": what we know in 2008. Part 1: overview," *Schizophrenia Research*, vol. 100, no. 1-3, pp. 4–19, 2008.

[9] R. Tandon, M. S. Keshavan, and H. A. Nasrallah, "Schizophrenia, "Just the Facts" what we know in 2008. 2. Epidemiology and etiology," *Schizophrenia Research*, vol. 102, no. 1-3, pp. 1–18, 2008.

[10] R. Tandon, H. A. Nasrallah, and M. S. Keshavan, "Schizophrenia, "just the facts" 4. Clinical features and conceptualization," *Schizophrenia Research*, vol. 110, no. 1-3, pp. 1–23, 2009.

[11] R. Tandon, H. A. Nasrallah, and M. S. Keshavan, "Schizophrenia, "Just the Facts" 5. Treatment and prevention past, present, and future," *Schizophrenia Research*, vol. 122, no. 1'3, pp. 1–23, 2010.

[12] M. S. Keshavan, H. A. Nasrallah, and R. Tandon, "Schizophrenia, "Just the Facts" 6: moving ahead with the schizophrenia concept: From the elephant to the mouse," *Schizophrenia Research*, vol. 127, no. 1-3, pp. 3–13, 2011.

[13] M. S. Keshavan, R. Tandon, and H. A. Nasrallah, "Renaming schizophrenia: keeping up with the facts," *Schizophrenia Research*, vol. 148, no. 1-3, pp. 1–2, 2013.

[14] G. A. Fava, "The intellectual crisis of psychiatric research," *Psychotherapy and Psychosomatics*, vol. 75, no. 4, pp. 202–208, 2006.

[15] R. Kendell and A. Jablensky, "Distinguishing between the validity and utility of psychiatric diagnoses," *The American Journal of Psychiatry*, vol. 160, no. 1, pp. 4–12, 2003.

[16] M. Maj, "Are psychiatrists an endangered species?" *World Psychiatry*, vol. 9, no. 1, pp. 1–2, 2010.

[17] M. Maj, "Mental disorders as "brain diseases" and Jaspers' legacy," *World Psychiatry*, vol. 2, no. 1, pp. 1–3, 2013.

[18] A. Jablensky and F. Waters, "RDoC: a roadmap to pathogenesis?" *World Psychiatry*, vol. 13, no. 1, pp. 43–44, 2014.

[19] J. Parnas, L. A. Sass, and D. Zahavi, "Rediscovering psychopathology: the epistemology and phenomenology of the psychiatric object," *Schizophrenia Bulletin*, vol. 39, no. 2, pp. 270–277, 2013.

[20] J. Parnas, "The RDoC program: psychiatry without psyche?" *World Psychiatry*, vol. 13, pp. 46–67, 2014.

[21] E. Kraepelin, "The German institute of psychiatric research," *Journal of Nervous and Mental Disease*, vol. 51, pp. 505–513, 1920.

[22] E. Kraepelin, "Die Erscheinungsformen des Irreseins," *Zeitschrift für die gesamte Neurologie und Psychiatrie*, vol. 62, no. 1, pp. 1–29, 1920 (German).

[23] W. Maier, "Psychiatrie als Beruf—wie sieht die Zukunft aus? Leserbrief zum Beitrag von H. Häfner in Der Nervenarzt (2002) 73: 33–40," *Nervenarzt*, vol. 73, pp. 96–99, 2002 (German).

[24] S. E. Hyman, "Can neuroscience be integrated into the DSM-V?" *Nature Reviews Neuroscience*, vol. 8, no. 9, pp. 725–732, 2007.

[25] B. N. Cuthbert, "The RDoC framework: facilitating transition from ICE/DSM to dimensional approaches that integrate neuroscience and psychopathology," *World Psychiatry*, vol. 13, no. 1, pp. 28–35, 2014.

[26] M. Maj, "Keeping an open attitude towards the RDoC project," *World Psychiatry*, vol. 13, pp. 1–4, 2014.

[27] G. A. Fava, C. Rafanelli, and E. Tomba, "The clinical process in psychiatry: a clinimetric approach," *Journal of Clinical Psychiatry*, vol. 73, no. 2, pp. 177–184, 2012.

[28] G. A. Fava, "Road to nowhere," *World Psychiatry*, vol. 13, no. 1, pp. 49–50, 2014.

[29] L. E. DeLisi, "The concept of progressive brain change in schizophrenia: implications for understanding schizophrenia," *Schizophrenia Bulletin*, vol. 34, no. 2, pp. 312–321, 2008.

[30] E. Kretschmer, *Körperbau und Charakter*, Springer, Berlin, Germany, 1921, (German).

[31] A. Jablensky, "Boundaries of mental disorders," *Current Opinion in Psychiatry*, vol. 18, no. 6, pp. 653–658, 2005.

[32] A. Jablensky, "The diagnostic concept of schizophrenia: its history, evolution, and future prospects," *Dialogues in Clinical Neuroscience*, vol. 12, no. 3, pp. 271–287, 2010.

[33] E. Kraepelin, *Psychiatrie. Ein Lehrbuch für Studierende und Ärzte*, Barth, Leipzig, Germany, 6th edition, 1899, (German).

[34] N. Craddock and M. J. Owen, "The Kraepelinian dichotomy—going, going... but still not gone," *The British Journal of Psychiatry*, vol. 196, no. 2, pp. 92–95, 2010.

[35] K. Jaspers, *Allgemeine Psychopathologie. Ein Leitfaden für Studierende, Ärzte und Psychologen*, Julius Springer, Berlin, Germany, 1913 (German).

[36] G. E. Berríos, "Psychiatry and its objects," *Revista de Psiquiatria y Salud Mental*, vol. 4, no. 4, pp. 179–182, 2011.

[37] G. E. Berrios, "Jaspers and the first edition of Allgemeine Psychopathologie," *The British Journal of Psychiatry*, vol. 202, p. 433, 2013.

[38] H. Häfner, "Karl Jaspers. 100 Jahre 'Allgemeine Psychopathologie'," *Der Nervenarzt*, vol. 84, no. 11, pp. 1281–1290, 2013 (German).

[39] K. Jaspers, "Die phänomenologische Forschungsrichtung in der Psychopathologie," *Zeitschrift für die gesamte Neurologie und Psychiatrie*, vol. 9, no. 1, pp. 391–408, 1912 (German).

[40] G. E. Berrios, "Phenomenology, psychopathology and Jaspers: a conceptual history," *History of psychiatry*, vol. 3, no. 11, pp. 303–327, 1992.

[41] W. Mayer-Gross, E. Slater, and M. Roth, Eds., *Clinical Psychiatry*, Baillière, Tindall & Cassell, London, UK, 1954.

[42] V. Roelcke and F. Schneider, "Psychiatrists under National Socialism. Biographies of perpetrators, Einführung zum Thema: Psychiater im Nationalsozialismus. Täterbiographien," *Der Nervenarzt*, vol. 83, no. 3, pp. 291–292, 2012.

[43] J. K. Wing, J. E. Cooper, and N. Sartorius, *Measurement and Classification of Psychiatric Symptoms: An Instruction Manual for the PSE and CATEGO Program*, Cambridge University Press, London, UK, 1974.

[44] J. K. Wing, T. Babor, T. Brugha et al., "SCAN: schedules for clinical assessment in neuropsychiatry," *Archives of General Psychiatry*, vol. 47, no. 6, pp. 589–593, 1990.

[45] K. Schneider, *Clinical Psychopathology*, translated by M. W. Hamilton, Grune & Stratton, New York, NY, USA, 1959.

[46] R. Warner and G. de Girolamo, *Schizophrenia*, Epidemiology of Mental Disorders and Psychological Problems, World Health Organization, Geneva, Switzerland, 1995.

[47] C. Arango and W. T. Carpenter, "The schizophrenia construct: symptomatic presentation," in *Schizophrenia*, D. R. Weinberger and P. J. Harrison, Eds., pp. 9–23, Wiley-Blackwell, Oxford, UK, 3rd edition, 2011.

[48] W. S. Fenton, L. R. Mosher, and S. M. Matthews, "Diagnosis of schizophrenia: a critical review of current diagnostic systems," *Schizophrenia Bulletin*, vol. 7, no. 3, pp. 452–476, 1981.

[49] A. Jablensky, N. Sartorius, G. Ernberg et al., "Schizophrenia: manifestations, incidence and course in different cultures. A World Health Organization ten-country study," *Psychological Medicine Monograph Supplement*, vol. 20, pp. 1–97, 1992.

[50] W. T. Carpenter Jr. and J. S. Strauss, "Cross cultural evaluation of Schneider's first rank symptoms of schizophrenia: a report from the International Pilot Study of Schizophrenia," *The American Journal of Psychiatry*, vol. 131, no. 6, pp. 682–687, 1974.

[51] H. G. Pope Jr. and J. F. Lipinski Jr., "Diagnosis in schizophrenia and manic-depressive illness. A reassessment of the specificity of "schizophrenic" symptoms in the light of current research," *Archives of General Psychiatry*, vol. 35, no. 7, pp. 811–828, 1978.

[52] M. A. Taylor and R. Abrams, "Manic-depressive illness and good prognosis schizophrenia," *The American Journal of Psychiatry*, vol. 132, no. 7, pp. 741–742, 1975.

[53] P. J. Möbius, *Abriss der Lehre von den Nervenkrankheiten*, Abel, Leipzig, Germany, 1893, (German).

[54] R. E. Kendell and I. F. Brockington, "The identification of disease entities and the relationship between schizophrenic and affective psychoses," *The British Journal of Psychiatry*, vol. 137, no. 4, pp. 324–331, 1980.

[55] A. Frances, "RDoC is necessary, but very oversold," *World Psychiatry*, vol. 13, no. 1, pp. 47–49, 2014.

[56] U. Ettinger, I. Meyhöfer, M. Steffens, M. Wagner, and N. Koutsouleris, "Genetics, cognition, and neurobiology of schizotypal personality: a review of the overlap with schizophrenia," *Frontiers in Psychiatry*, vol. 5, article 18, 2014.

[57] World Health Organization, *The ICD-10 Classification of Mental and Behavioural Disorders*, WHO, Geneva, Switzerland, 1992.

[58] World Health Organization, *International Statistical Classification of Diseases and Related Health Problems 10th Revision (ICD-10) Version for 2010*, 2010, http://apps.who.int/classifications/icd10/browse/2010/en#/F20-F29.

[59] American Psychiatric Association, *Diagnostic and Statistical Manual of Mental Disorders*, American Psychiatric Publishing, Washington, DC, USA, 4th edition, 2005.

[60] H. Häfner, K. Maurer, and W. an der Heiden, "Schizophrenie—eine einheitliche Krankheit?" *Der Nervenarzt*, vol. 84, no. 9, pp. 1093–1103, 2013 (German).

[61] I. F. Brockington, R. E. Kendell, and J. P. Leff, "Definitions of schizophrenia: concordance and prediction of outcome," *Psychological Medicine*, vol. 8, no. 3, pp. 387–398, 1978.

[62] H. Sass, "The classification of schizophrenia in the different diagnostic systems," in *Search for the Causes of Schizophrenia*, H. Häfner, W. F. Gattaz, and W. Janzarik, Eds., pp. 19–43, Springer, Berlin, Germany, 1987.

[63] J. Endicott, J. Nee, J. Fleiss, J. Cohen, J. B. Williams, and R. Simon, "Diagnostic criteria for schizophrenia: reliabilities and agreement between systems," *Archives of General Psychiatry*, vol. 39, no. 8, pp. 884–889, 1982.

[64] D. J. Castle, S. Wessely, and R. M. Murray, "Sex and schizophrenia: effects of diagnostic stringency, and associations with premorbid variables," *The British Journal of Psychiatry*, vol. 162, pp. 658–664, 1993.

[65] M. Kramer, "Cross-national study of diagnosis of the mental disorders: origin of the problem," *The American Journal of Psychiatry*, vol. 10, pp. 1–11, 1969.

[66] R. L. Spitzer and J. L. Fleiss, "A reanalysis of the reliability of psychiatric diagnosis," *The British Journal of Psychiatry*, vol. 125, no. 10, pp. 341–347, 1974.

[67] A. W. Loranger, "The impact of DSM-III on diagnostic practice in a university hospital. A comparison of DSM-II and DSM-III in 10,914 patients," *Archives of General Psychiatry*, vol. 47, no. 7, pp. 672–675, 1990.

[68] J. de Leon, "A post-DSM-III wake-up call to European psychiatry," *Acta Psychiatrica Scandinavica*, vol. 129, pp. 76–77, 2014.

[69] J. Zubin, "Crosss-national study of diagnosis of the mental disorders: methodology and planning," *The American Journal of Psychiatry*, vol. 10, pp. 12–20, 1969.

[70] B. J. Gurland, J. L. Fleiss, L. Sharpe, P. Roberts, J. E. Cooper, and R. E. Kendell, "Cross-national study of diagnosis of mental disorders: hospital diagnoses and hospital patients in New York and London," *Comprehensive Psychiatry*, vol. 11, no. 1, pp. 18–25, 1970.

[71] J. de Leon, "One hundred years of limited impact of Jaspers' General Psychopathology on US psychiatry," *The Journal of Nervous and Mental Disease*, vol. 202, no. 2, pp. 79–87, 2014.

[72] R. E. Kendell, J. E. Cooper, A. J. Gourlay, J. R. Copeland, L. Sharpe, and B. J. Gurland, "Diagnostic criteria of American and British psychiatrists," *Archives of General Psychiatry*, vol. 25, no. 2, pp. 123–130, 1971.

[73] J. E. Cooper, R. E. Kendell, B. J. Gurland, L. Sharpe, J. R. M. Copeland, and R. Simon, *Psychiatric Diagnosis in New York and London*, Maudsley Monograph no. 20, Oxford University Press, London, UK, 1972.

[74] J. P. Feighner, E. Robins, S. B. Guze, R. A. Woodruff Jr., G. Winokur, and R. Munoz, "Diagnostic criteria for use in psychiatric research," *Archives of General Psychiatry*, vol. 26, no. 1, pp. 57–63, 1972.

[75] R. L. Spitzer, N. C. Andreasen, and J. Endicott, "Schizophrenia and other psychotic disorders in DSM-III," *Schizophrenia Bulletin*, vol. 4, no. 4, pp. 489–511, 1978.

[76] R. L. Spitzer, J. Endicott, and E. Robins, "Research diagnostic criteria: rationale and reliability," *Archives of General Psychiatry*, vol. 35, no. 6, pp. 773–782, 1978.

[77] G. L. Klerman, "The evolution of a scientific nosology," in *Schizophrenia: Science and Practice*, J. C. Shershow, Ed., pp. 99–121, Harvard University Press, Cambridge, Mass, USA, 1978.

[78] R. K. Blashfield, "Feighner et al., invisible colleges, and the Matthew effect," *Schizophrenia Bulletin*, vol. 8, no. 1, pp. 1–12, 1982.

[79] H. S. Decker, "How Kraepelinian was Kraepelin? How Krae-pelinian are the neo-Kraepelinians?—from Emil Kraepelin to DSM-III," *History of Psychiatry*, vol. 18, no. 3, pp. 337–360, 2007.

[80] N. C. Andreasen, "DSM and the death of phenomenology in America: an example of unintended consequences," *Schizophrenia Bulletin*, vol. 33, no. 1, pp. 108–112, 2007.

[81] E. Robins and S. B. Guze, "Establishment of diagnostic validity in psychiatric illness: its application to schizophrenia," *The American Journal of Psychiatry*, vol. 126, no. 7, pp. 983–987, 1970.

[82] American Psychiatric Association, *Diagnostic and Statistical Manual of Mental Disorders (DSM-IIII)*, American Psychiatric Association, Washington, DC, USA, 3rd edition, 1980.

[83] N. C. Andreasen and M. Flaum, "Schizophrenia: the character-istic symptoms," *Schizophrenia Bulletin*, vol. 17, no. 1, pp. 27–50, 1991.

[84] G. E. Berrios and I. S. Marková, "Symptoms—historical per-spective and effect on diagnosis," in *Psychosomatic Medicine*, M. Blumenfield and J. J. Strain, Eds., pp. 27–38, Lippincott Williams & Wilkins, Philadelphia, Pa, USA, 2006.

[85] S. N. Ghaemi, "Nosologomania: DSM & Karl Jaspers' critique of Kraepelin," *Philosophy, Ethics, and Humanities in Medicine*, vol. 4, article 10, 2009.

[86] P. R. McHugh, "Rendering mental disorders intelligible: addressing psychiatry's urgent challenge," in *Philosophical Issues in Psychiatry II. Nosology: International Perspectives in Philoso-phy and Psychiatry*, K. S. Kendler and J. Parnas, Eds., pp. 269–280, Oxford University Press, Oxford, UK, 2012.

[87] P. R. McHugh and P. R. Slavney, "Methods of reasoning in psychopathology: conflict and resolution," *Comprehensive Psy-chiatry*, vol. 23, no. 3, pp. 197–215, 1982.

[88] P. R. Slavney and P. R. McHugh, "Explanation and understand-ing," in *Psychiatric Polarities*, P. R. Slavney and P. R. McHugh, Eds., pp. 29–44, The Johns Hopkins University Press, Baltimore, Md, USA, 1987.

[89] A. L. Stoll, M. Tohen, R. J. Baldessarini et al., "Shifts in diagnos-tic frequencies of schizophrenia and major affective disorders at six North American psychiatric hospitals, 1972–1988," *The American Journal of Psychiatry*, vol. 150, no. 11, pp. 1668–1673, 1993.

[90] L. N. Robins, J. E. Helzer, J. L. Croughan, J. B. W. Williams, and R. L. Spitzer, *NIMH Diagnostic Interview Schedule: Version III*, National Institute of Mental Health, Washington, DC, USA, 1981.

[91] A. Y. Tien and W. W. Eaton, "Psychopathologic precursors and sociodemographic risk factors for the schizophrenia syndrome," *Archives of General Psychiatry*, vol. 49, no. 1, pp. 37–46, 1992.

[92] J. R. M. Copeland, M. E. Dewey, and P. Saunders, "The epidemi-ology of dementia: GMS-AGECAT studies of prevalence and incidence, including studies in progress," *European Archives of Psychiatry and Clinical Neuroscience*, vol. 240, no. 4-5, pp. 212–217, 1991.

[93] J. J. McGrath and R. M. Murray, "Environmental risk factors for schizophrenia," in *Schizophrenia*, D. R. Weinberger and P. J. Harrison, Eds., pp. 226–233, Wiley-Blackwell, Oxford, UK, 3rd edition, 2011.

[94] E. L. Messias, C. Chen, and W. W. Eaton, "Epidemiology of schizophrenia: review of findings and myths," *Psychiatric Clinics of North America*, vol. 30, no. 3, pp. 323–338, 2007.

[95] W. W. Eaton, "Evidence for universitality and uniformity of schizophrenia around the world: assessment and implications," in *Search for the Causes of Schizophrenia, vol IV. Balance of*

[96] T. Helgason, "Epidemiology of mental disorders in Iceland," *Acta Psychiatrica Scandinavica*, supplement 173, 1964.

[97] C. Astrup, "The increase of mental disorders," The National Case Register of Mental Disorder, Gaustad Hospital, Oslo, Norway, 1982.

[98] J. Krupinski and L. Alexander, "Patterns of psychiatric morbid-ity in Victoria, Australia, in relation to changes in diagnostic criteria 1848–1978," *Social Psychiatry*, vol. 18, no. 2, pp. 61–67, 1983.

[99] H. Häfner, "Epidemiology of schizophrenia," in *Search for the Causes of Schizophrenia*, H. Häfner, W. F. Gattaz, and W. Janzarik, Eds., pp. 47–74, Springer, Berlin, Germany, 1987.

[100] E. G. Torrey, *Schizophrenia and Civilization*, Aronson, London, UK, 1980.

[101] E. H. Hare, "Was insanity on the increase?" *The British Journal of Psychiatry*, vol. 142, no. 5, pp. 439–455, 1983.

[102] G. Der, S. Gupta, and R. M. Murray, "Is schizophrenia disap-pearing?" *The Lancet*, vol. 335, no. 8688, pp. 513–516, 1990.

[103] G. Harrison, J. E. Cooper, and R. Gancarczyk, "Changes in the administrative incidence of schizophrenia," *The British Journal of Psychiatry*, vol. 159, pp. 811–816, 1991.

[104] H. Häfner and W. F. Gattaz, "Is schizophrenia disappearing? (letter)," *European Archives of Psychiatry and Clinical Neuro-science*, vol. 240, pp. 373–378, 1991.

[105] R. M. Murray, S. W. Lewis, and A. M. Reveley, "Towards an aetiological classification of schizophrenia," *The Lancet*, vol. 1, no. 8436, pp. 1023–1026, 1985.

[106] R. M. Murray, "Neurodevelopmental schizophrenia: the redis-covery of dementia praecox," *The British Journal of Psychiatry*, vol. 165, no. 25, pp. 6–12, 1994.

[107] R. E. Kendell, D. E. Malcolm, and W. Adams, "The problem of detecting changes in the incidence of schizophrenia," *The British Journal of Psychiatry*, vol. 162, pp. 212–218, 1993.

[108] R. E. Faris and W. Dunham, *Mental Disorders in Urban Areas. An Ecological Study of Schizophrenia and Other Psychoses*, Uni-versity of Chicago Press, Chicago, Ill, USA, 1939.

[109] H. W. Dunham, "Current status of ecological research in mental disorder," *Social Forces*, vol. 25, no. 3, pp. 321–326, 1947.

[110] H. W. Dunham, "Social class and schizophrenia," *American Journal of Orthopsychiatry*, vol. 34, pp. 634–642, 1964.

[111] H. W. Dunham, *Community and Schizophrenia. An Epidemio-logical Analysis*, Wayne Sstate University Press, Detroit, Mich, USA, 1965.

[112] C. W. Schroeder, "Mental disorders in cities," *American Journal of Sociology*, vol. 48, no. 1, pp. 40–48, 1942.

[113] E. A. Gardner and H. M. Babigian, "A longitudinal comparison of psychiatric service to selected socioeconomic areas of Mon-roe County, New York," *American Journal of Orthopsychiatry*, vol. 36, no. 5, pp. 818–828, 1966.

[114] G. D. Klee, E. Spiro, A. K. Bahn, and K. Gorwitz, "An ecological analysis of diagnosed mental illness in Baltimore," in *Psychiatric Epidemiology and Mental Health Planning*, R. P. Monroe, G. D. Klee and, and E. B. Brody, Eds., pp. 107–148, American Psychi-atric Association, Washington, DC, USA, 1967.

[115] H. W. Dunham, "City core and suburban fringe: distribution pattern of mental illness," in *Changing Perspectives in Mental Illness*, S. C. Plog and R. Edgerton, Eds., pp. 336–363, Holt, Rine-hard and Winstin, New York, NY, USA, 1969.

[116] H. Häfner, H. Reimann, H. Immich, and H. Martini, "Inzidenz seelischer Erkrankungen in Mannheim 1965," *Social Psychiatry*, vol. 4, no. 3, pp. 126–135, 1969 (German).

[117] S. Weyerer and H. Häfner, "The stability of the ecological distribution of the incidence of treated mental disorders in the city of Mannheim," *Social Psychiatry and Psychiatric Epidemiology*, vol. 24, no. 2, pp. 57–62, 1989.

[118] M. Marcelis, F. Navarro-Mateu, R. Murray, J. P. Selten, and J. van Os, "Urbanization and psychosis: a study of 1942–1978 birth cohorts in The Netherlands," *Psychological Medicine*, vol. 28, no. 4, pp. 871–879, 1998.

[119] W. Löffler and H. Häfner, "Ecological pattern of first admitted schizophrenics in two German cities over 25 years," *Social Science and Medicine*, vol. 49, no. 1, pp. 93–108, 1999.

[120] P. B. Mortensen, C. B. Pedersen, T. Westergaard et al., "Effects of family history and place and season of birth on the risk of schizophrenia," *The New England Journal of Medicine*, vol. 340, no. 8, pp. 603–608, 1999.

[121] C. B. Pedersen and P. B. Mortensen, "Family history, place and season of birth as risk factors for schizophrenia in Denmark: a replication and reanalysis," *The British Journal of Psychiatry*, vol. 178, pp. 46–52, 2001.

[122] C. B. Pedersen and P. B. Mortensen, "Evidence of a dose-response relationship between urbanicity during upbringing and schizophrenia risk," *Archives of General Psychiatry*, vol. 58, no. 11, pp. 1039–1046, 2001.

[123] C. B. Pedersen and P. B. Mortensen, "Are the cause(s) responsible for urban-rural differences in schizophrenia risk rooted in families or in individuals?" *American Journal of Epidemiology*, vol. 163, no. 11, pp. 971–978, 2006.

[124] J. B. Kirkbride, P. Fearon, C. Morgan et al., "Heterogeneity in incidence rates of schizophrenia and other psychotic syndromes: findings from the 3-center ÆSOP study," *Archives of General Psychiatry*, vol. 63, no. 3, pp. 250–258, 2006.

[125] L. Levy and L. Rowitz, "The spatial distribution of treated mental disorders in Chicago," *Social Psychiatry*, vol. 5, no. 1, pp. 1–11, 1970.

[126] L. Levy and L. Rowitz, *The Ecology of Mental Disorders in Chicago*, Behavioral Publications, New York, NY, USA, 1973.

[127] J. A. Giggs and J. E. Cooper, "Ecological structure and the distribution of schizophrenia and affective psychoses in Nottingham," *The British Journal of Psychiatry*, vol. 151, pp. 627–633, 1987.

[128] H. Häfner and H. Reimann, "Spatial distribution of mental disorders in Mannheim 1965," in *Psychiatric Epidemiology*, E. H. Hare and J. K. Wing, Eds., pp. 341–354, Oxford University Press, London, UK, 1970.

[129] J. A. Clausen and M. L. Kohn, "The ecological approach in social psychiatry," *American Journal of Sociology*, vol. 60, pp. 140–149, 1954.

[130] J. A. Clausen and M. L. Kohn, "Social isolation and schizophrenia," *American Sociological Review*, vol. 20, pp. 265–273, 1955.

[131] J. A. Clausen and M. L. Kohn, "Relation of schizophrenia to the social structure of a small city," in *Epidemiology of Mental Disorder*, B. Pasamanick, Ed., pp. 69–86, AAAS Publisher, Washington, DC, USA, 1959.

[132] L. Stein, "'Social class' gradient in schizophrenia," *British Journal Of Preventive & Social Medicine*, vol. 11, no. 4, pp. 181–195, 1957.

[133] D. Klusmann and M. C. Angermeyer, "Urban ecology and psychiatric admission rates: results from a study in the city of Hamburg," in *From Social Class to Social Stress*, M. C. Angermeyer and D. Klusmann, Eds., pp. 16–45, Springer, Berlin, Germany, 1987.

[134] R. E. L. Faris, "Cultural isolation and the schizophrenic personality," *American Journal of Sociology*, vol. 40, no. 2, pp. 155–164, 1934.

[135] E. G. Jaco, "The social isolation hypothesis and schizophrenia," *American Sociological Review*, vol. 19, pp. 567–577, 1954.

[136] A. Hollingshead and F. Redlich, *Social Class and Mental Illness*, Wiley, New York, NY, USA, 1958.

[137] E. H. Hare and G. K. Shore, *Mental Health on a New Housing Estate*, Oxford University Press, New York, NY, USA, 1965.

[138] D. L. Gerard and L. G. Houston, "Family setting and the social ecology of schizophrenia," *The Psychiatric Quarterly*, vol. 27, no. 1–4, pp. 90–101, 1953.

[139] R. Lapouse, M. A. Monk, and M. Terris, "Drift hypothesis and socioeconomic differentials in schizophrenia," *American Journal of Public Health*, vol. 46, pp. 978–986, 1956.

[140] B. P. Dohrenwend, I. Levav, P. E. Shrout et al., "Socioeconomic status and psychiatric disorders: the causation-selection issue," *Science*, vol. 255, no. 5047, pp. 946–952, 1992.

[141] K. Dauncey, J. Giggs, K. Baker, and G. Harrison, "Schizophrenia in Nottingham: lifelong residential mobility of a cohort," *The British Journal of Psychiatry*, vol. 163, pp. 613–619, 1993.

[142] Ö. Ödegård, "The incidence of psychoses in various occupations," *International Journal of Social Psychiatry*, vol. 2, pp. 85–104, 1956.

[143] Ö. Ödegård, "Hospitalized psychoses in Norway: time trends 1926–1965," *Social Psychiatry*, vol. 6, no. 2, pp. 53–58, 1971.

[144] W. W. Eaton, "Residence, social class, and schizophrenia," *Journal of Health and Social Behavior*, vol. 15, no. 4, pp. 289–299, 1974.

[145] E. F. Torrey, A. E. Bowler, and K. Clark, "Urban birth and residence as risk factors for psychoses: an analysis of 1880 data," *Schizophrenia Research*, vol. 25, no. 3, pp. 169–176, 1997.

[146] J. Allardyce, J. Boydell, J. van Os et al., "Comparison of the incidence of schizophrenia in rural Dumfries and Galloway and urban Camberwell," *The British Journal of Psychiatry*, vol. 179, pp. 335–339, 2001.

[147] P. B. Mortensen and C. B. Pedersen, "Urban/rural life as a risk factor?" in *Risk and Protective Factors in Schizophrenia*, H. Häfner, Ed., pp. 123–131, Steinkopff, Darmstadt, Germany, 2002.

[148] W. W. Eaton, P. B. Mortensen, and M. Frydenberg, "Obstetric factors, urbanization and psychosis," *Schizophrenia Research*, vol. 43, no. 2-3, pp. 117–123, 2000.

[149] F. J. Oher, A. Demjaha, D. Jackson et al., "The effect of the environment on symptom dimensions in the first episode of psychosis: a multilevel study," *Psychological Medicine*, vol. 44, no. 11, pp. 2419–2430, 2014.

[150] M. Hanssen, M. Bak, R. Bijl, W. Vollebergh, and J. van Os, "Outcome of self-reported psychotic experiences in the general population: a prospective study," in *Continuous Psychosis Phenotype: From Description to Prediction*, M. Hanssen, Ed., South-Limburg Mental Health Research and Teaching Network PHD Series, pp. 95–107, M.S.S. Hanssen, Maastricht, The Netherlands, 2004.

[151] F. Jacobi, M. Höfler, J. Siegert et al., "Twelve-month prevalence, comorbidity and correlates of mental disorders in Germany: the Mental Health Module of the German Health Interview and Examinatiion Survey for Adults (DEGS1-MH)," *International Journal of Methods in Psychiatric Research*, 2014.

[152] P. B. Mortensen, "Urban-Rural Differences in the Risk for Schizophrenia," *International Journal of Mental Health*, vol. 29, no. 3, pp. 101–110, 2000.

[153] R. Welz, "Räumliche Verteilung von Selbstmordversuchen in einer städtischen Region. Forschungsartefakte, Aggregierungseffekte und Clusterbildung," in *Raumbezogenheit sozialer Probleme (Beiträge zur sozialwissenschaftlichen Forschung, Bd. 35)*, L. A. Vaskovics, Ed., pp. 250–272, Westdeutscher, Opladen, Germany, 1982, (German).

[154] E. Silver, E. P. Mulvey, and J. W. Swanson, "Neighborhood structural characteristics and mental disorder: Faris and Dunham revisited," *Social Science and Medicine*, vol. 55, no. 8, pp. 1457–1470, 2002.

[155] Ö. Ödegård, *Emigration and Insanity: A Study of Mental Disease among the Norwegianborn Population of Minnesota*, Acta Psychiatrica et Neurologica Scandinavica, supplement 4, 1932.

[156] J. Van Os, M. Hanssen, M. Bak, R. V. Bijl, and W. Vollebergh, "Do urbanicity and familial liability coparticipate in causing psychosis?" *The American Journal of Psychiatry*, vol. 160, no. 3, pp. 477–482, 2003.

[157] J. van Os, C. B. Pedersen, and P. B. Mortensen, "Confirmation of synergy between urbanicity and familial liability in the causation of psychosis," *The American Journal of Psychiatry*, vol. 161, no. 12, pp. 2312–2314, 2004.

[158] J. Spauwen, L. Krabbendam, R. Lieb, H. Wittchen, and J. van Os, "Evidence that the outcome of developmental expression of psychosis is worse for adolescents growing up in an urban environment," *Psychological Medicine*, vol. 36, no. 3, pp. 407–415, 2006.

[159] M. Weiser, J. van Os, A. Reichenberg et al., "Social and cognitive functioning, urbanicity and risk for schizophrenia," *The British Journal of Psychiatry*, vol. 191, pp. 320–324, 2007.

[160] L. Krabbendam and J. van Os, "Schizophrenia and urbanicity: a major environmental influence—conditional on genetic risk," *Schizophrenia Bulletin*, vol. 31, no. 4, pp. 795–799, 2005.

[161] J. Van Os, R. J. Linscott, I. Myin-Germeys, P. Delespaul, and L. Krabbendam, "A systematic review and meta-analysis of the psychosis continuum: evidence for a psychosis proneness-persistence-impairment model of psychotic disorder," *Psychological Medicine*, vol. 39, no. 2, pp. 179–195, 2009.

[162] D. March, S. L. Hatch, C. Morgan et al., "Psychosis and place," *Epidemiologic Reviews*, vol. 30, no. 1, pp. 84–100, 2008.

[163] F. Lederbogen, P. Kirsch, L. Haddad et al., "City living and urban upbringing affect neural social stress processing in humans," *Nature*, vol. 474, no. 7352, pp. 498–501, 2011.

[164] M. Weiser, N. Werbeloff, T. Vishna et al., "Elaboration on immigration and risk for schizophrenia," *Psychological Medicine*, vol. 38, no. 8, pp. 1113–1119, 2008.

[165] C. Corcoran, S. Perrin, S. Harlap et al., "Incidence of schizophrenia among second-generation immigrants in the Jerusalem Perinatal Cohort," *Schizophrenia Bulletin*, vol. 35, no. 3, pp. 596–602, 2008.

[166] H. Häfner, G. Moschel, and M. Özek, "Psychische Störungen bei türkischen Gastarbeitern. Eine prospektive Studie zur Untersuchung der Reaktion auf Einwanderung und partielle Anpassung," *Nervenarzt*, vol. 48, pp. 268–275, 1977 (German).

[167] T. J. Gaber, S. Bouyrakhen, B. Herpertz-Dahlmann et al., "Migration background and juvenile mental health: a descriptive retrospective analysis of diagnostic rates of psychiatric disorders in young people," *Global Health Action*, vol. 6, Article ID 20187, 2013.

[168] R. Littlewood and M. Lipsedge, "Some social and phenomenological characteristics of psychotic immigrants," *Psychological Medicine*, vol. 11, no. 2, pp. 289–302, 1981.

[169] D. McGovern and R. V. Cope, "First psychiatric admission rates of first and second generation Afro Caribbeans," *Social Psychiatry*, vol. 22, no. 3, pp. 139–149, 1987.

[170] G. Harrison, D. Owens, A. Holton, D. Neilson, and D. Boot, "A prospective study of severe mental disorder in Afro-Caribbean patients," *Psychological Medicine*, vol. 18, no. 3, pp. 643–657, 1988.

[171] D. Castle, S. Wessely, G. Der, and R. M. Murray, "The incidence of operationally defined schizophrenia in Camberwell, 1965–84," *The British Journal of Psychiatry*, vol. 159, pp. 790–794, 1991.

[172] S. Wessely, D. Castle, G. Der, and R. Murray, "Schizophrenia and Afro-Caribbeans. A case-control study," *The British Journal of Psychiatry*, vol. 159, pp. 795–801, 1991.

[173] G. Harrison, J. J. Brewin, R. Cantwell et al., "The increased risk of psychosis in African-Caribbean migrants to the UK: a replication," *Schizophrenia Research*, vol. 18, p. 102, 1996.

[174] D. Bhugra, J. Leff, R. Mallett, G. Der, B. Corridan, and S. Rudge, "Incidence and outcome of schizophrenia in Whites, African-Caribbeans and Asians in London," *Psychological Medicine*, vol. 27, no. 4, pp. 791–798, 1997.

[175] W. Eaton and G. Harrison, "Ethnic disadvantage and schizophrenia," *Acta Psychiatrica Scandinavica, Supplement*, vol. 102, no. 407, pp. 38–43, 2000.

[176] P. Fearon, J. B. Kirkbride, C. Morgan et al., "Incidence of schizophrenia and other psychoses in ethnic minority groups: results from the MRC AESOP Study," *Psychological Medicine*, vol. 36, no. 11, pp. 1541–1550, 2006.

[177] J. P. Selten, J. P. J. Slaets, and R. S. Kahn, "Schizophrenia in Surinamese and Dutch Antillean immigrants to The Netherlands: evidence of an increased incidence," *Psychological Medicine*, vol. 27, no. 4, pp. 807–811, 1997.

[178] J. P. Selten, N. Veen, W. Feller et al., "Incidence of psychotic disorders in immigrant groups to the Netherlands," *The British Journal of Psychiatry*, vol. 178, pp. 367–372, 2001.

[179] W. Veling, J.-P. Selten, N. Veen, W. Laan, J. D. Blom, and H. W. Hoek, "Incidence of schizophrenia among ethnic minorities in the Netherlands: a four-year first-contact study," *Schizophrenia Research*, vol. 86, no. 1–3, pp. 189–193, 2006.

[180] E. Cantor-Graae, C. B. Pedersen, T. F. McNeil, and P. B. Mortensen, "Migration as a risk factor for schizophrenia: a Danish population-based cohort study," *The British Journal of Psychiatry*, vol. 182, pp. 117–122, 2003.

[181] K. Zolkowska, E. Cantor-Graae, and T. F. McNeil, "Increased rates of psychosis among immigrants to Sweden: is migration a risk factor for psychosis?" *Psychological Medicine*, vol. 31, no. 4, pp. 669–678, 2001.

[182] P. A. Sugarman and D. Craufurd, "Schizophrenia in the Afro-Caribbean community," *The British Journal of Psychiatry*, vol. 164, pp. 474–480, 1994.

[183] J. W. Coid, J. B. Kirkbride, D. Barker et al., "Raised incidence rates of all psychoses among migrant groups: findings from the East london first episode psychosis study," *Archives of General Psychiatry*, vol. 65, no. 11, pp. 1250–1258, 2008.

[184] J. B. Kirkbride, D. Barker, F. Cowden et al., "Psychoses, ethnicity and socio-economic status," *The British Journal of Psychiatry*, vol. 193, no. 1, pp. 18–24, 2008.

[185] A. Hjern, S. Wicks, and C. Dalman, "Social adversity contributes to high morbidity in psychoses in immigrants—a national

cohort study in two generations of Swedish residents," *Psychological Medicine*, vol. 34, no. 6, pp. 1025–1033, 2004.

[186] T. S. Leão, J. Sundquist, G. Frank, L. Johansson, S. Johansson, and K. Sundquist, "Incidence of schizophrenia or other psychoses in first- and second-generation immigrants: a national cohort study," *Journal of Nervous and Mental Disease*, vol. 194, no. 1, pp. 27–33, 2006.

[187] F. W. Hickling and P. Rodgers-Johnson, "The incidence of first contact schizophrenia in Jamaica," *The British Journal of Psychiatry*, vol. 167, pp. 193–196, 1995.

[188] G. E. Mahy, R. Mallett, J. Leff, and D. Bhugra, "First-contact incidence rate of schizophrenia on Barbados," *The British Journal of Psychiatry*, vol. 175, pp. 28–33, 1999.

[189] D. Bhugra, M. Hilwig, B. Hossein et al., "First-contact incidence rates of schizophrenia in Trinidad and one-year follow-up," *The British Journal of Psychiatry*, vol. 169, no. 5, pp. 587–592, 1996.

[190] J. Selten, E. Cantor-Graae, J. Slaets, and R. S. Kahn, "Ødegaard's selection hypothesis revisited: schizophrenia in Surinamese immigrants to the Netherlands," *The American Journal of Psychiatry*, vol. 159, no. 4, pp. 669–671, 2002.

[191] J. Allardyce, H. Gilmour, J. Atkinson, T. Rapson, J. Bishop, and R. G. McCreadie, "Social fragmentation, deprivation and urbanicity: relation to first-admission rates for psychoses," *The British Journal of Psychiatry*, vol. 187, pp. 401–406, 2005.

[192] J. Boydell, J. van Os, K. McKenzie et al., "Incidence of schizophrenia in ethnic minorities in London: ecological study into interactions with environment," *The British Medical Journal*, vol. 323, no. 7325, pp. 1336–1338, 2001.

[193] E. Cantor-Graae and J. Selten, "Schizophrenia and migration: a meta-analysis and review," *The American Journal of Psychiatry*, vol. 162, no. 1, pp. 12–24, 2005.

[194] W. Veling, J. Selten, J. P. Mackenbach, and H. W. Hoek, "Symptoms at first contact for psychotic disorder: comparison between native Dutch and ethnic minorities," *Schizophrenia Research*, vol. 95, no. 1–3, pp. 30–38, 2007.

[195] W. Veling, J. Selten, E. Susser, W. Laan, J. P. Mackenbach, and H. W. Hoek, "Discrimination and the incidence of psychotic disorders among ethnic minorities in The Netherlands," *International Journal of Epidemiology*, vol. 36, no. 4, pp. 761–768, 2007.

[196] W. Veling, E. Susser, J. van Os, J. P. Mackenbach, J. Selten, and H. W. Hoek, "Ethnic density of neighborhoods and incidence of psychotic disorders among immigrants," *The American Journal of Psychiatry*, vol. 165, no. 1, pp. 66–73, 2008.

[197] J. B. Kirkbride, C. Morgan, P. Fearon, P. Dazzan, R. M. Murray, and P. B. Jones, "Neighbourhood-level effects on psychoses: Re-examining the role of context," *Psychological Medicine*, vol. 37, no. 10, pp. 1413–1425, 2007.

[198] E. Essen-Möller, "Untersuchungen über die Fruchtbarkeit gewisser Gruppen von Geisteskranken," *Acta Psychiatrica et Neurologica Scandinavica*, vol. 8, 1935 (German).

[199] Ö. Ödegård, "Fertility of psychiatric first admissions in Norway 1936–1975," *Acta Psychiatrica Scandinavica*, vol. 62, no. 3, pp. 212–220, 1980.

[200] F. Haverkamp, P. Propping, and T. Hilger, "Is there an increase of reproductive rates in schizophrenics? I. Critical review of the literature," *Archiv für Psychiatrie und Nervenkrankheiten*, vol. 232, no. 5, pp. 439–450, 1982.

[201] T. Hilger, P. Propping, and F. Haverkamp, "Is there an increase of reproductive rates in schizophrenics? III. An investigation in Nordbaden (SW Germany): results and discussion," *Archiv für Psychiatrie und Nervenkrankheiten*, vol. 233, no. 3, pp. 177–186, 1983.

[202] P. Propping, T. Hilger, and F. Haverkamp, "Is there an increase of reproductive rates in schizophrenics? II. An investigation in Nordbaden (SW Germany): methods and description of the patient sample," *Archiv für Psychiatrie und Nervenkrankheiten*, vol. 233, no. 3, pp. 167–175, 1983.

[203] L. Fananas and J. Bertranpetit, "Reproductive rates in families of schizophrenic patients in a case-control study," *Acta Psychiatrica Scandinavica*, vol. 91, no. 3, pp. 202–204, 1995.

[204] J. J. McGrath, J. Hearle, L. Jenner, K. Plant, A. Drummond, and J. M. Barkla, "The fertility and fecundity of patients with psychoses," *Acta Psychiatrica Scandinavica*, vol. 99, no. 6, pp. 441–446, 1999.

[205] V. L. Nimgaonkar, S. E. Ward, H. Agarde, N. Weston, and R. Ganguli, "Fertility in schizophrenia: results from a contemporary US cohort," *Acta Psychiatrica Scandinavica*, vol. 95, no. 5, pp. 364–369, 1997.

[206] J. Haukka, J. Suvisaari, and J. Lönnqvist, "Fertility of patients with schizophrenia, their siblings, and the general population: a cohort study from 1950 to 1959 in Finland," *The American Journal of Psychiatry*, vol. 160, no. 3, pp. 460–463, 2003.

[207] J. H. MacCabe, I. Koupil, and D. A. Leon, "Lifetime reproductive output over two generations in patients with psychosis and their unaffected siblings: the Uppsala 1915–1929 Birth Cohort Multigenerational Study," *Psychological Medicine*, vol. 39, no. 10, pp. 1667–1676, 2009.

[208] D. Ropeter, *Fertilitätsraten schizophren Erkrankter—Trends über 5 Jahrzehnte und Versuche ihrer Erklärung (Doctoral thesis)*, Faculty of Clinical Medicine Mannheim, Ruprecht Karls University of Heidelberg, Heidelberg, Germany, 2006, (German).

[209] A. C. Svensson, P. Lichtenstein, S. Sandin, and C. M. Hultman, "Fertility of first-degree relatives of patients with schizophrenia: a three generation perspective," *Schizophrenia Research*, vol. 91, no. 1–3, pp. 238–245, 2007.

[210] B. Xu, J. L. Roos, P. Dexheimer et al., "Exome sequencing supports a *de novo* mutational paradigm for schizophrenia," *Nature Genetics*, vol. 43, no. 9, pp. 864–868, 2011.

[211] J. L. Waddington and H. A. Youssef, "Familial-genetic and reproductive epidemiology of schizophrenia in rural Ireland: age at onset, familial morbid risk and parental fertility," *Acta Psychiatrica Scandinavica*, vol. 93, no. 1, pp. 62–68, 1996.

[212] M. Avila, G. Thaker, and H. Adami, "Genetic epidemiology and schizophrenia: a study of reproductive fitness," *Schizophrenia Research*, vol. 47, no. 2-3, pp. 233–241, 2001.

[213] A. Jablensky, J. B. Kirkbride, and P. B. Jones, "Schizophrenia: the epidemiological horizon," in *Schizophrenia*, D. R. Weinberger and P. J. Harrison, Eds., pp. 185–225, Wiley-Blackwell, Oxford, UK, 3rd edition, 2011.

[214] H. Stefansson, R. A. Ophoff, S. Steinberg et al., "Common variants conferring risk of schizophrenia," *Nature*, vol. 460, pp. 744–747, 2009.

[215] J. R. Geddes and S. M. Lawrie, "Obstetric complications and schizophrenia: a meta-analysis," *The British Journal of Psychiatry*, vol. 167, pp. 786–793, 1995.

[216] C. M. Hultman, A. Öhman, S. Cnattingius, I. M. Wieselgren, and L. H. Lindstrom, "Prenatal and neonatal risk factors for schizophrenia," *The British Journal of Psychiatry*, vol. 170, pp. 128–133, 1997.

[217] M. Cannon, P. B. Jones, and R. M. Murray, "Obstetric complications and schizophrenia: historical and meta-analytic review," *The American Journal of Psychiatry*, vol. 159, no. 7, pp. 1080–1092, 2002.

[218] P. Rantakallio, P. Jones, J. Moring, and L. von Wendt, "Association between central nervous system infections during childhood and adult onset schizophrenia and other psychoses: a 28-year follow-up," *International Journal of Epidemiology*, vol. 26, no. 4, pp. 837–843, 1997.

[219] W. F. Gattaz, A. L. Abrahao, and R. Foccacia, "Childhood meningitis and adult schizophrenia," in *Search for the Causes of Schizophrenia*, W. F. Gattaz and H. Häfner, Eds., pp. 26–31, Steinkopff, Darmstadt, Germany, 2004.

[220] A. L. Abrahao, R. Focaccia, and W. F. Gattaz, "Childhood meningitis increases the risk for adult schizophrenia," *World Journal of Biological Psychiatry*, vol. 6, supplement 2, pp. 44–48, 2005.

[221] G. Harrison, C. Glazebrook, J. Brewin et al., "Increased incidence of psychotic disorders in migrants from the Caribbean to the United Kingdom," *Psychological Medicine*, vol. 27, no. 4, pp. 799–806, 1997.

[222] E. Kringlen, *Heredity and Environment in the Functional Psychoses: An Epidemiological-Clinical Study*, University Press, Oslo, Norway, 1967, reprinted by Heinemann, London, UK, 1968.

[223] E. Kringlen, "Twins: still our best method," *Schizophrenia Bulletin*, vol. 2, no. 3, pp. 429–433, 1976.

[224] I. I. Gottesman and J. Shields, *Schizophrenia: The Epigenetic Puzzle*, Sage, New York, NY, USA, 1982.

[225] P. McGuffin, A. E. Farmer, I. I. Gottesman, R. M. Murray, and A. M. Reveley, "Twin concordance for operationally defined schizophrenia. Confirmation of familiality and heritability," *Archives of General Psychiatry*, vol. 41, no. 6, pp. 541–545, 1984.

[226] A. E. Farmer, P. McGuffin, and I. I. Gottesman, "Twin concordance for DSM-III schizophrenia: scrutinizing the validity of the definition," *Archives of General Psychiatry*, vol. 44, no. 7, pp. 634–641, 1987.

[227] T. D. Cannon, J. Kaprio, J. Lönnqvist, M. Huttunen, and M. Koskenvuo, "The genetic epidemiology of schizophrenia in a Finnish twin cohort: a population-based modeling study," *Archives of General Psychiatry*, vol. 55, no. 1, pp. 67–74, 1998.

[228] S. Onstad, I. Skre, S. Torgersen, and E. Kringlen, "Twin concordance for DSM-III-R schizophrenia," *Acta Psychiatrica Scandinavica*, vol. 83, no. 5, pp. 395–401, 1991.

[229] A. G. Cardno and I. I. Gottesman, "Twin studies of schizophrenia: from bow-and-arrow concordances to STAR WARS Mx and functional genomics," *American Journal of Medical Genetics*, vol. 97, no. 1, pp. 12–17, 2000.

[230] W. Coryell and M. Zimmerman, "The heritability of schizophrenia and schizoaffective disorder. A family study," *Archives of General Psychiatry*, vol. 45, no. 4, pp. 323–327, 1988.

[231] E. S. Gershon, L. E. DeLisi, J. Hamovit et al., "A controlled family study of chronic psychoses. Schizophrenia and schizoaffective disorder," *Archives of General Psychiatry*, vol. 45, no. 4, pp. 328–336, 1988.

[232] W. Maier, D. Lichtermann, J. Minges et al., "Continuity and discontinuity of affective disorders and schizophrenia: results of a controlled family study," *Archives of General Psychiatry*, vol. 50, no. 11, pp. 871–883, 1993.

[233] J. Parnas, T. D. Cannon, B. Jacobsen, H. Schulsinger, F. Schulsinger, and S. A. Mednick, "Lifetime DSM-III-R diagnostic outcomes in the offspring of schizophrenic mothers: results from the Copenhagen high-risk study," *Archives of General Psychiatry*, vol. 50, no. 9, pp. 707–714, 1993.

[234] P. F. Sullivan, K. S. Kendler, and M. C. Neale, "Schizophrenia as a complex trait: evidence from a meta-analysis of twin studies," *Archives of General Psychiatry*, vol. 60, no. 12, pp. 1187–1192, 2003.

[235] I. I. Gottesman, *Schizophrenia Genesis: The Origins of Madness*, W. H. Freeman, New York, NY, USA, 1991.

[236] B. Riley and K. S. Kendler, "Classical genetic studies of schizophrenia," in *Schizophrenia*, D. R. Weinberger and P. J. Harrison, Eds., pp. 245–268, Wiley-Blackwell, Oxford, UK, 3rd edition, 2011.

[237] P. Tienari, L. C. Wynne, K. Läksy et al., "Genetic boundaries of the schizophrenia spectrum: evidence from the Finnish adoptive family study of schizophrenia," *The American Journal of Psychiatry*, vol. 160, no. 9, pp. 1587–1594, 2003.

[238] C. Wynne, P. Tienari, P. Nieminen et al., "I. Genotype-environment interaction in the schizophrenia spectrum: genetic liability and global family ratings in the Finnish adoption study," *Family Process*, vol. 45, no. 4, pp. 419–434, 2006.

[239] H. Wickham, C. Walsh, P. Asherson et al., "Familiality of clinical characteristics in schizophrenia," *Journal of Psychiatric Research*, vol. 36, no. 5, pp. 325–329, 2002.

[240] W. Maier, J. Hallmayer, J. Minges, and D. Lichtermann, "Morbid risks in relatives of affective, schizoaffective and schizophrenic patients. Results of a family study," in *Affective and Schizoaffective Disorders. Similarities and Differences*, A. Marneros and M. T. Tsuang, Eds., pp. 201–207, Springer, Berlin, Germany, 1990.

[241] J. X. van Snellenberg and T. de Candia, "Meta-analytic evidence for familial coaggregation of schizophrenia and bipolar disorder," *Archives of General Psychiatry*, vol. 66, no. 7, pp. 748–755, 2009.

[242] M. Baron and N. Risch, "The spectrum concept of schizophrenia: evidence for a genetic-environmental continuum," *Journal of Psychiatric Research*, vol. 21, no. 3, pp. 257–267, 1987.

[243] S. Ripke, C. O'Dushlaine, K. Chambert et al., "Genome-wide association analysis identifies 13 new risk loci for schizophrenia," *Nature Genetics*, vol. 45, pp. 1150–1159, 2013.

[244] Schizophrenia Working Group of the Psychiatric Genomics Consortium, "Biological insights from 108 schizophrenia-associated genetic loci," *Nature*, vol. 511, no. 7510, pp. 421–427, 2014.

[245] I. I. Gottesman and T. D. Gould, "The endophenotype concept in psychiatry: etymology and strategic intentions," *The American Journal of Psychiatry*, vol. 160, no. 4, pp. 636–645, 2003.

[246] C. Esslinger, H. Walter, P. Kirsch et al., "Neural mechanisms of a genome-wide supported psychosis variant," *Science*, vol. 324, no. 5927, p. 605, 2009.

[247] J. L. Hess and S. J. Glatt, "How might ZNF804A variants influence risk for schizophrenia and bipolar disorder? A literature review, synthesis, and bioinformatic analysis," *The American Journal of Medical Genetics B: Neuropsychiatric Genetics*, vol. 165, no. 1, pp. 28–40, 2014.

[248] International Schizophrenia Consortium, S. M. Purcell, N. R. Wray et al., "Common polygenic variation contributes to risk of schizophrenia and bipolar disorder," *Nature*, vol. 460, pp. 748–752, 2009.

[249] J. Yang, S. H. Lee, M. E. Goddard, and P. M. Visscher, "GCTA: a tool for genome-wide complex trait analysis," *The American Journal of Human Genetics*, vol. 88, no. 1, pp. 76–82, 2011.

[250] S. H. Lee, T. R. DeCandia, S. Ripke et al., "Estimating the proportion of variation in susceptibility to Schizophrenia captured by common SNPs," *Nature Genetics*, vol. 44, pp. 247–250, 2014.

[251] Cross-Disorder Group of the Psychiatric Genomics, S. H. Lee, S. Ripke et al., "Genetic relationship between five psychiatric disorders estimated from genome-wide SNPs," *Nature Genetics*, vol. 45, no. 9, pp. 984–994, 2013.

[252] J. Frank, M. Lang, S. H. Witt et al., "Identification of increased genetic risk scores for schizophrenia in treatment-resistant patients," *Molecular Psychiatry*, 2014.

[253] T. Lencz, E. Knowles, and G. Davies, "Molecular genetic evidence for overlap between general cognitive ability and risk for schizophrenia: a report from the Cognitive Genomics consortium (COGENT)," *Molecular Psychiatry*, vol. 19, pp. 168–174, 2014.

[254] A. Hoischen, N. Krumm, and E. E. Eichler, "Priorization of neurodevelopmental disease genes by discovery of new mutations," *Nature Neuroscience*, vol. 17, pp. 764–772, 2014.

[255] J. P. Szatkiewicz, C. O'Dushlaine, G. Chen et al., "Copy number variation in schizophrenia in Sweden," *Molecular Psychiatry*, vol. 19, pp. 762–773, 2014.

[256] J. L. Doherty and M. J. Owen, "Genomic insights into the overlap between psychiatric disorders: implications for research and clinical practice," *Genome Medicine*, vol. 6, pp. 29–42, 2014.

[257] H. Stefansson, A. Meyer-Lindenberg, S. Steinberg et al., "CNVs conferring risk of autism or schizophrenia affect cognition in controls," *Nature*, vol. 505, no. 7483, pp. 361–366, 2014.

[258] T. F. McNeil, "Perinatal risk factors and schizophrenia: selective review and methodological concerns," *Epidemiologic Reviews*, vol. 17, no. 1, pp. 107–112, 1995.

[259] J. R. Geddes, H. Verdoux, N. Takei et al., "Schizophrenia and complications of pregnancy and labor: an individual patient data meta-analysis," *Schizophrenia Bulletin*, vol. 25, no. 3, pp. 413–423, 1999.

[260] C. McDonald and R. M. Murray, "Early and late environmental risk factors for schizophrenia," *Brain Research Reviews*, vol. 31, no. 2-3, pp. 130–137, 2000.

[261] T. D. Cannon, I. M. Rosso, J. M. Hollister, C. E. Bearden, L. E. Sanchez, and T. Hadley, "A prospective cohort study of genetic and perinatal influences in the etiology of schizophrenia," *Schizophrenia Bulletin*, vol. 26, no. 2, pp. 351–366, 2000.

[262] P. B. Jones, P. Rantakallio, A. Hartikainen, M. Isohanni, and P. Sipilä, "Schizophrenia as a long-term outcome of pregnancy, delivery, and perinatal complications: a 28-year follow-up of the 1966 North Finland general population birth cohort," *The American Journal of Psychiatry*, vol. 155, no. 3, pp. 355–364, 1998.

[263] M. Isohanni, E. Lauronen, K. Moilanen et al., "Predictors of schizophrenia: evidence from the Northern Finland 1966 Birth Cohort and other sources," *The British Journal of Psychiatry*, vol. 187, no. 48, pp. s4–s7, 2005.

[264] A. Heck, M. Fastenrath, S. Ackermann et al., "Converging genetic and functional brain imaging evidence links neural excitability to working memory, psychiatric disease, and brain activity," *Neuron*, vol. 81, no. 5, pp. 1203–1213, 2014.

[265] L. J. Seidman, S. L. Buka, J. M. Goldstein, and M. T. Tsuang, "Intellectual decline in schizophrenia: evidence from a prospective birth cohort 28 year follow-up study," *Journal of Clinical and Experimental Neuropsychology*, vol. 28, no. 2, pp. 225–242, 2006.

[266] S. A. Mednick and F. Schulsinger, "A longitudinal study of children with a high risk for schizophrenia: a preliminary report," in *Methods and Goal in Human Behavior Genetics*, S. Vangenberg, Ed., pp. 255–296, Academic Press, New York, NY, USA, 1965.

[267] S. A. Mednick and F. Schulsiger, "Some premorbid characteristics related to breakdown in children with schizophrenic mothers," in *Transmission of Schizophrenia*, D. Rosenthal and S. S. Kety, Eds., pp. 267–291, Pergamon Press, New York, NY, USA, 1968.

[268] J. R. Asarnow, "Children at risk for schizophrenia: converging lines of evidence," *Schizophrenia Bulletin*, vol. 14, no. 4, pp. 613–631, 1988.

[269] L. Erlenmeyer-Kimling, D. Rock, E. Squires-Wheeler, S. Roberts, and J. Yang, "Early life precursors of psychiatric outcomes in adulthood in subjects at risk for schizophrenia or affective disorders," *Psychiatry Research*, vol. 39, no. 3, pp. 239–256, 1991.

[270] L. Erlenmeyer-Kimling, B. A. Cornblatt, D. Rock, S. Roberts, M. Bell, and A. West, "The New York high-risk project: anhedonia, attentional deviance, and psychopathology," *Schizophrenia Bulletin*, vol. 19, no. 1, pp. 141–153, 1993.

[271] L. Erlenmeyer-Kimling, E. Squires-Wheeler, U. H. Adamo, and A. S. Bassett, "The New York high-risk project," *Archives of General Psychiatry*, vol. 52, pp. 857–865, 1995.

[272] L. Erlenmeyer-Kimling, U. H. Adamo, D. Rock et al., "The New York high-risk project," *Archives of General Psychiatry*, vol. 54, pp. 1096–1102, 1997.

[273] M. Dragovic, F. A. V. Waters, and A. Jablensky, "Estimating premorbid intelligence in schizophrenia patients: demographically based approach," *Australian & New Zealand Journal of Psychiatry*, vol. 42, no. 9, pp. 814–818, 2008.

[274] V. A. Morgan, H. Leonard, J. Bourke, and A. Jablensky, "Intellectual disability co-occurring with schizophrenia and other psychiatric illness: population-based study," *The British Journal of Psychiatry*, vol. 193, no. 5, pp. 364–372, 2008.

[275] B. Cornblatt, M. Obuchowski, S. Roberts, S. Pollack, and L. Erlenmeyer-Kimling, "Cognitive and behavioral precursors of schizophrenia," *Development and Psychopathology*, vol. 11, no. 3, pp. 487–508, 1999.

[276] J. Marcus, J. Auerbach, L. Wilkinson, and C. M. Burack, "Infants at risk for schizophrenia: the Jerusalem Infant Development Study," *Archives of General Psychiatry*, vol. 38, no. 6, pp. 703–713, 1981.

[277] J. Marcus, S. L. Hans, E. Lewow, L. Wilkinson, and C. M. Burack, "Neurological findings in high-risk children: childhood assessment and 5-year followup," *Schizophrenia Bulletin*, vol. 11, no. 1, pp. 85–100, 1985.

[278] B. Fish, J. Marcus, S. L. Hans, J. G. Auerbach, and S. Perdue, "Infants at risk for schizophrenia: sequelae of a genetic neurointegrative defect. A review and replication analysis of pandysmaturation in the Jerusalem infant development study," *Archives of General Psychiatry*, vol. 49, no. 3, pp. 221–235, 1992.

[279] E. F. Walker, T. Savoie, and D. Davis, "Neuromotor precursors of schizophrenia," *Schizophrenia Bulletin*, vol. 20, no. 3, pp. 441–451, 1994.

[280] E. E. Walker, J. Weinstein, K. Baum, and C. S. Neumann, "Antecedents of schizophrenia: Moderating effects of development and biological sex," in *Search for the Causes of Schizophrenia*, H. Häfner and W. F. Gattaz, Eds., vol. 3, pp. 21–42, Springer, Berlin, Germany, 1995.

[281] O. D. Howes, C. McDonald, M. Cannon, L. Arseneault, J. Boydell, and R. M. Murray, "Pathways to schizophrenia: the impact of environmental factors," *International Journal of Neuropsychopharmacology*, vol. 7, no. 1, pp. S7–S13, 2004.

[282] P. H. Connell, *Amphetamine Psychosis*, Chapman & Hall, London, UK, 1958.

[283] K. Nakamura, C. Chen, Y. Sekine et al., "Association analysis of SOD2 variants with methamphetamine psychosis in Japanese and Taiwanese populations," *Human Genetics*, vol. 120, no. 2, pp. 243–252, 2006.

[284] R. Näkki, J. Koistinaho, F. R. Sharp, and S. M. Sagar, "Cerebellar toxicity of phencyclidine," *Journal of Neuroscience*, vol. 15, part 2, no. 3, pp. 2097–2108, 1995.

[285] S. Andreasson, P. Allebeck, A. Engstrom, and U. Rydberg, "Cannabis and schizophrenia. A longitudinal study of Swedish conscripts," *The Lancet*, vol. 2, no. 8574, pp. 1483–1486, 1987.

[286] P. Allebeck, C. Adamsson, and A. Engstrom, "Cannabis and schizophrenia: a longitudinal study of cases treated in Stockholm county," *Acta Psychiatrica Scandinavica*, vol. 88, no. 1, pp. 21–24, 1993.

[287] M. Hambrecht and H. Häfner, "Substance abuse and the onset of schizophrenia," *Biological Psychiatry*, vol. 40, no. 11, pp. 1155–1163, 1996.

[288] L. Arseneault, M. Cannon, R. Poulton, R. Murray, A. Caspi, and T. E. Moffitt, "Cannabis use in adolescence and risk for adult psychosis: longitudinal prospective study," *British Medical Journal*, vol. 325, no. 7374, pp. 1212–1213, 2002.

[289] S. Zammit, P. Allebeck, S. Andreasson, I. Lundberg, and G. Lewis, "Self reported cannabis use as a risk factor for schizophrenia in Swedish conscripts of 1969: historical cohort study," *The British Medical Journal*, vol. 325, no. 7374, pp. 1199–1201, 2002.

[290] C. Henquet, R. Murray, D. Linszen, and J. van Os, "The environment and schizophrenia: the role of cannabis use," *Schizophrenia Bulletin*, vol. 31, no. 3, pp. 608–612, 2005.

[291] T. H. Moore, S. Zammit, A. Lingford-Hughes et al., "Cannabis use and risk of psychotic or affective mental health outcomes: a systematic review," *The Lancet*, vol. 370, no. 9584, pp. 319–328, 2007.

[292] D. J. Foti, R. Kotov, L. T. Guey, and E. J. Bromet, "Cannabis use and the course of schizophrenia: 10-year follow-up after first hospitalization," *The American Journal of Psychiatry*, vol. 167, no. 8, pp. 987–993, 2010.

[293] E. Manrique-Garcia, S. Zammit, C. Dalman, T. Hemmingsson, S. Andreasson, and P. Allebeck, "Prognosis of schizophrenia in persons with and without a history of cannabis use," *Psychological Medicine*, 2014.

[294] P. Jones, B. Rodgers, R. Murray, and M. Marmot, "Child developmental risk factors for adult schizophrenia in the British 1946 birth cohort," *The Lancet*, vol. 344, no. 8934, pp. 1398–1402, 1994.

[295] P. Jones and D. J. Done, "From birth to onset: a developmental perspective of schizophrenia in two national birth cohorts," in *Neurodevelopmental Models of Psychopathology*, M. S. Keshavan and R. M. Murray, Eds., pp. 119–136, Cambridge University Press, Cambridge, UK, 1997.

[296] P. B. Jones and C. J. Tarrant, "Vorläufersymptome funktioneller Psychosen," *ZNS Journal*, vol. 18, pp. 4–15, 1998 (German).

[297] D. J. Done, T. J. Crow, E. C. Johnstone, and A. Sacker, "Childhood antecedents of schizophrenia and affective illness: social adjustment at ages 7 and 11," *British Medical Journal*, vol. 309, no. 6956, pp. 699–703, 1994.

[298] R. Poulton, A. Caspi, T. E. Moffitt, M. Cannon, R. Murray, and H. Harrington, "Children's self-reported psychotic symptoms and adult schizophreniform disorder: a 15-year longitudinal study," *Archives of General Psychiatry*, vol. 57, no. 11, pp. 1053–1058, 2000.

[299] M. Cannon, T. E. Moffitt, A. Caspi, R. M. Murray, H. Harrington, and R. Poulton, "Neuropsychological performance at the age of 13 years and adult schizophreniform disorder: prospective birth cohort study," *The British Journal of Psychiatry*, vol. 189, pp. 463–464, 2006.

[300] M. Isohanni, P. Rantakallio, P. Jones et al., "The predictors of schizophrenia in the 1966 Northern Finland Birth Cohort study," *Schizophrenia Research*, vol. 29, p. 11, 1998.

[301] I. Isohanni, M.-R. Järvelin, P. Nieminen et al., "School performance as a predictor of psychiatric hospitalization in adult life. A 28-year follow-up in the Northern Finland 1966 Birth Cohort," *Psychological Medicine*, vol. 28, no. 4, pp. 967–974, 1998.

[302] M. Isohanni, P. B. Jones, S. Räsänen et al., "Early developmental milestones in adult schizophrenia. A 28-year follow-up of the North Finland birth cohort," *Schizophrenia Research*, vol. 52, pp. 1–19, 2001.

[303] P. B. Jones, R. M. Murray, and B. Rodgers, "Childhood risk factors for schizophrenia in a general population birth cohort at age 43 years," in *Neural Development in Schizophrenia: Theory and Practice*, S. A. Mednick and J. M. Hollister, Eds., pp. 151–176, Plenum Press, New York, NY, USA, 1995.

[304] P. B. Jones, "Risk factors for schizophrenia in childhood and youth," in *Risk and Protective Factors in Schizophreni*, H. Häfner, Ed., pp. 141–162, Steinkopff, Darmstadt, Germany, 2002.

[305] M. Solomon, E. Olsen, T. Niendam et al., "From lumping to splitting and back again: atypical social and language development in individuals with clinical-high-risk for psychosis, first episode schizophrenia, and autism spectrum disorders," *Schizophrenia Research*, vol. 131, no. 1–3, pp. 146–151, 2011.

[306] A. Piton, J. Gauthier, F. F. Hamdan et al., "Systematic resequencing of X-chromosome synaptic genes in autism spectrum disorder and schizophrenia," *Molecular Psychiatry*, vol. 16, no. 8, pp. 867–880, 2011.

[307] R. Waltereit, T. Banaschewski, A. Meyer-Lindenberg, and L. Poustka, "Interaction of neurodevelopmental pathways and synaptic plasticity in mental retardation, autism spectrum disorder and schizophrenia: Implications for psychiatry," *World Journal of Biological Psychiatry*, 2013.

[308] A. S. David, A. Malmberg, L. Brandt, P. Allebeck, and G. Lewis, "IQ and risk for schizophrenia: A population-based cohort study," *Psychological Medicine*, vol. 27, no. 6, pp. 1311–1323, 1997.

[309] A. Malmberg, G. Lewis, A. David, and P. Allebeck, "Premorbid adjustment and personality in people with schizophrenia," *The British Journal of Psychiatry*, vol. 172, pp. 308–313, 1998.

[310] M. Davidson, A. Reichenberg, J. Rabinowitz, M. Weiser, Z. Kaplan, and M. Mark, "Behavioral and intellectual markers for schizophrenia in apparently healthy male adolescents," *The American Journal of Psychiatry*, vol. 156, no. 9, pp. 1328–1335, 1999.

[311] M. Weiser, "Association between cognitive and behavioral functioning, non-psychotic psychiatric diagnoses, and drug abuse in adolescence, with later hospitalization for schizophrenia," in *Risk and Protective Factors in Schizophrenia*, H. Häfner, Ed., pp. 163–175, Steinkopff, Darmstadt, Germany, 2002.

[312] I. Isohanni, M.-R. Järvelin, P. Jones, J. Jokelainen, and M. Isohanni, "Can excellent school performance be a precursor of schizophrenia? A 28-year follow-up in the Northern Finland 1966 birth cohort," *Acta Psychiatrica Scandinavica*, vol. 100, no. 1, pp. 17–26, 1999.

[313] J. Bertranpetit and L. Fananas, "Parental age in schizophrenia in a case-controlled study," *The British Journal of Psychiatry*, vol. 162, p. 574, 1993.

[314] D. Malaspina, S. Harlap, S. Fennig et al., "Advancing paternal age and the risk of schizophrenia," *Archives of General Psychiatry*, vol. 58, no. 4, pp. 361–367, 2001.

[315] A. S. Brown, C. A. Schaefer, R. J. Wyatt et al., "Paternal age and risk of schizophrenia in adult offspring," *The American Journal of Psychiatry*, vol. 159, no. 9, pp. 1528–1533, 2002.

[316] A. Jung, H. C. Schuppe, and W. B. Schill, "Are children of older fathers at risk for genetic disorders?" *Andrologia*, vol. 35, no. 4, pp. 191–199, 2003.

[317] M. C. Perrin, A. S. Brown, and D. Malaspina, "Aberrant epigenetic regulation could explain the relationship of paternal age to schizophrenia," *Schizophrenia Bulletin*, vol. 33, no. 6, pp. 1270–1273, 2007.

[318] J. J. McGrath, L. Petersen, E. Agerbo, O. Mors, P. B. Mortensen, and C. B. Pedersen, "A comprehensive assessment of parental age and psychiatric disorders," *The Journal of the American Medical Association Psychiatry*, vol. 71, no. 3, pp. 301–309, 2014.

[319] A. E. Jaffe, W. W. Eaton, R. E. Straub, S. Marenco, and D. R. Weinberger, "Paternal age, de novo mutations and schizophrenia," *Molecular Psychiatry*, vol. 19, pp. 274–283, 2014.

[320] B. Miller, E. Messias, J. Miettunen et al., "Meta-analysis of paternal age and schizophrenia risk in male versus female offspring," *Schizophrenia Bulletin*, vol. 37, no. 5, pp. 1039–1047, 2011.

[321] A. Kong, M. L. Frigge, G. Masson et al., "Rate of de novo mutations and the importance of father's age to disease risk," *Nature*, vol. 488, no. 7412, pp. 471–475, 2012.

[322] L. Petersen, P. B. Mortensen, and C. B. Pedersen, "Paternal age at birth of first child and risk of schizophrenia," *The American Journal of Psychiatry*, vol. 168, pp. 82–88, 2011.

[323] H. Häfner, K. Maurer, W. Löffler et al., "Onset and early course of schizophrenia," in *Search for the Causes of Schizophrenia III*, H. Häfner and W. F. Gattaz, Eds., pp. 43–66, Springer, Berlin, Germany, 1995.

[324] N. C. Stefanis, M. Hanssen, N. K. Smirnis et al., "Evidence that three dimensions of psychosis have a distribution in the general population," *Psychological Medicine*, vol. 32, no. 2, pp. 347–358, 2002.

[325] J. van Os, H. Verdoux, S. Maurice-Tison et al., "Self-reported psychosis-like symptoms and the continuum of psychosis," *Social Psychiatry and Psychiatric Epidemiology*, vol. 34, no. 9, pp. 459–463, 1999.

[326] H.-U. Wittchen, M. Höfler, R. Lieb, J. Spauwen, and J. van Os, "Depressive und psychotische Symptome in der Bevölkerung—Eine prospektiv-longitudinale Studie (EDSP) an 2.500 Jugendlichen und jungen Erwachsenen," *Nervenarzt*, vol. 75, supplement 2, p. 87, 2004 (German).

[327] R. L. Loewy, J. K. Johnson, and T. D. Cannon, "Self-report of attenuated psychotic experiences in a college population," *Schizophrenia Research*, vol. 93, no. 1–3, pp. 144–151, 2007.

[328] T. D. Cannon, "Prediction of psychosis through the prodromal syndrome," in *Advances in Schizophrenia Research 2009*, W. F. Gattaz and G. G. Busatto, Eds., pp. 251–266, Springer, New York, NY, USA, 2010.

[329] J. van Os, M. Hanssen, R. V. Bijl, and A. Ravelli, "Strauss (1969) revisited: a psychosis continuum in the general population?" *Schizophrenia Research*, vol. 45, no. 1-2, pp. 11–20, 2000.

[330] J. Van Os, M. Hanssen, R. V. Bijl, and W. Vollebergh, "Prevalence of psychotic disorder and community level of psychotic symptoms: An urban-rural comparison," *Archives of General Psychiatry*, vol. 58, no. 7, pp. 663–668, 2001.

[331] J. Spauwen, L. Krabbendam, R. Lieb, H. Wittchen, and J. van Os, "Sex differences in psychosis: normal or pathological?" *Schizophrenia Research*, vol. 62, no. 1-2, pp. 45–49, 2003.

[332] M. Hanssen, M. Bak, R. Bijl, W. Vollebergh, and J. van Os, "The incidence and outcome of subclinical psychotic experiences in the general population," *British Journal of Clinical Psychology*, vol. 44, no. 2, pp. 181–191, 2005.

[333] J. Allardyce and J. van Os, "The natural history of the course and outcome of Schizophrenia," in *Advances in Schizophrenia Research 2009*, W. F. Gattaz and G. Busatto, Eds., pp. 51–66, Springer, New York, NY, USA, 2010.

[334] M. D. G. Dominguez, M. Wichers, R. Lieb, H. Wittchen, and J. van Os, "Evidence that onset of clinical psychosis is an outcome of progressively more persistent subclinical psychotic experiences: an 8-year cohort study," *Schizophrenia Bulletin*, vol. 37, no. 1, pp. 84–93, 2011.

[335] M. S. S. Hanssen, M. Bak, R. Bijl, W. Vollebergh, and J. Os, "Is prediction of psychosis in the general population feasible?" *European Psychiatry*, vol. 17, supplement 1, p. 74, 2002.

[336] N. Haroun, L. Dunn, A. Haroun, and K. S. Cadenhead, "Risk and protection in prodromal schizophrenia: ethical implications for clinical practice and future research," *Schizophrenia Bulletin*, vol. 32, no. 1, pp. 166–178, 2006.

[337] T. D. Cannon, K. Cadenhead, B. Cornblatt et al., "Prediction of psychosis in youth at high clinical risk: a multisite longitudinal study in North America," *Archives of General Psychiatry*, vol. 65, no. 1, pp. 28–37, 2008.

[338] J. Lyne, L. Renwick, K. Madigan et al., "Do psychosis prodrome onset negative symptoms predict first presentation negative symptoms?" *European Psychiatry*, vol. 29, pp. 153–159, 2014.

[339] I. van Rossum, M. Dominguez, R. Lieb, H. Wittchen, and J. van Os, "Affective dysregulation and reality distortion: a 10-year prospective study of their association and clinical relevance," *Schizophrenia Bulletin*, vol. 37, no. 3, pp. 561–571, 2011.

[340] L. Krabbendam, I. Myin-Germeys, M. Hanssen et al., "Development of depressed mood predicts onset of psychotic disorder in individuals who report hallucinatory experiences," *The British Journal of Clinical Psychology*, vol. 44, no. 1, pp. 113–125, 2005.

[341] J. Klosterkötter, M. Hellmich, and F. Schultze-Lutter, "Ist die Diagnose schizophrener Störungen schon in der initialen Prodromalphase vor der psychotischen Erstmanifestation möglich?" *Fortschritte der Neurologie Psychiatrie*, vol. 68, Sonderheft 1, pp. S13–S21, 2000 (German).

[342] J. Klosterkötter, M. Hellmich, E. M. Steinmeyer, and F. Schultze-Lutter, "Diagnosing schizophrenia in the initial prodromal phase," *Archives of General Psychiatry*, vol. 58, no. 2, pp. 158–164, 2001.

[343] G. Gross, G. Huber, J. Klosterkötter, and M. Linz, *Bonner Skala für die Beurteilung von Basissymptomen (BSABS)*, Springer, Berlin, Germany, 1987 (German).

[344] J. Addington, K. S. Cadenhead, T. D. Cannon et al., "North American prodrome longitudinal study: a collaborative multisite approach to prodromal schizophrenia research," *Schizophrenia Bulletin*, vol. 33, no. 3, pp. 665–672, 2007.

[345] P. Fusar-Poli, I. Bonoldi, A. R. Yung et al., "Predicting psychosis: Meta-analysis of transition outcomes in individuals at high clinical risk," *Archives of General Psychiatry*, vol. 69, no. 3, pp. 220–229, 2012.

[346] A. R. Yung, L. J. Phillips, H. P. Yuen, and P. D. McGorry, "Risk factors for psychosis in an ultra high-risk group: psychopathology and clinical features," *Schizophrenia Research*, vol. 67, no. 2-3, pp. 131–142, 2004.

[347] P. Fusar-Poli, S. Borgwardt, A. Bechdolf et al., "The psychosis high-risk state: a comprehensive state-of-the-art review," *The Journal of the American Medical Association Psychiatry*, vol. 70, no. 1, pp. 107–120, 2013.

[348] P. F. Liddle and T. R. E. Barnes, "Syndromes of chronic schizophrenia," *The British Journal of Psychiatry*, vol. 157, pp. 558–561, 1990.

[349] P. F. Liddle, "Syndromes of schizophrenia on factor analysis," *The British Journal of Psychiatry*, vol. 161, p. 861, 1992.

[350] H. Häfner, K. Maurer, W. Löffler, W. an der Heiden, M. Hambrecht, and F. Schultze-Lutter, "Modeling the early course of schizophrenia," *Schizophrenia Bulletin*, vol. 29, no. 2, pp. 325–340, 2003.

[351] A. Serretti and P. Olgiati, "Dimensions of major psychoses: a confirmatory factor analysis of six competing models," *Psychiatry Research*, vol. 127, no. 1-2, pp. 101–109, 2004.

[352] M. Ruggeri, M. Koeter, A. Schene et al., "Factor solution of the BPRS-expanded version in schizophrenic outpatients living in five European countries," *Schizophrenia Research*, vol. 75, no. 1, pp. 107–117, 2005.

[353] S. Z. Levine and J. Rabinowitz, "Revisiting the 5 dimensions of the positive and negative syndrome scale," *Journal of Clinical Psychopharmacology*, vol. 27, no. 5, pp. 431–436, 2007.

[354] A. Picardi, C. Viroli, L. Tarsitani et al., "Heterogeneity and symptom structure of schizophrenia," *Psychiatry Research*, vol. 198, no. 3, pp. 386–394, 2012.

[355] N. C. Andreasen, *The Scale for the Assessment of Negative Symptoms (SANS)*, University of Iow, Iowa City, Iowa, USA, 1983.

[356] M. J. Cuesta and V. Peralta, "Psychopathological dimensions in schizophrenia," *Schizophrenia Bulletin*, vol. 21, no. 3, pp. 473–482, 1995.

[357] W. P. Horan, A. M. Kring, and J. J. Blanchard, "Anhedonia in schizophrenia: a review of assessment strategies," *Schizophrenia Bulletin*, vol. 32, no. 2, pp. 259–273, 2006.

[358] G. Foussias and G. Remington, "Negative symptoms in schizophrenia: avolition and Occam's razor," *Schizophrenia Bulletin*, vol. 36, no. 2, pp. 359–369, 2010.

[359] S. M. Stahl and P. F. Buckley, "Negative symptoms of schizophrenia: a problem that will not go away," *Acta Psychiatrica Scandinavica*, vol. 115, no. 1, pp. 4–11, 2007.

[360] W. Löffler and H. Häfner, "Dimensionen der schizophrenen Symptomatik. Vergleichende Modellprüfung an einem Erstepisodensample," *Der Nervenarzt*, vol. 70, no. 5, pp. 416–429, 1999 (German).

[361] S. R. Kay and S. Sevy, "Pyramidical model of schizophrenia," *Schizophrenia Bulletin*, vol. 16, no. 3, pp. 537–545, 1990.

[362] A. Arora, A. Avasthi, and P. Kulhara, "Subsyndromes of chronic schizophrenia: a phenomenological study," *Acta Psychiatrica Scandinavica*, vol. 96, no. 3, pp. 225–229, 1997.

[363] L. Davidson and T. H. McGlashan, "The varied outcomes of schizophrenia," *Canadian Journal of Psychiatry*, vol. 42, no. 1, pp. 34–43, 1997.

[364] R. K. R. Salokangas, "Structure of schizophrenic symptomatology and its changes over time: prospective factor-analytical study," *Acta Psychiatrica Scandinavica*, vol. 95, no. 1, pp. 32–39, 1997.

[365] L. White, P. D. Harvey, L. Opler, and J. P. Lindenmayer, "Empirical assessment of the factorial structure of clinical symptoms in schizophrenia. A multisite, multimodel evaluation of the factorial structure of the positive and negative syndrome scale. The PANSS Study Group," *Psychopathology*, vol. 30, no. 5, pp. 263–274, 1997.

[366] D. Freeman, "Cognitive and social processes in psychosis: recent developments," in *Advances in Schizophrenia Research 2009*, W. F. Gattaz and G. Busatto, Eds., pp. 283–298, Springer, New York, NY, USA, 2010.

[367] I. Myin-Germeys, M. Birchwood, and T. Kwapil, "From environment to therapy in psychosis: a real-world momentary assessment approach," *Schizophrenia Bulletin*, vol. 37, no. 2, pp. 244–247, 2011.

[368] J. J. Blanchard, M. Aghevli, A. Wilson, and M. Sargeant, "Developmental instability in social anhedonia: an examination of minor physical anomalies and clinical characteristics," *Schizophrenia Research*, vol. 118, no. 1–3, pp. 162–167, 2010.

[369] T. Laughren and R. Levin, "Food and drug administration commentary on methodological issues in negative symptom trials," *Schizophrenia Bulletin*, vol. 37, no. 2, pp. 255–256, 2011.

[370] P. D. Harvey, D. Koren, A. Reichenberg, and C. R. Bowie, "Negative symptoms and cognitive deficits: what is the nature of their relationship?" *Schizophrenia Bulletin*, vol. 32, no. 2, pp. 250–258, 2006.

[371] K. H. Nuechterlein, M. F. Green, and R. S. Kern, "Schizophrenia as a cognitive disorder. Recent approaches to identifying its core cognitive components to aid treatment development," in *Advances in Schizophrenia Research 2009*, W. F. Gattaz and G. Busatto, Eds., pp. 267–282, Springer, New York, NY, USA, 2010.

[372] T. E. Goldberg, A. David, and J. M. Gold, "Neurocognitive impairments in schizophrenia: their character and role in symptom formation," in *Schizophrenia*, D. R. Weinberger and P. J. Harrison, Eds., pp. 142–162, Wiley-Blackwell, Oxford, UK, 3rd edition, 2011.

[373] R. S. E. Keefe, "Should cognitive impairment be included in the diagnostic criteria for schizophrenia?" *World Psychiatry*, vol. 7, no. 1, pp. 22–28, 2008.

[374] American Psychiatric Association, *Diagnostic and Statistical Manual of Mental Disorders (DSM-5)*, American Psychiatric Publishing, Washington, DC, USA, 5th edition, 2013.

[375] J. M. Kane and T. Lencz, "Cognitive deficits in schizophrenia: short-term and long-term," *World Psychiatry*, vol. 7, no. 13, pp. 29–30, 2008.

[376] A. Simning, Y. Conwell, and E. van Wijngaarden, "Cognitive impairment in public housing residents living in Western New York," *Social Psychiatry and Psychiatric Epidemiology*, vol. 49, no. 3, pp. 477–485, 2014.

[377] S. R. Marder, D. G. Daniel, L. Alphs, A. G. Awad, and R. S. E. Keefe, "Methodological issues in negative symptom trials," *Schizophrenia Bulletin*, vol. 37, no. 2, pp. 250–254, 2011.

[378] J. M. Gold, "Cognitive deficits as treatment targets in Schizophrenia," *Schizophrenia Research*, vol. 72, no. 1, pp. 21–28, 2004.

[379] S. E. Hyman and W. S. Fenton, "Medicine: what are the right targets for psychopharmacology?" *Science*, vol. 299, no. 5605, pp. 350–351, 2003.

[380] W. Wölwer, N. Frommann, S. Halfmann, A. Piaszek, M. Streit, and W. Gaebel, "Remediation of impairments in facial affect recognition in schizophrenia: Efficacy and specificity of a new training program," *Schizophrenia Research*, vol. 80, no. 2-3, pp. 295–303, 2005.

[381] D. N. Allen, G. P. Strauss, B. Donohue, and D. P. van Kammen, "Factor analytic support for social cognition as a separable

cognitive domain in schizophrenia," *Schizophrenia Research*, vol. 93, no. 1–3, pp. 325–333, 2007.

[382] M. F. Green, D. L. Penn, R. Bentall et al., "Social cognition in schizophrenia: an NIMH workshop on definitions, assessment, and research opportunities," *Schizophrenia Bulletin*, vol. 34, no. 6, pp. 1211–1220, 2008.

[383] W. P. Horan, R. S. Kern, K. Shokat-Fadai, M. J. Sergi, J. K. Wynn, and M. F. Green, "Social cognitive skills training in schizophrenia: an initial efficacy study of stabilized outpatients," *Schizophrenia Research*, vol. 107, no. 1, pp. 47–54, 2009.

[384] W. Gaebel, W. Wölwer, M. Riesbeck, and J. Zilasek, "The cross-sectional and longitudinal architecture of schizophrenia: significance for diagnosis and intervention," in *Advances in Schizophrenia Research 2009*, W. F. Gattaz and G. Busatto, Eds., pp. 317–330, Springer, New York, NY, USA, 2010.

[385] G. Fervaha, G. Foussias, O. Agid, and G. Remington, "Impact of primary negative symptoms on functional outcomes in schizophrenia," *European Psychiatry*, 2014.

[386] R. Bottlender, T. Sato, M. Jäger et al., "Does considering duration of negative symptoms increase their specificity for schizophrenia?" *Schizophrenia Research*, vol. 60, no. 2-3, pp. 321–322, 2003.

[387] A. K. Malla, R. M. G. Norman, J. Takhar et al., "Can patients at risk for persistent negative symptoms be identified during their first episode of psychosis?" *Journal of Nervous and Mental Disease*, vol. 192, no. 7, pp. 455–463, 2004.

[388] H. Häfner, W. an der Heiden, and K. Maurer, "Evidence for separate diseases? Stages of one disease or different combinations of symptom dimensions?" *European Archives of Psychiatry and Clinical Neuroscience*, vol. 258, no. 2, pp. 85–96, 2008.

[389] J. Mäkinen, J. Miettunen, M. Isohanni, and H. Koponen, "Negative symptoms in schizophrenia: a review," *Nordic Journal of Psychiatry*, vol. 62, no. 5, pp. 334–341, 2008.

[390] J. A. Husted, M. Beiser, and W. G. Iacono, "Negative symptoms and the early course of schizophrenia," *Psychiatry Research*, vol. 43, no. 3, pp. 215–222, 1992.

[391] W. an der Heiden, R. Könnecke, K. Maurer, D. Ropeter, and H. Häfner, "Depression in the long-term course of schizophrenia," *European Archives of Psychiatry and Clinical Neuroscience*, vol. 255, no. 3, pp. 174–184, 2005.

[392] W. an der Heiden and H. Häfner, "Course and outcome," in *Schizophrenia*, D. R. Weinberger and P. J. Harrison, Eds., pp. 104–141, Wiley-Blackwell, Oxford, UK, 3rd edition, 2011.

[393] M. F. Pogue-Geile and J. Zubin, "Negative symptomatology and schizophrenia: a conceptual and empirical review," *International Journal of Mental Health*, vol. 16, no. 4, pp. 3–45, 1988.

[394] J. M. Gold and M. F. Green, "Neurocognition in schizophrenia," in *Kaplan & Sadocks Comprehensive Textbook of Psychiatry*, B. J. Sadock and V. A. Sadock, Eds., vol. 8, Baltimore, Md, USA, pp. 1436–1448, Kaplan Lippincott, Williams & Williams, 2005.

[395] G. P. Strauss, D. N. Allen, P. Miski, R. W. Buchanan, B. Kirkpatrick, and W. T. Carpenter, "Differential patterns of premorbid social and academic deterioration in deficit and nondeficit schizophrenia," *Schizophrenia Research*, vol. 135, no. 1–3, pp. 134–138, 2012.

[396] H. Häfner, K. Maurer, and W. an der Heiden, "ABC Schizophrenia study: an overview of results since 1996," *Social Psychiatry and Psychiatric Epidemiology*, vol. 48, no. 7, pp. 1021–1031, 2013.

[397] V. A. Morgan, J. J. McGrath, A. Jablensky et al., "Psychosis prevalence and physical, metabolic and cognitive co-morbidity: data from the second Australian national survey of psychosis," *Psychological Medicine*, vol. 23, pp. 1–14, 2013.

[398] J. J. Blanchard, A. M. Kring, W. P. Horan, and R. Gur, "Toward the next generation of negative symptom assessments: The collaboration to advance negative symptom assessment in schizophrenia," *Schizophrenia Bulletin*, vol. 37, no. 2, pp. 291–299, 2011.

[399] L. Schwarz, T. P. Roskos, and G. T. Grossberg, "Answers to 7 questions about using neuropsychological testing in your practice," *Current Psychiatry*, vol. 13, pp. 33–39, 2014.

[400] K. H. Nuechterlein, R. E. Asarnow, K. L. Subotnik et al., "Neurocognitive vulnerability factors for schizophrenia: convergence across genetic risk studies and longitudinal trait/state studies," in *Origins and Development of Schizophrenia: Advances in Experimental Psychopathology*, M. F. Lenzenweger and R. H. Dworkin, Eds., pp. 299–327, American Psychological Association, Washington, DC, USA, 1998.

[401] R. E. Gur, M. E. Calkins, R. C. Gur et al., "The consortium on the genetics of schizophrenia: neurocognitive endophenotypes," *Schizophrenia Bulletin*, vol. 33, no. 1, pp. 49–68, 2007.

[402] B. E. Snitz, A. W. MacDonald III, and C. S. Carter, "Cognitive deficits in unaffected first-degree relatives of schizophrenia patients: a meta-analytic review of putative endophenotypes," *Schizophrenia Bulletin*, vol. 32, no. 1, pp. 179–194, 2006.

[403] A. L. Hoff, M. Sakuma, M. Wieneke, R. Horon, M. Kushner, and L. E. DeLisi, "Longitudinal neuropsychological follow-up study of patients with first-episode schizophrenia," *The American Journal of Psychiatry*, vol. 156, no. 9, pp. 1336–1341, 1999.

[404] A. Reichenberg, M. Weiser, M. A. Rapp et al., "Premorbid intra-individual variability in intellectual performance and risk for schizophrenia: a population-based study," *Schizophrenia Research*, vol. 85, no. 1-3, pp. 49–57, 2006.

[405] A. Reichenberg, P. D. Harvey, C. R. Bowie et al., "Neuropsychological function and dysfunction in schizophrenia and psychotic affective disorders," *Schizophrenia Bulletin*, vol. 35, no. 5, pp. 1022–1029, 2009.

[406] M. Albus, W. Hubmann, J. Scherer et al., "A prospective 2-year follow-up study of neurocognitive functioning in patients with first-episode schizophrenia," *European Archives of Psychiatry and Clinical Neuroscience*, vol. 252, no. 6, pp. 262–267, 2002.

[407] K. Maurer and H. Häfner, "Negativsymptomatik im Frühverlauf der Schizophrenie und im Verlauf über drei Jahre nach Ersthospitalisation," in *Befunderhebung in der Psychiatrie: Lebensqualität, Negativsymptomatik und andere aktuelle Entwicklungen*, H.-J. Möller, R. R. Engel, and P. Hoff, Eds., pp. 225–240, Springer, Vienna, Austria, 1996, (German).

[408] P. D. Harvey, E. Howanitz, M. Parrella et al., "Symptoms, cognitive functioning, and adaptive skills in geriatric patients with lifelong schizophrenia: a comparison across treatment sites," *The American Journal of Psychiatry*, vol. 155, no. 8, pp. 1080–1086, 1998.

[409] P. D. Harvey, M. Parrella, L. White, R. C. Mohs, M. Davidson, and K. L. Davis, "Convergence of cognitive and adaptive decline in late-life schizophrenia," *Schizophrenia Research*, vol. 35, no. 1, pp. 77–84, 1999.

[410] D. M. Barch, J. Bustillo, W. Gaebel et al., "Logic and justification for dimensional assessment of symptoms and related clinical phenomena in psychosis: relevance to DSM-5," *Schizophrenia Research*, vol. 150, no. 1, pp. 20–25, 2013.

[411] W. T. Carpenter Jr., D. W. Heinrichs, and A. M. I. Wagman, "Deficit and nondeficit forms of schizophrenia: the concept," *The American Journal of Psychiatry*, vol. 145, no. 5, pp. 578–583, 1988.

[412] A. Marneros, N. C. Andreasen, and M. T. Tsuang, Eds., *Negative versus Positive Schizophrenia*, Springer, Berlin, Germany, 1991.

[413] W. T. Carpenter, R. W. Buchanan, B. Kirkpatrick, G. Thaker, and C. Tamminga, "Negative symptoms: a critique of current approaches," in *Negative Versus Positive Schizophrenia*, A. Marneros, N. C. Andreasen, and M. T. Tsuang, Eds., pp. 126–133, Springer, Berlin, Germany, 1991.

[414] B. Kirkpatrick and S. Galderisi, "Deficit schizophrenia: an update," *World Psychiatry*, vol. 7, no. 3, pp. 143–147, 2008.

[415] W. T. Carpenter Jr. and B. Kirkpatrick, "The heterogeneity of the long-term course of schizophrenia," *Schizophrenia Bulletin*, vol. 14, no. 4, pp. 645–652, 1988.

[416] J. K. Wing and G. W. Brown, *Institutionalism and Schizophrenia. A Comparative Study of Three Mental Hospitals 1960-1968*, Cambridge University Press, Cambridge, UK, 1970.

[417] W. W. Eaton, R. Thara, B. Federman, B. Melton, and K. Y. Liang, "Structure and course of positive and negative symptoms in schizophrenia," *Archives of General Psychiatry*, vol. 52, no. 2, pp. 127–134, 1995.

[418] E. S. Herbener and M. Harrow, "Longitudinal assessment of negative symptoms in schizophrenia/schizoaffective patients, other psychotic patients, and depressed patients," *Schizophrenia Bulletin*, vol. 27, no. 3, pp. 527–537, 2001.

[419] R. M. Murray and S. W. Lewis, "Is schizophrenia a neurodevelopmental disorder?" *British Medical Journal*, vol. 295, no. 6600, pp. 681–682, 1987.

[420] D. R. Weinberger, "Schizophrenia as a neurodevelopmental disorder," in *Schizophrenia*, S. R. Hirsch and D. R. Weinberger, Eds., pp. 293–323, Blackwell, Oxford, UK, 1995.

[421] T. H. McGlashan and R. E. Hoffman, "Schizophrenia as a disorder of developmentally reduced synaptic connectivity," *Archives of General Psychiatry*, vol. 57, no. 7, pp. 637–648, 2000.

[422] M. V. Zanetti, M. S. Schaufelberger, and J. A. S. Crippa, "Brain anatomical abnormalities in schizophrenia: neurodevelopmental origins and patterns of progression over time," in *Advances in Schizophrenia Research 2009*, W. F. Gattaz and G. Busatto, Eds., pp. 113–148, Springer, New York, NY, USA, 2010.

[423] M. K. Stachowiak, A. Kucinski, R. Curl et al., "Schizophrenia: a neurodevelopmental disorder—integrative genomic hypothesis and therapeutic implications from a transgenic mouse model," *Schizophrenia Research*, vol. 143, no. 2-3, pp. 367–376, 2013.

[424] T. J. Crow, "The two-syndrome concept: origins and current status," *Schizophrenia Bulletin*, vol. 11, no. 3, pp. 471–486, 1985.

[425] T. J. Crow, "Discussion: The genetics of psychosis is the genetics of the speciation of Homo sapiens," in *Search for the Causes of Schizophrenia*, W. F. Gattaz and H. Häfner, Eds., vol. 5, pp. 297–312, Steinkopff, Darmstadt, Germany, 2004.

[426] S. R. Kay, A. Fiszbein, and L. A. Opler, "The positive and negative syndrome scale (PANSS) for schizophrenia," *Schizophrenia Bulletin*, vol. 13, no. 2, pp. 261–276, 1987.

[427] B. Kirkpatrick, W. S. Fenton, W. T. Carpenter Jr., and S. R. Marder, "The NIMH-MATRICS consensus statement on negative symptoms," *Schizophrenia Bulletin*, vol. 32, no. 2, pp. 214–219, 2006.

[428] C. Forbes, J. J. Blanchard, M. Bennett, W. P. Horan, A. Kring, and R. Gur, "Initial development and preliminary validation of a new negative symptom measure: the Clinical Assessment Interview for Negative Symptoms (CAINS)," *Schizophrenia Research*, vol. 124, no. 1-3, pp. 36–42, 2010.

[429] S. R. Marder and B. Kirkpatrick, "Defining and measuring negative symptoms of schizophrenia in clinical trials," *European Neuropsychopharmacology*, vol. 24, no. 5, pp. 737–743, 2014.

[430] W. S. Fenton and T. H. McGlashan, "Natural history of schizophrenia subtypes: II. Positive and negative symptoms and long-term course," *Archives of General Psychiatry*, vol. 48, no. 11, pp. 978–986, 1991.

[431] T. E. Goldberg, T. M. Hyde, J. E. Kleinman, and D. R. Weinberger, "Course of schizophrenia: neuropsychological evidence for a static encephalopathy," *Schizophrenia Bulletin*, vol. 19, no. 4, pp. 797–804, 1993.

[432] T. W. Weickert and T. E. Goldberg, "Neuropsychologie der Schizophrenie," in *Psychiatrie der Gegenwart*, H. Helmchen, F. Henn, H. Lauter et al., Eds., vol. 5, pp. 163–180, Springer, New York, NY, USA, 4th edition, 2000, (German).

[433] C. L. Marvel and S. Paradiso, "Cognitive and neurological impairment in mood disorders," *Psychiatric Clinics of North America*, vol. 27, no. 1, pp. 19–36, 2004.

[434] S. H. Sullivan, "The onset of schizophrenia," *The American Journal of Psychiatry*, vol. 6, pp. 105–134, 1927.

[435] D. E. Cameron, "Early schizophrenia," *The American Journal of Psychiatry*, vol. 95, pp. 567–578, 1938.

[436] K. Conrad, *Die beginnende Schizophrenie. Versuch einer Gestaltanalyse des Wahns*, Thieme-Verlag, Stuttgart, Germany, 1958 (German).

[437] J. P. Docherty, D. P. van Kammen, S. G. Siris, and S. R. Marder, "Stages of onset of schizophrenic psychosis," *The American Journal of Psychiatry*, vol. 135, no. 4, pp. 420–426, 1978.

[438] M. Hambrecht and H. Häfner, ""Trema, Apophänie, Apokalypse"—Ist Conrads Phasenmodell empirisch begründbar?" *Fortschritte der Neurologie Psychiatrie*, vol. 61, no. 12, pp. 418–423, 1993 (German).

[439] F. Schultze-Lutter, W. Löffler, and H. Häfner, "Testing models of the early course of schizophrenia," in *Risk and Protective Factors in Schizophrenia*, H. Häfner, Ed., pp. 229–241, Steinkopff, Darmstadt, Germany, 2002.

[440] P. D. McGorry, J. Edwards, C. Mihalopoulos, S. M. Harrigan, and H. J. Jackson, "EPPIC: an evolving system of early detection and optimal management," *Schizophrenia Bulletin*, vol. 22, no. 2, pp. 305–326, 1996.

[441] P. D. McGorry, A. R. Yung, and L. J. Phillips, "The "close-in" or ultra high-risk model: a safe and effective strategy for research and clinical intervention in prepsychotic mental disorder," *Schizophrenia Bulletin*, vol. 29, no. 4, pp. 771–790, 2003.

[442] A. R. Yung, L. J. Phillips, and P. McGorry, *Treating Schizophrenia in the Prodromal Phase*, Taylor & Francis, London, UK, 2004.

[443] A. R. Yung, H. P. Yuen, P. D. McGorry et al., "Mapping the onset of psychosis: the comprehensive assessment of at-risk mental states," *Australian & New Zealand Journal of Psychiatry*, vol. 39, no. 11-12, pp. 964–971, 2005.

[444] H. Häfner, K. Maurer, W. Löffler et al., "Onset and prodromal phase as determinants of the course," in *Search for the Causes of Schizophrenia, Vol. IV: Balance of the Century*, W. F. Gattaz and H. Häfner, Eds., pp. 1–24, Steinkopff, Darmstadt, Germany, 1999.

[445] D. O. Perkins, H. Gu, K. Boteva, and J. A. Lieberman, "Relationship between duration of untreated psychosis and outcome in first-episode schizophrenia: a critical review and meta-analysis," *The American Journal of Psychiatry*, vol. 162, no. 10, pp. 1785–1804, 2005.

[446] F. Schultze-Lutter, S. Ruhrmann, H. Picker, H. G. von Reventlow, A. Brockhaus-Dumke, and J. Klosterkötter, "Basic symptoms in early psychotic and depressive disorders," *The British Journal of Psychiatry*, vol. 191, no. 51, supplement, pp. s31–s37, 2007.

[447] F. Schultze-Lutter, S. Ruhrmann, J. Berning, W. Maier, and J. Klosterkötter, "Basic symptoms and ultrahigh risk criteria: symptom development in the initial prodromal state," *Schizophrenia Bulletin*, vol. 36, no. 1, pp. 182–191, 2010.

[448] F. Schultze-Lutter, J. Klosterkötter, and S. Ruhrmann, "Improving the clinical prediction of psychosis by combining ultrahigh risk criteria and cognitive basic symptoms," *Schizophrenia Research*, vol. 154, no. 1–3, pp. 100–106, 2014.

[449] R. K. R. Salokangas and T. McGlashan, "Early detection and intervention of psychosis. A review," *Nordic Journal of Psychiatry*, vol. 62, no. 2, pp. 92–105, 2008.

[450] J. Rietdijk, S. J. Hogerzeil, A. M. van Hemert, P. Cuijpers, D. H. Linszen, and M. van der Gaag, "Pathways to psychosis: Help-seeking behavior in the prodromal phase," *Schizophrenia Research*, vol. 132, no. 2-3, pp. 213–219, 2011.

[451] W. Rössler, M. P. Hengartner, V. Ajdacic-Gross, H. Haker, A. Gamma, and J. Angst, "Sub-clinical psychosis symptoms in young adults are risk factors for subsequent common mental disorders," *Schizophrenia Research*, vol. 131, no. 1–3, pp. 18–23, 2011.

[452] J. Addington and R. Heinssen, "Prediction and prevention of psychosis in youth at clinical high risk," *Annual Review of Clinical Psychology*, vol. 8, pp. 269–289, 2012.

[453] H. Häfner, K. Maurer, G. Trendler, W. an der Heiden, M. Schmidt, and R. Könnecke, "Schizophrenia and depression: challenging the paradigm of two separate diseases—a controlled study of schizophrenia, depression and healthy controls," *Schizophrenia Research*, vol. 77, no. 1, pp. 11–24, 2005.

[454] T. H. McGlashan, "Duration of untreated psychosis in first-episode schizophrenia: marker or determinant of course?" *Biological Psychiatry*, vol. 46, no. 7, pp. 899–907, 1999.

[455] R. M. G. Norman and A. K. Malla, "Duration of untreated psychosis: a critical examination of the concept and its importance," *Psychological Medicine*, vol. 31, no. 3, pp. 381–400, 2001.

[456] E. C. Johnstone, T. J. Crow, A. L. Johnson, and J. F. MacMillan, "The Northwick Park study of first episodes of schizophrenia. I. Presentation of the illness and problems relating to admission," *The British Journal of Psychiatry*, vol. 148, pp. 115–120, 1986.

[457] J. P. McEvoy, N. R. Schooler, and W. H. Wilson, "Predictors of therapeutic response to haloperidol in acute schizophrenia," *Psychopharmacology Bulletin*, vol. 27, no. 2, pp. 97–101, 1991.

[458] M. Birchwood and F. Macmillan, "Early intervention in schizophrenia," *Australian & New Zealand Journal of Psychiatry*, vol. 27, no. 3, pp. 374–378, 1993.

[459] A. D. Loebel, J. A. Lieberman, J. M. J. Alvir, D. I. Mayerhoff, S. H. Geisler, and S. R. Szymanski, "Duration of psychosis and outcome in first-episode schizophrenia," *The American Journal of Psychiatry*, vol. 149, no. 9, pp. 1183–1188, 1992.

[460] D. Linszen, M. Lenior, L. De Haan, P. Dingemans, and B. Gersons, "Early intervention, untreated psychosis and the course of early schizophrenia," *The British Journal of Psychiatry*, vol. 172, no. 33, pp. 84–89, 1998.

[461] H. Häfner and K. Maurer, "Early detection of schizophrenia: current evidence and future perspectives," *World Psychiatry*, vol. 5, pp. 130–138, 2006.

[462] A. C. Altamura, R. Bassetti, F. Sassella, D. Salvadori, and E. Mundo, "Duration of untreated psychosis as a predictor of outcome in first-episode schizophrenia: a retrospective study," *Schizophrenia Research*, vol. 52, no. 1-2, pp. 29–36, 2001.

[463] A. R. Yung, E. J. Kollackey, B. Nelson, and P. McGorry, "The impact of early intervention in schizophrenia," in *Advances in Schizophrenia Research 2009*, W. F. Gattaz and G. Busatto, Eds., pp. 299–316, Springer, New York, NY, USA, 2010.

[464] C. Rapp, E. Studerus, H. Bugra et al., "Duration of untreated psychosis and cognitive functioning," *Schizophrenia Research*, vol. 145, no. 1–3, pp. 43–49, 2013.

[465] R. J. Wyat, "Neuroleptics and the natural course of schizophrenia," *Schizophrenia Bulletin*, vol. 17, no. 2, pp. 325–351, 1991.

[466] R. J. Wyatt, "Early intervention with neuroleptics may decrease the long-term morbidity of schizophrenia," *Schizophrenia Research*, vol. 5, no. 3, pp. 201–202, 1991.

[467] J. A. Lieberman, B. B. Sheitman, and B. J. Kinon, "Neurochemical sensitization in the pathophysiology of schizophrenia: deficits and dysfunction in neuronal regulation and plasticity," *Neuropsychopharmacology*, vol. 17, no. 4, pp. 205–229, 1997.

[468] J. A. Lieberman, G. Tollefson, and M. Tohen, "Comparative efficacy and safety of atypical and coventional antipsychotic drugs in first-episode psychosis: a randomized, double-blind trial of olanzapine versus haloperidol," *The American Journal of Psychiatry*, vol. 160, pp. 1396–1404, 2003.

[469] R. J. Wyatt and I. D. Henter, "The effects of early and sustained intervention on the long-term morbidity of schizophrenia," *Journal of Psychiatric Research*, vol. 32, no. 3-4, pp. 169–177, 1998.

[470] N. Tandon, J. Shah, M. S. Keshavan, and R. Tandon, "Attenuated psychosis and the schizophrenia prodrome: current status of risk identification and psychosis prevention," *Neuropsychiatry*, vol. 2, pp. 345–353, 2012.

[471] M. T. Tsuang, J. van Os, R. Tandon et al., "Attenuated psychosis syndrome in DSM-5," *Schizophrenia Research*, vol. 150, pp. 31–35, 2013.

[472] J. O. Johannessen, T. K. Larsen, M. Horneland et al., "The TIPS Project. A systematized program ro reduce duration of untreated psychosis in first episode psychosis," in *Early Intervention in Psychotic Disorders*, T. Miller, S. A. Mednick, T. H. McGlashan, J. Libiger, and J. O. Johannessen, Eds., pp. 151–166, Kluwer Academic Pubishers, Dordrecht, The Netherlands, 2001.

[473] P. McGorry, "A stitch in time . . . the scope for preventive strategies in early psychosis," in *The Recognition and Management of Early Psychosis*, P. D. McGorry and H. J. Jackson, Eds., pp. 3–23, Cambridge University Press, Cambridge, UK, 1999.

[474] P. D. McGorry, A. R. Yung, L. J. Phillips et al., "Randomized controlled trial of interventions designed to reduce the risk of progression to first-episode psychosis in a clinical sample with subthreshold symptoms," *Archives of General Psychiatry*, vol. 59, no. 10, pp. 921–928, 2002.

[475] S. Ruhrmann, K. U. Kühn, M. Streit, R. Bottlender, W. Maier, and J. Klosterkötter, "Pharmakologische und psychologische Frühintervention bei Risikopersonen mit psychosenahen Prodromen: erste Ergebnisse einer kontrollierten Studie," *Nervenarz*, vol. 73, no. 1, p. 9, 2002 (German).

[476] T. H. McGlashan, R. B. Zipursky, D. Perkins et al., "The PRIME North America randomized double-blind clinical trial of olanzapine versus placebo in patients at risk of being prodromally symptomatic for psychosis: I. Study rationale and design," *Schizophrenia Research*, vol. 61, no. 1, pp. 7–18, 2003.

[477] J. Klosterkötter, "Prävention psychotischer Störungen," *Nervenarzt*, vol. 84, pp. 1299–1309, 2013 (German).

[478] M. Hambrecht, M. Wagner, A. Bechdolf, S. Maier, and C. Schröder, *Psychologische Frühintervention bei Risikopersonen/ Personen mit psychosefernen Prodromen. Manual für die Durchführung der Studieninterventionen im Projekt 1.1.2 des Kompetenznetz Schizophrenie*, (KNS-Zentrale, Rheinische Landes- und

Hochschulklinik Düsseldorf, Postfach 12 05 10, D-40605 Düs-s eldorf), 2000 (German).

[479] S. Lewis, N. Tarrier, G. Haddock et al., "Randomised controlled trial of cognitive-behavioural therapy in early schizophrenia: acute-phase outcomes," *The British Journal of Psychiatry*, vol. 181, no. 43, pp. s91–s97, 2002.

[480] V. Bird, P. Premkumar, T. Kendall, C. Whittington, J. Mitchell, and E. Kuipers, "Early intervention services, cognitive-behavioural therapy and family intervention in early psychosis: systematic review," *The British Journal of Psychiatry*, vol. 197, no. 5, pp. 350–356, 2010.

[481] G. Lee, C. Barrowclough, and F. Lobban, "Positive affect in the family environment protects against relapse in first-episode psychosis," *Social Psychiatry and Psychiatric Epidemiology*, vol. 49, no. 3, pp. 367–376, 2014.

[482] A. Bechdolf, D. Köhn, B. Knost, R. Pukrop, and J. Klosterkötter, "A randomized comparison of group cognitive-behavioural therapy and group psychoeducation in acute patients with schizophrenia: outcome at 24 months," *Acta Psychiatrica Scandinavica*, vol. 112, no. 3, pp. 173–179, 2005.

[483] A. Bechdolf, V. Veith, D. Schwarzer et al., "Cognitive-behavioral therapy in the pre-psychotic phase: an exploratory study," *Psychiatry Research*, vol. 136, no. 2-3, pp. 251–255, 2005.

[484] A. P. Morrison, P. French, L. Walford et al., "Cognitive therapy for the prevention of psychosis in people at ultra-high risk: randomised controlled trial," *The British Journal of Psychiatry*, vol. 185, pp. 291–297, 2004.

[485] S. J. Bartels and R. E. Drake, "Depressive symptoms in schizophrenia: comprehensive differential diagnosis," *Comprehensive Psychiatry*, vol. 29, no. 5, pp. 467–483, 1988.

[486] S. G. Siris and C. Bench, "Depression and schizophrenia," in *Schizophrenia*, S. R. Hirsch and D. R. Weinberger, Eds., pp. 142–167, Blackwell Publishing Company, Oxford, UK, 2nd edition, 2003.

[487] H. Häfner, "The early Kraepelin's dichotomy of schizophrenia and affective disorder—evidence for separate diseases?" *European Journal of Psychiary*, vol. 24, no. 2, pp. 98–113, 2010.

[488] E. Kraepelin, *Psychiatrie*, vol. 1–4, Barth, Leipzig, Germany, 8th edition, 1909-1915 (German).

[489] A. Jablensky, H. Hugler, M. von Cranach, and K. Kalinov, "Kraepelin revisited: a reassessment and statistical analysis of dementia praecox and manic-depressive insanity in 1908," *Psychological Medicine*, vol. 23, no. 4, pp. 843–858, 1993.

[490] M. C. Angermeyer and L. Kühn, "Gender differences in age at onset of schizophrenia: an overview," *European Archives of Psychiatry and Neurological Sciences*, vol. 237, no. 6, pp. 351–364, 1988.

[491] R. R. J. Lewine, "Gender and Schizophrenia," in *Handbook of Schizophrenia*, H. A. Nasrallah, Ed., vol. 3, pp. 379–397, Elsevier, Amsterdam, The Netherlands, 1988.

[492] J. M. Goldstein, "The impact of gender on understanding the epidemiology of schizopohrenia," in *Gender and Psychopathology*, M. W. Seeman, Ed., pp. 159–199, American Psychiatric Press, Washington, DC, USA, 1995.

[493] D. J. Castle, "Women and schizophrenia: an epidemiological perspective," in *Women and Schizophrenia*, D. J. Castle, J. McGrath, and J. Kulkarni, Eds., pp. 19–34, Cambridge University Press, Cambridge, UK, 2000.

[494] H. Häfner, A. Riecher-Rössler, W. an der Heiden, K. Maurer, B. Fätkenheuer, and W. Löffler, "Generating and testing a causal explanation of the gender difference in age at first onset of schizophrenia," *Psychological Medicine*, vol. 23, no. 4, pp. 925–940, 1993.

[495] H. Häfner, K. Maurer, W. Löffler et al., "The epidemiology of early schizophrenia. Influence of age and gender on onset and early course," *The British Journal of Psychiatry*, vol. 164, no. 23, pp. 29–38, 1994.

[496] H. Häfner, A. Riecher, K. Maurer, W. Löffler, P. Munk-Jörgensen, and E. Strömgren, "How does gender influence age at first hospitalization for schizophrenia? A transnational case register study," *Psychological Medicine*, vol. 19, no. 4, pp. 903–918, 1989.

[497] S. V. Eranti, J. H. MacCabe, H. Bundy, and R. M. Murray, "Gender difference in age at onset of schizophrenia: a meta-analysis," *Psychological Medicine*, vol. 43, no. 1, pp. 155–167, 2013.

[498] B. N. Gangadhar, C. Panner Selvan, D. K. Subbakrishna, and N. Janakiramaiah, "Age-at-onset and schizophrenia: reversed gender effect," *Acta Psychiatrica Scandinavica*, vol. 105, no. 4, pp. 317–319, 2002.

[499] G. V. S. Murthy, N. Janakiramaiah, B. N. Gangadhar, and D. K. Subbakrishna, "Sex difference in age at onset of schizophrenia: discrepant findings from India," *Acta Psychiatrica Scandinavica*, vol. 97, no. 5, pp. 321–325, 1998.

[500] G. Stöber, E. Franzek, I. Haubitz, B. Pfuhlmann, and H. Beckmann, "Gender differences and age of onset in the catatonic subtypes of schizophrenia," *Psychopathology*, vol. 31, no. 6, pp. 307–312, 1998.

[501] K. Leonhard, *Aufteilung der endogenen Psychosen*, Akademie-Verlag, Berlin, Germany, 5th edition, 1980 (German).

[502] M. Hambrecht, K. Maurer, H. Häfner, and N. Sartorius, "Transnational stability of gender differences in schizophrenia? An analysis based on the WHO study on determinants of outcome of severe mental disorders," *European Archives of Psychiatry and Clinical Neuroscience*, vol. 242, no. 1, pp. 6–12, 1992.

[503] M. Hambrecht, K. Maurer, and H. Häfner, "Gender differences in schizophrenia in three cultures. Results of the WHO collaborative study on psychiatric disability," *Social Psychiatry and Psychiatric Epidemiology*, vol. 27, no. 3, pp. 117–121, 1992.

[504] S. O. Moldin, "Gender and schizophrenia," in *Gender and Its Effects on Psychopathology*, E. Frank, Ed., pp. 169–186, American Psychiatric Press, Washington, DC, USA, 2000.

[505] S. V. Faraone, W. J. Chen, J. M. Goldstein, and M. T. Tsuang, "Gender differences in age at onset of schizophrenia," *The British Journal of Psychiatry*, vol. 164, pp. 625–629, 1994.

[506] W. F. Gattaz, S. Behrens, J. de Vry, and H. Häfner, "Estradiol inhibits dopamine mediated behavior in rats—an animal model of sex-specific differences in schizophrenia," *Fortschritte der Neurologie Psychiatrie*, vol. 60, pp. 8–16, 1992.

[507] H. Häfner, S. Behrens, J. De Vry, and W. F. Gattaz, "An animal model for the effects of estradiol on dopamine-mediated behavior: implications for sex differences in schizophrenia," *Psychiatry Research*, vol. 38, no. 2, pp. 125–134, 1991.

[508] M. Laruelle, A. Abi-Dargham, C. H. van Dyck et al., "Single photon emission computerized tomography imaging of amphetamine-induced dopamine release in drug-free schizophrenic subjects," *Proceedings of the National Academy of Sciences of the United States of America*, vol. 93, no. 17, pp. 9235–9240, 1996.

[509] A. Breier, T. P. Su, R. Saunders et al., "Schizophrenia is associated with elevated amphetamine-induced synaptic dopamine concentrations: Evidence from a novel positron emission tomography method," *Proceedings of the National Academy of Sciences of the United States of America*, vol. 94, no. 6, pp. 2569–2574, 1997.

[510] A. Abi-Dargham, R. Gil, J. Krystal et al., "Increased striatal dopamine transmission in schizophrenia: confirmation in a second cohort," *The American Journal of Psychiatry*, vol. 155, no. 6, pp. 761–767, 1998.

[511] L. H. Lindström, O. Gefvert, G. Hagberg et al., "Increased dopamine synthesis rate in medial prefrontal cortex and striatum in schizophrenia indicated by L-(β-11C) DOPA and PET," *Biological Psychiatry*, vol. 46, no. 5, pp. 681–688, 1999.

[512] S. Kapur and D. Mamo, "Half a century of antipsychotics and still a central role for dopamine D2 receptors," *Progress in Neuro-Psychopharmacology & Biological Psychiatry*, vol. 27, no. 7, pp. 1081–1090, 2003.

[513] G. J. Lyon, A. Abi-Dargham, H. Moore, J. A. Lieberman, J. A. Javitch, and D. Sulzer, "Presynaptic regulation of dopamine transmission in schizophrenia," *Schizophrenia Bulletin*, vol. 37, no. 1, pp. 108–117, 2011.

[514] D. Eyles, J. Feldon, and U. Meyer, "Schizophrenia: Do all roads lead to dopamine or is this where they start? Evidence from two epidemiologically informed developmental rodent models," *Translational Psychiatry*, vol. 2, article e81, 2012.

[515] J. Kulkarni and G. Fink, "Hormones and psychoses," in *Women and Schizophrenia*, D. J. Castle, J. McGrath, and J. Kulkarni, Eds., pp. 51–66, Cambridge University Press, Cambridge, UK, 2000.

[516] S. Akhondzadeh, A. A. Nejatisafa, H. Amini et al., "Adjunctive estrogen treatment in women with chronic schizophrenia: a double-blind, randomized, and placebo-controlled trial," *Progress in Neuro-Psychopharmacology and Biological Psychiatry*, vol. 27, no. 6, pp. 1007–1012, 2003.

[517] J. Kulkarni, A. De Castella, P. B. Fitzgerald et al., "Estrogen in severe mental illness: a potential new treatment approach," *Archives of General Psychiatry*, vol. 65, no. 8, pp. 955–960, 2008.

[518] J. Kulkarni, E. Gavrilidis, W. Wang et al., "Estradiol for treatment-resistant schizophrenia: a large-scale randomized-controlled trial in women of child-bearing age," *Molecular Psychiatry*, 2014.

[519] L. E. DeLisi, N. Bass, A. Boccio, G. Shields, C. Morganti, and A. Vita, "Age of onset in familial schizophrenia," *Archives of General Psychiatry*, vol. 51, no. 4, pp. 334–335, 1994.

[520] M. Albus and W. Maier, "Lack of gender differences in age at onset in familial schizophrenia," *Schizophrenia Research*, vol. 18, no. 1, pp. 51–59, 1995.

[521] M. Alda, B. Ahrens, W. Lit et al., "Age of onset in familial and sporadic schizophrenia," *Acta Psychiatrica Scandinavica*, vol. 93, no. 6, pp. 447–450, 1996.

[522] R. Könnecke, H. Häfner, K. Maurer, W. Löffler, and W. an der Heiden, "Main risk factors for schizophrenia: increased familial loading and pre- and peri-natal complications antagonize the protective effect of oestrogen in women," *Schizophrenia Research*, vol. 44, no. 1, pp. 81–93, 2000.

[523] R. L. Spitzer, J. Endicott, and E. Robins, *Research Diagnostic Criteria (RDC) for a Selected Group of Functional Disorders*, New York State Psychiatric Institute, New York, NY, USA, 3rd edition, 1977.

[524] J. van Os, R. Howard, N. Takei, and R. Murray, "Increasing age is a risk factor for psychosis in the elderly," *Social Psychiatry and Psychiatric Epidemiology*, vol. 30, no. 4, pp. 161–164, 1995.

[525] D. J. Castle, S. Wessely, J. van Os, and R. M Murray, *Psychosis in the Inner City*, Psychology Press, East Sussex, UK, 1998.

[526] H. Häfner, W. an der Heiden, S. Behrens et al., "Causes and consequences of the gender difference in age at onset of schizophrenia," *Schizophrenia Bulletin*, vol. 24, no. 1, pp. 99–113, 1998.

[527] D. J. Castle, "Preface," in *Women and Schizophrenia*, D. J. Castle, J. McGrath, and J. Kulkarni, Eds., p. 11, Cambridge University Press, Cambridge, UK, 2000.

[528] P. Jörgensen and P. Munk-Jörgensen, "Paranoid psychoses in the elderly," *Acta Psychiatrica Scandinavica*, vol. 72, pp. 358–363, 1985.

[529] D. J. Castle and R. M. Murray, "The epidemiology of late-onset schizophrenia," *Schizophrenia Bulletin*, vol. 19, no. 4, pp. 691–700, 1993.

[530] O. P. Almeida, R. J. Howard, R. Levy, and A. S. David, "Psychotic states arising in late life (Late paraphrenia): psychopathology and nosology," *The British Journal of Psychiatry*, vol. 166, pp. 205–214, 1995.

[531] H. Häfner, W. Löffler, A. Riecher-Rössler, and W. Häfner-Ranabauer, "Schizophrenie und Wahn im höheren und hohen Lebensalter," *Nervenarzt*, vol. 72, pp. 347–357, 2001 (German).

[532] M. Roth, "The natural history of mental disorder in old age," *Journal of Mental Science*, vol. 101, pp. 281–301, 1955.

[533] D. W. K. Kay and M. Roth, "Environmental and hereditary factors in the schizophrenia of old age ("late paraphrenia") and their bearing on the general problem of causation in schizophrenia," *Journal of Mental Science*, vol. 107, pp. 649–686, 1961.

[534] M. J. Harris and D. V. Jeste, "Late-onset schizophrenia: an overview," *Schizophrenia Bulletin*, vol. 14, no. 1, pp. 39–55, 1988.

[535] H. Häfner, M. Hambrecht, W. Löffler, P. Munk-Jørgensen, and A. Riecher-Rössler, "Is schizophrenia a disorder of all ages? A comparison of first episodes and early course across the lifecycle," *Psychological Medicine*, vol. 28, no. 2, pp. 351–365, 1998.

[536] H. Remschmidt, *Schizophrene Erkrankungen im Kindes-und Jugendalter*, Schattauer, Stuttgart, Germany, 2004 (German).

[537] S. Luoma, H. Hakko, T. Ollinen, M. R. Jarvelin, and S. Lindeman, "Association between age at onset and clinical features of schizophrenia," *European Psychiatry*, vol. 23, pp. 331–335, 2008.

[538] C. Eggers, *Schizophrenie des Kindes—und Jugendalters*, MWV Medizinisch Wissenschaftliche Verlagsgesellschaft, Berlin, Germany, 2011, (German).

[539] R. P. Bentall, R. Corcoran, R. Howard, N. Blackwood, and P. Kinderman, "Persecutory delusions: a review and theoretical integration," *Clinical Psychology Review*, vol. 21, no. 8, pp. 1143–1192, 2001.

[540] H. Häfner and W. an der Heiden, "Epidemiology of schizophrenia," *The Canadian Journal of Psychiatry*, vol. 42, no. 2, pp. 139–151, 1997.

[541] T. H. McGlashan, "The Chestnut Lodge follow-up study. I. Follow-up methodology and study sample," *Archives of General Psychiatry*, vol. 41, no. 6, pp. 573–585, 1984.

[542] T. H. McGlashan, "The Chestnut Lodge follow-up study. II. Long-term outcome of schizophrenia and the affective disorders," *Archives of General Psychiatry*, vol. 41, no. 6, pp. 586–601, 1984.

[543] C. M. Harding, G. W. Brooks, T. Ashikaga, J. S. Strauss, and A. Breier, "The Vermont longitudinal study of persons with severe mental illness, I: methodology, study sample, and overall status 32 years later," *The American Journal of Psychiatry*, vol. 144, no. 6, pp. 718–726, 1987.

[544] C. M. Harding, G. W. Brooks, T. Ashikaga, J. S. Strauss, and A. Breier, "The Vermont longitudinal study of persons with severe mental illness. II: long-term outcome of subjects who retrospectively met DSM-III criteria for schizophrenia," *The American Journal of Psychiatry*, vol. 144, no. 6, pp. 727–735, 1987.

[545] W. T. Carpenter Jr. and J. S. Strauss, "The prediction of outcome in schizophrenia IV: eleven-year follow-up of the Washington IPSS cohort," *Journal of Nervous and Mental Disease*, vol. 179, no. 9, pp. 517–525, 1991.

[546] A. Breier, J. L. Schreiber, J. Dyer, and D. Pickar, "National Institute of Mental Health longitudinal study of chronic schizophrenia: prognosis and predictors of outcome," *Archives of General Psychiatry*, vol. 48, no. 3, pp. 239–246, 1991.

[547] J. Leff, N. Sartorius, A. Jablensky, A. Korten, and G. Ernberg, "The International Pilot Study of Schizophrenia: five-year follow-up findings," *Psychological Medicine*, vol. 22, no. 1, pp. 131–145, 1992.

[548] W. an der Heiden, B. Krumm, S. Müller, I. Weber, H. Biehl, and M. Schäfer, "The Mannheim long-term schizophrenia project: initial results on course and outcome 14 years after first admission," *Nervenarzt*, vol. 66, no. 11, pp. 820–827, 1995.

[549] W. an der Heiden, B. Krumm, S. Müller, I. Weber, H. Biehl, and M. Schäfer, "Eine prospektive Studie zum Langzeitverlauf schizophrener Psychosen: Ergebnisse der 14-Jahres-Katamnese," *Zeitschrift für Medizinische Psychologie*, vol. 5, pp. 66–75, 1996 (German).

[550] W. an der Heiden, "Der Langzeitverlauf schizophrener Psychosen—eine Literaturübersicht," *Zeitschrift für Medizinische Psychologie*, vol. 5, pp. 8–21, 1996 (German).

[551] K. Hopper, G. Harrison, A. Janca, and N. Sartorius, *Recovery from Schizophrenia—An International Perspective. A Report from the WHO Collaborative Project, the International Study of Schizophrenia*, Oxford University Press, Oxford, UK, 2007.

[552] E. Jääskeläinen, P. Juola, N. Hirvonen et al., "A systematic review and meta-analysis of recovery in schizophrenia," *Schizophrenia Bulletin*, vol. 39, no. 6, pp. 1296–1306, 2013.

[553] J. Marengo, M. Harrow, J. Sands, and C. Galloway, "European versus U.S. data on the course of schizophrenia," *The American Journal of Psychiatry*, vol. 148, no. 5, pp. 606–611, 1991.

[554] A. Marneros, A. Deister, and A. Rohde, *Affektive, schizoaffektive und schizophrene Psychosen. Eine vergleichende Langzeitstudie*, Springer, Berlin, Germany, 1991 (German).

[555] M. Bleuler, *Die schizophrenen Geistesstörungen im Lichte langjähriger Kranken- und Familiengeschichten*, Thieme, Stuttgart, Germany, 1972, (German).

[556] H. Hinterhuber, "Zur Katamnese der Schizophrenien," *Fortschritte der Neurologie Psychiatrie*, vol. 41, no. 10, pp. 527–558, 1973 (German).

[557] L. Ciompi and C. H. Müller, *Lebensweg und Alter der Schizophrenen. Eine katamnestische Langzeitstudie bis ins Senium*, vol. 12 of *Monographien aus dem Gesamtgebiet der Psychiatrie*, Springer, Berlin, Germany, 1976, (German).

[558] G. Huber, G. Gross, and R. Schüttler, *Schizophrenie. Eine Verlaufs- und sozialpsychiatrische Langzeitstudie*, Springer, Berlin, Germany, 1979 (German).

[559] H. Häfner and W. an der Heiden, "The course of schizophrenia in the light of modern follow-up studies: the ABC and WHO studies," *European Archives of Psychiatry and Clinical Neuroscience*, vol. 249, supplement 4, pp. IV14–IV26, 1999.

[560] N. Sartorius, W. Gulbinat, G. Harrison, E. Laska, and C. Siegel, "Long-term follow up of schizophrenia in 16 countries: a description of the International Study of Schizophrenia conducted by the World Health Organization," *Social Psychiatry and Psychiatric Epidemiology*, vol. 31, no. 5, pp. 249–258, 1996.

[561] P. Mason, G. Harrison, C. Glazebrook, I. Medley, and T. Croudace, "The course of schizophrenia over 13 years: a report from the International Study on Schizophrenia (ISoS) coordinated by the World Health Organization," *The British Journal of Psychiatry*, vol. 169, no. 5, pp. 580–586, 1996.

[562] D. Wiersma, F. J. Nienhuis, C. J. Slooff, and R. Giel, "Natural course of schizophrenic disorders: a 15-year followup of a Dutch incidence cohort," *Schizophrenia Bulletin*, vol. 24, no. 1, pp. 75–85, 1998.

[563] N. Sartorius, A. Jablensky, A. Korten et al., "Early manifestations and first-contact incidence of schizophrenia in different cultures," *Psychological Medicine*, vol. 16, no. 4, pp. 909–928, 1986.

[564] G. Harrison, K. Hopper, T. Craig et al., "Recovery from psychotic illness: a 15- and 25-year international follow-up study," *The British Journal of Psychiatry*, vol. 178, pp. 506–517, 2001.

[565] N. M. Menezes, T. Arenovich, and R. B. Zipursky, "A systematic review of longitudinal outcome studies of first-episode psychosis," *Psychological Medicine*, vol. 36, no. 10, pp. 1349–1362, 2006.

[566] H. Häfner, W. Löffler, K. Maurer, A. Riecher-Rössler, and A. Stein, *Interview für die retrospektive Erfassung des Erkrankungsbeginns und -verlaufs bei Schizophrenie und anderen Psychosen*, Huber, Bern, Switzerland, 1999 (German).

[567] H. Häfner, W. Löffler, K. Maurer, A. Riecher-Rössler, and A. Stein, *IRAOS—Interview for the Retrospective Assessment of the Onset and Course of Schizophrenia and Other Psychoses*, Hogrefe & Huber, Göttingen, Germany, 2003.

[568] A. Jablensky, "The epidemiological horizon," in *Schizophrenia*, S. R. Hirsch and D. Weinberger, Eds., pp. 203–231, Blackwell, Oxford, UK, 2nd edition, 2003.

[569] R. A. Bressan, A. C. Chaves, L. S. Pilowsky, I. Shirakawa, and J. J. Mari, "Depressive episodes in stable schizophrenia: critical evaluation of the DSM-IV and ICD-10 diagnostic criteria," *Psychiatry Research*, vol. 117, no. 1, pp. 47–56, 2003.

[570] C. M. Harding, "Course types in schizophrenia: an analysis of European and American studies," *Schizophrenia Bulletin*, vol. 14, no. 4, pp. 633–643, 1988.

[571] H. Häfner and W. an der Heiden, "Course and outcome of schizophrenia," in *Schizophrenia*, S. R. Hirsch and D. Weinberger, Eds., pp. 124–147, Blackwell Science, Oxford, UK, 2nd edition, 2003.

[572] M. Shepherd, D. Watt, I. Falloon, and N. Smeeton, *The Natural History of Schizophrenia: A Five-Year Follow-up Study of Outcome and Prediction in a Representative Sample of Schizophrenics*, Psychological Medicine Monograph, supplement 15, Cambridge University Press, London, UK, 1989.

[573] J. W. Newcomer and S. Leucht, "Metabolic adverse effects associated with antipsychotic medications," in *Schizophrenia*, D. R. Weinberger and P. J. Harrison, Eds., pp. 577–598, Wiley-Blackwell, Oxford, UK, 3rd edition, 2011.

[574] S. Brown, "Excess mortality of schizophrenia. A meta-analysis," *The British Journal of Psychiatry*, vol. 171, pp. 502–508, 1997.

[575] S. Brown, M. Kim, C. Mitchell, and H. Inskip, "Twenty-five year mortality of a community cohort with schizophrenia," *The British Journal of Psychiatry*, vol. 196, no. 2, pp. 116–121, 2010.

[576] M. V. Seeman, "An outcome measure in schizophrenia: mortality," *The Canadian Journal of Psychiatry*, vol. 52, no. 1, pp. 55–60, 2007.

[577] C. W. Colton and R. W. Manderscheid, "Congruencies in increased mortality rates, years of potential life lost, and causes of death among public mental health clients in eight states," *Preventing Chronic Disease*, vol. 3, no. 2, article A42, 2006.

[578] T. M. Laursen, "Life expectancy among persons with schizophrenia or bipolar affective disorder," *Schizophrenia Research*, vol. 131, no. 1–3, pp. 101–104, 2011.

[579] H. Häfner and S. Kasper, "Akute lebensbedrohliche Katatonie: epidemiologische und klinische Befunde," *Nervenarzt*, vol. 53, pp. 385–394, 1982 (German).

[580] J. Höffler and P. Bräunig, "Abnahme der Häufigkeit katatoner Schizophrenien im Epochenvergleich," in *Differenzierung Katatoner und Neuroleptika-Induzierter Bewegungsstörungen*, P. Bräunig, Ed., pp. 32–35, Thieme, Stuttgart, Germany, 1995, (German).

[581] Ö. Ödegård, "Mortality in Norwegian psychiatric hospitals 1950–1962," *Acta Genetica et Statistica Medica*, vol. 17, no. 1, pp. 137–153, 1967.

[582] P. Allebeck, "Schizophrenia: a life-shortening disease," *Schizophrenia Bulletin*, vol. 15, no. 1, pp. 81–89, 1989.

[583] D. Healy, J. Le Noury, M. Harris et al., "Mortality in schizophrenia and related psychoses: data from two cohorts," *British Medical Journal*, vol. 2, Article ID e001810, 2012.

[584] S. Leucht, T. Burkard, J. Henderson, M. Maj, and N. Sartorius, "Physical illness and schizophrenia: a review of the literature," *Acta Psychiatrica Scandinavica*, vol. 116, no. 5, pp. 317–333, 2007.

[585] T. M. Laursen, T. Munk-Olsen, E. Agerbo, C. Gasse, and P. B. Mortensen, "Somatic hospital contacts, invasive cardiac procedures, and mortality from heart disease in patients with severe mental disorder," *Archives of General Psychiatry*, vol. 66, no. 7, pp. 713–720, 2009.

[586] T. M. Laursen, T. Munk-Olsen, and C. Gasse, "Chronic somatic comorbidity and excess mortality due to natural causes in persons with schizophrenia or bipolar affective disorder," *PLoS ONE*, vol. 6, no. 9, Article ID e24597, 2011.

[587] B. G. Druss and T. H. Bornemann, "Improving health and health care for persons with serious mental illness: the window for US federal policy change," *The Journal of the American Medical Association*, vol. 303, no. 19, pp. 1972–1973, 2010.

[588] J. W. Newcomer and C. H. Hennekens, "Severe mental illness and risk of cardiovascular disease," *The Journal of the American Medical Association*, vol. 298, no. 15, pp. 1794–1796, 2007.

[589] S. M. Grundy, "Obesity, metabolic syndrome, and coronary atherosclerosis," *Circulation*, vol. 105, no. 23, pp. 2696–2698, 2002.

[590] D. E. Casey, D. W. Haupt, J. W. Newcomer et al., "Antipsychotic-induced weight gain and metabolic abnormalities: implications for increased mortality in patients with schizophrenia," *Journal of Clinical Psychiatry*, vol. 65, no. 7, pp. 4–18, 2004.

[591] J. P. Despres, I. Lemieuz, and J. Bergeron, "Abdominal obesity and the metabolic syndrome: contribution to global cardiometabolic risk," *Arteriosclerosis, Thrombosis, and Vascular Biology*, vol. 28, pp. 1039–1049, 2008.

[592] D. B. Allison, K. R. Fontaine, J. E. Manson, J. Stevens, and T. B. VanItallie, "Annual deaths attributable to obesity in the United States," *The Journal of the American Medical Association*, vol. 282, no. 16, pp. 1530–1538, 1999.

[593] M. T. Susce, N. Villanueva, F. J. Diaz, and J. de Leon, "Obesity and associated complications in patients with severe mental illnesses: a cross-sectional survey," *Journal of Clinical Psychiatry*, vol. 66, no. 2, pp. 167–273, 2005.

[594] R. G. McCreadie, "Diet, smoking and cardiovascular risk in people with schizophrenia: descriptive study," *The British Journal of Psychiatry*, vol. 183, pp. 534–539, 2003.

[595] T. Cohn, D. Prud'homme, D. Streiner, H. Kameh, and G. Remington, "Characterizing coronary heart disease risk in chronic schizophrenia: high prevalence of the metabolic syndrome," *The Canadian Journal of Psychiatry*, vol. 49, no. 11, pp. 753–760, 2004.

[596] K. Hawton, L. Sutton, C. Haw, J. Sinclair, and J. J. Deeks, "Schizophrenia and suicide: systematic review of risk factors," *The British Journal of Psychiatry*, vol. 187, pp. 9–20, 2005.

[597] C. B. Caldwell and I. I. Gottesman, "Schizophrenics kill themselves too: a review of risk factors for suicide," *Schizophrenia Bulletin*, vol. 16, no. 4, pp. 571–590, 1990.

[598] S. J. Bartels, R. E. Drake, and G. J. McHugo, "Alcohol abuse, depression, and suicidal behavior in schizophrenia," *The American Journal of Psychiatry*, vol. 149, no. 3, pp. 394–395, 1992.

[599] A. McGirr, M. Tousignant, D. Routhier et al., "Risk factors for completed suicide in schizophrenia and other chronic psychotic disorders: a case-control study," *Schizophrenia Research*, vol. 84, no. 1, pp. 132–143, 2006.

[600] H. Häfner and W. an der Heiden, "Schizophrenia and depression—challenging the paradigm of two separate diseases," in *Textbook of Schizophrenia Spectrum Disorders*, M. S. Ritsner, Ed., pp. 389–402, Springer, London, UK, 2011.

[601] W. S. Fenton, "Depression, suicide, and suicide prevention in schizophrenia," *Suicide and Life-Threatening Behavior*, vol. 30, no. 1, pp. 34–49, 2000.

[602] N. Crumlish, P. Whitty, M. Kamali et al., "Early insight predicts depression and attempted suicide after 4 years in first-episode schizophrenia and schizophreniform disorder," *Acta Psychiatrica Scandinavica*, vol. 112, no. 6, pp. 449–455, 2005.

[603] J. D. López-Moríñigo, R. Ramos-Ríos, A. S. David, and R. Dutta, "Insight in schizophrenia and risk of suicide: a systematic update," *Comprehensive Psychiatry*, vol. 53, no. 4, pp. 313–322, 2012.

[604] J. van Os, "Is there a continuum of psychotic experiences in the general population?" *Epidemiologia e Psichiatria Sociale*, vol. 12, no. 4, pp. 242–252, 2003.

[605] J. Allardyce, R. G. McCreadie, G. Morrison, and J. van Os, "Do symptom dimensions or categorical diagnoses best discriminate between known risk factors for psychosis?" *Social Psychiatry and Psychiatric Epidemiology*, vol. 42, no. 6, pp. 429–437, 2007.

[606] W. Gaebel and J. Zielasek, "The DSM-V initiative "deconstructing psychosis" in the context of Kraepelin's concept on nosology," *European Archives of Psychiatry and Clinical Neuroscience*, vol. 258, no. 2, pp. 41–47, 2008.

[607] S. Arndt, N. C. Andreasen, M. Flaum, D. Miller, and P. Nopoulos, "A longitudinal study of symptom dimensions in schizophrenia: prediction and patterns of change," *Archives of General Psychiatry*, vol. 52, no. 5, pp. 352–360, 1995.

[608] H. Häfner, "Psychose, Depression und manische Symptomatik—Leitsyndrome eigener Krankheiten oder Kontinuum?" in *Schizophrenie—Zukunftsperspektiven in Klinik und Forschung*, H.-J. Möller and N. Müller, Eds., pp. 3–30, Springer, Vienna, Germany, 2010 (German).

[609] N. Sartorius, "Stigma: what can psychiatrists do about it?" *The Lancet*, vol. 352, no. 9133, pp. 1058–1059, 1998.

[610] B. G. Link, J. C. Phelan, M. Bresnahan, A. Stueve, and B. A. Pescosolido, "Public conceptions of mental illness: labels, causes, dangerousness, and social distance," *American Journal of Public Health*, vol. 89, no. 9, pp. 1328–1333, 1999.

[611] B. Mueller, C. Nordt, C. Lauber, P. Rueesch, P. C. Meyer, and W. Roessler, "Social support modifies perceived stigmatization in the first years of mental illness: a longitudinal approach," *Social Science & Medicine*, vol. 62, no. 1, pp. 30–49, 2006.

[612] V. Gentil, "More for the same?" *Revista Brasileira de Psiquiatria*, vol. 29, no. 2, pp. 193–194, 2007.

[613] W. Rössler, "Does stigma impair treatment response and rehabilitation in schizophrenia? The "contribution" of mental health professionals," in *Advances in Schizophrenia Research 2009*, W. F. Gattaz and G. Busatto, Eds., pp. 429–439, Springer, New York, NY, USA, 2010.

[614] M. Sato, "Renaming schizophrenia: a Japanese perspective," *World Psychiatry*, vol. 5, no. 1, pp. 53–55, 2006.

[615] H. Takahashi, T. Ideno, S. Okubo et al., "Impact of changing the Japanese term for "schizophrenia" for reasons of stereotypical beliefs of schizophrenia in Japanese youth," *Schizophrenia Research*, vol. 112, no. 1–3, pp. 149–152, 2009.

[616] M. C. Angermeyer, H. Matschinger, M. G. Carta, and C. Schomerus, "Changes in the perception of mental illness stigma in Germany over the last two decades," *European Psychiatry*, 2013.

[617] C. Thornicroft, A. Wyllie, G. Thornicroft, and N. Mehta, "Impact of the "Like Minds, Like Mine" anti-stigma and discrimination campaign in New Zealand on anticipated and experienced discrimination," *Australian & New Zealand Journal of Psychiatry*, vol. 48, no. 4, pp. 360–370, 2014.

23

Emotional Intelligence and Personality in Anxiety Disorders

Nathalie P. Lizeretti,[1,2,3] **María Vázquez Costa,**[1,3] **and Ana Gimeno-Bayón**[4]

[1]*Center for Research and Development of Emotional Intelligence (CIDIE), C/Marià Fortuny, 26-28, 1°-6ª, 08301 Mataró, Spain*
[2]*FPCEE Blanquerna, Ramon Llull University, C/Císter 34, 08022 Barcelona, Spain*
[3]*Maresme Health Consortium C/Prolongació Cirera, s/n, 08304 Mataró, Spain*
[4]*Erich Fromm Institute of Humanist Psychotherapy, C/Madrazo, 113 Entlo. 2°, 08021 Barcelona, Spain*

Correspondence should be addressed to Nathalie P. Lizeretti; nathaliepl@blanquerna.url.edu

Academic Editor: Takahiro Nemoto

Anxiety disorders (AD) are by far the most frequent psychiatric disorders, and according to epidemiologic data their chronicity, comorbidities, and negative prognostic constitute a public health problem. This is why it is necessary to continue exploring the factors which contribute to the incidence, appearance, and maintenance of this set of disorders. The goal of this study has been to analyze the possible relationship between Emotional Intelligence (EI) and personality disorders (PersD) in outpatients suffering from AD. The sample was made up of 146 patients with AD from the Mental Health Center at the Health Consortium of Maresme, who were evaluated with the STAI, MSCEIT, and MCMI-II questionnaires. The main findings indicate that 89,4% of the patients in the sample met the criteria for the diagnosis of some PersD. The findings also confirm that patients with AD present a low EI, especially because of difficulties in the skills of emotional comprehension and regulation, and the lack of these skills is related to a higher level of anxiety and the presence of PersD. These findings suggest the need to consider emotional skills of EI and personality as central elements for the diagnosis and treatment of AD.

1. Introduction

1.1. Anxiety Disorders. Due to their high population prevalence, their tendency to become chronic, comorbidities, and bad prognostic, anxiety disorders (AD) constitute an important public health problem [1]. Thus, generalized anxiety disorder (GAD) and substance abuse disorder are the most frequent psychiatric pathologies in the general population [2]. In the specific realm of phobic psychopathology, the rate of lifetime prevalence of panic disorder is around 4% and agoraphobia is about 2%, and 1% of the population is diagnosed with panic disorder with agoraphobia (PDA) [3, 4]. All of these emotional problems linked to high levels of anxiety are frequently complicated due to the presence of medical and psychiatric comorbidities, where depressive disorders and substance abuse from Axis I of DSM-IV are most commonly associated with anxiety disorders [3].

1.2. Personality Disorders. Between 33.9% and 95% of patients with anxiety disorder meet the criteria for a personality disorder (PersD) [3, 5, 6], and 20.5% of patients meet criteria for more than one personality disorder simultaneously [7]. The most prevalent personality disorders are those in cluster C (especially Avoidant and Dependent), but it is also frequent to find personality disorders from cluster B (Borderline and Histrionic) and even Narcissist and Antisocial [1, 7]. It is less frequent to find cluster A personality disorders associated with anxiety disorders, although they have been found in some research [3].

PersD are a factor of bad prognostic of AD, affecting its clinical course, severity, and dysfunction level. For example, patients with AD and comorbid PersD have higher levels of anxiety, depression, and agoraphobic symptoms [7]. Some studies explore the relationship between AD and personality traits (which may not meet the disorder criteria *per se*) and conclude that even these personality traits are risk predictors for AD, and the more extreme these traits, the higher the level of dysfunction [8].

In order to evaluate PersD, the most commonly used research instrument is the MCMI-II test [9]. In Theodore

Millon's perspective, personality is understood as an organizing principle which would explain both psychopathology (PersD) and the context to interpret the clinical disorders in Axis I of DSM [9]. According to this model, the comorbidity between Axes I and II is not surprising, and the high prevalence of PersD in clinical samples is explained by the aggravation of nonadaptive behavior patterns when they concur with emotional alterations. However, on some occasions this finding has been interpreted as a tendency of the test instrument to overdiagnose PersD; thus the data must be interpreted carefully [10].

1.3. IE in Anxiety and Personality Disorders. Emotional Intelligence (IE) has been described as a set of skills to identify, facilitate, understand, and regulate emotions, which allows use of emotional knowledge to achieve a higher adjustment and psychological wellbeing [11]. In order to evaluate Emotional Intelligence, the model has developed self-completion scales and a multidimensional measure based on execution tasks, the Mayer-Salovey-Caruso Emotional Intelligence Test V2.0 (MSCEIT) [12] which requires the resolution of problems with emotions. Studies performed on these instruments show that people with a high EI tend to have a more positive frame of mind; they are more able to redress their mood after unpleasant emotions and score lower on anxiety, depression, and stress [13, 14]. However, given that emotional regulation is crucial for the development and maintenance of adequate mental health [15] there is still insufficient research on the relationship between EI, psychopathological disorders, and PersD.

Recent studies prove that patients with several clinical disorders present deficits in EI, as measured with the MSCEIT skill test [16–19] and with self-assessment measures [20–22]. The studies which explore EI in patients with AD show that the deficit in any of these emotional skills can somehow contribute to the development and maintenance of the AD. A finding is that for patients with social anxiety there is a strong correlation between the gravity of symptoms and the difficulty to adequately perceive emotions and use them to facilitate their thinking [17]. Patients with PDA have significantly lower scores in emotional comprehension and regulation skills than healthy control group participants, which indicates that deficits in emotional comprehension and integration are involved in the phenomenology of panic disorder [19]. Another observation is that patients with GAD pay excessive attention to their emotions and have important difficulties in repairing their negative moods, as well as the fact that the presence and gravity of this disorder's symptoms are related to their incapacity to clearly distinguish between different emotional states. This implies that the perceived incapacity to manage one's emotions could be a vulnerability factor in the development of GAD [20].

The difficulty in managing emotional states is also a key factor in personality disorders. Some pathological personality traits have been associated with important deficits in EI in nonclinical subjects, such as Psychopathic [23], Schizotypal [24], and Borderline [25, 26] traits. Thus, we think that the presence of PersD in patients with AD could be associated with higher deficits in EI. The goal of this research has been to analyze the relationship between EI and PersD in patients with AD, with the initial hypothesis that the presence of PersD will be associated with deficits in emotional skills and a higher severity of AD.

2. Method

2.1. Participants. The participants were 153 patients from the Mental Health Center of the Maresme Health Consortium (in Mataró, Spain) diagnosed with AD by the reference psychiatrist or psychologist and referred over to psychotherapy services. The period of data collection was from February 2007 to July 2009. Those who presented a severe psychotic disorder ($n = 1$), mental retardation, literacy difficulties ($n = 3$), or difficulties in understanding the language ($n = 3$) were excluded from the study. None of the patients had an organic brain disorder or a history of substance abuse. The sample was made up of 146 Caucasian patients (84.2% women), of which 54.8% ($n = 80$) met DSM-IV-TR diagnostic criteria for PDA, and 45.2% ($n = 66$) met the diagnostic criteria for GAD. All patients included in the study provided written informed consent. The age of patients was between 18 and 65 years ($M = 38.05$; SD $= 10.72$), and the average time span of disorder progression was 6.77 years (SD $= 5.36$). The anxiety level of the sample was high ($M = 37.73$; SD $= 10.40$), thus standing within percentiles 95 and 96, as measured with the STAI-R [27].

2.2. Materials and Procedure. After being diagnosed, the patients who met the inclusion criteria were informed of the research purposes and expressed their informed consent to participate. This research was approved by the ethical review board. The evaluation of participants was preformed through two 90-minute individual interviews (within 10 days apart) prior to psychotherapeutic treatment. The Structured Clinical Interview for Axis I DSM-IV (SCID-I Clinical Version) [28] was used in the first session in order to confirm the diagnosis for Axis I. Millon's Multiaxial Clinical Inventory (MCMI-II) [9] was also administered for the diagnosis of disorders on Axis II of DSM-IV. Throughout the 176 items of dichotomic response, MCMI-II gathers aspects of pathological personality in 26 scales (4 reliability scales, 10 basic personality scales, 3 pathologic personality scales, and 9 clinical syndrome scales). The validity indexes range between 0.71 for major depression scale and 0.85 for the Dependent PersD scale. For the present study, the most conservative criteria were chosen, considering as PersD the scores over TB > 84 [6].

During the second interview, EI was evaluated using MSCEIT V2.0 [12]. This test has 141 items with five response choices which measure the subject's skills in different emotional tasks. Test questions are grouped in four branches and two fields of construct: the experiential field which includes perception skills and use of emotions to facilitate thinking and the field of reasoning, which includes emotional comprehension and regulation. This test allows us to obtain a total EI coefficient, scores for two fields, and the four branches of skills. The alpha indexes of reliability for the main scales under the general scoring criteria range between

TABLE 1: Patients with clinical significant punctuations in the personality scales.

	PersD (>84) % (n)	PDA % (n)	GAD % (n)	χ^2	P value
Schizoid	**43.3% (61)**	40.8% (31)	46.2% (30)	.411	.319
Avoidant	22.0% (31)	25.0% (19)	18.5% (12)	.873	.233
Dependent	**48.2% (68)**	47.4% (36)	49.2% (32)	.049	.479
Histrionic	21.3% (30)	21.1% (16)	21.5% (14)	.005	.553
Narcissistic	24.1% (34)	23.7% (18)	24.6% (16)	.017	.526
Antisocial	27.7% (39)	27.6% (21)	27.7% (18)	.000	.571
Aggressive-Sadistic	23.4% (33)	18.4% (14)	29.2% (19)	2.284	.095
Compulsive	**60.3% (85)**	52.6% (40)	69.2% (45)	4.032	**.033***
Passive-Aggressive	14.4% (26)	15.8% (12)	21.5% (14)	.770	.254
Self-Defeating	28.4% (40)	27.6% (21)	29.2% (19)	.044	.490
Schizotypal	28.4% (40)	27.6% (21)	29.2% (19)	.044	.490
Borderline	26.2% (37)	25.0% (19)	27.7% (18)	.131	.432
Paranoid	34.0% (48)	30.3% (23)	36.5% (25)	1.049	.199

χ^2 significance value; $^*P < 0.050$.

0.93 for total EI and 0.79 for emotional facilitation. Out of the different scales in the test, age and gender were jointly used. The scores obtained were standardized according to the normative sample ($M = 100$; SD = 15). Score ranges for all scales are the following: *Improve* (0–<70), *Consider developing* (≥70–<90), *Competent* (≥90–<110), *Skilled* (≥110–<130), and *Expert* (≥130).

2.3. Analysis. A frequency analysis for PersD was preformed, to prove whether there were differences between patients with PDA and GAD in comparison with the demographic variables, the level of anxiety, and EI in the chi-squared and Student's t-test. After this, a covariance analysis was preformed, in order to control the effect of demographic variables on the scores for EI skills and the personality scales. To finish, a Pearson correlation analysis was preformed between the subscales of the MSCEIT and the scales of the MCMI-II. These analyses were carried out with the statistical software package SPSS version 15.0.

3. Results

3.1. PersD Frequency Analysis. The frequency of clinically significant scores is high for all the personality scales (see Table 1). The result in the Compulsive scale is extreme, since 60.3% of the sample exceeds the cutoff point; thus it is found more frequently amongst patients with GAD. The analysis also indicated that 83.7% of the sample met criteria for more than one PersD, according to the MCMI-II ($M = 4.23$; SD = 2.633), where the presence of two PersD was the most frequent test result (17.1% of patients).

3.2. Descriptive Statistics. Among the personality scales, apart from the high scores in the Compulsive scale (which exceed the TB > 84), the scores in the Dependent and

Schizoid scales (above TB > 74) also stand out, indicating an important presence of these PersD amongst the participants (see Table 2). Low EI coefficient scores also appear in the four skills branches, where the greatest difficulties are in the area of reasoning (comprehension and regulation), scoring more than one standard deviation below the standardized mean. Student's t-test shows that amongst patients with PDA and GAD there are differences in age, and patients with GAD obtain higher scores in the Aggressive-Sadistic scale ($P = 0.028$) and Compulsive scale ($P = 0.044$), but no significant EI differences were found between both diagnoses.

3.3. Variance Analysis. ANOVA models were thereafter preformed to compare the mean scores of the MCMI-II and MSCEIT between patients with PDA and patients with GAD, checking for possible confounding effects of age, gender, and years of disorder progression. The results indicate a significant positive effect of years of disorder progression on the Phobic scale scores ($F = 6.507$; $P = 0.012$) for PDA patients. There is also a significant positive effect of years of disorder progression on the Aggressive-Sadistic scale ($F = 4.404$; $P = 0.038$) and on the identification of emotions skills ($F = 4.174$; $P = 0.043$) for the GAD patients.

3.4. Correlations. Table 3 shows several statistically significant correlations between personality scales, anxiety scales, and EI skills. Anxiety correlated positively with PersD, except for cluster B and Compulsive patients. Emotional facilitation correlated negatively with the Schizotypal, Dependent, and Self-Defeating scales. Emotional comprehension correlated negatively with Schizoid, Phobic, Self-Defeating, Borderline, and Dependent scales, but it correlated positively with the scales in cluster B (Histrionic, Narcissistic, and Antisocial). The emotional regulation skills also correlated negatively with most of the personality scales. However, emotion identification did not correlate with any of the personality scales, and

TABLE 2: Descriptive statistics in the MCMI-II and the MSCEIT scales.

Variables			Women 84.2 (123)		PDA 85 (68)		GAD 83.3 (55)		Statistics $\chi^2 = .822$	P value $P = .479$
	% (n)		Mean	SD	Mean	SD	Mean	SD	$t_{(144)}$	P
Age			38.05	10.72	35.03	985	41.73	10.64	-3.994	.000**
Time of disorder progression			6.77	5.36	6.45	5.05	7.03	5.64	-.584	.560
STAI-T			37.73	10.4	36.33	11.24	38.85	9.63	-1.305	.195
		1. Schizoid	76.69	26.30	75.45	28.25	74.14	23.96	-.604	.547
		2A. Avoidant	61.30	26.85	63.84	26.77	58.34	26.83	1.215	.226
		3. Dependent	79.14	28.84	78.09	29.82	80.37	27.82	-.466	.642
		4. Histrionic	51.09	32.93	50.53	32.77	51.75	33.36	-.220	.826
		5. Narcissistic	55.49	30.86	52.91	31.50	58.51	30.05	-1.075	.284
		6A. Antisocial	54.20	32.74	54.47	32.29	53.88	33.50	.108	.915
PersD		6B. Aggressive	55.89	31.88	50.45	32.27	62.26	30.44	-2.224	.028*
		7. Compulsive	85.15	29.01	80.61	29.23	90.46	28.04	-2.033	.044*
		8A. Passive-Aggressive	55.40	27.41	53.58	28.19	57.54	26.52	-.854	.394
		8B. Self-Defeating	62.05	28.42	61.21	29.36	63.03	27.47	-.378	.706
		S. Schizotypal	67.33	25.82	67.91	25.72	66.65	26.11	.288	.774
		C. Borderline	61.34	25.90	61.39	25.98	61.28	26.00	.027	.979
		P. Paranoid	67.05	28.84	63.89	29.89	70.74	27.36	-1.409	.161
		Perceiving Emotions	94.21	15.22	95.65	15.84	92.45	14.35	1.256	.211
		Facilitating Thought	90.26	12.99	91.20	12.20	89.12	13.90	.956	.341
		Understanding Emotions	78.84	9.66	78.33	9.26	79.47	10.15	-.705	.482
MSCEIT		Managing Emotions	84.54	10.48	84.44	10.21	84.66	10.88	-.705	.482
		Experiential area	91.20	13.64	92.78	13.11	89.27	14.12	1.545	.125
		Strategic area	79.05	9.07	78.73	8.28	79.45	10.01	.470	.639
		EI coefficient	81.45	11.84	82.06	11.25	80.72	12.58	.673	.502

Significance value ** $P < 0.010$; * $P < 0.050$.

TABLE 3: Correlations between personality, anxiety, and IE's skills.

Variables	Anx.	Emotional Intelligence				
PersD	STAI-T	Perceiving Emotions	Facilitating Thought	Understanding Emotions	Managing Emotions	EI coefficient
1. Schizoid	.400**	−.116	−.011	−.228**	−.146	−.169*
2A. Avoidant	.426**	−.125	−.086	−.236**	−.220**	−.228**
3. Dependent	.335**	−.030	−.198*	−.208*	−.282**	−.261**
4. Histrionic	−.098	.122	.000	.211*	.007	.126
5. Narcissistic	−.064	−.038	.033	.210*	.012	.081
6A. Antisocial	−.075	.052	.061	.282**	.060	.124
6B. Aggressive	.032	−.101	−.037	.153	.049	−.014
7. Compulsive	.106	−.014	−.052	−.072	.030	−.054
8A. Passive-Aggressive	.306**	−.067	−.046	−.107	−.224**	−.147
8B. Self-Defeating	.478**	−.076	−.208*	−.334**	−.323**	−.324**
S. Schizotypal	.452**	−.192	−.254**	−.351**	−.366**	−.405**
C. Borderline	.387**	−.087	−.165	−.317**	−.307**	−.292**
P. Paranoid	.203**	−.147	−.120	−.028	−.200*	−.192*

Significance value ** $P < 0.010$; * $P < 0.050$.

none of the EI skills correlated with the Aggressive-Sadistic scale and Compulsive scale.

4. Discussion and Conclusions

No studies were found that investigated the relationship between EI with the skills model and PersD in patients with psychopathology. In response to the need for research in this realm, the goal of the present research has been to analyze the relationship between EI and PersD for patients with AD. Our hypothesis stated that the patients with AD would present difficulties managing their emotions, which would translate into a low level of EI, and that this would be related to more anxiety and the presence of PersD.

The results indicate that 89.4% of the patients in the sample met the criteria for the diagnosis of some PersD (according to the MCMI-II). This data is superior to that found in some previous studies, which found a frequency of PersD approximately at 33.9% [7] and 46% [5], but it is similar to some other studies that found that up to 95% of patients with AD meet criteria for a PersD, and 20.5% meet criteria for more than one [3, 6].

The most prevalent PersD were Compulsive, Dependent, and Schizoid. The high prevalence of these PersD has also been noted by numerous researches [7], but the prevalence of Schizoid PersD has been higher in this case than in other studies [3, 29]. The Schizoid PersD could be related to the severity of the AD, being more frequent amongst patients with a severe PDA. Avoidance and progressive isolation to which it leads could accentuate these personality traits.

In terms of prevalence, the only significant differences found between PDA and GAD were in the Compulsive scale. Previous studies have found higher rates of obsessive-compulsive personality disorder (OCPD) in patients with GAD than in patients with PDA [30].

Our results also confirm that patients with AD present a low EI, without finding significant differences between PDA and GAD. Specifically, patients show sufficient competence in identification and facilitation skills but have difficulties in the skills of emotional comprehension and regulation (which imply greater processing complexity). These results are consistent with the studies performed within the Emotional Intelligence paradigm [17, 19, 20] and outside of this paradigm [31], which show that in AD the symptoms are associated with a higher emotional intensity, low emotional comprehension capacity, negative reactions towards one's own emotions, and difficulties in emotional management.

Also, we have observed that the years of AD progression have a significant impact on personality and EI, indicating that chronicity of the disorder is related with lower emotional management skills. The longer the time of disorder progression is, the more the Phobic personality traits are accentuated in PDA and the Aggressive-Sadistic traits are accentuated in GDA, decreasing the emotional identification skills. These data could lead to two complementary explanatory hypotheses. The first hypothesis is that baseline PersD is a vulnerability factor [9], which increases the severity and risk of chronicity of the AD [7]. The second hypothesis is that anxiety symptoms experienced for a long time can modify personality structure. This hypothesis offers a circular view of the interaction between disorders in Axis I and Axis II for the patients with AD and suggests the need to contemplate personality in the evaluation and treatment of AD.

In accordance with our hypothesis, the correlation analysis indicates that the presence of PersD is associated with a higher anxiety and a lower EI. Among the most prevalent ones, the Dependent PersD is related to difficulties in the use of emotion to facilitate thinking but, especially in the comprehension and regulation of emotional experiences. The Dependent person tends to disconnect her own emotions, and her thought and behavior are guided by significant others (on whom she depends) rather than her own emotional needs. For the Schizoid PersD it is unsurprising to find an association with a high anxiety and a difficulty in understanding emotional states in self and others. It is surprising to find a total absence of correlation between obsessive-compulsive PersD and EI. Possibly this lack of correlation could be explained due to the rationalizing tendency of this OCPD, which acts as a control mechanism at the expense of spontaneity and authenticity of emotional experience.

It is also interesting to find a positive relation between the Histrionic, Narcissistic, and Antisocial scales with emotional comprehension, although it is true that these personality types show a certain emotional dominance through their manipulative and seductive behaviors. The pioneers of the EI concept, Salovey and Mayer [32], already warned that "those whose [emotional] skills are channeled antisocially may create manipulative scenes or lead others sociopathically to nefarious ends" (p.198). So, emotion-regulation knowledge "has a dark side as well"; that is, it facilitates both prosocial and interpersonally deviant behavior by enhancing the motivational effects of traits [33]. In a person with Narcissistic or Antisocial traits (which imply an egocentric attitude of despising others' needs and social norms), a high emotional comprehension could be a powerful manipulation weapon. For example, it has been noted that the school bullies scored higher on emotion understanding than did nonbullies [34].

Referring to these results and keeping in mind the intrinsic goodness of authentic emotions (in their instinctive and adaptive character) [35] one may wonder whether the emotional skills assessed with the MSCEIT are really referring to an authentic, natural, and deep EI or, on the contrary, they refer to a set of emotional manipulation skills or manipulative EI. In any case, it is necessary to discriminate between one and the other type of EI, and for this matter personality is a key factor to keep in mind.

In this research, we have analyzed the relationship between different dimensions of EI and PersD in patients with AD. Our results offer two possible hypotheses which could occur simultaneously: first, that deficits in EI skills are an important factor in the etiology of personality disorders and, second, that the pathological personality traits tamper the development of emotional skills, which could partly explain the incidence of these clinical disorders in Axis I. In any case, it seems obvious that the patients with AD need to develop their emotional reasoning skills to attain an adequate emotional competence, and this suggests that interventions aimed at the development of these emotional skills can contribute to a higher efficacy of the current treatments. However, more research will be necessary to clarify the relationship between EI and the different PersD in clinical patients.

Limitations and Future Research Directions

One of the strong points of this study is the use of the MSCEIT skill test to measure IE. Most studies on EI discussing clinical issues rely on self-report measures. Our study also presents some limitations such as the reduced sample size or the exclusive use of MCMI-II for the diagnosis of PersD. On the other hand, the cross-sectional study design does not allow establishing causal relationship between the observed associations. Further longitudinal research is needed to clarify causal relation between deficits in EI and PersD in AD patients.

Highlights

We highlight the following points: (i) almost 90% of patients suffering AD present a Compulsive, Dependent, or Schizoid PersD, (ii) patients with AD present an EI level which is lower than the general population, (iii) patients with AD have greater difficulties in emotional comprehension and regulation, and (iv) suffering an AD together with a PersD indicates that fewer emotional management skills are available.

Conflict of Interests

The authors declare that there is no conflict of interests regarding the publication of this paper.

References

[1] B. L. Milrod, A. C. Leon, J. P. Barber, J. C. Markowitz, and E. Graf, "Do comorbid personality disorders moderate panic-focused psychotherapy? An exploratory examination of the American psychiatric association practice guideline," *The Journal of Clinical Psychiatry*, vol. 68, no. 6, pp. 885–891, 2007.

[2] J. Alonso, M. C. Angermeyer, S. Bernert et al., "Prevalence of mental disorders in Europe: results from the European Study of the Epidemiology of Mental Disorders (ESEMeD) project," *Acta Psychiatrica Scandinavica, Supplement*, vol. 109, no. 420, pp. 21–27, 2004.

[3] B. F. Grant, D. S. Hasin, F. S. Stinson et al., "The epidemiology of DSM-IV panic disorder and agoraphobia in the United States: results from the National epidemiologic survey on alcohol and related conditions," *The Journal of Clinical Psychiatry*, vol. 67, no. 3, pp. 363–374, 2006.

[4] R. C. Kessler, A. M. Ruscio, K. Shear, and H.-U. Wittchen, "Epidemiology of anxiety disorders," *Current Topics in Behavioral Neurosciences*, vol. 2, pp. 21–35, 2010.

[5] R. C. Durham, T. Murphy, T. Allan, K. Richard, L. R. Treliving, and G. W. Fenton, "Cognitive therapy, analytic psychotherapy and anxiety management training for generalised anxiety disorder," *The British Journal of Psychiatry*, vol. 165, pp. 315–323, 1994.

[6] S. Wetzler, R. S. Kahn, W. Cahn, H. M. van Praag, and G. M. Asnis, "Psychological test characteristics of depressed and panic patients," *Psychiatry Research*, vol. 31, no. 2, pp. 179–192, 1990.

[7] M. Ozkan and A. Altindag, "Comorbid personality disorders in subjects with panic disorder: do personality disorders increase clinical severity?" *Comprehensive Psychiatry*, vol. 46, no. 1, pp. 20–26, 2005.

[8] M. Brandes and O. J. Bienvenu, "Personality and anxiety disorders," *Current Psychiatry Reports*, vol. 8, no. 4, pp. 263–269, 2006.

[9] T. Millon, *Millon Multiaxial Clinical Inventory II (MCMI-II)*, TEA, Madrid, Spain, 1987, Spanish adaptation by Ávila-Espada, 1997.

[10] F. M. Martín, A. J. Cangas, and M. E. Pozo, "Personality disorders in patients with eating disorders," *Psicothema*, vol. 21, pp. 33–38, 2009.

[11] J. D. Mayer and P. Salovey, "What is emotional intelligence?" in *Emotional Development and Emotional Intelligence Educational Implications*, P. Salovey and D. J. Sluyter, Eds., pp. 3–31, Basic Books, New York, NY, USA, 1997.

[12] J. D. Mayer, P. Salovey, D. Caruso, and G. Sitarenios, *Mayer-Salove -Caruso Emotional Intelligence Test (MSCEIT) User's Manual*, MHS, Ontario, Canada, 2005.

[13] P. Fernández-Berrocal and N. Extremera, "Emotional intelligence and emotional reactivity and recovery in laboratory context," *Psicothema*, vol. 18, no. 1, pp. 72–78, 2006.

[14] P. Salovey, L. R. Stroud, A. Woolery, and E. S. Epel, "Perceived emotional intelligence, stress reactivity, and symptom reports: further explorations using the trait meta-mood scale," *Psychology and Health*, vol. 17, no. 5, pp. 611–627, 2002.

[15] A. Aldao and S. Nolen-Hoeksema, "Specificity of cognitive emotion regulation strategies: a transdiagnostic examination," *Behaviour Research and Therapy*, vol. 48, no. 10, pp. 974–983, 2010.

[16] J. Hertel, A. Schütz, and C. H. Lammers, "Emotional intelligence and mental disorder," *Journal of Clinical Psychology*, vol. 65, no. 9, pp. 942–954, 2009.

[17] M. Jacobs, J. Snow, M. Geraci et al., "Association between level of emotional intelligence and severity of anxiety in generalized social phobia," *Journal of Anxiety Disorders*, vol. 22, no. 8, pp. 1487–1495, 2008.

[18] S. Kee, P. Horan, P. Salovey et al., "Emotional intelligence in schizophrenia," *Schizophrenia Research*, vol. 107, no. 1, pp. 61–68, 2009.

[19] G. Perna, R. Menotti, G. Borriello, P. Cavedini, L. Bellodi, and D. Caldirola, "Emotional intelligence in panic disorder," *Rivista di Psichiatria*, vol. 45, no. 5, pp. 320–325, 2010.

[20] N. P. Lizeretti and N. Extremera, "Emotional intelligence and clinical symptoms in outpatients with Generalized Anxiety Disorder (GAD)," *Psychiatric Quarterly*, vol. 82, no. 3, pp. 253–260, 2011.

[21] N. P. Lizeretti, N. Extremera, and A. Rodríguez, "Perceived emotional intelligence and clinical symptoms in outpatiens with mental disorders," *Psychiatry Quaterly*, vol. 83, pp. 407–418, 2012.

[22] N. P. Lizeretti and A. Rodríguez, "Perceived emotional intelligence in patients diagnosed with panic disorder with agoraphobia," *Anxiety and Stress*, vol. 18, no. 1, pp. 43–53, 2012.

[23] M. B. Malterer, S. J. Glass, and J. P. Newman, "Psychopathy and trait emotional intelligence," *Personality and Individual Differences*, vol. 44, no. 3, pp. 735–745, 2008.

[24] F. Aguirre, M. J. Sergi, and C. A. Levy, "Emotional intelligence and social functioning in persons with schizotypy," *Schizophrenia Research*, vol. 104, no. 1–3, pp. 255–264, 2008.

[25] K. Gardner and P. Qualter, "Emotional intelligence and Borderline personality disorder," *Personality and Individual Differences*, vol. 47, no. 2, pp. 94–98, 2009.

[26] T. L. Leible and W. E. Snell Jr., "Borderline personality disorder and multiple aspects of emotional intelligence," *Personality and Individual Differences*, vol. 37, no. 2, pp. 393–404, 2004.

[27] C. D. Spielberger, R. L. Gorsuch, and R. F. Lushene, *State-Trait Anxiety Inventory*, TEA, Madrid, Spain, 1970.

[28] M. B. First, R. L. Spitzer, M. Gibbon, and J. B. Williams, *Structured Clinical Interview for DSM-IV Axis I disorders (SCID-I) Clinical Version*, Masson, Barcelona, Spain, 1997, Spanish adaptation by Blanch and Andreu 1999.

[29] I. R. Dyck, K. A. Phillips, M. G. Warshaw et al., "Patterns of personality pathology in patients with generalized anxiety disorder, panic disorder with and without agoraphobia, and social phobia," *Journal of Personality Disorders*, vol. 15, no. 1, pp. 60–71, 2001.

[30] J. E. Grant, M. E. Mooney, and M. G. Kushner, "Prevalence, correlates, and comorbidity of DSM-IV obsessive-compulsive personality disorder: results from the National Epidemiologic Survey on Alcohol and Related Conditions," *Journal of Psychiatric Research*, vol. 46, no. 4, pp. 469–475, 2012.

[31] D. S. Mennin, R. G. Heimberg, C. L. Turk, and D. M. Fresco, "Preliminary evidence for an emotion dysregulation model of generalized anxiety disorder," *Behaviour Research and Therapy*, vol. 43, no. 10, pp. 1281–1310, 2005.

[32] P. Salovey and J. D. Mayer, "Emotional intelligence," *Imagination, Cognition and Personality*, vol. 9, pp. 185–211, 1990.

[33] S. Côté, K. A. DeCelles, J. M. McCarthy, G. A. van Kleef, and I. Hideg, "The jekyll and hyde of emotional intelligence: emotion-regulation knowledge facilitates both prosocial and interpersonally deviant behavior," *Psychological Science*, vol. 22, no. 8, pp. 1073–1080, 2011.

[34] J. Sutton, P. K. Smith, and J. Swettenham, "Social cognition and bullying: social inadequacy or skilled manipulation?" *British Journal of Developmental Psychology*, vol. 17, no. 3, pp. 435–450, 1999.

[35] N. P. Lizeretti, *Emotional Intelligence Based Therapy. Treatment Manual*, Milenio, Lérida, Spain, 2012.

Permissions

List of Contributors

Ulrich Palm, Rabee Mokhtari-Nejad, Susanne Rospleszcz, Larissa de la Fontaine, Felix M. Segmiller and Daniela Eser-Valeri
Department of Psychiatry, Psychotherapy and Psychosomatics, Ludwig-Maximilians University Munich, Nußbaumstraße 7, 80336 Munich, Germany

Wolfgang E. Thasler and Peter Rittler
Department of General, Visceral, Transplantation, Vascular, andThoracic Surgery, Ludwig-Maximilians University Munich, Marchioninistraße 15, 81377 Munich, Germany

Ann Natascha Epple
KBO Heckscher Clinic for Childhood and Adolescent Psychiatry, Deisenhofener Straße 28, 81539 Munich, Germany

Martin Lieb
Privatklinik Meiringen, Willigen, 3860 Meiringen, Switzerland

Hala Mahmoud Obeidat
Maternal Child Health Nursing Department, Princess Muna College of Nursing, Mutah University, Amman, Jordan

Adlah M. Hamlan
Jordan University, Amman, Jordan

Lynn Clark Callister
Brigham Young University College of Nursing, Provo, UT 84602, USA

Hidehiro Sugisawa
Graduate School of Gerontology, J. F. Oberlin University, Machida-shi 194-0294, Japan

Hiroaki Sugisaki
Hachioji Azumacho Clinic, Hachioji-shi 192-0082, Japan

Seiji Ohira
Sapporo Kita Clinic, Sapporo-shi 001-0018, Japan

Toshio Shinoda
Kawakita General Hospital, Suginami-ku 166-0001, Japan

Yumiko Shimizu
School of Nursing, Jikei University, Chofu-shi 182-08570, Japan

Tamaki Kumagai
Faculty of Health Care and Nursing, Juntendo University, Urayasu-shi 279-0023, Japan

Nicholas J. K. Breitborde and CindyWoolverton
Department of Psychiatry, The University of Arizona, Tucson, AZ 85713, USA

R. Brock Frost
Department of Psychiatry, University of New Mexico, Albuquerque, NM 87131, USA

Nicole A. Kiewel
Department of Psychiatry, Cleveland Clinic, Cleveland, OH 44195, USA

Abyot Endale Gurmu, Esileman Abdela, Bashir Allele, Ermias Cheru and Bemnet Amogne
School of Pharmacy, College of Medicine and Health Sciences, University of Gondar, P.O. Box 196, Gondar, Ethiopia

Frauke Schultze-Lutter and Benno G. Schimmelmann
University Hospital of Child and Adolescent Psychiatry and Psychotherapy, University of Bern, Bolligenstrasse 111, Haus A, 3000 Bern 60, Switzerland

Peter Wennberg
Centre for Social Research on Alcohol and Drugs, Stockholm University, 10691 Stockholm, Sweden

Kristina Berglund and Claudia Fahlke
Department of Psychology, University of Gothenburg, 405 30 Gothenburg, Sweden

Ulf Berggren and Jan Balldin
Department of Psychiatry and Neurochemistry, Institute of Neuroscience and Physiology, University of Gothenburg, 413 45 Gothenburg, Sweden

Sadao Otsuka, Mie Matsui, Takatoshi Hoshino and Kayoko Miura
Department of Psychology, Graduate School of Medicine and Pharmaceutical Sciences, University of Toyama, Toyama 930-0194, Japan

Yuko Higuchi and Michio Suzuki
Department of Neuropsychiatry, Graduate School of Medicine and Pharmaceutical Sciences, University of Toyama, Toyama 930-0194, Japan

Dimitre H. Dimitrov, Shuko Lee, Jesse Yantis, Craig Honaker, and Nicole Braida
South Texas Veterans Health Care Systems, San Antonio, TX 78229-4404, USA

Åsa Daremo
Department of Psychiatry, University Hospital, 581 85 Linköping, Sweden
Department of Social and Welfare Studies, Faculty of Health Sciences, Linköping University, Linköping, Sweden

Anette Kjellberg and Lena Haglund
Department of Social and Welfare Studies, Faculty of Health Sciences, Linköping University, Linköping, Sweden

Andrew Soundy and Carolyn Roskell
School of Sport, Exercise and Rehabilitation Sciences, University of Birmingham, Birmingham B15 2TT, UK

Paul Freeman
School of Biological Sciences, University of Essex, Essex CO4 3SQ, UK

Brendon Stubbs
School of Health and Social Care, University of Greenwich, London SE10 9LS, UK

Michel Probst and Davy Vancampfort
Department of Neurosciences, University Psychiatric Centre, KU Leuven, Leuvensesteenweg 517, 3070 Kortenberg, Belgium
Department of Rehabilitation Sciences, KU Leuven, Tervuursevest 101, 3001 Leuven, Belgium

Glenn Shean
College of William & Mary, P.O. Box 8795, Williamsburg, VA 23187-8795, USA

Harini Atturu
Pennine Care NHS Foundation Trust, Royal Oldham Hospital, Oldham, Lancashire OL1 2JH, UK

Adedeji Odelola
Pennine Care NHS Foundation Trust, Birch Hill Hospital, Rochdale OL12 9QB, UK

Ádám Takács
Institute of Psychology, Eötvös Loŕ and University, Izabella u. 46., Budapest 1064, Hungary
Brain Imaging Centre, Research Centre for Natural Sciences, Hungarian Academy of Sciences, Magyar Tudósok Körùtja 2., Budapest 1117, Hungary

Zsanett Tárnok
Vadaskert Child Psychiatry Hospital, Hűvösvölgyi ùt 116., Budapest 1021, Hungary
Institute of Psychology, Károli Gáspár University, Bécsi ùt 324., Budapest 1037, Hungary

Andrea Kóbor
Institute of Psychology, Eötvös Loŕ and University, Izabella u. 46., Budapest 1064, Hungary
Brain Imaging Centre, Research Centre for Natural Sciences, Hungarian Academy of Sciences, Magyar Tudósok Körùtja 2., Budapest 1117, Hungary

András Vargha
Institute of Psychology, Eötvös Loŕ and University, Izabella u. 46., Budapest 1064, Hungary
Institute of Psychology, Károli Gáspár University, Bécsi íut 324., Budapest 1037, Hungary

Ravi Philip Rajkumar
Department of Psychiatry, Disaster Management Committee, Jawaharlal Institute of Postgraduate Medical Education and Research (JIPMER), Puducherry 605 006, India

Balaji Bharadwaj
Department of Psychiatry, Jawaharlal Institute of Postgraduate Medical Education and Research (JIPMER), Puducherry 605 006, India

Jan Volavka
New York University School of Medicine, P.O. Box 160663, Big Sky, MT 59716, USA

Eleni Jelastopulu and Evangelia Giourou
Department of Public Health, School of Medicine, University of Patras, 26500 Rio Patras, Greece

Argyropoulos
Department of Public Health, School of Medicine, University of Patras, 26500 Rio Patras, Greece
Psychiatric Hospital of Tripoli, 5th Km Tripolis-Kalamatas, 22100 Tripoli, Greece

Konstantinos Eleftheria Kariori
Health Center of Erymanthia, 25015 Erymanthia, Greece

Eleftherios Moratis and Angeliki Mestousi
Department of Medical Affairs, Janssen-Cilag, 56 Eirinis Avenue, Pefki, 15121 Athens, Greece

John Kyriopoulos
Department of Health Economics, National School of Public Health, 196 Alexandras Avenue, 11521 Athens, Greece

Ragnfrid Kogstad and Jan Kaare Hummelvoll
Hedmark University College, 2418 Elverum, Norway

Tor-Johan Ekeland
Volda University College, 6101 Volda, Norway

Andrea R. Durrant
Research and Psychiatry Departments, Ezrath Nashim-Herzog Memorial Hospital, P.O. Box 3900, 91035 Jerusalem, Israel

Uriel Heresco-Levy
Research and Psychiatry Departments, Ezrath Nashim-Herzog Memorial Hospital, P.O. Box 3900, 91035 Jerusalem, Israel
Hadassah Medical School, Hebrew University, Jerusalem, Israel

Enrica Marzola, Secondo Fassino, Federico Amianto and Giovanni Abbate-Daga
Eating Disorders Center, Department of Neuroscience, University of Turin, Via Cherasco 15, 10126 Turin, Italy

Sophie van Rijn, Tim Ziermans and Hanna Swaab
Clinical Child and Adolescent Studies, Leiden University, Wassenaarseweg 52, 2333 AK Leiden, Netherlands
Leiden Institute for Brain and Cognition, P.O. Box 9600, 2300 RC Leiden, Netherlands
Pieter Kroonenberg
Family Studies, Leiden University, Wassenaarseweg 52, 2333 AK Leiden, Netherlands

Heinz Häfner
Schizophrenia Research Group, Central Institute of Mental Health, Mannheim Faculty of Medicine, University of Heidelberg, J5, 68159Mannheim, Germany

Nathalie P. Lizeretti
Center for Research and Development of Emotional Intelligence (CIDIE), C/Marià Fortuny, 26-28, 1o-6a, 08301Mataró, Spain
FPCEE Blanquerna, Ramon Llull University, C/Císter 34, 08022 Barcelona, Spain
Maresme Health ConsortiumC/Prolongació Cirera, s/n, 08304 Mataró, Spain

María Vázquez Costa
Center for Research and Development of Emotional Intelligence (CIDIE), C/Mariá Fortuny, 26-28, 1o-6a, 08301Mataró, Spain
Maresme Health ConsortiumC/Prolongació Cirera, s/n, 08304 Mataró, Spain

Ana Gimeno-Bayón
Erich Fromm Institute of Humanist Psychotherapy, C/Madrazo, 113 Entlo. 2o, 08021 Barcelona, Spain

www.ingramcontent.com/pod-product-compliance
Lightning Source LLC
Chambersburg PA
CBHW070152240326
41458CB00126B/4442